# Human Diseases

## A Systemic Approach

**Seventh Edition**

**Mark Zelman, PhD**
Associate Professor
Aurora University
Aurora, Illinois

**Elaine Tompary, PharmD**
Outcomes Research
McNeil Consumer and Specialty Pharma
Fort Washington, Pennsylvania

**Jill Raymond, PhD**
Professor
Rock Valley College
Rockford, Illinois

**Paul Holdaway, MA**
Professor
William Rainey Harper College
Palatine, Illinois

**Mary Lou Mulvihill, PhD**
Professor Emeritus
William Rainey Harper College
Palatine, Illinois

Upper Saddle River, New Jersey 07458

**Library of Congress Cataloging-in-Publication Data**

Human diseases : a systemic approach. — 7th ed. / Mark Zelman
. . . [et al.].
    p. ; cm.
  Includes bibliographical references and index.
  ISBN-13: 978-0-13-515556-1
  ISBN-10: 0-13-515556-8
  1. Pathology.   I. Zelman, Mark.
  [DNLM: 1.  Disease. QZ 140 H9185 2010]
  RB111.M83 2010
  616—dc22

                                2008043019

To Mary Lou Mulvihill,
friend, colleague, and
educator, whose vision
began this work

and

To our students,
who inspired us to continue it

**Publisher:** Julie Levin Alexander
**Assistant to Publisher:** Regina Bruno
**Executive Editor:** Mark Cohen
**Associate Editor:** Melissa Kerian
**Assistant Editor:** Nicole Ragonese
**Development Editor:** Kim Wyatt
**Managing Production Editor:** Patrick Walsh
**Production Liaison:** Christina Zingone
**Production Editor:** Jessica Balch, Pine Tree Composition
**Manufacturing Manager:** Ilene Sanford
**Manufacturing Buyer:** Pat Brown
**Creative Design Director:** Christy Mahon
**Senior Art Director:** Maria Guglielmo
**Design Coordinator:** Christopher Weigand
**Cover/Interior Design:** Jill Little
**Director of Marketing:** Karen Allman

**Executive Marketing Manager:** Katrin Beacom
**Marketing Specialist:** Michael Sirinides
**Marketing Assistant:** Judy Noh
**Senior Media Editor:** Amy Peltier
**Media Project Manager:** Lorena Cerisano
**Developer:** All Things Media LLC
**IRC Manager, Rights and Permissions:** Zina Arabia
**Manager, Visual Research:** Beth Brenzel
**Manager, Cover Visual Research & Permissions:**
  Karen Sanatar
**Image Permission Coordinator:** Angelique Sharps
**Composition:** Pine Tree Composition, Inc.
**Printer/Binder:** CJK
**Cover Printer:** Lehigh Phoenix
**Cover Images:** Courtesy of the CDC—*Left*: Stacy
  Howard, 1994; *Right*: Sherry Brinkman, 1963

Pearson Education Ltd., London
Pearson Education Singapore, Pte. Ltd.
Pearson Education Canada, Inc.
Pearson Education—Japan
Pearson Education Australia PTY, Limited

Pearson Education North Asia, Ltd., Hong Kong
Pearson Educación de Mexico, S.A. de C.V.
Pearson Education Malaysia, Pte. Ltd.
Pearson Education Upper Saddle River, New Jersey

10 9 8 7 6 5 4 3 2 1
ISBN-13: 978-0-13-515556-1
ISBN-10:    0-13-515556-8

# Brief Contents

# Contents

## Welcome to the Seventh Edition

The seventh edition of *Human Diseases: A Systemic Approach* has been thoroughly updated and revised for accuracy, currency, and consistency, and to better meet the needs of students and instructors. A complete set of multimedia ancillaries accompany the text and provide a multidimensional learning experience. The book retains the organization and engaging, readable style that have made it a success throughout the years.

## Organization

The text is organized into two parts. Part I, *Mechanisms of Disease,* introduces students to terminology, immunity and inflammation, inheritance, cancer, and infectious diseases. Part II, *Diseases of the Systems,* discusses the major diseases of the body systems. Also returning is the popular *Side by Side* feature; *Prevention Plus!* boxes; *Diseases at a Glance* charts; and expanded *Interactive Exercises,* including case studies and multiple-choice, true/false, fill-in-the-blank, and labeling exercises.

## Enhancements to the Seventh Edition

- **Expanded *Diseases at a Glance* charts.** These popular and effective study guides now include information from the text on prevention and diseases across the lifespan.
- **Expanded diseases across lifespan.** Discussion of age-related diseases is expanded to include material on diseases across the lifespan.
- **Expanded pharmacology.** Common pharmacologic treatments of disease have been incorporated throughout the text. Readers will recognize the names and uses of common over-the-counter and prescription medicines.
- **Consistent coverage of disease topics.** Throughout the text, the authors attempted to include, for each disease, information on incidence, prevalence, risk factors, symptoms, etiology, diagnosis, treatment, and prevention.
- **Nutrition incorporated throughout.** The material on nutrition that was covered in a single chapter has been integrated into relevant areas throughout the text.
- **Trauma included.** More trauma-related disorders and diseases have been added throughout.
- **Addition of diseases of the eyes and ears.** This material has been included in an expanded Chapter 13, *Diseases of the Nervous System and Special Senses.*
- **Resources/references.** Updated professional resources have been included at the end of each chapter.
- **A better fit for one-semester courses.** By incorporating nutrition information throughout, the seventh edition now has 16 chapters, making this text adaptable to most semester-long courses.

## Teaching and Learning Package

### Student DVD-ROM

The interactive student DVD-ROM packaged in the back of the book contains a host of interactive study aids. The videos and animations help the students to visualize the content they are learning. Interactive exercises, games, and activities provide students with extra practice to master the chapter content.

### Companion Website

The Companion Website (www.pearsonhighered .com/zelman) is a text-specific, interactive, online workbook that provides student activities and practice quizzes—complete with instant scoring and immediate feedback. This website may be used to enrich the students' learning, and comes complete with Internet links, an audio glossary, and case studies. The website scores the student's results and allows those results to be sent to instructors via e-mail.

## Instructor's Resource Manual

This manual (0-13-515558-4) contains a wealth of material to help faculty plan and manage the human disease course. It includes lecture suggestions and content abstracts, learning objectives, a 1,289-question test bank, worksheets, and more for each chapter.

## Instructor's Resource DVD-ROM

The DVD-ROM (0-13-515559-2) provides many resources in an electronic format. It includes the complete 1,289-question test bank that allows instructors to design customized quizzes and exams. It also includes a PowerPoint™ lec-ture package that contains key discussion points along with color images, animations, and videos. This package allows instructors to customize the materials to meet their specific course needs.

The Instructor's Resource DVD-ROM also includes a collection of 212 images available for instructors to download for presentation purposes. This image library encompasses each of the high-quality images contained in the text and may be used in any way that instructors wish.

## Online Course Management Systems

**Online Course Options** are available for schools using course management systems. The online course solutions feature interactive assessment modules, electronic test banks, PowerPoint™ lectures, animations and video clips, and more. For more information about adopting an online course management system to accompany *Human Diseases, 7/e,* please contact your local Pearson Health Science representative.

**James Aumer, MS, C(ASCP)**
Program Director, Department of Medical Sciences
Rochester Institute of Technology
Rochester, New York

**Carole Berube, MA, MSN, BSN, RN**
Instructor, Health Sciences
Bristol Community College
Fall River, Massachusetts

**Glenn Bower, BA, MS, Ed**
Department Coordinator, Mortuary Science
Cypress College
Cypress, California

**Paula Cantwell, BS, RN, BSN, MA**
Associate Professor, Technical Science Department
New England Institute of Technology
Warwick, Rhode Island

**Michael P. Covone, MEd, RT(R), CT**
Assistant Professor, School of Health Sciences
Pennsylvania College of Technology
Williamsport, Pennsylvania

**Debra Downs, LPN, RMA**
Program Director, Medical Assisting
Okefenokee Technical College
Waycross, Georgia

**Ruby Fogg, MA/MAT**
Professor, Math and Science
New Hampshire Community Technical College
Manchester, New Hampshire

**Suzanne B. Garrett, MSA, RHIA**
Associate Professor, Health Information Management
Central Florida Community College
Ocala, Florida

**Rebecca Gibson Lee, MSTE, CMA, ASPT**
Professor/Program Director, Medical Assisting Technology
The University of Akron
Akron, Ohio

**Karen E. Gieseker, PhD, MS**
Assistant Professor, Institute of Public Health
Georgia State University
Atlanta, Georgia

**Naomi S. Greenberg, OTR, MPH, PhD**
Program Director, Occupational Therapy Assisting
LaGuardia Community College
Long Island City, New York

**Sandra Johnson, RHIT**
Instructor, Health Information Technology
San Juan College
Farmington, New Mexico

**Cherie Mattson, CMA, LPN**
Instructor, Medical Assisting
Ridgewater College
Willmar, Minnesota

**Ryan D. Morris, BS, MS**
Instructor, Life Sciences
Pierce College
Lakewood, Washington

**Brigitte Niedzwiecki, RN, MSN**
Program Director, Medical Assisting
Chippewa Valley Technical College
Eau Claire, Wisconsin

**Pamela K. Terry, PhD, CHES, CADP CIPS, FASHA**
Associate Professor, Health Sciences
Western Illinois University
Macomb, Illinois

**Connie Werner, RHIA, MS**
Coordinator, Healthcare Coding Program
York College of Pennsylvania
York, Pennsylvania

**Judy Williams, PhD**
Professor, Biological Sciences
Southeastern Oklahoma State University
Durant, Oklahoma

**Kari Williams, DC**
Program Director, Medical Office Technology
Front Range Community College
Longmont, Colorado

**Mark Zelman, PhD,** is Associate Professor of Biology and Chair of Natural Sciences and Mathematics at Aurora University in Aurora, Illinois. A native of Chicago, Mark received his BS in Biology, with minors in Psychology and Chemistry, at Rockford College. Mark received his PhD from the Department of Microbiology and Immunology at Loyola University Chicago, where he studied bacterial and mammalian antigens in a mouse model for human autoimmune disease. Mark was a postdoctoral fellow at University of Chicago, where he studied molecular cell physiology. Before coming to AU, Mark was a biology professor, a college administrator, and a medical writer. Mark pursues a wide range of interests in biology and he is especially interested in enhancing K–12 science education. He enjoys bird-watching and camping with his sons, Joe and Tom, and wears out quite a few shoes training for marathons and triathlons. Mark dedicates the seventh edition to Joe and Tom.

**Elaine Tompary, PharmD,** received her Doctor of Pharmacy Degree from the University of Illinois at Chicago. Dr. Tompary taught courses in pharmacology, pathophysiology, pharmacy law, and pharmaceutical calculations at William Rainey Harper College and the College of Lake County in Illinois. She has served as mentor and preceptor for pharmacy students at the University of Illinois and Drake University. She currently works for McNeil Consumer and Specialty Pharmaceuticals as a manager of medical science and outcomes research. She is a dedicated wife to Drew and mother and teacher to her children, Christopher and Andriana.

**Jill Raymond, PhD,** received her PhD in Microbiology from the University of California at Davis. She received and completed a postdoctoral fellowship in infectious diseases at the University of California at San Diego, where she studied the parasite *Giardia lamblia.* She has been teaching for thirteen years at Rock Valley College in Rockford, Illinois. In addition to teaching numerous biology courses, both traditional and online, Dr. Raymond teaches a human sexuality course and lectures at community education outreach programs. Dr. Raymond enjoys gardening, working with dogs, and European travel. Dr. Raymond would like to thank her wonderful husband and family for their continuing support through the craziness of writing a textbook.

**Paul Holdaway, MA,** a native Hoosier, is a graduate of Indiana State University and was an instructor there for two years. He is currently the senior member of the Biology Department at Harper College in Palatine, Illinois, where Dr. Mary Lou Mulvihill was an admired fellow biologist and friend. Dr. Zelman and Dr. Tompary are also former departmental colleagues and longstanding friends. Upon Dr. Mulvihill's retirement, Professor Holdaway assumed the teaching schedule of Dr. Mulvihill, and he has been involved in the anatomy, physiology, and human disease curriculum since that time. Paul takes pleasure in a wide range of biological and clinical interests, as well as sports and family activities.

# Part I

## Mechanisms of Disease

How do we define and describe disease? What causes disease? In Part I, we discuss the manifestations, terminology, diagnosis, and mechanisms of disease.

### Chapters

# Introduction to Disease

## Learning Objectives

After studying this chapter, you should be able to

- Define disease and disease-related terms
- Define and discuss the manifestations of disease
- Define terms used to describe disease
- Explain diagnosis of disease
- Define and discuss the chief causes of disease
- Identify risk factors related to disease

## Fact or Fiction?

Plague does not occur in the United States.

**Fiction:** Plague first reached the western United States around 1900. Plague now occurs at low levels in the American southwest, particularly in Arizona, Colorado, and New Mexico. Rats, mice, foxes, squirrels, marmots, prairie dogs, and even house cats have been identified as carriers.

# Disease Chronicle

## The Black Death

... If one were to seek to establish one generalization ... to catch the mood of the Europeans in the second half of the fourteenth century, it would be that they were enduring a crisis of faith. Assumptions which had been taken for granted for centuries were now in question, the very framework of men's reasoning seemed to be breaking up. And though the Black Death was far from being the only cause, the anguish and disruption which it had inflicted made the greatest single contribution to the disintegration of an age.

—P. Ziegler, *The Black Death*

The Black Death, also known as the plague, has killed and terrified people through the ages. For much of human history, understanding of disease and knowledge of normal human physiology was extremely limited. Effective control and treatment of most diseases awaited a systematic, scientific approach and a body of medical knowledge and technology.

# ▶ Introduction

The human body possesses a remarkable capacity to maintain health. Changes constantly occur within and outside the body, and yet a steady state called **homeostasis** is generally maintained. Although pH, temperature, blood composition, and fluid levels fluctuate, organ systems normally correct these changes before they threaten the body's health. A significant disturbance in the homeostasis of the body triggers a variety of responses that often produce disease. If we consider homeostasis to be a state of equilibrium, **disease** can be defined as a state of functional disequilibrium, a change in function or structure that is considered to be abnormal. Clearly, knowledge of normal structure (**anatomy**) and normal function (**physiology**) are essential to the study of disease. **Pathology** is the study of disease in general, and **pathophysiology** is the study of the physiological processes leading up to disease.

# ▶ Manifestations of Disease

A disease manifests itself through certain signs and symptoms. **Signs** are objective evidence of disease observed on physical examination, such as abnormal pulse or respiratory rate, fever, sweating, and pallor; **symptoms** are subjective indications of disease reported by the patient, such as pain, dizziness, and itching. Certain sets of signs and symptoms occur concurrently in some diseases, and their combination is called a **syndrome**. These include acquired immunodeficiency syndrome, malabsorption syndrome, and Down's syndrome.

# ▶ Diagnosis

**Diagnosis** is the use of scientific or clinical methods to determine the nature of a disease. A diagnosis provides the basis for rational and effective treatment of disease and is based on many factors, including the physical exam, signs and symptoms, patient history, laboratory data, and specific diagnostic tests. Signs and symptoms, discussed previously, are familiar manifestations of disease and can be ascertained through physical examination and interviews with a patient or with a patient's family. Frequently the course and history of the signs and symptoms yields important diagnostic information. Likewise, family disease history may give insight into genetic risk for developing certain diseases. Laboratory data are derived from procedures such as urinalysis, blood chemistry, electrocardiography, and radiography. Diagnostic-imaging techniques such as computed tomography (CT scan), magnetic resonance imaging (MRI), ultrasound, and nuclear medicine allow physicians to visualize structural and functional changes. A biopsy, surgical removal and analysis of tissue samples, yields information about changes at the cellular level.

# ▶ Describing Disease

The physician, having made a diagnosis, may state the **prognosis** of the disease, or the predicted course and outcome of the disease. The prognosis may state the chances for complete recovery, predict the permanent loss of function, or give probability of survival. The course of a disease varies; it may have a sudden onset and short duration, in which case it is an **acute** disease. Influenza, measles, and the common cold are examples. A disease may have a slower, less severe onset and a long duration of months or years; such a disease is **chronic**. Such diseases include diabetes, cancers, and osteoarthritis. Diseases that will end in death are called **terminal**.

The signs and symptoms of disease at times subside, during a period known as **remission**. They may recur in all their severity in a period of **exacerbation**. Certain diseases (leukemia and ulcerative colitis, for example) are characterized by periods of remission and exacerbation. A **relapse** occurs when a disease returns weeks or months after its apparent cessation.

A **complication** is a disease or other abnormal state that develops in a person already suffering from a disease. The complication may negatively affect the prognosis or course of the original disease. For example, a person confined to bed with a serious fracture may develop pneumonia as a complication of the inactivity. Infection of the testes may be a complication of mumps, particularly after puberty. Anemia generally accompanies leukemia, cancer, and chronic kidney disease. The aftermath of a particular disease is called the **sequela**, a sequel. The permanent damage to the heart after rheumatic fever is an example of a sequela, as is the paralysis of polio. Sterility may be a sequela of pelvic inflammatory disease and sexually transmitted infections.

Public health agencies monitor the impact diseases have on populations by gathering mortality and morbidity data. **Mortality** is a measure of the number of deaths attributed to a disease in a given population over a given period of time. **Morbidity** is a measure of the disability and extent of illness caused by a disease. Each gives public health officials and physicians an idea of how serious a disease is and thus helps direct resources toward prevention and cure. Table 1–1▶ lists the 10 leading causes of death in the United States.

Disease occurrence is also described in terms of prevalence and incidence. **Prevalence** describes the number of cases of a disease occurring at a given time in a specified population. Prevalence data allow the determination of the impact and significance of a disease for a given population and these data are used to direct healthcare resources and research. Certain diseases, such as cancer, heart disease, and diabetes, are more prevalent in older adults than in adolescents. **Incidence** describes the number of new cases of a disease at a given time in a specified population. Incidence data allow tracking of changes in the occurrence of disease. A disease may increase in incidence seasonally, as influenza does during winter.

**Epidemiology** is the study of the occurrence, transmission, distribution, and control of disease. Epidemiologists use prevalence and incidence data and information about the geo-graphic distribution of disease to develop methods to prevent and control diseases. The Centers for Disease Control and Prevention in Atlanta, Georgia (www.cdc.gov) is the chief epidemiologic institution in the United States.

## ▶ Causes of Disease

An important aspect of any disease is its **etiology**, or cause. The source or cause of a disease, together with its development, is its **pathogenesis**. If the cause of a disease is not known, it is said to be **idiopathic**. Most causes of disease fall into one or more categories. At the root of most causes, however, is a **lesion** of some sort. A lesion could be a damaged gene or enzyme, or abnormal cells, tissues, or organs. The major causes and mechanisms of disease are

| Table 1–1 ▶ Ten Leading Causes of Death, 2004, U.S. | |
| --- | --- |
| **Disease** | **Number of Deaths** |
| Heart disease | 654,092 |
| Cancer | 550,270 |
| Stroke | 150,147 |
| Chronic lower respiratory disease | 123,884 |
| Accidents | 108,694 |
| Diabetes | 72,815 |
| Alzheimer's disease | 65,829 |
| Influenza/pneumonia | 61,472 |
| Nephritis, nephrotic syndrome, and nephrosis | 42,762 |
| Septicemia | 33,464 |

*Source:* CDC National Vital Statistics Report, vol. 54, no. 19, June 28, 2006

## Prevention ✚ Plus!

### Centers for Disease Control and Prevention

Credible, accurate information about disease is critical to maintaining personal health. Students of human disease should become familiar with appropriate professional resources and organizations. The mission of the Centers for Disease Control and Prevention in Atlanta, Georgia is "to promote health and quality of life by preventing and controlling disease, injury, and disability." First founded by the U.S. government in 1946 as the Communicable Disease Center, with a focus on controlling malaria and other infectious diseases, the CDC has become part of the Department of Health and Human Services and has been dedicated to promoting both public health and personal health. It is of interest to note CDC's own objectives for promoting public health:

- Promote social and physical environments that are accessible; that support health, safety, and quality of life; and that promote healthy behaviors.
- Promote access to and receipt of recommended quality, effective, evidence-based preventive and healthcare services, including dental and mental health care.
- Promote social, emotional, and mental well-being.
- Promote reproductive and sexual health.
- Prevent chronic diseases and their consequences.
- Prevent infectious diseases and their consequences.
- Prevent injury, violence, suicide, and their consequences.
- Improve behaviors that promote health and well-being.

Visit the CDC website, www.cdc.gov, for information on disease control and prevention, healthy living, traveler's health, vaccinations, workplace health and safety, most diseases and conditions, disease statistics, and health across the lifespan. The website provides educational documents and links to research on many diseases.

discussed in the remaining chapters in Part I of the text. These causes include inflammatory or immune disorders, including allergy; infection; abnormal cell growth (neoplasms); heredity; nutrition; environmental factors; and stress. Table 1–2► lists major causes and examples of associated diseases.

## ► Risk Factors

**Risk factors** predispose an individual to the development of a disease. Note that a risk factor is not equivalent to a **cause**. While an individual with a risk factor for a certain disease has an increased chance of developing that disease, it

| Table 1–2 ► Major Causes of Disease | |
|---|---|
| **Cause** | **Disease** |
| Inflammation/autoimmunity/allergy | Asthma, systemic lupus erythematosus |
| Infection | Tuberculosis, influenza |
| Neoplasm | Lung cancer, malignant melanoma |
| Heredity | Sickle cell anemia, cystic fibrosis |
| Malnutrition | Pernicious anemia, iron-deficiency anemia |
| Stress | Hypertension, heart disease |

may not necessarily cause the disease. Risk factors may be environmental, chemical, physiological, psychological, or genetic. A well-known risk factor for lung cancer is cigarette smoking. The development of coronary artery disease has multiple well-established risk factors, such as high blood cholesterol and lipids, a history of hypertension, cigarette smoking, physical inactivity, obesity, diabetes, and a family history. Knowledge of disease risk factors is important; while eliminating known risk factors for a disease may not prevent disease, it may reduce the chance of developing disease.

## ▶ Treatment of Disease

Treatment includes procedures for the cure or reduction of symptoms of disease. Treatment depends on the nature of the disease, the characteristics of the patient, and goals of the patient and physician. Treatment may be aimed at curing a disease and/or removing its cause if possible. Not all diseases are curable, and in some cases, the causes are unknown. Thus some treatments are **palliative**, or **symptomatic**, designed to relieve and manage the symptoms of the disease without addressing the cause.

Treatment includes medical (pharmacologic) procedures, which use specific drugs to cure or relieve symptoms. Other diseases may require surgery to correct anatomical and physiological abnormalities related to the disease. Some diseases require psychiatric and psychological treatments. In some cases, effective treatment requires the use of several procedures simultaneously.

Readers will apply disease terms and concepts learned in Chapter 1 throughout their study of the text. In Part I, general processes of disease will be discussed, including the roles of heredity, infection, abnormal cell growth (cancer), inflammation, and immunity. In Part II of the text, readers will apply concepts and terms from Part I to the study of specific diseases of the body systems.

## RESOURCES

Centers for Disease Control and Prevention: www.cdc.gov

United States Department of Health and Human Services: www.dhhs.gov

# Interactive Exercises

## Cases for Critical Thinking

1. Some athletes may develop abnormally high red blood cell counts. Why? In the athlete's case, is this a sign of disease?

2. A patient reports to her physician that she feels weak and dizzy. Is this enough information to make a diagnosis? What other sources of information can her physician consult?

3. Consult Table 1–1. How can this information be used to direct healthcare research and resources? What is the significance of the information about accidents?

## Multiple Choice

1. A skin rash is an example of a _____.
   a. sign                     b.    symptom
   c. laboratory result        d.    syndrome

2. A(n) _____ disease has a sudden onset and short course.
   a. acute                    b.    terminal
   c. chronic                  d.    idiopathic

3. The cause of a disease is known as its _____.
   a. pathogensis              b.    complication
   c. sequela                  d.    etiology

4. A steady state maintained within the body is called _____.
   a. homeostasis              b.    disease
   c. disequilibrium           d.    pathology

5. The worsening of signs and symptoms is known as _____.
   a. remission                b.    exacerbation
   c. relapse                  d.    complication

## True or False

_____ 1. Anatomy is the study of normal body function.

_____ 2. Mortality refers to the number of deaths caused by a disease.

_____ 3. Symptoms are objective evidence of a disease.

_____ 4. Signs may be perceived by the physician.

_____ 5. Exacerbation and remission may characterize a chronic disease.

## Fill-Ins

1. The predicted outcome of a disease is its _____.

2. Damaged tissue, DNA, or enzymes are examples of _____ that cause a disease.

3. If the cause of a disease is not known, it is said to be _____.

4. Return of symptoms after their apparent cessation is _____.

5. The signs and symptoms of a chronic disease at times subside during a period known as _____.

# Multimedia Preview

Additional interactive resources and activities for this chapter can be found on the Companion Website. For videos, audio glossary, and review, access the accompanying DVD-ROM in this book.

## ▶ DVD-ROM Highlights

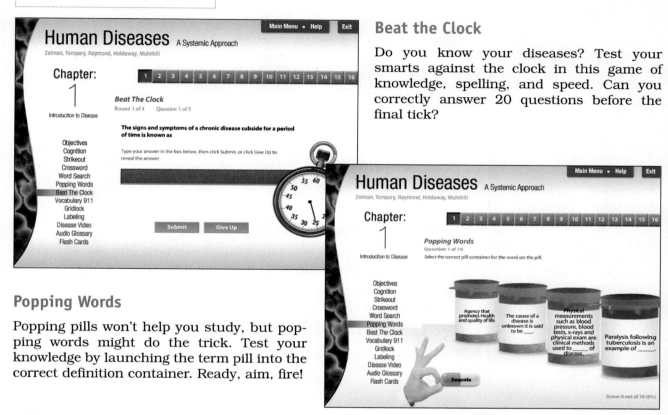

### Beat the Clock

Do you know your diseases? Test your smarts against the clock in this game of knowledge, spelling, and speed. Can you correctly answer 20 questions before the final tick?

### Popping Words

Popping pills won't help you study, but popping words might do the trick. Test your knowledge by launching the term pill into the correct definition container. Ready, aim, fire!

## ▶ Website Highlights—www.pearsonhighered.com/zelman

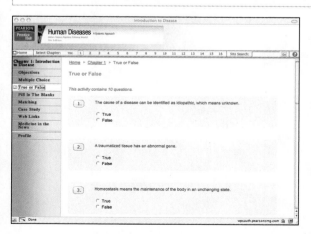

### True or False Quiz

Take advantage of the free-access online study guide that accompanies your textbook. You'll find a true or false quiz that provides instant feedback and allows you to check your score to see what you got right or wrong. By clicking on this URL you'll also access links to current news articles and an audio glossary.

In these renal glomeruli, there is proliferation of cells representing proliferative glomerulonephritis. (Courtesy of the National Toxicology Program.)

CHAPTER

2

# Immunity and the Lymphatic System

## Learning Objectives

After studying this chapter, you should be able to

- Define immunity
- Compare and contrast nonspecific and specific immunity
- Describe the normal structure and function of the lymphatic system
- Identify the four types of hypersensitivities
- Define autoimmunity and autoantibodies
- Describe the etiology, incidence, symptoms, diagnosis, and treatment for selected autoimmune diseases
- Describe the etiology, incidence, symptoms, diagnosis, and treatment for HIV and AIDS
- Explain AIDS as it relates to immunodeficiency
- Compare and contrast active and passive immunity

## Fact or Fiction?

HIV can be transmitted through saliva.

*Fiction: HIV is found in saliva, but in quantities too small to cause infection.*

## Inflammation

Throughout history, humans undoubtedly have observed the inflammatory response even if they understood little of its causes or treatment. Around 1500 B.C., Egyptians used dried myrtle leaves to relieve back pain. In 200 B.C., the Greek physician Hippocrates prescribed willow bark leaves to relieve fever and pain. One of the early systemic descriptions of inflammation came from the Roman physician Aulus Cornelius Celsus (25 B.C.– 50 A.D.), who recorded its cardinal signs: heat, redness, swelling, and pain. Today, the active ingredient in aspirin, acetylsalicylic acid, is derived from a related anti-inflammatory chemical (salicylic acid) found in myrtle leaves and willow tree bark.

# ▶ Immunity

**Immunity** is the ability of the body to defend itself against infectious agents, foreign cells, and even abnormal body cells, such as cancer cells. Immunity can be acquired naturally by infection, as when chicken pox confers protection against acquiring it again. Immunity can be artificially acquired by immunization, as when the polio vaccine induces immunity against polio. Immunity includes nonspecific and specific immunity. Nonspecific immunity, also known as innate immunity, is present at birth and provides immediate but general protection against any foreign agent that enters the body. **Specific immunity**, also known as acquired immunity, is effective against particular identified foreign agents and develops in response to contact with that agent. Once established against a foreign agent, specific immunity is able to respond to future exposures to the same agent.

## Nonspecific Immunity

*Physical and Chemical Barriers*   Intact skin is the body's first line of defense. A physical barrier, skin also produces chemical barriers to infection. Secretions such as tears, saliva, sweat, and oil contain chemicals that destroy foreign invaders. Mucous membranes that line body passages open to the exterior produce mucus, which traps foreign material and forms a barrier to invasion. Microscopic cilia hairs that line the respiratory tract sweep out debris and impurities trapped in mucus.

*Phagocytosis*   White blood cells (**leukocytes**) can destroy infectious agents through phagocytosis. In phagocytosis, which means cell eating, leukocytes engulf and digest bacteria or other material. This process is fairly nonspecific, unable to discriminate among or remember past encounters with various types of infectious agents. While some leukocytes travel in the blood to target foreign material, others remain in tissues.

*Natural Killer Cells*   Natural killer cells are a type of leukocyte that recognizes body cells with abnormal membranes. Cell membranes can become altered from cells being infected with foreign invaders like viruses. Natural killer cells can destroy abnormal cells on contact by secreting a protein that destroys the cell membrane.

*Fever*   Fever can be a sign that the body is defending itself. When phagocytes find and destroy foreign invaders, they release substances that raise body temperature. Fever aids the immune system by stimulating phagocytes, increasing metabolism, and inhibiting the multiplication of some microorganisms. Hence, fever is a symptom arising from the normal interplay between the immune system and microorganisms, and can be beneficial. Fever should not always be eliminated; however, fever should be monitored closely.

*Interferon*   **Interferon** is a group of substances that stimulate the immune system. Because interferon boosts the immune system, it has been used to treat infections and cancer. Interferon was first found in cells infected with the flu virus and was named for its ability to interfere with viral multiplication. Virus-infected cells and other agents produce interferon.

*Inflammation*   The cause of inflammation may be a trauma or injury, such as a sprained ankle or a severe blow. A physical irritant in the tissue—a piece of glass, a wasp sting, or an ingrown toenail—will trigger the response. Pathogenic organisms such as bacteria, viruses, fungi, or parasites will do the same. Figure 2–1 ▶ shows various agents that are capable of stimulating an inflammatory response.

The signs and symptoms of inflammation are redness, swelling, heat, and pain. Inflammation is a protective tissue response to injury or invasion. Vascular changes occur when tissue is traumatized or irritated. Local blood vessels, arterioles, and capillaries dilate, increasing blood flow to the injured area. This increased amount of blood, **hyperemia**, causes the heat and redness associated with inflammation. As the blood flow to the site of the injury or infection increases, more and more leukocytes reach the

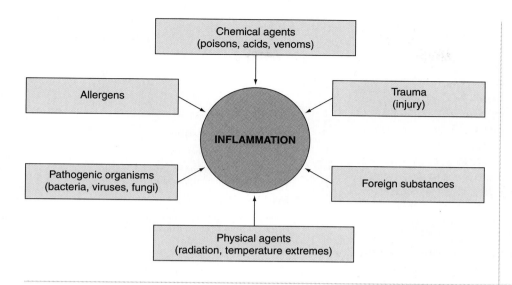

Figure 2–1 ► Agents capable of stimulating an inflammatory response.

area. Leukocytes called **neutrophils** line up within the capillary walls. Neutrophils are specialized cells that defend the body against invading microorganisms and speed healing by engulfing cell debris in injured tissues. The damaged tissue releases a substance called **histamine** that causes the capillary walls to become more permeable. This increased permeability enables plasma and neutrophils to move out of the blood vessels into the tissue. The attraction of the white blood cells to the site of inflammation is called **chemotaxis**. The plasma and white blood cells that escape from the capillaries comprise the **inflammatory exudate** (Figure 2–2 ►). This exudate in the tissues causes the swelling associated with inflammation. The excess of fluid in the tissues puts pressure on sensitive nerve endings, causing pain.

Bacterial infection may cause inflammation. The presence of toxin-producing bacteria such as *Staphylococci* and *Streptococci* triggers an inflammatory response. To increase the effectiveness of the inflammatory and immune response, the bone marrow and lymph nodes release very large quantities of leukocytes. The white cell count may rise to 30,000 or more from the normal range of 4000 to 10,000 per cubic microliter of blood. The excessive production of white cells is called **leukocytosis** and

is a sign of infection or inflammation, such as appendicitis.

The neutrophils die soon after ingesting bacteria and toxins, and release substances that liquefy the surrounding tissue, forming pus, a thick yellow fluid consisting of liquefied tissue, dead neutrophils, and inflammatory exudate. Other phagocytic white cells, the **monocytes** or **macrophages**, follow the neutrophils in the process of clearing debris. Inflammatory exudate contains a plasma protein, **fibrin**, essential for the blood-clotting mechanism. Fibrin forms a clot in the damaged tissue, walling off the infection and preventing its spread.

Bacteria that cause pus formation are called **pyogenic** bacteria. An inflammation associated with pus formation is a **suppurative** inflammation. Abscesses, boils, and styes are examples of inflammations with suppuration.

The inflammatory agent may damage tissue. Wound healing occurs in two ways: by regeneration and fibrosis. Whether one or both processes occurs depends on the type of tissue damaged and the severity of the injury. Regeneration is the replacement of destroyed tissue with the same kind of cells. In fibrosis, **fibroblasts**, a type of connective tissue cell, produce collagen fibers. The fibers contract, drawing the cut surfaces together. The healed site

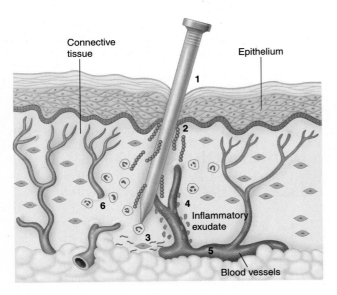

Connective tissue

Epithelium

1. Dirty nail punctures skin.

2. Bacteria enter and multiply.

3. Injured cells release histamine.

4. Blood vessels dilate and become permeable, releasing inflammatory exudate.

5. Blood flow to the damaged site increases.

6. Neutrophils (polymorph) move toward bacteria (chemotaxis) and destroy them (phagocytosis).

Inflammatory exudate

Blood vessels

**Figure 2–2** ▶ Vascular changes that occur with inflammation.

consists of a meshwork of collagen fibers known as scar tissue. A scar after surgery or a severe burn is often raised and hard. This development is known as keloid healing and is really a benign tumor (Figure 2–3 ▶). Surgery to remove such a scar is usually ineffective, as the subsequent incision will have a tendency to heal in the same way. Sometimes the collagen fibers anchor together adjacent structures, causing **adhesions**, which can interfere with organ functions. The problems associated with adhesions are explained in later chapters.

**Figure 2–3** ▶ Keloid. (© JCD/ Custom Medical Stock Photo.)

## ▶ Specific Immunity and the Lymphatic System

Specific immunity or the immune system is connected to the body via the lymphatic system. The lymphatic system includes a network of **lymphatic vessels**, **lymph nodes**, and other **lymphoid organs** (Figure 2–4 ▶). Without the lymphatic system the cardiovascular system would cease to function and body defenses would be seriously impaired. Because the cardiovascular system is a high-pressure system, fluid leaks out of the capillary beds into tissues. Most of this fluid is reabsorbed, but some, up to 3 liters a day, remains behind in the tissues. The fluid, called **lymph**, must be returned to the bloodstream or it will accumulate in the tissues, producing swelling or edema, and there will be insufficient blood volume for cardiovascular functioning. Lymphedema occurs when tissues swell because lymphatic vessels are blocked.

As lymph is transported in the lymphatic vessels toward the heart, it is filtered by lymph nodes. Within lymph nodes, macrophages phagocytize or engulf and digest bacteria, viruses,

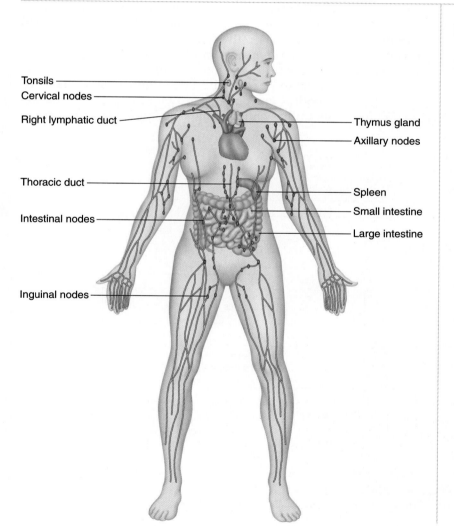

**Figure 2–4** ▶ The lymphatic system.

Tonsils

Cervical nodes

Right lymphatic duct

Thoracic duct

Intestinal nodes

Inguinal nodes

Thymus gland

Axillary nodes

Spleen

Small intestine

Large intestine

and other foreign material. Swelling of lymph nodes during infection is a result of this filtration function. Lymph nodes produce **lymphocytes**, a type of white blood cell that responds to bacteria, viruses, and foreign material in lymph. Lymphocytes play a critical role in specific immunity.

Specific immunity is based on the ability to recognize and respond to foreign elements. The foreign element that triggers the immune response is known as an **antigen**, which often is a protein from microorganisms or other foreign cells. Antigens differ from each other in structure and are unique. The specificity of acquired immunity is its ability to recognize these different antigens.

Specific immunity against antigens includes humoral and cell-mediated immunity. **Humoral immunity** includes **antibodies**, and **cell-mediated immunity** includes activated lymphocytes. Antibodies and activated lymphocytes comprise acquired immunity (Figure 2–5▶). Both humoral and cell-mediated immunity work to-

gether to fight a foreign invader. Both are activated by an antigen, such as *Salmonella* bacteria from an undercooked chicken breast. The antigen interacts with lymphocytes in tissues, in lymph, or in blood.

Two types of lymphocytes provide immunity: the T and B lymphocytes. The lymphocytes responsible for cell-mediated immunity are processed by the thymus gland; hence they are called **T lymphocytes**. The other type of lymphocyte, **B lymphocytes**, are responsible for humoral immunity. Antibodies and T lymphocytes are each highly specific for one type of antigen.

B lymphocytes can play different roles in humoral immunity. Some B lymphocytes interact with antigens and become activated. Some other activated B lymphocytes are transformed into **plasma cells**, which divide rapidly and produce large numbers of antibodies. These agents are secreted into the lymph and travel to the blood to be circulated through the body. The antibodies are plasma proteins, which are gamma globulins called **immunoglobulins** (Ig). Antibodies

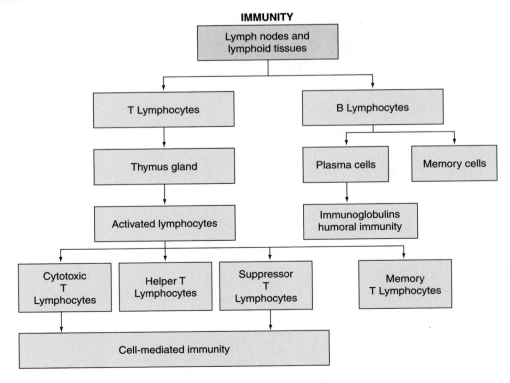

Figure 2–5 ▶ Cell-mediated immunity versus humoral immunity.

| Table 2–1 ► Types of Immunoglobulins | | |
| --- | --- | --- |
| **Type** | **Function** | **Location** |
| IgG | Produced in primary and secondary immune responses, neutralizes toxins, bacteria, and viruses | Blood plasma; crosses the placenta from mother to fetus |
| IgM | Protects newborns | Bound to B lymphocytes in circulation; usually the first to increase in the immune response |
| IgA | Localized protection at mucosal surfaces | Mucosal secretions, colostrum (early breast milk) |
| IgE | Allergy | Trace amounts in serum; secreted by sensitized plasma cells in tissues and locally attached to mast cells |
| IgD | Activates B lymphocytes | Attached to B lymphocytes |

bind to antigens and tag the antigen for destruction by the immune system. There are several types of immunoglobulins: IgG neutralizes toxins and viruses; IgM protects newborns; IgA offers localized protection at mucosal surfaces; IgE is involved in allergy; and IgD activates B lymphocytes. See Table 2–1 ► for a summary of Ig functions.

Other B lymphocytes do not become plasma cells but remain dormant until reactivated by the same antigen. These lymphocytes are called **memory cells** and are responsible for a more potent and rapid antibody response during subsequent exposures to the same antigen. This secondary response to the antigen produces antibodies faster and in larger quantities, and lasts longer than the initial response. This strong secondary response explains why a vaccine protects a person from a subsequent exposure to an infectious agent. The secondary immune response also is the basis for the effectiveness of booster shots, which are given at intervals after initial vaccinations in order to increase levels of memory cells (Figure 2–6 ►).

**Figure 2–6** ► Secondary response begins more rapidly after exposure to antigen, produces more antibodies, and lasts for a longer time than initial exposure.

There are several different kinds of T lymphocytes, each with different functions: **cytotoxic** or **CD8 T lymphocytes**, **helper** or **CD4 T lymphocytes**, memory T lymphocytes, and **suppressor T lymphocytes**. The cytotoxic T lymphocytes are often called killer lymphocytes because they are capable of killing invading organisms. They have on their surfaces receptor proteins that bind tightly to cells or organisms that contain a specific antigen. Once bound, the cytotoxic T lymphocytes release poisonous substances into the attacked cell. Many organisms can be killed by one killer lymphocyte. The cytotoxic lymphocytes are important in killing cells that have been invaded by viruses. These T lymphocytes also can destroy cancer cells.

The helper T lymphocytes are named for their ability to help the immune system in many ways. They increase the activity of killer lymphocytes and stimulate B lymphocytes. Activated helper T lymphocytes secrete lymphokines that increase the response of other types of lymphoid cells to the antigen. In addition, lymphokines activate macrophages to destroy large numbers of invaders by phagocytosis. After an infection or vaccination, some of the T lymphocytes that participated in the response remain as memory T lymphocytes that can rapidly mobilize should the same antigen be encountered again. Suppressor T lymphocytes are believed to dampen or suppress the immune response.

▶ Hypersensitivity—Allergies

Closely related to the concept of immunity is **allergy**, or **hypersensitivity**. Some diseases result from an individual's immune response, which causes tissue damage and disordered function rather than immunity. The immune phenomena are destructive rather than defensive in the individual who is hypersensitive or allergic to an antigen. Hypersensitivity diseases or allergic diseases may manifest themselves locally or systemically.

Abnormal sensitivity to allergens such as pollens, dust, dog hair, and certain foods or chemicals is the result of overproduction of IgE and its interaction with the allergens. IgE attaches one end to cells called **basophils** and **mast cells**; its other end points away from the cells, where the IgE can bind to the allergens. Mast cells are found in connective tissue and contain the chemicals **heparin**, **serotonin**, **bradykinin**, prostaglandin, and histamine.

When allergens enter the body and bind to the IgE antibodies located on the mast cells, the cells break down and release their chemicals. Histamine causes the dilation of the blood vessels, making them leak plasma into the tissues. This tissue fluid causes edema, or swelling, which when localized in the nasal passages results in the familiar congestion and irritation of hay fever. If the tissue damage and edema are near the skin, the welts and itching of hives may appear. Antihistamines inhibit the effects of histamine and are quite effective in the treatment of hives but less so for hay fever. A typical allergic reaction is illustrated in Figure 2–7 ▶.

Skin tests can determine the specific cause of an allergy. This procedure involves injecting a minute amount of antigen intradermally and observing any redness, which indicates a positive skin reaction. Allergy shots can desensitize the hypersensitive person. Small amounts of the offending allergen are administered, and concentrations are gradually increased. Desensitization inoculations work by causing an increase of IgG in the bloodstream. The IgG coats the allergen in the blood, blocking it from binding to IgE in the tissues, subsequently reducing the amount of tissue damage.

Local allergies occur in confined areas such as skin and mucous membranes and are exemplified by the development of a stuffy nose after inhaling pollen. In contrast, systemic allergy (anaphylaxis) occurs throughout the body and may be life threatening.

The underlying cellular mechanisms of the systemic anaphylactic reaction are the same as in the local response. However, during the systemic response, mast cells and basophils throughout the body become involved, triggering a generalized change in capillary permeability that leads to hypotension (low blood pressure) and shock. Smooth muscle contraction in the respiratory tract causes respiratory distress resembling asthma. Fluid in the larynx may obstruct the airways and necessitate a tracheotomy, a surgical opening into the trachea to facilitate passage of air or evacuation of secretions.

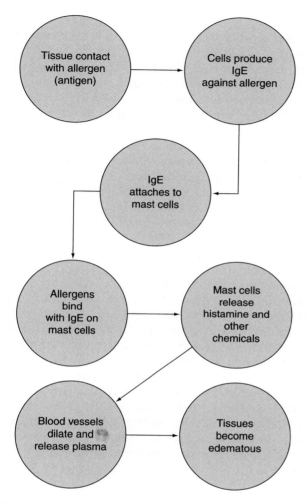

**Figure 2–7** ▶ Typical allergic reaction.

Epinephrine, glucocorticoids, or cortisone derivatives may be used to reduce the immune response and stabilize the vascular system.

Four types of hypersensitivities are recognized. Type I hypersensitivities are labeled allergic or anaphylactic hypersensitivity. These are triggered by allergen binding to IgE on mast cells, which produces either local severe inflammation or systemic severe inflammation (anaphylactic shock) (Figure 2–8▶). These are produced by bee venom, foods, or pollen.

Type II hypersensitivities are labeled cytotoxic or cytolytic and involve IgM or IgG interacting with foreign cells to cause their destruction. An example of a type II response is an incompatible blood transfusion. A person with type A blood has A antigens on the red cells and antibodies against type B blood in the serum. If such a person receives a type B transfusion, the antigens and antibodies interact. The red blood cells agglutinate, or clump together, and massive hemolysis (rupture) occurs.

Cross-matching for a blood transfusion must match blood type and **Rh factor**. In addition to antigens that determine blood type, Rh positive (Rh⁺) individuals have another antigen, the Rh factor, on their red blood cells. Rh negative (Rh⁻) individuals lack the Rh antigen. Another example of the cytolytic allergic response involves the transfusion of Rh⁺ blood to an Rh⁻ recipient. No problems would arise for the Rh⁻ recipient if it were the first such transfusion received, but if the Rh⁻ recipient was previously exposed or sensitized to the Rh factor, the recipient may form antibodies against this foreign protein, causing clumping and rupture of red blood cells.

Rh incompatibility during pregnancy is also a type II hypersensitivity. An Rh⁻ mother can become sensitized to the Rh antigen if the fetus is Rh⁺. However, maternal antibodies do not form

Less severe signs may include skin flush, hives, swelling of lips or tongue, wheezing, and abdominal cramps. Life-threatening signs include weakness and collapse due to low blood pressure, inability to breathe, and seizures.

## Prevention ✚ PLUS!

### Epinephrine Treatment for Anaphylaxis

The most vital therapy for systemic anaphylaxis is prompt intramuscular injection of epinephrine (adrenalin). Certain allergic individuals must carry epinephrine at all times in an EpiPen®, which can be self-injected in an emergency.

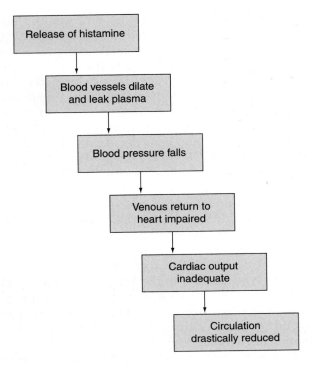

**Figure 2–8** ▶ Sequence of vascular events in anaphylactic shock.

and damage the fetus during the first such pregnancy, because the maternal and fetal blood do not mix. But during birth there may be mixing of blood, exposing the mother to the Rh⁺ antigen. The mother's immune system can recognize this antigen as foreign and produce antibodies against it, which would threaten subsequent pregnancies with an Rh⁺ fetus. To prevent this, RhoGAM®, an injectable medication, is given to Rh⁻ women after the delivery of Rh⁺ babies.

Type III hypersensitivities are labeled immune complex. In this type of hypersensitivity, antigens combine with antibodies, forming immune complexes. These immune complexes deposit in tissues and blood vessels, causing inflammation and tissue destruction. Immune complexes may form in the kidneys (causing glomerulonephritis, triggered after a streptococcal infection) or the lungs (causing farmer's lung, triggered by mold spore inhalation). Types I, II, and III are all immediate hypersensitivities; they develop within about 30 minutes of exposure to antigens or allergens.

Type IV hypersensitivities are called cell-mediated or delayed. Initial exposure to an antigen results in activation of a T lymphocyte-mediated immune response, which is slow to develop (delayed). For example, no reaction occurs the first time one contacts the oil of poison ivy. However, T cells may become sensitized to it. On the next exposure, the typical rash and irritation appear, caused by T lymphocyte secretion of cytokines that damage the tissues where the ivy oil has been absorbed. This delayed development is the type of reaction found in contact dermatitis and the significant tuberculin test (Figure 2–9▶). Table 2–2▶ summarizes the four types of hypersensitivities.

Organ transplantation can be a desirable treatment option for those suffering from serious organ disease. There are currently over 95,000 Americans waiting for an organ, and 4000 new patients are added to the list every month while 17 people die every day waiting for an organ. Organs that can be transplanted include heart, kidney, lung, liver, intestine, and pancreas. In an **autograft,** tissue grafts are transplanted from one site to another in the same patient; for example, a skin graft. **Isografts** are tissues donated by an identical twin. Autografts and isografts are highly successful because the immune system does not

**Figure 2–9** ▶ Induration measurement in a tuberculin skin test, a type IV hypersensitivity. (Courtesy of the CDC.)

| Table 2–2 ► Types of Hypersensitivities | | |
|---|---|---|
| **Type** | **Mechanism** | **Effect** |
| I | Excess IgE bound to mast cells and activated by allergens | Inflammation |
| II | IgM or IgG cause destruction of foreign cells | Cell lysis |
| III | Immune complexes are deposited in tissue and vessels | Inflammation and tissue destruction |
| IV | Sensitized T lymphocytes release cytokines | Inflammation and tissue damage |

view the graft as foreign. **Xenografts** are tissue grafts harvested from a different animal species; the use of pig heart valves in humans is an example.

The most common type of graft is an **allograft**, in which tissue is transplanted from one person to another, but the transplant donor and recipient are not identical twins. Before an allograft is attempted, the blood type of both the donor and recipient must be determined and must match. In addition, cell membrane antigens of their tissue cells are typed to determine how closely they match. At least a 75% match in cell membrane antigens is needed to attempt an allograft. Good tissue matches between unrelated people are difficult to find.

Tissue and organ rejections are examples of type IV or delayed hypersensitivity reactions. Organs could be easily transplanted if it were not for the immune system. The immune system recognizes the transplanted organ as foreign, and lymphocytes attack it, eventually destroying the transplanted organ. Compounding the problem is that the transplanted organ carries with it donor lymphocytes that react against the recipient's tissues (a graft versus host reaction). For these reasons, donor and recipient antigens are matched as closely as possible to lessen possible rejection. To prevent immune system rejection, the transplant patient receives medications, which may include corticosteroids to suppress inflammation and immunosuppressants. These drugs have severe side effects, including the suppressed immune system being unable to protect the body against other foreign agents and leaving the patient open to infection.

## ► Autoimmunity

The immune response normally recognizes the difference between the individual's own tissues and those of invaders; this is known as *tolerance.* When tolerance fails, an **autoimmune disease** may be the result. **Autoimmunity** occurs when individuals develop antibodies called autoantibodies to their own tissues or self-antigens. Almost all patients presenting with autoimmunity have some autoantibodies present in their serum. It is not always known whether the autoantibodies play an important role in the disease or are a secondary result of the tissue damage which has been caused by the disease process itself. Autoimmune patients also have autoreactive T cells. Several of these autoimmune diseases are described elsewhere in this book. **Lupus**, **scleroderma**, and **Sjögren's syndrome** are considered here.

### Lupus

Lupus is chronic inflammatory disease that can affect various parts of the body, including the skin, joints, heart, lungs, blood, kidneys, and brain. The National Women's Health Information Center estimates that 1.4 million, or 1 in 85, Americans have a form of lupus. Over 90% of lupus patients are women, and symptoms and diagnosis usually occur between the ages of 15 and 45. There are four types of lupus: systemic, discoid, drug induced, and neonatal.

Seventy percent of people with lupus have **systemic lupus erythematosis (SLE)**. In SLE, autoantibodies against DNA and RNA can damage any body cell, so many body systems can be involved. About half of SLE patients have an organ-threatening disease involving the heart, lungs, kidneys, liver, and blood; the other half of SLE patients have a non-organ-threatening disease. Common signs and symptoms of SLE include arthritis, low-grade fever, butterfly rash over the cheeks and bridge of the nose or more widespread rash, fatigue, photosensitivity, hair loss, and Raynaud's phenomenon (fingers turning white and blue in the cold). Raynaud's disease is discussed in Chapter 6. Figure 2–10► shows lupus skin rashes.

**Discoid** or **cutaneous lupus** is limited to the skin. It is identified by a rash that may appear on the face, neck, and scalp. Approximately 10% of discoid lupus patients develop systemic lupus. **Drug-induced lupus erythematosus (DILE)** can be brought on by more than 70 different prescription drugs; however, only about 4% of the people who take these drugs will develop DILE. The signs and symptoms of DILE are similar to those of SLE. Signs and symptoms disappear within days to months after discontinuing the drug. **Neonatal lupus** is a rare condition acquired from passage of maternal autoantibodies which can affect the skin, heart, and blood of the fetus and newborn. It is associated with a rash that appears within several weeks of life and may persist for about six months before disappearing.

The cause(s) of lupus is unknown, but there are environmental and genetic factors involved. Some environmental factors which may trigger the disease include infections, antibiotics (especially those in the sulfa and penicillin groups), ultraviolet light, extreme stress, certain drugs, and hormones. Genetics may play a role in lupus. Genes on chromosomes 1 and 6 have been associated with lupus, and 10% of lupus patients will have a parent or a sibling who already has or may develop lupus. Five percent of children born to lupus patients will develop lupus. Scientists recently found a genetic tie between rheumatoid arthritis and lupus; some patients share a variation in the STAT4 gene of chromosome 2. Hormonal factors may explain why lupus occurs more frequently in women than in men. The increase of disease signs and symptoms before menstrual periods or during pregnancy supports that hormones, particularly estrogen, may in some way influence the progression of lupus.

Because lupus signs and symptoms mimic those of other illnesses, are sometimes vague, and may come and go, lupus can be difficult to diagnose. Currently there is no single laboratory test that can determine whether someone has lupus. Diagnosis is based on a careful review of the patient's entire medical history, current signs and symptoms, and laboratory tests, including blood and chemistry panels, measure-

**A**

**B**

Figure 2–10 ► (A) Butterfly-shaped lupus rash. Lupus is the Latin word for wolf; the face rash was thought to look like the face markings of a wolf (NMSB/Custom Medical Stock Photo). (B) Lupus rash on the trunk (Phototake NYC).

ment of general levels of inflammation, and autoantibody testing. To assist physicians in the diagnosis of lupus, the American College of Rheumatology (ACR) in 1982 issued a list of 11 symptoms or signs that help distinguish lupus from other diseases.

Lupus patients should limit their exposure to the sun, control fatigue, maintain a good diet and exercise routine, apply moist heat to painful joints, avoid smoking, and take care of fevers over 99.6°F promptly. Medications, including anti-inflammatory drugs (nonsteroidal and corticocosteroids), antimalarials, and immunosuppressive drugs, may be necessary. Anti-inflammatory drugs relieve the symptoms of lupus by reducing the inflammation responsible for pain and discomfort, but in high doses corticosteroids also suppress immune function. Antimalarial drugs are used to treat lupus arthritis, skin rashes, and mouth ulcers. Immunosuppressive drugs are used to suppress the immune system of lupus patients and are generally reserved for patients with more serious manifestations (kidney or neurological involvement) when corticosteroid treatment has failed.

Lupus tends to be chronic and relapsing, often with symptom-free periods that can last for years. Flare-ups occur less often after menopause. Because many people are being diagnosed earlier than in the past and better treatment is available, the prognosis has improved markedly over the last two decades. However, because the course of lupus is unpredictable, the prognosis varies widely. Usually, if the initial inflammation is controlled, the long-term prognosis is good. Early detection and treatment of kidney damage reduces the incidence of severe kidney disease.

## Scleroderma

Derived from the Greek words *sclerosis*, meaning "hardness," and *derma*, meaning "skin," scleroderma literally means "hard skin." Scleroderma or systemic sclerosis is an autoimmune disease of the connective tissue. Scleroderma is characterized by the formation of scar tissue (fibrosis) in the skin and organs of the body. The National Women's Health Information Center estimates that 300,000, or 1 in 906, Americans have scleroderma. Scleroderma is four times more common in women than in men. Scleroderma is categorized into two major classes, localized scleroderma and systemic scleroderma. Both groups include subgroups (Figure 2–11 ▶).

Localized types of scleroderma are those limited to the skin and related tissues and, in some cases, the muscle below. Internal organs are not affected by localized scleroderma, and localized scleroderma can never progress to the systemic forms of the diseases. There are two generally recognized types of localized scleroderma: **morphea** and **linear scleroderma**. Morphea comes from a Greek word that means "form" or "structure." The word refers to local patches of scleroderma. The first signs of the disease are reddish patches

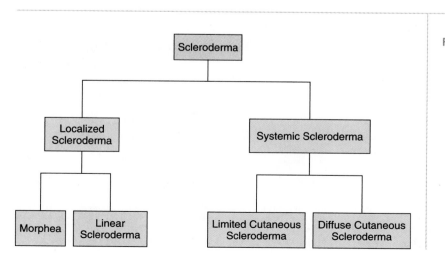

Figure 2–11 ▶ Types of scleroderma.

of skin that thicken into firm, oval-shaped areas. The center of each patch becomes ivory colored with violet borders. These patches sweat very little and have little hair growth. Patches appear most often on the chest, stomach, and back. Morphea can be localized or generalized. Localized morphea limits itself to one or several patches, ranging in size from half an inch to 12 inches in diameter. The disease is referred to as generalized morphea when the skin patches become very hard and dark and spread over large areas of the body. Regardless of the type, morphea generally fades out in 3 to 5 years; however, some people are left with darkened skin patches and, in rare cases, muscle weakness. Linear scleroderma is characterized by a single line or band of thickened skin. It usually runs down an arm or leg, but in some patients it runs down the forehead.

**Systemic scleroderma** involves the skin, tissues under the skin, blood vessels, and the major organs. Systemic scleroderma is typically broken down into **limited cutaneous scleroderma** and **diffuse cutaneous scleroderma**. Limited cutaneous scleroderma typically comes on gradually and affects the skin of the fingers, hands, face, lower arms, and legs. People with limited disease often have all or some of the signs and symptoms that are referred to as CREST: calcinosis, Raynaud's phenomenon, esophageal dysfunction, sclerodactyly, and telangiectasia. Calcinosis refers to the formation of calcium deposits in the connective tissue. They are typically found on the fingers, hands, face, and trunk. When the deposits break through the skin, painful ulcers can result. Raynaud's is a condition in which the small blood vessels of the hands and/or feet contract in response to cold or anxiety; see Chapter 6 for further information. Esophageal dysfunction refers to impaired function of the esophagus that occurs when smooth muscles in the esophagus lose normal movement. In the upper and lower esophagus, the result can be swallowing difficulties; in the lower esophagus, the result can be chronic heartburn or inflammation. Sclerodactyly refers to thick and tight skin on the fingers, resulting from deposits of excess collagen within skin layers. The condition makes it more difficult to bend and straighten the fingers. The skin may also appear

shiny and darkened. Telangiectasia is a condition caused by the swelling of tiny blood vessels, in which red spots appear on the hands and face. While not painful, these red spots can create cosmetic problems.

Diffuse cutaneous scleroderma comes on suddenly; skin thickening begins in the hands and spreads quickly over much of the body in a symmetrical fashion. Skin changes can cause the skin to swell, appear shiny, and feel tight and itchy (Figure 2–12 ►). Internally it can damage key organs such as the intestines, lungs, heart, and kidneys; however less than one-third of patients develop severe organ problems. Patients are often tired, lose appetite and weight, and have joint swelling or pain. The damage of diffuse cutaneous scleroderma occurs over a few years, and patients often have periods of exacerbation and remission.

The cause(s) of scleroderma is unknown, but there are immune, genetic, environmental, and hormonal factors involved. The immune system is thought to stimulate fibroblasts so they produce too much collagen. The collagen forms thick connective tissue that builds up within the skin and internal organs. Genetics may put certain people at risk for scleroderma. Although no environmental agent has been shown to cause scleroderma, research suggests that exposure to viral infections and certain chemicals may trigger scleroderma in those who are genetically predisposed. By middle to late childbearing years (ages 30 to 55), women develop sclero-

Figure 2–12 ► Scleroderma of the hand. (Phototake NYC)

derma 7 to 12 times more often than men; this suggests that the disease may be linked to estrogen production.

Diagnosis of scleroderma begins with a thorough medical history and physical exam. Finding one or more of the following can aid in the diagnosis: changes in skin appearance and texture; swollen fingers and hands; tight skin around the hands, face, mouth, or elsewhere; calcium deposits developing under the skin; changes in the capillaries at the base of the fingernails; thickened skin patches. Autoantibodies against DNA are found in the blood of some scleroderma patients. In some cases a skin biopsy is performed.

Scleroderma has no known cure, and there is no treatment to stop the overproduction of collagen. Scleroderma patients should not smoke and should avoid exposure to cold and stress, protect their skin, and moisturize frequently.

Physical therapy and exercise can help to maintain muscle strength but cannot totally prevent joints from freezing in permanent (usually flexed) positions. Medications, including anti-inflammatory drugs (nonsteroidal and cortiocosteroids) and immunosuppressive drugs, may be necessary. Light therapy may be helpful in treating skin lesions. For some people, scleroderma (particularly the localized forms) is fairly mild and resolves with time. But for others, living with the disease and its effects day to day has a significant impact on their quality of life. A negative prognosis is more likely for those who have early symptoms of heart, lung, or kidney damage.

## Sjögren's Syndrome

Sjögren's syndrome is a chronic autoimmune inflammatory disease of glands and other tissues. The National Institute of Health estimates that 1 to 4 million Americans have Sjögren's syndrome, and 90% of Sjögren's patients are women. About half the time, Sjögren's occurs alone and is known as primary Sjögren's, and the other half it occurs with a disease like rheumatoid arthritis, lupus, or scleroderma and is called secondary Sjögren's. Sjögren's can be a systemic disease affecting the entire body, including kidneys, gastrointestinal system, blood vessels, lungs, liver, pancreas, and nervous sys-

tem. The most common symptoms of Sjögren's syndrome are dry eyes, dry mouth, dry skin, and vaginal dryness.

The cause(s) of Sjögren's syndrome are not known. Genetic factors, hormones, and environmental triggers like viral infections may play a role. A first-degree relative with autoimmunity increases the risk for Sjögren's syndrome sevenfold. Sjögren's syndrome often affects women during their childbearing years, suggesting a link between Sjögren's syndrome and female hormones. Sjögren's syndrome is often underdiagnosed or misdiagnosed because the signs and symptoms of Sjögren's syndrome may mimic those of menopause, drug side effects, or diseases like lupus, rheumatoid arthritis, and multiple sclerosis. The average time from the onset of symptoms to diagnosis is over 6 years. No single test will confirm the diagnosis of Sjögren's syndrome. Tear and salivary gland function are measured. Laboratory tests, including blood and chemistry panels, measurement of general levels of inflammation, and autoantibody testing, may be performed. Lip or salivary gland biopsy may also be performed.

Currently there is no cure for Sjögren's syndrome. Medications may be used to alleviate different types of dryness. Medications, including anti-inflammatory drugs (nonsteroidal and cortiocosteroids), anti-malarials, and immunosuppressive drugs, may be necessary. Sjögren's patients should be aware that the incidence of lymphoma (cancer of the lymph nodes) is significantly higher in Sjögren's patients. The prognosis is generally good. However, if the lungs, kidneys, or lymph nodes are damaged by the antibodies, pneumonia, kidney failure, or lymphoma may result.

## ▶ Immune Deficiency

## Acquired Immunodeficiency Syndrome (AIDS)

One of the most deadly diseases to affect today's population is **acquired immunodeficiency syndrome (AIDS)**. AIDS destroys the individual's immune system, making the person remarkably susceptible to infection. AIDS was first noted in the early 1980s among men with multiple sexual contacts with other men and drug users who shared hypodermic needles.

AIDS is now a pandemic. According to the Joint United Nations Programme on HIV/AIDS, at the end of 2007, an estimated 30.8 million adults and 2.5 million children worldwide were living with HIV/AIDS, 2.5 million people worldwide became infected with HIV, and 2.1 million people died of AIDS-related death. Heterosexual transmission accounts for two-thirds of new infections. Mother-to-infant transmission and IV drug use each account for approximately 10% of HIV infections. Homosexual transmission and healthcare transmission each account for approximately 5 to 10% of HIV infections. Ninety-five percent of people living with HIV live in the developing world, with over 60% in sub-Saharan Africa. An estimated 1.3 million adults in North America were living with HIV/AIDS; at the end of 2007, 46,000 people in North America became infected with HIV and 21,000 people died of AIDS-related deaths.

The causative agent of AIDS is the **human immunodeficiency virus (HIV)**, a retrovirus; that is, it carries its genetic information as RNA rather than DNA (Figure 2–13►). HIV is transmitted via contaminated body fluids, including blood, semen, vaginal secretions, and breast milk. Therefore, HIV is transmitted by unprotected anal, oral, or vaginal intercourse; birth; breastfeeding; and the sharing of needles. The virus infects primarily helper or CD4 T lymphocytes. The virus replicates within these lymphocytes, killing them and spreading to others. These lymphocytes normally activate B-cell lymphocytes; thus, the body's immune response is crippled, and the body is susceptible to infections and tumors that a healthy immune system could easily control.

Many people do not develop signs or symptoms immediately after HIV infection. Some people develop signs and symptoms within several days to weeks after infection, and these usually disappear within a few weeks. The length of an asymptomatic period may last a few months or more than 10 years. The long latent period increases the risk of spreading the infection because individuals may not be aware they have the disease. During this period the virus continues to multiply, infecting and killing CD4 lymphocytes. Once the immune system is weakened by the virus,

**Figure 2–13** ► Colored scanning electron micrograph (SEM) of a T lymphocyte (green) infected with the HIV virus (red). The virus has infected the T lymphocyte and instructed the lymphocyte to reproduce many more viruses. Small spherical virus particles (red) are budding away from the T lymphocyte membrane. Viral budding destroys the T lymphocyte. Depletion in the blood of CD4 lymphocytes through HIV infection is the main reason for the destruction of the immune system in AIDS. (National Institute for Biological Standards and Control (U.K.)/Science Photo Library/Photo Researchers, Inc.)

an HIV-positive person may develop signs and symptoms. Eventually, a threshold is crossed and the HIV-infected person develops AIDS. To move from an HIV-positive diagnosis to an AIDS diagnosis, the patient must have one of the AIDS indicator diseases and have a CD4 T lymphocyte count of less than 200. Table 2–3► shows common signs and symptoms for initial HIV infection, the asymptomatic period, and AIDS.

The presence of HIV antibodies in the blood can be detected with the enzyme-linked immunosorbent assay (ELISA), as most people produce antibodies against HIV within 3 months of being infected. If the ELISA test is positive, the test is usually repeated and the result confirmed using a Western blot test. A positive P24 antigen test indicates circulating HIV antigen. Polymerase chain reaction (PCR) can also be used to test for HIV RNA. Anonymous free testing for HIV antibodies is available at local health departments throughout the United States.

| Table 2–3 ▸ | Possible Signs and Symptoms of Initial HIV Infection, Asymptomatic Period, and AIDS | | |
|---|---|---|---|
| | **Initial HIV Infection** | **Asymptomatic Period** | **AIDS** |
| **Signs and Symptoms** | HIV + | HIV+ | HIV + |
| | Fever | Lack of energy | One of AIDS indicator diseases |
| | Headache | Weight loss | CD4 T lymphocyte count less than 200 |
| | Fatigue | Frequent fever and sweats | Cough and shortness of breath |
| | Enlarged lymph nodes | Persistent or frequent yeast infection | Seizures and lack of coordination |
| | | Persistent skin rashes or flaky skin | Difficult or painful swallowing |
| | | Short-term memory loss | Confusion and forgetfulness |
| | | Mouth, genital, or anal herpes sores | Severe and persistent diarrhea |
| | | | Fever |
| | | | Vision loss |
| | | | Nausea |
| | | | Abdominal cramps and vomiting |
| | | | Weight loss |
| | | | Extreme fatigue |
| | | | Severe headache with stiff neck |
| | | | Coma |

Drug therapy that begins shortly after infection increases the chances that the immune system will not be destroyed by HIV. While there is no cure for AIDS, medications may hinder HIV replication to the extent that the viral load becomes undetectable in some individuals. Anti-HIV medications are used to control replication of the virus and to slow the progression of HIV-related disease. Anti-HIV medications do not cure HIV infection, and individuals taking these medications can still transmit HIV to others. Highly active antiretroviral therapy (HAART) is the recommended treatment for HIV infection. HAART combines three or more anti-HIV medications in a daily regimen. HAART medications target HIV replication and entry. These drugs are very expensive, cause side effects, and the regimen of pill-taking throughout the day is very demanding. If the drugs are not taken as prescribed or if the therapy is stopped, resistance or relapse may occur. AIDS-related deaths in the United States have declined nearly 70% since 1995 as a result of HAART. Most people living with HIV in the developing world have no access to HAART.

There are some exciting experimental HIV drugs on the horizon that target HIV DNA integration, transcription, and viral assembly. Development of a vaccine to prevent the spread of AIDS has not yet been possible. The genetic makeup of the AIDS virus varies greatly from strain to strain; HIV tends to mutate quickly, which complicates the attempt to develop an AIDS vaccine; and vaccines to date have not been successful in stimulating HIV antibody production. A new area of research involves attempting to stimulate and train killer T cells to quickly recognize and destroy HIV.

The Global HIV Prevention Working Group estimates that by delivering comprehensive HIV prevention to those who need it, annual HIV incidence would be nearly two-thirds lower in 2015. This would mean 4 million fewer infections each year by the middle of the next decade. Sexual transmission can be prevented by abstinence, monogamy, and use of condoms. Blood transmission can be prevented by needle exchange programs and screening of blood. Healthcare workers should use personal protective equipment and safe administration of injections (as discussed in Chapter 3) to protect themselves. Mother to child transmission can be prevented by antiretroviral medication. Unfortunately, most people at risk of HIV infection have little or no access to these prevention tools.

## ▶ Vaccination

Two types of artificial immunity can be administered: active and passive immunity. In **active immunity**, the person receives a **vaccine** or a **toxoid** as the antigen, and he or she forms antibodies to counteract it. A vaccine is a suspension of whole organisms or pieces of organisms that is used to induce immunity. Attenuated whole-agent vaccines use living but attenuated (weakened) organisms. Organisms can be attenuated by aging or altering their growing conditions. Because the organisms have been specially treated to deactivate them, they cannot cause disease. As proteins foreign to the body, these antigens do trigger antibody production against them. Examples of attenuated vaccines include the Sabin polio vaccine and the MMR (measles, mumps, and rubella) vaccine. Inactivated whole-agent vaccines use organisms that have been killed, usually by formalin or phenol. Examples of inactivated whole-agent vaccines include rabies, influenza, and the Salk polio vaccine. A **toxoid** works similarly. It consists of a chemically altered toxin, the poisonous material produced by a pathogenic organism. Having been treated chemically, the toxin will not cause disease. It will, however, stimulate the immune response. Examples of toxoid vaccines include tetanus and diphtheria. Subunit vaccines use only those antigenic fragments of organisms that best stimulate an immune response. Genes for specific disease antigens are inserted into the genetic material of harmless organisms. The antigens produced by these organisms are extracted, purified, and used for immunization. The hepatitis B vaccine is produced in this manner. Active immunity is long lived. Time is required to build up immunity, and for some vaccines, a booster shot is necessary. Once cells have been sensitized to these viruses, bacteria, or toxins, they retain the ability to produce antibodies against them when encountered again.

What if a person is exposed to a serious disease such as hepatitis, tetanus, or rabies and has no immunity against it? It takes too much time to build antibodies in response to a vaccination. In this case, the person is given **passive immunity**, doses of preformed antibodies from immune serum of an animal, usually a horse. This type of immunity is short lived but acts immediately. Table 2–4 ▶ contrasts active and passive immunity.

| Table 2–4 ▶ Differences between Active and Passive Immunity | |
|---|---|
| **Active Immunity** | **Passive Immunity** |
| Person forms antibodies | Preformed antibodies received |
| Vaccine (deactivated bacteria or virus) | Immune horse serum |
| or | or |
| Toxoid (chemically altered toxin) | Antibodies, cells in breast milk |
| Long-lived immunity (requires time to act) | Short-lived immunity (acts immediately) |

# Prevention ✚ PLUS!

## Disease Prevention through Vaccination

Without appropriate immunization, children are susceptible to many serious and life-threatening infections, such as measles, whooping cough, hepatitis, and meningitis. Vaccines are effective, particularly when a high proportion of people in a population are immunized. Reactions to the vaccines are usually mild and rarely serious. The risks from these childhood diseases far outweigh the risk of a serious reaction from a vaccine. The following charts include childhood immunization recommendations from the American Academy of Pediatrics.

### Recommended Immunization Schedule for Persons Aged 0–6 Years—UNITED STATES • 2008
*For those who fall behind or start late, see the catch-up schedule*

| Vaccine ▼ Age ▶ | Birth | 1 month | 2 months | 4 months | 6 months | 12 months | 15 months | 18 months | 19–23 months | 2–3 years | 4–6 years |
|---|---|---|---|---|---|---|---|---|---|---|---|
| Hepatitis B[1] | HepB | HepB | see footnote 1 | | HepB | | | | | | |
| Rotavirus[2] | | | Rota | Rota | Rota | | | | | | |
| Diphtheria, Tetanus, Pertussis[3] | | | DTaP | DTaP | DTaP | see footnote 3 | DTaP | | | | DTaP |
| Haemophilus influenzae type b[4] | | | Hib | Hib | Hib[4] | Hib | | | | | |
| Pneumococcal[5] | | | PCV | PCV | PCV | PCV | | | | PPV | PPV |
| Inactivated Poliovirus | | | IPV | IPV | IPV | | | | | | IPV |
| Influenza[6] | | | | | Influenza (Yearly) | | | | | | |
| Measles, Mumps, Rubella[7] | | | | | | MMR | | | | | MMR |
| Varicella[8] | | | | | | Varicella | | | | | Varicella |
| Hepatitis A[9] | | | | | | HepA (2 doses) | | | | HepA Series | |
| Meningococcal[10] | | | | | | | | | | MCV4 | MCV4 |

Range of recommended ages

Certain high-risk groups

This schedule indicates the recommended ages for routine administration of currently licensed childhood vaccines, as of December 1, 2007, for children aged 0 through 6 years. Additional information is available at www.cdc.gov/vaccines/recs/schedules. Any dose not administered at the recommended age should be administered at any subsequent visit, when indicated and feasible. Additional vaccines may be licensed and recommended during the year. Licensed combination vaccines may be used whenever any components of the combination are indicated and other components of the vaccine are not contraindicated and if approved by the Food and Drug Administration for that dose of the series. Providers should consult the respective Advisory Committee on Immunization Practices statement for detailed recommendations, including for **high-risk conditions:** http://www.cdc.gov/vaccines/pubs/ACIP-list.htm. Clinically significant adverse events that follow immunization should be reported to the Vaccine Adverse Event Reporting System (VAERS). Guidance about how to obtain and complete a VAERS form is available at www.vaers.hhs.gov or by telephone, 800-822-7967.

### Recommended Immunization Schedule for Persons Aged 7–18 Years—UNITED STATES • 2008
*For those who fall behind or start late, see the green bars and the catch-up schedule*

| Vaccine ▼ Age ▶ | 7–10 years | 11–12 years | 13–18 years |
|---|---|---|---|
| Diphtheria, Tetanus, Pertussis[1] | see footnote 1 | Tdap | Tdap |
| Human Papillomavirus[2] | see footnote 2 | HPV (3 doses) | HPV Series |
| Meningococcal[3] | MCV4 | MCV4 | MCV4 |
| Pneumococcal[4] | | PPV | |
| Influenza[5] | | Influenza (Yearly) | |
| Hepatitis A[6] | | HepA Series | |
| Hepatitis B[7] | | HepB Series | |
| Inactivated Poliovirus[8] | | IPV Series | |
| Measles, Mumps, Rubella[9] | | MMR Series | |
| Varicella[10] | | Varicella Series | |

Range of recommended ages

Catch-up immunization

Certain high-risk groups

This schedule indicates the recommended ages for routine administration of currently licensed childhood vaccines, as of December 1, 2007, for children aged 7–18 years. Additional information is available at www.cdc.gov/vaccines/recs/schedules. Any dose not administered at the recommended age should be administered at any subsequent visit, when indicated and feasible. Additional vaccines may be licensed and recommended during the year. Licensed combination vaccines may be used whenever any components of the combination are indicated and other components of the vaccine are not contraindicated and if approved by the Food and Drug Administration for that dose of the series. Providers should consult the respective Advisory Committee on Immunization Practices statement for detailed recommendations, including for **high risk conditions:** http://www.cdc.gov/vaccines/pubs/ACIP-list.htm. Clinically significant adverse events that follow immunization should be reported to the Vaccine Adverse Event Reporting System (VAERS). Guidance about how to obtain and complete a VAERS form is available at www.vaers.hhs.gov or by telephone, 800-822-7967.

## ▶ Stress and the Immune System

Stressors such as trauma, infection, surgery, pain, and emotional distress all have significant effects on the immune system's ability to function. Stress causes an increased production of the hormone **cortisol**. Cortisol decreases production of antibodies and substances released by leukocytes that stimulate other cells of the immune system.

Cortisol production occurs when norepinephrine and epinephrine are released by the sympathetic nervous system, as happens during the fight-or-flight response. The combined effect of these three hormones increases the total number of neutrophils in the circulation. Lymphocyte maturation in the lymph nodes stops because epinephrine decreases blood flow to the lymph nodes as it increases blood flow to the heart, lungs, brain, and muscles. These changes in the immune response brought on by stress leave the body less capable of fighting off the effects of injury, disease, and other stress causes.

## ▶ Age and the Immune System

The immune system simply does not function as efficiently in older adults as in younger people. The body becomes less able to distinguish self from nonself and, as a result, autoimmune disorders become more common among the elderly. Common problems related to the immune system in older people include increased infection risk and decreased ability to fight disease. By middle age, the thymus is only about 15% of its maximum size. The total number of T lymphocytes does not decrease with age, but the diversity of T lymphocytes is reduced. This decrease in T-lymphocyte population diversity in older adults leads to less effective locating and eliminating of pathogens. There are fewer lymphocytes capable of responding to new antigens; therefore, when older people encounter a new antigen, the body is less able to recognize and defend against it. It takes longer for macrophages to destroy bacteria, viruses, cancer cells, and other antigens. The amount of antibody produced in response to an antigen and the antibody's ability to attach to the antigen are reduced. Because of the reduction in antibody production, vaccines are less likely to produce immunity in older people. While vaccines do not work as well in older adults, vaccinations for diseases such as influenza, pneumonia, hepatitis B, tuberculosis, diphtheria, and tetanus have been found to reduce mortality in the elderly and are still worthwhile.

## RESOURCES

American Academy of Allergy Asthma and Immunology: www.aaaai.org

American Academy of Pediatrics: www.aap.org

Global HIV Prevention Working Group: www.globalhivprevention.org/index.html

Joint United Programme on HIV/AIDS: www.unaids.org/en

Lupus Foundation of America: www.lupus.org

Scleroderma Foundation: www.scleroderma.org

Sjögren's Syndrome Foundation: www.sjogrens.org

# Interactive Exercises

## Cases for Critical Thinking

1. Tetanus is caused by bacteria that enter the body through wounds in the skin. The bacteria produce a toxin that causes spastic muscle contraction. Death often results from failure of the respiratory muscles. A patient comes to the emergency room after stepping on a nail. If the patient has been vaccinated against tetanus, he or she is given a tetanus booster shot, which consists of the toxin altered so that it is harmless. If the patient has never been vaccinated against tetanus, he or she is given an antiserum shot against tetanus. Explain the rationale for this treatment.

2. Explain why identical twins are an ideal case for organ transplantation.

3. A crime scene investigator finds a body of a woman and discovers animal bites on the victim's body. The investigator examines the bites and sees they are not inflamed. Did the animal bites happen before or after the woman died?

4. A baby receives his first dose of oral polio vaccine from his pediatrician. Is this active or passive immunity? What does the polio virus trigger in the body?

5. Some people with decreased IgA exhibit recurrent sinus and respiratory infections. Why?

6. Explain why HIV's attack on helper CD4 T lymphocytes devastates the entire immune system.

## Multiple Choice

1. Passive immunity is achieved artificially by injection of _____.
   a. preformed antibodies
   b. autoantibodies
   c. deactivated viruses and bacteria
   d. toxoids
   e. bacterial toxins

2. Long-lived lymphocytes, which remain dormant until reactivated after an immune response, are the _____.
   a. helper lymphocytes
   b. cytotoxic lymphocytes
   c. suppressor lymphocytes
   d. memory lymphocytes
   e. plasma cells

3. Defense against antigens via antibodies is called _____.
   a. humoral immunity
   b. cell-mediated immunity
   c. plasma cells
   d. adhesion
   e. suppression

4. Which of the following agents is/are capable of causing an inflammatory response?
   a. allergen          b. trauma
   c. chemical agents    d. all of the above

5. Which is a foreign substance that triggers an immune response?
   a. antigen      b. antibody
   c. antibiotic   d. adhesion

6. Which cells secrete antibodies during the immune response?
   a. T helper    b. B
   c. plasma      d. T killer

7. The response to poison ivy is an example of which type of hypersensitivity?
   a. I      b. II
   c. III    d. IV

8. Which antibody is produced in excess during an allergic response?
   a. IgE    b. IgG
   c. IgM    d. IgA

9. The virus of acquired immune deficiency syndrome invades and damages leukocytes, especially targeting the _____.
   a. B lymphocytes
   b. cytotoxic or CD8 T lymphocytes
   c. helper or CD4 lymphocytes
   d. suppressor lymphocytes

10. Which cells are involved in both cellular and humoral reactions during an immune response?
   a. cytotoxic T cells    b. natural killer cells
   c. plasma cells         d. helper cells

## True or False

_____  1.  HIV can be transmitted through saliva.

_____  2.  Fever is an example of specific immunity.

_____  3.  Inflammation is an undesirable reaction to injury.

_____  4.  Antibodies provide humoral immunity.

_____  5.  Cell-mediated immunity depends on the activities of B lymphocytes.

_____  6.  T lymphocytes produce antibodies.

_____  7.  The release of histamine increases the permeability of capillary walls.

_____  8.  Failure of immune tolerance creates an autoimmune disease.

_____  9.  Anaphylactic shock is a moderately serious allergic reaction.

_____ 10.  Type I hypersensitivities involve IgM or IgG and cause destruction of foreign cells.

## Fill-Ins

1. Bacteria that cause pus formation are called _____ bacteria.

2. _____ is a group of substances that stimulate the immune system.

3. A substance that triggers an immune response is an _____.

4. A _____ consists of a low dose of dead or deactivated bacteria or viruses.

5. _____ immunity is effective against any foreign agent.

6. Damaged tissue releases _____.

7. Ig _____ protects newborns.

8. _____ are a type of leukocyte that recognizes body cells with abnormal membranes.

9. The causative agent of AIDS is the _____.

10. In _____ immunity, the person is given preformed antibodies.

# Multimedia Preview

Additional interactive resources and activities for this chapter can be found on the Companion Website. For videos, audio glossary, and review, access the accompanying DVD-ROM in this book.

## ▶ DVD-ROM Highlights

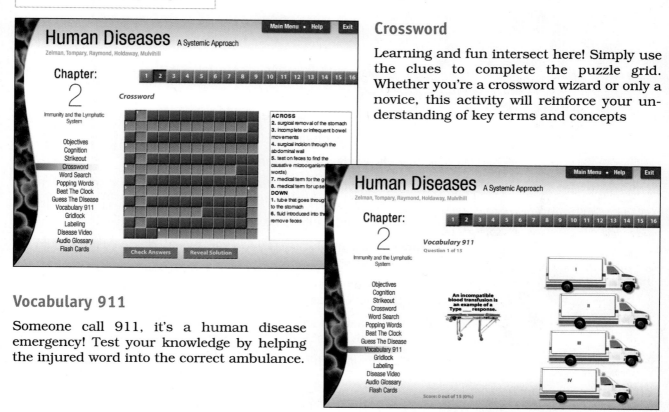

### Crossword

Learning and fun intersect here! Simply use the clues to complete the puzzle grid. Whether you're a crossword wizard or only a novice, this activity will reinforce your understanding of key terms and concepts

### Vocabulary 911

Someone call 911, it's a human disease emergency! Test your knowledge by helping the injured word into the correct ambulance.

## ▶ Website Highlights—www.pearsonhighered.com/zelman

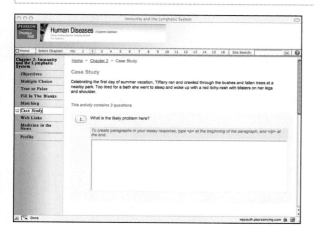

### Case Study

Take advantage of the free-access online study guide that accompanies your textbook. Put your understanding of human diseases to the test with this real world-scenario. You'll be presented with a clinical case followed by a series of questions that challenge your grasp of the situation. By clicking on this URL you'll also access links to current news articles and an audio glossary.

CHAPTER

# 3

# Infectious Diseases

## Learning Objectives

After studying this chapter, you should be able to

- Define infectious disease and its terminology
- Explain how infectious diseases are transmitted
- Describe and compare the characteristics of prions, viruses, bacteria, protozoa, fungi, and helminths
- Define nosocomial infections
- Explain treatment for bacterial, viral, fungal, and parasitic infectious diseases
- Understand the appropriate use of antibiotics and explain the problem of antibiotic resistance
- Describe examples and causes of emerging and re-emerging infectious diseases
- Identify common childhood vaccine-preventable infectious diseases

## Fact or Fiction?

Thanks to modern medicine, notorious infectious diseases like tuberculosis are things of the past.

*Fiction: Population growth, climate and weather change, human behavior, and other factors are responsible for the re-emergence of many infectious diseases, including tuberculosis.*

# Disease Chronicle

## Spanish Flu Pandemic

If the epidemic continues its mathematical rate of acceleration, civilization could easily disappear from the face of the earth within a few weeks.

Victor Vaughan, Surgeon General of the Army
October, 1918

The influenza pandemic of 1918–1919 has been called the most devastating pandemic in recorded world history. Known as Spanish Flu, the influenza pandemic of 1918–1919 was a global disaster. The pandemic killed an estimated 20 to 40 million people worldwide and 675,000 in the United States; one-quarter of the United States and one-fifth of the world was infected. The mortality rate was 2.5% compared to the previous influenza pandemics, which had mortality rates of 0.1%. One of the great unsolved mysteries surrounding the 1918 pandemic is why it tended to kill healthy adults between the ages of 20 and 40. During normal seasonal influenza outbreaks, deaths are most common among the young, elderly, and those with chronic health conditions. Scientists believe that even with modern antiviral and antibacterial drugs, vaccines, and prevention knowledge, the return of a pandemic virus equivalent in pathogenicity to the virus of 1918 would likely kill more 100 million people worldwide.

# ▶ Introduction

Despite medical advances that have produced drugs and vaccines that are safe and effective against bacteria, viruses, fungi, and parasites, **infectious diseases** are still a major cause of death, disability, and social and economic upheaval for millions around the world. Illness and death from infectious diseases are particularly tragic because they are largely preventable and treatable. More than 90% of deaths from infectious diseases worldwide are caused by a few diseases (Table 3–1 ▶). In developed countries, infectious disease accounts for 1 out of 10 deaths; in developing countries, infectious disease accounts for 6 out of 10 deaths. Poverty, lack of access to health care, antibiotic resistance, evolving human migration patterns, new infectious agents, and changing environmental and developmental activities all contribute to the expanding impact of infectious diseases. How many more victims could a lethal strain of influenza similar to the 1918 pandemic claim today with half a billion passengers traveling on planes?

The world's population now exceeds 6 billion people, and most of the growth has occurred in the most densely populated and poorest cities. Crowding, chronic disease, malnutrition, and lack of medical resources will become dire. Infectious diseases thrive on these conditions. Scientists must continue research into the cause, transmission, prevention, and treatment of infectious diseases for future generations. This chapter describes the nature of infectious diseases, surveys the types of microorganisms responsible for infections, explains their transmission, and discusses treatment.

# ▶ Principles of Infectious Disease

Some infectious diseases described in this book have been in existence for centuries whereas others have emerged as new pathologies. It is important to have a framework for understanding infectious diseases. Most microorganisms do not cause disease. A **pathogen** or infectious agent is a disease-causing organism.

Infectious diseases are caused by a pathogen which subsequently grows and multiplies in the body. Diseases transmitted by human contact are said to be **contagious** or **communicable**. Measles and influenza are well-known contagious diseases. Infectious diseases are classified as **noncommunicable** if they cannot be transmitted directly from person to person. For example, rabies can be transmitted by the bite of a rabid raccoon, and cholera is transmitted by drinking fecal-contaminated water.

**Epidemiology** is the study of the transmission, occurrence, distribution, and control of disease. Study of the distribution and frequency of diseases can help predict and prevent disease. The number of new cases of a disease in a population is its **incidence**. Disease incidence may follow a pattern, as when influenza incidence increases in winter and subsides in summer or when Lyme disease increases in summer and subsides in winter. The number of existing cases of a disease is known as its **prevalence**, and this information can tell how significant the disease is in a certain population. When a disease always occurs at low levels in a population, it is said to be **endemic**. Sexually transmitted infections (Chapter 11) are endemic diseases. If a disease occurs in unusually large numbers over a specific area, it is said to be **epidemic**. Influenza

| Table 3–1 ▶ Leading Causes of Death Due to Infectious Diseases | |
|---|---|
| **Disease** | **Number of Deaths** |
| Lower respiratory infections | 3.9 million |
| HIV/AIDS | 2.8 million |
| Diarrheal diseases | 1.8 million |
| Tuberculosis | 1.6 million |
| Malaria | 1.2 million |
| Measles | 0.6 million |

*Source:* World Health Report, 2004, World Health Organization (WHO)

occurs as epidemics. When an epidemic has spread to include several large areas worldwide, it is said to be **pandemic**. AIDS is considered to be pandemic. When a disease suddenly occurs in unexpected numbers in a limited area and then subsides, this is described as an **outbreak**. Certain diseases are under constant surveillance in the United States and are called **notifiable diseases**. Physicians are required to report the occurrence of these diseases to the Centers for Disease Control and Prevention. This ensures tracking and identification of disease occurrence and patterns. Chlamydia infections were not notifiable before 1998. After these infections were classified as notifiable, it was discovered that the number of chlamydial infections surpassed gonorrhea. Other notifiable infectious diseases include measles, mumps, polio, tuberculosis, Legionnares' disease, and tetanus.

The 100 trillion microorganisms in and on our bodies make up our **normal flora** or **microbiota**. Normal flora does not harm us and in some cases helps us by preventing overgrowth of harmful microorganisms and producing vitamins. Normal flora may become harmful if an opportunity to do so arises. In this case, normal flora becomes opportunistic pathogens or opportunists. Opportunists typically do not cause disease in their usual location in a healthy person but may cause disease in a different location or if the host is weakened or immunocompromised (for example, a patient with an HIV infection or AIDS).

## ▶ Transmission of Infectious Diseases

The source of an infectious agent is known as a **reservoir**. Reservoirs include humans, animals, insects, soil, and water. For example, humans are the reservoir for the measles virus because it does not infect other organisms. Those who harbor an infectious agent but do not have signs or symptoms are known as carriers. Carriers play an important role in the transmission of pathogens like HIV (Chapter 2). Infectious diseases can be transmitted directly from an infected human to a susceptible human. This route is called **horizontal transmission**. Influenza

and gonorrhea are transmitted this way. Other infectious diseases are transmitted from one generation to the next, as when syphilis (Chapter 11), HIV (Chapter 2), or ophthalmia neonatorum (an eye infection; see Chapter 13) are transmitted to newborns from infected mothers. This route is called **vertical transmission**.

To cause disease, microorganisms must enter the human host. The respiratory tract is the easiest and most frequently used portal of entry for pathogens. Microbes that use the respiratory tract as their portal of entry include the common cold, influenza, and tuberculosis. Microbes also use the gastrointestinal and genitourinary tracts as portals of entry. Punctures, injections, bites, and surgery can allow microorganisms to be deposited directly into the tissues below the skin. This is known as the **parenteral** route, and microorganisms like HIV and hepatitis B can use this portal of entry.

Infectious agents may be transmitted from the reservoir to the host through either direct or indirect contact. Direct contact occurs when an individual is infected by contact with the reservoir (for example, by touching an infected person, kissing, engaging in sexual contact, or being bitten by an infected animal or insect). Some diseases that are transmitted primarily by direct contact with the reservoir include ringworm (Chapter 16), AIDS (Chapter 2), influenza, rabies, and malaria. Transmission by direct contact also includes inhaling the infectious agent in droplets emitted by sneezing or coughing. The droplets may travel as much as 3 feet. Diseases spread by droplet transmission include pneumonia and influenza.

Indirect contact occurs when a pathogen can withstand the environment outside its host for a long period of time before infecting another individual. In airborne transmission, droplets containing infectious agents are small enough to remain airborne for prolonged periods and travel more than 3 feet from the reservoir to the host; tuberculosis and measles can be transmitted by airborne droplets. Inanimate objects or **fomites** that are contaminated by direct contact with the reservoir (e.g., a tissue used to wipe the nose of an individual who has a cold, syringes, or utensils) may be the indirect contact for a susceptible individual. Intravenous drug users who share needles can transmit infectious agents like hepatitis and HIV via indirect contact transmission.

Ingesting food and beverages contaminated by contact with a disease reservoir is another example of disease transmission by indirect contact. The fecal-oral route of transmission, in which sewage-contaminated water is used for drinking, washing, or preparing foods, is a significant form of indirect transmission, especially for gastrointestinal diseases such as cholera, rotavirus infection, and giardiasis. Every year there are 1.8 million diarrheal deaths related to unsafe water, sanitation, and hygiene worldwide. More than 1 billion people lack access to an improved water source. The CDC estimates that 76 million people get sick, more than 300,000 are hospitalized, and 5000 die each year from illnesses caused by contaminated foods or beverages in the United States.

Control of infectious diseases can be achieved by preventing transmission. **Isolation** of infected persons in hospitals and self-imposed isolation, such as when a person with influenza remains home in bed, can be effective. **Quarantine** is the separation of persons who may or may not be infected from healthy people until the period of infectious risk is passed. **Disinfection** of potentially infectious materials is necessary to prevent transmission. Medical and dental implements need disinfection to remove human pathogens after use.

## ▶ Survey of Infectious Agents and Pathogenic Microorganisms

Humans can be infected by a variety of pathogens, ranging from tiny, single-celled bacteria to macroscopic, complex worms (Figure 3–1 ▶).

## Prions

A **prion**, short for proteinaceous infectious particle, is an infectious agent composed only of protein. Prions cause a number of diseases in animals and humans known as spongiform encephalopathies, in which the brain becomes riddled with holes. All known prion diseases affect the structure of the brain or other neural tissue by inducing abnormal folding of normal cellular proteins in the brain, leading to brain damage. Prion diseases usually progress rapidly and are currently untreatable and fatal. Human prion diseases include Creutzfeldt-Jakob disease (CJD), familial Creutzfeldt-Jakob disease (fCJD), and kuru. Although CJD is the most common human prion disease, it is still rare and only occurs in about one out of every one million people.

## Viruses

Viruses are infectious particles made of a core of genetic material (either RNA or DNA) wrapped in a protein coat (**capsid**). Some viruses also have a lipid membrane surrounding their capsid that plays a role in host cell recognition and spikes that aid in attachment. Viruses may be classified into several different morphological types, including helical or rod shaped, polyhedral or many sided, enveloped, or complex. Viruses are not considered living organisms because they do not independently grow, metabolize, or reproduce. Viruses must carry out their life processes by entering cells and directing the cells' energy, materials, and organelles for these purposes.

Certain viruses infect and grow in only certain types of human cells. Some viruses, like cold viruses, target only cells of the respiratory epithelium. Others, like herpes viruses, reproduce in nervous tissue. Signs and symptoms of infection result from the way these viruses reproduce in cells or from the way the immune system responds to viral infection. Some viruses cause the cells they infect to lyse, or rupture. This is the case when HIV infects and reproduces within T cells. The resultant T-cell deficiency leads to the immunodeficiency in AIDS. Other viruses sustain a **latent infection**, whereby the viruses insert themselves in cells and do not reproduce. At this time, no signs and symptoms may be present. Later, a trigger, such as stress, infection with another pathogen, or a weakened immune defense, activates the viruses. Signs and symptoms of the disease then manifest themselves as the viruses reproduce. This pattern is seen in the recurrence of herpes infec-

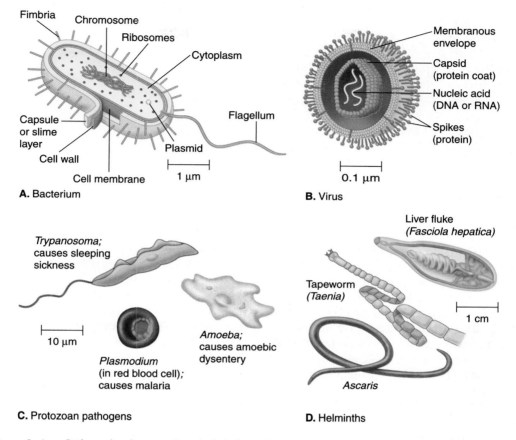

**Figure 3–1** ► Pathogenic microorganisms include bacteria (A), viruses (B), protozoa (C), and helminths (D).

tions. Other viruses cause abnormal cell growth because the viral genetic material interferes with the cell's growth-control genes. Abnormal growth of tissues is discussed further in Chapter 4. Such growth may be benign, as in a dermal wart (Chapter 16). However, the result may be a malignant growth; that is, a cancer. For example, human papillomavirus infection is linked to cervical cancer (Chapter 11).

## Bacteria

Bacteria are microscopic, single-celled organisms. A simple structure (no nucleus or membranous organelles) and small size (1 to 10 μm) are key characteristics that differentiate bacteria from other single-celled organisms. Although often described as simple, they are far from primitive, for they have adapted to a wide variety of habitats and have evolved complex strategies for infecting and surviving in the human body.

Bacteria have **cell walls**, a rigid layer of organic material surrounding their delicate cell membranes. These walls give bacteria their characteristic shapes. Bacteria may have spherical, round cells called **cocci**, rod-shaped cells called **bacilli**, spiral-shaped cells called **spirilla**, corkscrew-shaped cells called **spirochetes**, or comma-shaped cells called **vibrios**. The walls protect these cells; should walls be disrupted, cells are susceptible to bursting. This is the action of the antibiotic penicillin. Penicillin interferes with correct cell wall construction of certain types of bacteria. The bacteria cell walls may be thick, thin, or absent. The thickness and chemical composition of the cell wall accounts for the way certain cells stain during the **gram stain** procedure. During the gram stain,

**A**

**B**

Figure 3–2 ► Gram-stained bacteria on a microscope slide. (A) Red rod-shaped cells are *Escherichia coli* (Courtesy of the CDC, 1979). (B) Blue-purple cocci are *Staphylococcus aureus* (© SIU BioMed/Custom Medical Stock Photo).

thick-walled cells turn blue-purple and thin-walled cells become red; thus, bacteria can be identified using this technique (Figure 3–2 ►). Identification is critical to obtain an accurate diagnosis and effective treatment of an infection. Other bacteria that do not fit into the above categories of shape and gram stain properties include the chlamydias and rickettsias, which are intracellular parasites. *Chlamydia trachomatis* causes a sexually transmitted infection (Chapter 11). Rickettsias are transmitted by ticks and cause diseases such as typhus and Rocky Mountain spotted fever.

Many bacteria secrete on their surface a substance called **glycocalyx** or sugar coat. The bacterial glycocalyx is sticky and lies outside the wall. If the glycocalyx is organized and firmly attached to the wall, it is described as a **capsule**. Capsules often protect bacteria from phagocytosis by host cells. If the glycocalyx is unorganized and loosely attached to the wall, it is described as a **slime layer**. Slime layers aid in attachment to surfaces. *Streptococcus mutans,* an important cause of dental decay, attaches itself to the surface of teeth using a slime layer.

Some bacteria, like *E. coli,* have **flagella** that can be used for locomotion. Motility enables bacteria to move toward a favorable environment or away from an adverse environment. Many gram-negative bacteria contain short, hairlike appendages called **fimbrae** and **pili**. Fimbrae can occur at the ends of bacteria or they can cover the entire surface of the bacteria. Fimbrae enable bacteria to attach to surfaces;

*Neisseria gonorrhoeae* uses fimbrae to attach to the reproductive tract (Chapter 11). Pili are usually longer than fimbrae, and bacteria have only one or two pili. Pili join bacteria in preparation for the transfer of DNA from one cell to another; because of this they are also called sex pili. Transfer of DNA between bacteria can aid in antibiotic resistance.

Some bacteria produce **endospores**, commonly called spores. The endospore contains the genetic material of the cell packaged in a tough outer coat that is resistant to desication, acid, extreme temperature, and even radiation. Endospores germinate and form growing cells when conditions are correct. Certain diseases, like tetanus and botulism, can be caused by endospores that contaminate food, water, or wounds.

Bacteria cause illness in humans in a variety of ways. A particularly potent toxin called **endotoxin** causes life-threatening shock. This toxin is released into tissues when gram-negative cells die. Some bacteria produce other types of toxins that interfere with normal physiology. For example, tetanus is caused by the toxin produced by the bacterium *Clostridium tetani*. The tetanus toxin interferes with the ability of muscle cells to relax, resulting in frozen, rigid muscles characteristic of the disease. Other toxins are enzymes that enable the bacteria to spread through tissues and to obtain nutrients.

In addition to the bacterial chromosome, bacteria often contain small circular, double-stranded DNA molecules called **plasmids**. Plasmids contain extra genetic material that replicates independently of the bacterial chromosome. Plasmids may carry genetic information for antibiotic resistance, the production of toxins, tolerance to toxic metals, and the synthesis of enzymes.

Bacteria grow rapidly and reproduce by splitting in half, a process known as **binary fission**. Under favorable conditions, this process may take only 30 minutes, which means that a small number of cells may increase to a very large number in a relatively short time. The reproduction of a cell and its genetic material occurs with very few errors or mutations. Still, this rapid growth rate virtually guarantees that mutations will arise, and some of these will favor survival of the bacteria under certain conditions.

## Protozoa

Protozoa are single-celled eukaryotic microorganisms. They are much larger than bacteria and have complex internal structures, including a nucleus and membranous organelles. Protozoa are found in nearly every habitat, and most do not cause disease; however, they may invade and destroy certain tissues, or they may provoke damaging inflammatory responses. Protozoa are classified as **amoeboids**, **flagellates**, **ciliates**, and **sporozoans**.

Amoeboids move by means of cell membrane extensions called **pseudopodia**. An amoeba of great health concern is *Entamoeba histolytica,* the cause of amoebic dysentery (Chapter 9), an intestinal infection acquired from feces-contaminated food or water. The flagellates swim by using one or more whiplike appendages called flagella. Pathogens in this group include *Trichomonas vaginalis,* the cause of trichomoniasis, a sexually transmitted infection (Chapter 11), and *Giardia,* the cause of giardiasis, an intestinal infection. Ciliates move by means of numerous short, hair-like projections called **cilia**. There are few pathogens among the ciliates.

Sporozoans are not mobile. *Plasmodium* is the most notorious among them because it causes malaria. Every year, more than 500 million people worldwide become severely ill with malaria and more than 1 million people die as a result. Malaria kills mostly infants, young children, and pregnant women, largely in Africa.

*Plasmodium* is transmitted via the bites of infected mosquitoes.

## Fungi

Fungi are single-celled or multicelled organisms with cell walls that contain a special polysaccharide called **chitin**. Fungi use specialized filaments called **mycelia** to absorb nutrients from their surroundings. They also have reproductive structures bearing **spores**, which are known allergens.

Fungal infections are known as **mycoses**. Healthy human tissue is relatively resistant to fungal infections but may be susceptible under certain circumstances. Fungi can more easily infect damaged tissue than intact healthy tissue. Also, immunocompromised hosts may be unable to resist fungal infections. Fungi cause disease by producing toxins, interfering with normal organ structure or function, or inducing inflammation or allergy. Some common fungal diseases include candidiasis, an infection of skin or mucous membranes caused by the yeast *Candida* (Chapter 16); *Pneumocystis,* an opportunistic pathogen and one of the diagnostic indicator diseases for AIDS (Chapter 2); and a variety of ringworm infections of the skin, hair, and nails (Chapter 16).

## Helminths

Helminths are parasitic worms. Like other animals, helminths are complex multicellular motile organisms. They often have well-developed reproductive systems capable of producing large numbers of offspring. Many helminths have also evolved complex life cycles and strategies for infecting new hosts. Infections with these organisms are often called **infestations**.

**Ascaris** infects an estimated 1.4 billion people (Figure 3–3 ▶). Ascariasis is found worldwide, but the largest numbers of cases occur in tropical and subtropical regions. The eggs of the worm are found in soil contaminated by human feces or in uncooked food contaminated by soil. A person becomes infected by ingesting the eggs. The eggs hatch into larvae in the small intestine and mature into adult worms. The female adult worm lays eggs that are then passed into feces. Infections are usually asymptomatic.

Figure 3–3 ► Ascaris. (Sinclair Stammers/Science Photo Library/Photo Researchers, Inc.)

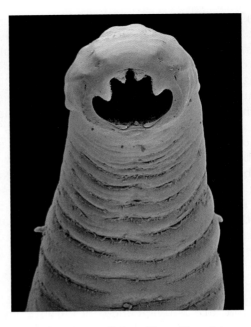

Figure 3–4 ► *Necator americanus*. The cutting plates around the mouth are used to tear open blood vessels of the host. (© David Scharf/Peter Arnold, Inc.)

Stool samples are used for diagnosis, and drugs are available for treatment. Prevention includes the use of toilet facilities, hand washing, safe stool disposal, protection of food from dirt and soil, and thorough washing of produce.

**Hookworms** like *Necator americanus* are a leading cause of anemia and protein malnutrition, afflicting an estimated 740 million people in the developing nations of the tropics (Figure 3–4 ►). The largest numbers of cases occur in sub-Saharan Africa, Latin America, Southeast Asia, and China. Larvae of the hookworm penetrate the skin of the foot, hand, arm, or leg. The larvae travel to the small intestine and mature into adult worms.

Females lay several thousand eggs per day. The eggs are shed in feces and hatch out into larvae in water. There are no specific symptoms or signs of hookworm infection. Stool samples are used for diagnosis, and drugs are available for treatment. Prevention includes not walking barefoot, using toilet facilities, and not using human excrement or raw sewage as fertilizer in agriculture.

*Enterobius vermicularis* infects an estimated 200 million people worldwide and is the most common worm infection in the United States (Figure 3–5 ►). The female pinworm migrates to the anus to deposit her eggs on the skin around the anus. She then secretes a substance that

causes a very strong itching sensation, inciting the host to scratch the area and thus transfer some of the eggs to the fingers. Eggs can also be transferred to cloth, toys, and the bathtub and can survive from 2 to 3 weeks outside of the

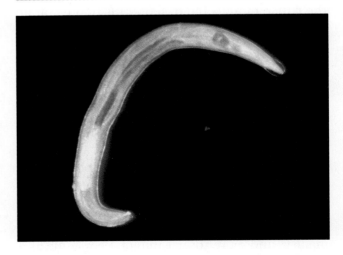

Figure 3–5 ► Adult *Enterobius vermicularis*. (Newscom/Custom Medical Stock Photo)

human body. Humans ingest the eggs, which hatch into larvae in the small intestine. The larvae then migrate to the large intestine and mate. *Enteroboiasis* infections are diagnosed by the Graham sticky-tape method. A piece of transparent tape is placed on the skin around the anus so it can pick up eggs that were laid earlier. The tape is microscopically examined for the presence of eggs. Treatment includes drugs and thorough washing of clothing and linens to kill eggs. Prevention includes practicing proper personal hygiene, frequent changing and washing of linens and clothing, keeping nails trimmed, and not scratching the bare anal area.

## ▶ Nosocominal Infections

**Nosocomial** or hospital-acquired infections are infections acquired in a healthcare facility. The Centers for Disease Control and Prevention estimates that 1.7 million patients in the United States contract a nosocomial infection each year and 99,000 die as a result; 32% of nosocomial infections are urinary tract infections, 22% are infections at the surgical site, 15% are lung infections like pneumonia, and 14% are infections of the bloodstream. Rates of nosocomial infections are markedly higher in developing countries due to lack of supervision, poor infection practices, inappropriate use of limited resources, and overcrowding of hospitals. The microorganisms that cause nosocomial infections can come from the patient's normal flora, contact with healthcare staff, contaminated instruments or needles, and the healthcare environment. Because hospital stays are short, patients are often discharged before the infection becomes apparent. As a consequence, it is often difficult to determine the source of the infection.

Healthcare facilities are a major reservoir for a variety of opportunistic pathogens that can cause nosocomial infections. A weakened patient is an ideal target for an opportunistic pathogen. The weakened patient's resistance to infection can be reduced as a result of disease, compromised nonspecific defenses, and a suppressed immune system. Burns, surgical wounds, injections, invasive diagnostic procedures, ventilators, intravenous therapy, and catheters increase the risk of infection. The principal routes of transmission of nosocomial infections are direct contact transmission from healthcare staff to patient and indirect contact transmission through fomites and the hospital's ventilation system.

According to the Centers for Disease Control and Prevention, handwashing is the single most important means of preventing the spread of nosocomial infections. Education of healthcare facility staff and visitors about basic infection control measures, isolation of patients, sterilization of equipment, use of disposable materials, and prescription of antibiotics only when necessary can help control nosocomial infections.

### Occupational Exposure to Blood

The Occupation Safety and Heath Administration (OSHA) estimates that 5.6 million workers in the healthcare industry and related occupations are at risk of occupational exposure to bloodborne pathogens, including human immunodeficiency virus (HIV), hepatitis B virus (HBV), and hepatitis C virus (HCV). Precise data are not available on the annual number of needlestick and other percutaneous injuries among U.S. healthcare workers; however, estimates indicate

## Prevention ➕PLUS!

### Advice for Travelers

Traveling out of the country? Have you considered how you will protect yourself and your family from infectious diseases? In a different country, you will be faced with different infectious diseases to which you are unlikely to be immune. Will you need vaccinations or prophylactic medications? The Centers for Disease Control and Prevention in Atlanta, Georgia, maintains a website to advise travelers. Before you book your flight, go to www.cdc.gov for the latest information on infectious diseases at your destination.

## Prevention ┿ PLUS!

### Handwashing

According to the Centers for Disease Control and Prevention, handwashing is the single most important means of preventing the spread of infection. The CDC provides the following instructions for correct handwashing:

- Wet hands.
- Apply soap and rub vigorously for at least 15 seconds.
- Rinse with water.
- Dry thoroughly with disposable paper towel.
- Use paper towel to turn off faucet.

that 600,000 to 800,000 such injuries occur annually and about half of these injuries go unreported.

The rate of HBV transmission to susceptible healthcare workers ranges from 6% to 30% after a single needlestick exposure to an HBV-infected patient. However, such exposures are a risk only for healthcare workers who are not immune to HBV; healthcare workers who have antibodies to HBV either from pre-exposure vaccination or prior infection are not at risk. In addition, if a susceptible worker is exposed to HBV, post-exposure prophylaxis with hepatitis B immune globulin and initiation of hepatitis B vaccine is more than 90% effective in preventing HBV infection. The average risk for infection after a needlestick or cut exposure to HCV-infected blood is approximately 1.8%. There is no vaccine against HCV, and there is no postexposure prophylaxis treatment available that reduces transmission. The average risk of HIV infection after needlestick exposure or cut exposure to HIV-infected blood is 0.3%. There is no vaccine against HIV; however, the use of antiretroviral drugs after occupational exposures may reduce the chance of HIV transmission.

## ▶ Treatment of Infectious Disease

The effective treatment of an infectious disease depends on the type of causative pathogen. Bacterial infections can be treated with a variety of **antibiotics**. Penicillin and related drugs act on the cell wall, and they are especially useful in controlling gram-positive bacteria. Some antibiotics target the bacterial cell membrane, causing lysis. Other antibiotics target the protein synthesis machinery of the cell; this is effective because the ribosomes and enzymes involved in bacterial protein synthesis are sufficiently different from those in human cells. Other antibiotics interfere with bacterial metabolism or with DNA and RNA synthesis. Antibiotic resistance plays an important role in the increased incidence of bacterial infections.

Correct use of antibiotics can prevent the development of **antibiotic resistance**. Some *Staphylococcus* species, *Streptococcus* species, and *Enterococcus* species among others have developed resistance to several antibiotics. Resistance arises when bacteria adapt to antibiotics and the adaptation becomes common in the bacterial population, soon rendering the antibiotics ineffective. An antibiotic should be used only for bacterial infections. A number of infections, like influenza and the common cold, are viral and are not treatable with antibiotics. Some viral ailments closely mimic bacterial infections. For example, it turns out that group A *streptococci* cause only 15% of pharyngitis cases, so only a small proportion of sore throats are really strep throat. Most sore throats are really caused by viral infections, some of which closely mimic strep throat because the signs and symptoms include swelling and exudate. If antibiotics are used for many of these viral infections, bacterial populations will more likely evolve resistance to those antibiotics. The Centers for Disease Control and Prevention has asked physicians to take a throat swab and perform the rapid strep antigen test to confirm the presence of group A *streptococci* before prescribing antibiotics. If prescribed, the appropriate antibiotic must be selected. Guidelines are shared and updated for physicians so that the most effective types and dosages are used for certain infections. Patients need to follow through on the prescription and use the antibiotics for the entire time prescribed, should not end treatment early, and should not save antibiotics for use in subsequent illnesses.

Viruses do not have the cell walls and cell membranes of bacteria, nor do they have metabolic or protein synthesis machinery. Viruses are not susceptible to antibiotics. Viruses need human cells to reproduce and decode their genetic material. Some antiviral drugs interfere with this process by acting as **nucleic acid analogues**, substances that mimic the correct DNA or RNA bases. These analogues are used to manufacture the viral genetic material but, in fact, do not function as the normal DNA or RNA bases. Viruses are not replicated correctly and are eventually reduced in number or eliminated. Other antiviral drugs interfere with the assembly of new virus particles inside cells or interfere with the attachment of viruses to host cells and thus prevent infection before disease begins.

Antifungal drugs target fungal walls and membranes but can affect human cells as well, leading to serious toxic side effects. Topical agents are effective for skin infections, such as infections of nails or ringworm, and pose fewer adverse effects. A systemic infection, however, requires systemic treatment, which entails the risk of serious side effects. Systemic treatment requires careful dosing and monitoring for side effects.

Protozoa are treated with drugs that interfere with protein synthesis and metabolism. Certain antibiotics may be used to treat protozoal infections. Helminths are susceptible to drugs that paralyze their muscles or interfere with their carbohydrate metabolism.

Although effective treatments have been discovered and used for many important infections, certain problems remain. One complication is that resistant microorganisms can evolve, rendering existing treatments useless. Another difficulty is that some treatments are accompanied by unacceptable toxic side effects or allergies. For these reasons, preventive measures are the best choice for long-term control of certain diseases.

## ▶ Emerging and Re-Emerging Infectious Diseases

In 1963, the respected physician and anthropologist T. Aidan Cockburn said, "We can look forward with confidence to a considerable degree of freedom from infectious diseases at a time not too far in the future. Indeed … it seems reasonable to anticipate that within some measurable time … all the major infections will have disappeared." Infectious diseases are not only spreading faster, they appear to be emerging more quickly than ever before. Since the 1970s, newly emerging diseases have been identified at the unprecedented rate of one or more per year.

**Emerging infectious diseases** include outbreaks of previously unknown diseases or known diseases whose incidence in humans has significantly increased in the past two decades Table 3–2 ▶ lists emerging infectious diseases. **Re-emerging infectious diseases** are known diseases that have reappeared after a significant decline in incidence. Table 3–3 ▶ lists re-emerging infectious diseases. Human demographics and behavior, technology and industry, economic development and land use, international travel and commerce, microbial adaptation and change, breakdown of public health measures, and climate change can play a role in emergence or re-emergence of infectious diseases.

Human behavior (failing to vaccinate, for example) can play a role in the re-emergence of infectious diseases. Worldwide more than 20 million people are affected each year by measles. In 2005, it was estimated that there were 345,000 measles deaths globally; the primary reason for continuing high childhood measles morbidity and mortality is the failure to deliver at least one dose of measles vaccine to all infants. In countries that are able to keep vaccination coverage high, around 95%, measles is very rare. Because immunization controls most infectious diseases in the United States, many parents no longer fear the vaccine-preventable diseases. However, a small but growing number of parents in the United States are claiming religious exemptions

**Table 3–2 ► Examples of Pathogenic Microbes Identified since 1973**

| Microbe | Type | Disease |
|---|---|---|
| Rotavirus | Bacterium | Infantile diarrhea |
| Ebola virus | Virus | Acute hemorrhagic fever |
| *Legionella pneumophila* | Bacterium | Legionnaires' disease |
| Human T-lymphotrophic virus I | Virus | T-cell lymphoma/leukemia |
| Toxin-producing *Staphylococcus aureus* | Bacterium | Toxic shock syndrome |
| *Escherichia coli* 0157:H7 | Bacterium | Hemorrhagic colitis; hemolytic uremic syndrome |
| *Borrelia burgdorferi* | Bacterium | Lyme disease |
| Human immunodeficiency virus | Virus | Acquired immunodeficiency syndrome |
| *Helicobacter pylori* | Bacterium | Peptic ulcer disease |
| Hepatitis C | Virus | Hepatitis |
| *Vibrio cholerae* 0139 | Bacterium | Cholera |
| Hanatvirus | Virus | Respiratory distress syndrome |
| Cryptosporidium | Protozoa | Enteric disease |
| nvCJD | Prion | New variant Creutzfeldt-Jakob disease |
| HVN1 | Virus | Influenza |
| Nipah | Virus | Severe encephalitis |
| SARS coronavirus | Virus | Severe acute respiratory syndrome |

**Table 3–3 ► Re-emerging Pathogens**

| Microbe | Type | Disease |
|---|---|---|
| Paramyxovirus | Virus | Mumps |
| Prion | Prion | Prion disease |
| *Streptococcus*, group A | Bacterium | Strep throat, impetigo |
| *Staphylococcus aureus* | Bacterium | Pneumonia, meningitis |
| *Clostridium difficile* | Bacterium | Colitis |
| Enterovirus 71 | Virus | Hand, foot, mouth disease |
| *Coccidioides immitis* | Fungus | Valley fever |
| *Mycobacterium tuberculosis* | Bacterium | Tuberculosis |
| *Vibrio cholerae* | Bacterium | Cholera |
| *Plasmodium* | Protozoa | Malaria |
| Dengue virus | Virus | Dengue hemorrhagic fever |

to avoid vaccinating their children. In 1991, a religious group in Philadelphia that chose not to immunize its children was the cause of an outbreak of measles that claimed at least 8 lives and made more than 700 people, mostly children, sick.

Climate changes can alter the breeding ranges of arthropod vectors like mosquitoes and flies. Malaria, Dengue fever, and yellow fever, all mosquito-borne infections, show sensitivity to climate. Even in areas where malaria is endemic, it occurs with less frequency in higher and cooler elevations.

After a change in land use brought humans and deer in close proximity, Lyme disease became prominent in northeastern United States. Much of that area was cleared for farms, driving out deer and their predators. Forest and deer have reclaimed the farmland, but the predators have not returned. As urban centers grow, the human and deer populations inevitably come in contact with more frequency, giving the Lyme disease ticks ample opportunity to attach to humans and their pets.

Emerging antimicrobial resistance demonstrates the potential of microbial adaptation. XDR-TB is the abbreviation for extensively drug-resistant tuberculosis (TB). One in three people in the world is infected with dormant TB bacteria; only when the bacteria become active do people become ill with TB. Bacteria become active as a result of anything that can reduce the person's immunity, such as HIV, advancing age, or some medical conditions. TB can usually be treated with a course of four standard, or first-line, anti-TB drugs. If these drugs are misused or mismanaged, multidrug-resistant TB (MDR-TB) can develop. MDR-TB takes longer to treat with second-line drugs, which are more expensive and have more side effects. XDR-TB can develop when these second-line drugs are also misused or mismanaged and therefore also become ineffective. Because XDR-TB is resistant to first- and second-line drugs, treatment options are seriously limited. It is therefore vital that TB control is managed properly. Multi-drug-resistant strains of *Enterococcus, Staphylococcus, Streptococcus,* HIV, and *Plasmodium* are growing global threats.

International travel aids in the emergence of infectious disease. Severe acute respiratory syndrome (SARS) is a viral respiratory illness caused by a coronavirus, called SARS-associated coronavirus (SARS-CoV), first reported in Asia in February 2003. Over the next few months, the illness spread to more than two dozen countries in North America, South America, Europe, and Asia before the SARS global outbreak of 2003 was contained.

## ▶ Common Childhood Vaccine-Preventable Infectious Diseases

Vaccine-preventable childhood infectious disease levels are at or near record lows in the United States. The global picture is very different. Every year 1.4 million children worldwide die from vaccine-preventable diseases before they reach age 5.

Measles is a highly contagious disease caused by the rubeola virus. The rubeola virus is spread by respiratory droplets or airborne transmission. Early signs and symptoms include fever, cough, runny nose, and fatigue, followed by a rash that usually begins on the head and spreads to cover the body (Figure 3–6▶). Grayish spots, called Koplik spots, often develop inside the mouth before the rash appears. Diagnosis is

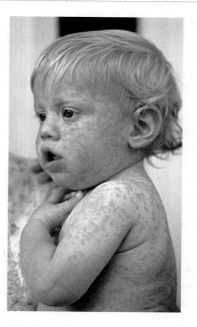

**Figure 3–6** ▶ Measles rash. (© Lowell Georgia/Science Source/ Photo Researchers, Inc.)

based on history of exposure, Koplik spots, and rash. There is no cure for measles, and it usually runs its course in 7 to 10 days. Treatment is supportive and may include pain relievers and fever reducers. Measels is part of the MMR (measles, mumps, rubella) vaccine.

Mumps is caused by the paramyxovirus and is spread by direct contact with respiratory secretions or saliva or through fomites. Cases of mumps may start with a fever of up to 103°F as well as a headache and loss of appetite. The well-known hallmark of mumps is swelling and pain in the parotid glands, the largest of the salivary glands. Mumps in adolescent and adult males may also result in the development of orchitis, an inflammation of the testicles. Diagnosis is based on history of exposure and signs and symptoms. Treatment is supportive and may include pain relievers and fever reducers. Mumps is part of the MMR vaccine.

Rubella (German measles or 3-day measles) is caused by the rubella virus. The rubella virus is highly contagious and is spread by respiratory droplets, by airborne transmission, and can also be transmitted from pregnant women to their fetus. When rubella occurs in a pregnant woman, it may cause congenital rubella syndrome, with potentially devastating consequences for the developing fetus. Many people with rubella have few or no signs or symptoms. Some rubella patients develop a rash that appears as either pink or light red spots, which may merge to form evenly colored patches. Other signs and symptoms of rubella, which are more common in teens and adults, may include headache; loss of appetite; mild conjunctivitis (inflammation of the lining of the eyelids and eyeballs); a stuffy or runny nose; swollen lymph nodes in other parts of the body; and pain and swelling in the joints (especially in young women). Diagnosis is based on history of exposure, signs and symptoms, and throat culture for the rubella virus. Treatment is supportive and may include pain relievers and fever reducers. Rubella is part of the MMR vaccine.

Whooping cough is a highly contagious bacterial infection caused by *Bordetella pertussis*. The bacteria is spread by direct contact with respiratory droplets. The first signs and symptoms of whooping cough include runny nose, sneezing, mild cough, and low-grade fever. After

1 to 2 weeks, the cough develops into coughing spells that ends with a whooping sound when the patient breathes in. Diagnosis is based on signs and symptoms and bacterial cultures of the nose and throat. Antiobiotics are used for treatment. Pertussis is part of the diphtheria, tetanus, pertussis vaccine.

Diphtheria is a highly contagious bacterial disease caused by *Corynebacterium diptheriae*, which is primarily spread by respiratory droplets; transmission by fomites is rare. Early signs and symptoms include low-grade fever and a sore throat. The bacteria produce a toxin that can cause a thick coating in the nose, throat, or airway that may hinder breathing and swallowing. In the bloodstream the toxin can cause damage to the heart, kidneys, and nervous system. Up to 50% of patients who do not get treatment die. Diagnosis is based on a throat culture. Treatment includes antibiotics and antitoxin. Diphtheria is part of the diphtheria, tetanus, pertussis vaccine.

Tetanus is a bacteria infection caused by *Clostridium tetani*. The bacteria is found in contaminated soil and animal excrement and enters the body via wounds. Once the bacteria are in the body, they produce a toxin that affects the nervous system, causing stiff neck, lock jaw, muscle spasms, and difficulty swallowing. Diagnosis is based on history of exposure, signs, and symptoms. Treatment includes antiobiotics and injection of tetanus immunoglobulin to neutralize the tetanus toxin. Tetanus is part of the diphtheria, tetanus, pertussis vaccine.

Chickenpox is a highly contagious viral infection caused by the varicella zoster virus. There are an estimated 60 million cases worldwide each year. The virus is spread by direct contact, droplet transmission, and airborne transmission. Symptoms begin with a runny or stuffy nose, sneezing, fever, and a cough. A few days later an itchy rash appears usually on the chest and face (Figure 3–7 ▶). At first, the rash looks like pinkish dots that quickly develop a small blister on top. After about 24 to 48 hours, the fluid in the blisters gets cloudy and the blisters begin to crust over. Chickenpox blisters show up in waves, so after some begin to crust over, a new group of spots may appear. A person is contagious from up to 48 hours before the initial rash occurs until all blisters have burst and

Figure 3–7 ▶ Chickenpox rash. (Ace Photo Agency/Phototake NYC)

crusted over. Diagnosis is based on history of exposure and the rash. Treatment is supportive and can include treatments to control scratching (corn starch dusting, calamine lotion, and baking soda baths), pain relievers, and fever reducers. A vaccine is available for varicella zoster.

*Haemophilus influenzae* type b (Hib) is a bacterium that causes diseases including meningitis and pneumonia. There are an estimated 3 million cases and nearly 400,000 deaths worldwide each year. The bacterium lives in the human respiratory tract and can be recovered from the nasal and throat passages of up to 90% of all healthy individuals. Hib disease is spread by respiratory droplets, and signs and symptoms include cough, fever, chills, lack of appetite, extreme sleepiness, severe headache, and stiff neck or back. More serious signs are mental confusion, convulsions, shock, and coma. Diagnosis is based on signs and symptoms, lumbar puncture, and bacterial culture. Antibiotics are used for treatment, and there is a vaccine available for Hib.

Poliomyelitis is caused by the polio virus. Transmission of the virus occurs either by direct person-to-person contact or by indirect contact with infectious saliva or feces or with contaminated sewage or water. Polio is asymptomatic in approximately 95% of cases. In the cases in which there are symptoms, the illness appears in two forms, nonparalytic polio and paralytic polio. Patients with nonparalytic polio do not develop paralysis. Signs and symptoms can include sore throat, fever, nausea, vomiting, and constipation. Nonparalytic aseptic meningitis is another type of nonparalytic polio. In addition to the flu-like signs and symptoms just mentioned, it causes stiffness of neck, back, or legs. Paralytic polio occurs in 0.1% to 2% of polio cases. Paralytic polio usually begins with fever; other symptoms, including headache, neck and back stiffness, and constipation, generally appear a few days later. Acute flaccid paralysis, which causes the limbs to appear loose and floppy, often comes on suddenly and usually affects only one side; if both sides are affected, typically one side is worse than the other. Diagnosis is based on history of exposure, signs and symptoms, isolation of the virus from the throat or feces, and lumbar puncture if the nervous system is involved. Treatment is supportive and may include pain relief. A vaccine is available for polio.

*Steptococcus pneumoniae* is a bacterium that causes diseases including meningitis and upper and lower respiratory disease. Worldwide each year *S. pneumoniae* is estimated to kill approximately 1 million children under age 5. *S. pneumoniae* is present in the upper respiratory tract of about half the population and is transmitted by respiratory droplets. Signs and symptoms may include fever, chills, headache, ear pain, cough, chest pain, disorientation, shortness of breath, and occasionally stiff neck. Diagnosis is based on bacterial culture of body fluids. Antibiotics are used for treatment, although antibiotic resistance is a problem. There is a vaccine available for *S. pneumoniae*.

## RESOURCES

Centers for Disease Control and Prevention: www.cdc.gov

Occupational Safety and Health Administration (OSHA): www.osha.org

National Institute of Allergy and Infectious Disease: www.niaid.nih.gov

World Health Organization: www.who.org

# DISEASES AT A GLANCE

## Pathogens

| PATHOGEN | DISEASE | SIGNS AND SYMPTOMS |
|---|---|---|
| Ascaris | Ascariasis | Asymptomatic |
| Necator americanus | Anemia and protein malnutrition | Asymptomatic |
| Enterobius vermicularis | Enterobiasis | Itching |
| Rubeola virus | Measles | Fever, cough, runny nose, fatigue, Koplik spots, rash |
| Paramyxovirus | Mumps | Fever, headache, loss of appetite, swelling and pain in parotid glands |
| Rubella virus | Rubella or German measles | May be asymptomatic; rash; other symptons in teens and adults may include headache; loss of appetite; mild conjunctivitis; a stuffy or runny nose; swollen lymph nodes in other parts of the body; and pain and swelling in the joints |
| *Bordetella pertussis* | Whooping cough | Runny nose, sneezing, low-grade fever, coughing spells with whooping sound when breathing in |
| *Corynebacterium diptheriae* | Diphtheria | Low-grade fever, sore throat, coating in the nose, throat or airway |
| *Clostridium tetani* | Tetanus | Stiff neck, lock jaw, muscle spasms, and difficulty swallowing |
| Varicella zoster virus | Chickenpox | Stuffy nose, sneezing, fever, cough, rash |
| *Haemophilus influenzae* type b | Meningitis and pneumonia | Cough, fever, chills, lack of appetite, extreme sleepiness, severe headache, and stiff neck or back. More serious signs are mental confusion, convulsions, shock, and coma. |
| Polio virus | Poliomyelitis | Nonparalytic polio: sore throat, fever, nausea, vomiting, and constipation. Nonparalytic aseptic meningitis: sore throat, fever, nausea, vomiting, and constipation, stiffness of neck, back, or legs. Paralytic polio: fever, headache, neck and back stiffness, constipation, acute flaccid paralysis |
| *Steptococcus pneumoniae* | Meningitis and lower respiratory diseases | Fever, chills, headache, ear pain, cough, chest pain, disorientation, shortness of breath, and occasionally stiff neck |

| DIAGNOSIS | TREATMENT | PREVENTION |
|---|---|---|
| Stool sample | Medication to paralyze helminth muscles or interfere with their carbohydrate metabolism | Use of toilet facilities, handwashing, safe stool disposal, protection of food from dirt and soil, thorough washing of produce |
| Stool sample | Medication to paralyze helminth muscles or interfere with their carbohydrate metabolism | Not walking barefoot, use of toilet facilities, not using human excrement or raw sewage as fertilizer in agriculture |
| Graham sticky-tape method | Medication to paralyze helminth muscles or interfere with their carbohydrate metabolism | Personal hygiene, frequent changing and washing of linens and clothing, keeping nails trimmed, not scratching the bare anal area |
| History of exposure, Koplik spots, rash | Supportive pain relievers, fever reducers | Vaccine |
| History of exposure, signs and symptoms | Supportive pain relievers, fever reducers | Vaccine |
| History of exposure, signs and symptoms, throat culture | Supportive pain relievers, fever reducers | Vaccine |
| Signs and symptoms, bacterial culture of nose and throat | Antibiotics | Vaccine |
| Throat culture | Antibiotics and antitoxin | Vaccine |
| History of exposure, signs and symptoms | Antibiotics and Tetanus immunoglobulin | Vaccine |
| History of exposure, rash | Supportive to control itching, pain relievers, fever reducers | Vaccine |
| Signs and symptoms, lumbar puncture, bacterial culture | Antibiotics | Vaccine |
| History of exposure, signs and symptoms, isolation of the virus from the throat or feces, and lumbar puncture if the nervous system is involved | Supportive pain relief | Vaccine |
| Culture of body fluids | Antibiotics | Vaccine |

# Interactive Exercises

## Cases for Critical Thinking

1. Based upon what you learned about transmission and control of infectious diseases, compare how one would approach the control of influenza with the control of malaria. Explain which methods would be useful for each disease.

2. Explain why antibiotics are ineffective against viral infections. What problems can arise when viral infections are treated with antibiotics?

3. Explain why vaccination is a particularly effective method for controlling infectious disease.

4. About a week or two ago, Joe, a 3-year-old boy, had a runny nose, a mild cough, and a low fever. Joe is now having coughing spells and he is having a difficult time inhaling during these coughing spells. What is your diagnosis? How is this transmitted? What treatment is available? Is a vaccine available?

5. Mason, a 5-year-old boy, had a runny nose, fever, and cough after attending a birthday party. A few days later a rash appeared on his chest and face. The rash began as pinkish dots but quickly developed a small blister on top. The blisters are appearing in waves. What is your diagnosis? How is this transmitted? What treatment is available? Is a vaccine available?

6. Marion, a 3-year-old girl, has a thick coating in her throat that hinders her breathing and swallowing. What is your diagnosis? How can this diagnosis be confirmed? What treatment is available?

## Multiple Choice

1. A glycocalyx that is organized and firmly attached to the wall is a _____.
   a. flagella
   b. pili
   c. capsule
   d. slime layer

2. These contain the genetic material of a bacteria packaged in a tough outer coat.
   a. pili
   b. toxins
   c. endospores
   d. fimbrae

3. Small, circular DNA molecules that some bacteria have in addition to the bacterial chromosome are called _____.
   a. pili
   b. endospore
   c. plasmid
   d. glycocalyx

4. Bacteria reproduce by _____.
   a. mitosis
   b. meiosis
   c. binary fission
   d. none of the above

5. Single-celled eukaryotic organisms are called _____.
   a. bacteria
   b. helminths
   c. viruses
   d. protozoa

6. German measles is caused by _____.
   a. *Bordetella pertussis*
   b. rubeola virus
   c. rubella virus
   d. varicella zoster virus

7. Whooping cough is caused by _____.
   a. *Bordetella pertussis*
   b. rubeola virus
   c. rubella virus
   d. varicella zoster virus

8. The protein coat of a virus is its _____.
   a. nucleus
   b. capsid
   c. core
   d. mycelia

9. The most common worm infection in the United States is _____.
   a. *Enterobius vermicularis*
   b. Lymphatic filariasis
   c. Ascariasis
   d. Shistosomiasis

10. Which of the following is not an example of contact transmission?
   a. kissing
   b. touching
   c. sexual contact
   d. a needlestick

## True or False

_____ 1. Infectious diseases are not a major cause of death and disability in the world today.

_____ 2. Rabies is a communicable disease.

_____ 3. Antibiotics are effective against viruses.

_____ 4. The respiratory system is the most frequently used portal of entry.

_____ 5. Ascariasis is the most common type of roundworm infection in humans.

_____ 6. More than 90% of deaths from infectious diseases worldwide are caused by a few diseases.

_____ 7. Prions are composed of protein and nucleic acid.

_____ 8. Handwashing is the single most important means of preventing the spread of nosocomial infections.

_____ 9. Antibiotics are effective treatments for helminth infestations.

_____ 10. Chickenpox is transmitted by the parenteral route.

## Fill-Ins

1. Microorganisms in and on our bodies make up our _____.

2. _____ diseases are known diseases that have reappeared after a significant decline in incidence.

3. Measles is caused by the _____ virus.

4. _____ infections are acquired in a hospital.

5. In _____ transmission, infectious diseases can be transmitted directly from an infected human to a susceptible human.

6. The bacterial _____ is sticky and lies outside the cell wall.

7. _____ are short, hair-like appendages that enable bacteria to attach to surfaces.

8. _____ are infectious agents composed only of protein.

9. Mumps is caused by the _____.

10. Chickenpox is caused by the _____ virus.

## Labeling Exercise

Fill in the blanks below to label the protozoan pathogens and helminths pictured.

**Protozoan pathogens**

**Helminths**

1 _____

2 _____

3 _____

4 _____

5 _____

6 _____

# Multimedia Preview

Additional interactive resources and activities for this chapter can be found on the Companion Website. For videos, audio glossary, and review, access the accompanying DVD-ROM in this book.

## ▶ DVD-ROM Highlights

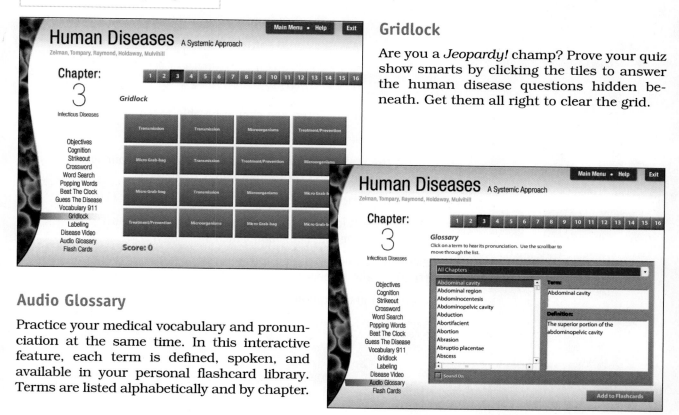

### Gridlock

Are you a *Jeopardy!* champ? Prove your quiz show smarts by clicking the tiles to answer the human disease questions hidden beneath. Get them all right to clear the grid.

### Audio Glossary

Practice your medical vocabulary and pronunciation at the same time. In this interactive feature, each term is defined, spoken, and available in your personal flashcard library. Terms are listed alphabetically and by chapter.

## ▶ Website Highlights—www.pearsonhighered.com/zelman

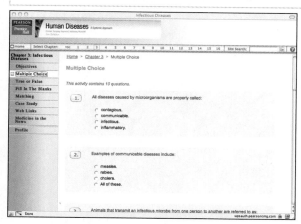

### Multiple Choice Quiz

Take advantage of the free-access online study guide that accompanies your textbook. You'll find a multiple-choice quiz that provides instant feedback and allows you to check your score to see what you got right or wrong. By clicking on this URL you'll also access links to current news articles and an audio glossary.

CHAPTER

4

# Cancer

## Learning Objectives

After studying this chapter, you should be able to

- Describe cancer classification

- Explain the biology of human cancer and the role of oncogenes, tumor suppressor genes, and DNA repair genes

- Identify the etiologies of cancer

- Describe the epidemiology, symptoms, etiology, diagnosis, and treatment of the most common cancers

- Demonstrate understanding of the value of cancer prevention, early detection, and screening in reducing cancer

- Develop an understanding of cancer staging

## Fact or Fiction?

From a public health perspective, there is an overwhelming case to justify the development of a human papillomavirus (HPV) vaccine.

**Fact:** At least 50% of sexually active adults have had a genital HPV infection. Low-risk HPV infections cause benign lesions or genital warts, whereas high-risk HPV infection is the main cause of cervical cancer.

## Disease Chronicle

### Peter Jennings: Lung Cancer

Peter Jennings was one of America's most distinguished journalists and reported on many important worldwide events. He was in Berlin in the 1960s when the Berlin Wall was going up, and there in the 1990s when it came down. He covered the civil rights movement in the southern United States during the 1960s and the struggle for equality in South Africa during the 1970s and 1980s. He was there when the Voting Rights Act was signed in the United States in 1965, and on the other side of the world when black South Africans voted for the first time.

In late March 2005, viewers started noticing that Jennings's voice sounded grave and unhealthy during evening newscasts. On April 1, 2005, he anchored *World News Tonight* for the last time. On April 5, 2005, Jennings informed viewers through a taped message on *World News Tonight* that he had been diagnosed with lung cancer and was starting chemotherapy. "As some of you know, I have learned in the last couple of days that I have lung cancer," he said. "Yes, I was a smoker until about 20 years ago, and I was weak and smoked over 9/11." Although he stated his intention to continue anchoring whenever possible, the message was his last appearance on television.

On August 7, 2005, Peter Jennings died from lung cancer in his New York apartment with his wife, two children, and sister at his side.

# ▶ Introduction

Cancer or **malignancy** is not a single disease. Over 100 different types and subtypes of human cancer affect the young and old and involve nearly every tissue or organ in the body. Cancer has a profound emotional and physical impact for the patient and is associated with significant **morbidity** or complications and possible **mortality** or death.

Cancer is the leading cause of death worldwide and afflicts two of every three families. Of a total of 58 million deaths worldwide in 2005, cancer claimed the lives of 7.6 million people. The main types of cancer leading to overall cancer mortality include

- Lung (1.3 million deaths/year)
- Stomach (almost 1 million deaths/year)
- Liver (662,000 deaths/year)
- Colon (665,000 deaths/year)
- Breast (502,000 deaths/year)

Deaths from cancer worldwide are projected to continue to rise, with an estimated 9 million deaths projected in 2015 and 11.4 million deaths in 2030, according to the World Health Organization.

In the United States, approximately one of every two men and one of every three women will be diagnosed with an invasive cancer in his or her lifetime. The National Institutes of Health estimated the overall costs for cancer in 2006 at $206.3 billion, which includes medical costs, costs due to losses in productivity, and premature death.

# ▶ Classification of Cancer

Other terms used to describe cancer are **tumors** and **neoplasms.** A **tumor** fundamentally means swelling, and **neoplasia** refers to new growth. A tumor or neoplasm can be either **benign** or **malignant.** A benign neoplasm is noncancerous and usually localized to a tissue or organ. Malignant neoplasms, or cancer, consist of rapidly dividing cells that accumulate uncontrollably, invade normal tissue, and have the ability to **metastasize** or generate tumors at distant sites. See Table 4–1▶.

Both benign and malignant tumors are classified according to the tissue in which they develop (Table 4–2▶). Benign tumors are generally encapsulated with clearly defined edges, which make their removal from surrounding tissues relatively easy. Benign tumors do not metastasize, nor do they recur after surgical removal. Unlike benign tumors, cancer cells continue to grow and form abnormal cells.

| Table 4–1 ▶ Classification of Tumors | |
|---|---|
| **T (Tumor)** | |
| Tx | Tumor cannot be adequately assessed |
| T0 | No evidence of primary tumor |
| Tis | Carcinoma in situ |
| T1–4 | Size and/or extent of primary tumor |
| **N (nodes)** | |
| Nx | Regional lymph nodes cannot be assessed |
| N0 | No evidence of regional lymph node involvement |
| N1–3 | Involvement of regional lymph nodes (number and/or extent of spread) |
| **M (metastasis)** | |
| Mx | Distant metastasis cannot be evaluated |
| M0 | No distant metastasis |
| M1 | Distant metastasis (cancer has spread to different parts of the body) |

## Table 4–2 ► Nomenclature of Selected Benign and Malignant Tumors

| Tissue of Origin | Benign | Malignant |
|---|---|---|
| Epithelial cells | Adenoma | Adenosarcoma |
| | Papilloma | Papillary adenocarcinoma |
| | Squamous cell papilloma | Squamous cell carcinoma |
| | Liver cell adenoma | Hepatocellular carcinoma |
| | Renal tubular adenoma | Renal cell carcinoma |
| Connective tissue | Fibroma | Fibrosarcoma |
| | Lipoma | Liposarcoma |
| | Chondroma | Chondrosarcoma |
| | Osteoma | Osteosarcoma |
| | Hemangioma | Angiosarcoma |
| | Rhabdomyoma | Rhabdomyosarcoma |
| | Leiomyoma | Leiomyosarcoma |

## ► Biology of Cancer

### Normal Cell Growth

In normal tissues, cells are reproduced according to the need of the organism. Four factors regulate cell growth: growth factors, growth inhibitors, cell cycle proteins called **cyclins,** and programmed cell death or **apoptosis**. In response to injury, cell growth is accelerated by growth factors. Once damaged tissue has been repaired, inhibitory growth factors decrease cell growth. Cell cycle proteins, or cyclins, regulate specific phases of the cell cycle. If a cell has not completely and accurately replicated its DNA or does not have the full complement of substances required to complete cell division, the cell is either repaired or undergoes or cell death.

### Carcinogenesis

**Carcinogenesis**, the development of cancer, is a multistep process that involves a complex sequence of genetic mutations. A **mutation** is a change in the biochemistry of a gene, resulting in the production of abnormal cells. Genes within DNA and its product RNA hold key information for cell replication. Most invasive cancers develop only when several genes are mutated. Generally, mutations in three classes of genes are responsible for the development of cancer: oncogenes, tumor suppressor genes, and DNA repair genes. See Table 4–3►.

*Oncogenes* An oncogene is a gene that when mutated or expressed at abnormally high levels contributes to converting a normal cell into a cancer cell. Oncogenes are derived from proto-oncogenes or growth-promoting genes and are activated genetic alterations induced by retroviruses. Normally, oncogenes encode for proteins that regulate cell growth, differentiation, and apoptosis. Activation or overproduction of an oncogene leads to dysregulation of cell growth, increased proliferation, and a loss of apoptosis. Over 100 different types of oncogenes have been identified.

### Table 4–3  ▶  Cancers Associated with Selected Genetic Mutations

| Gene | Major Tumor Type |
|---|---|
| **Oncogene** | |
| BCR_ABL translocation | Chronic myelogenous leukemia |
| BCL-2 | Chronic lymphocytic leukemia |
| KT, PDGFRA | Gastrointesinal tumors |
| **Tumor suppressor gene** | |
| P53 | Breast cancer, sarcoma, brain |
| APC | Colon, stomach, intestine |
| VHL | Kidney |
| **DNA repair gene** | |
| BRCA1 | Breast, ovary |
| MSH2, MLH1 | Colon, uterus, stomach |

*Source: Andreoli and Carpenter's Cecil Essentials of Medicine, 7th ed., 2007, Elsevier.*

*Tumor Suppressor Genes*  The transformation of a normal cell to a malignant cell takes place not only by activation of oncogenes but also by inactivation or deletion of tumor suppressor genes, or TSGs. The protein products of TSGs are involved in a number of cellular functions, such as cell cycle control, checkpoint control, cell signaling, promotion of apoptosis, and DNA repair. Inactivation or loss of TSGs by a mutation or deletion leads to a loss of function; reduced restrictions on cell growth and division, ultimately causing genetic instability and loss of apoptosis; and enhanced possibility of malignant behavior.

*DNA Repair Genes*  DNA repair genes, also known as caretaker genes, are responsible for the repair of errors in normal DNA replication. Mutations in DNA repair genes result in persistent DNA damage and consequent further mutations and genetic instability. This may lead to a loss of tumor repair genes and conversion of a proto-oncogene to an oncogene, resulting in an increased susceptibility to cancer.

## ▶ Etiology of Cancer

Understanding the causes of human cancer requires both laboratory or **in vitro** research and **epidemiological** or population-based studies. Laboratory research provides information on the development of cancer after exposure to a carcinogen, whereas epidemiological studies provide measures of cancer rates in relation to people and their environment. Population measures of cancer rates in epidemiological studies identify **endogenous** and **environmental** etiologies of cancer.

### Endogenous

The genetic makeup of the individual, including age, sex, race, heredity, hormones, and immunity, is among the endogenous nonmodifiable etiologies associated with cancer. Cancer can occur at any age; however, carcinomas are more common around the fifth to seventh decades of life. Sex differences in the etiology of cancer are often due to differences in hormone levels among males and females. Hereditary differences in cancer occur in both males and females, with either autosomal dominant or autosomal recessive inheritance. See Table 4–4 ▶.

### Environmental

The variations among different types of cancer as well as differential rates of cancer based on geography explain the importance of environmental factors in the development of cancer. Tobacco, industrial chemicals, and radiation are among the most significant environmental human carcinogens. Other causes of human cancer include diet, alcohol consumption, chronic infections, and certain medicinal drugs.

*Tobacco*  Cigarette smoke is the major cause of lung cancer throughout the world. The risk of cancer is 20-fold greater in long-term heavy

### Table 4–4 ▶ Autosomal Genes and Associated Cancers

| Inheritance | Associated Cancer |
| --- | --- |
| **Autosomal Dominant** | |
| Familial adenomatous polyposis of the colon | Carcinoma of the colon |
| Familial retinoblastoma | Retinoblastoma and osteogenic sarcoma |
| Von-Hippel-Lindau syndrome | Renal cell carcinoma |
| **Autosomal Recessive** | |
| Xeroderma pigmentosum | Skin cancer |
| Bloom syndrome | Lymphoid malignancies |
| Fanconi's anemia | Leukemia |

smokers than it is in nonsmokers. Smoking cessation decreases the risk of cancer to one-third the risk observed in continuing smokers. Smoking and chewing tobacco are the leading causes of head and neck cancer. Tobacco exposure is also a major factor in the development of cancers of the stomach, pancreas, kidney, bladder, and cervix. Exposure to secondhand smoke is also associated with an increased risk of lung cancer in nonsmoking women married to heavy smokers.

***Industrial Chemicals*** Asbestos exposure is the most common cause of occupational cancer. Exposure to asbestos increases the risk for **mesothelioma** (cancer of the membrane that covers and protects most of the internal organs of the body), lung cancer, and other cancers, such as those of the larynx and kidney. Rates of asbestos-related cancers are declining with a decrease in workplace-related exposure.

Miners exposed to radon are at a 20-fold increased risk for lung cancer. Other chemical compounds linked to human cancer include benzene (leukemia); benzidine (bladder cancer); arsenic, soot, and coal tars (lung and skin cancer); and wood dust (nasal cancer). Chemical carcinogens have also been identified in water and air pollution.

***Radiation*** Exposure to ionizing radiation from natural, industrial, and medical sources can cause a variety of neoplasms, including **leukemia** (cancer of white blood cells), breast cancer, and thyroid cancer.

Sunlight is the most significant source of ultraviolet radiation and causes several types of skin cancer. The development of skin cancers depends on the level of skin exposure, the position of the sun, and skin type. Highly exposed populations, those experiencing acute sunburn, and those with fair skin are particularly at risk for skin cancers.

***Diet*** After smoking, diet and obesity is the next largest contributor to cancer deaths. There is evidence that eating more than five portions of fruits or vegetables per day reduces cancer risk, especially colon and stomach cancer. Physical exercise reduces cancer risk, especially colon cancer, and is helpful in reducing obesity.

## Prevention ✚PLUS!

### Cigarettes and Cancer

It is estimated that nearly one-third of all cancers can be prevented by lifestyle modification. Cigarette smoking accounts for at least 30% of all cancer deaths. It is a major cause of cancers of the lung, larynx (voice box), oral cavity, pharynx (throat), and esophagus and is a contributing cause in the development of cancers of the bladder, pancreas, liver, uterine cervix, kidney, stomach, colon and rectum, and some leukemias. A lifestyle without smoking is a life with a significantly reduced risk of cancer.

*Source:* American Cancer Society, www.cancer.org

*Alcohol* Alcohol abuse, along with tobacco use, has been strongly associated with the development of cancers in the mouth, pharynx, larynx, and esophagus. Alcohol has also been linked to liver, rectal, and breast cancers.

*Chronic Infections* Almost 20% of cancers are associated with chronic infections. The most frequently associated organ sites are the liver, cervix, lymphoid tissue, and stomach. Chronic hepatitis B and C viral infections have been linked with the development of liver cancer. A universal vaccination program directed against hepatitis B has been shown to decrease the incidence of childhood hepatic cancer in Taiwan. Human papillomaviruses have been linked with cervical cancers, and a vaccine has been recently developed. The human immunodeficiency virus can lead to Kaposi's sarcoma and certain lymphomas. Chronic infection with the bacterium *Helicobacter pylori* can cause certain gastric lymphomas and gastric adenocarcinoma.

*Medicines* Various medicines have been associated with an increased risk of specific cancers. For example, synthetic estrogens such as diethylstilbestrol, which was given to mothers during pregnancy in the 1960s and 1970s, was strongly associated with the development of vaginal cancer in their offspring. Cancer chemotherapy agents not only fight cancer but can also be carcinogenic. Successful treatment of primary malignancies with cancer chemotherapy and radiation has been associated with the development of secondary cancers.

## ► Human Cancers by Organ Site

### Lung

Lung cancer is the most common malignant disease worldwide and is the major cause of death from cancer. It was a rare disease until the beginning of the twentieth century due to an increase in the consumption of tobacco. In both men and women, the incidence of lung cancer is low before age 40 and increases up to at least age 70. In the United States, an estimated 213,380 new cases of lung cancer are expected in 2007, accounting for about 15% of cancer diagnoses.

Tobacco smoke accounts for more than 90% of all lung cancers. Secondhand smoke is also associated with a high risk of lung cancer in the general population. In addition to cigarette smoke, household exposure to radon as well as industrial exposures to asbestos and other airborne chemicals increase lung cancer risk.

Most lung cancers are clinically silent, with symptoms presenting once the disease is advanced. Cough is the most common presenting symptom in lung cancer and is reported along with shortness of breath, blood in sputum, chest pain, and loss of appetite. Additional symptoms include wheezing; **stridor**, or a high pitch during respiration; hoarseness; and **dysphagia**, or difficulty speaking.

The two major types of lung cancer include non–small cell lung cancer (NSCLC) and small cell lung cancer (SCLC). NSCLC includes different cellular types, such as squamous cell carcinomas, adenocarcinomas, and large cell tumors. Squamous cell carcinomas are usually located in the bronchi and are commonly associated with abnormal increases in blood calcium. Adenocarcinomas are the most common lung cancers and the type most often diagnosed in nonsmokers. Large cell tumors are the least common form of lung cancer. SCLC is significantly linked to exposure to cigarette smoke. SCLCs often occur as large central tumors and are associated with endocrine abnormalities such as syndrome of inappropriate antidiuretic hormone production and Cushing's syndrome.

A number of different medical tests are required to accurately diagnose lung cancer. A screening diagnosis of lung cancer begins with a patient history, chest x-ray, sputum analysis, and various blood tests. CT scans are essential tools for **staging** or evaluating the extent of disease and for surgical evaluation for removal of the tumor. Positron emission tomography (PET) scans are useful for assessing metastases or distant dissemination of the disease. Bronchoscopy provides a tool for obtaining local tissue, or **biopsy**, for examination under a microscope for assessment of the **histology**, or cell structural abnormalities.

Early stage tumors are treated with surgery. Radiation therapy is also used to treat early stage tumors in patients who are considered poor candidates for surgery. More advanced stages of lung cancer may be treated with a combination of chemotherapy and radiation therapy. Using multiple chemotherapy agents often provides better treatment outcomes than using each respective agent alone. Chemotherapy agents commonly used to treat lung cancer include cisplatin, etopside, cyclophosphamide, doxorubicin, paclitaxel, vincristine, and vinblastine.

Despite the availability of multiple agents to treat lung cancer, relapse rates occur frequently and survival rates are poor. In light of poor survival rates, prevention of lung cancer remains a global priority. Lung cancer is a largely preventable disease that has declined due to anti-smoking campaigns and cancer prevention programs. According to the World Health Organization, decreasing current smoking rates by half could prevent 20 to 30 million deaths before 2025 and 150 million deaths by 2050.

## Breast

Breast cancer is the most frequently diagnosed cancer in women, with more than one million cases occurring worldwide annually. In the United States, an estimated 178,480 new cases of invasive breast cancer are expected to occur among women in 2007. In addition, an estimated 40,910 breast cancer deaths are expected in 2007.

The earliest sign of breast cancer is often an abnormality detected on a mammogram or breast self-examination. Large tumors are usually felt as a mass on or around the breast. Less common symptoms include changes to the breast such as thickening, swelling, distortion, tenderness, and skin irritation, and nipple changes such as spontaneous discharge or ulceration.

Age, female gender, and personal family history are the most important risk factors for breast cancer. Reproductive factors such as a long menstrual history, oral contraceptive use, never having children, or having a first child after age 30 have also been linked to breast cancer. Being overweight, obesity after menopause, postmenopausal hormone replacement therapy, physical inactivity, and excess consumption of alcohol are risk factors that can be modified to potentially reduce risk. Changes in certain genes increase the risk of breast cancer, including BRCA1, BRCA2, and others. Tests may show the presence of specific gene changes in families with a history of breast cancer.

The diagnosis of breast cancer is currently made by assessment of breast lumps, clinical history and physical exam, mammography and/or breast ultrasound, plus a fine needle aspiration biopsy. Breast cancer screening has been associated with a 30% reduction in breast cancer mortality in populations where mammography has been adopted. Treatment of breast cancer depends on the tumor size, stage, as well as patient preferences. Surgical treatment may involve a lumpectomy (surgical removal of a tumor) or mastectomy (surgical removal of the breast) with removal of some of the axillary (underarm) lymph nodes. In early stages of the disease, lumpectory followed by radiation therapy will allow for breast conservation. Mastectomies are often necessary for large tumors. Chemotherapy, hormone therapy, or targeted biologic therapy are also used alone or in combination with surgery and radiation.

## Stomach

Stomach cancer was the fourth most common malignancy in the world in 2000 and is steadily becoming less common. The incidence of stomach cancer in Europe, for example, has fallen by more than 60% during the past 50 years. There is good evidence that the advent of refrigeration of food protects against stomach cancer by facilitating year-round consumption of fruits and vegetables. Vitamin C, contained in fruits and vegetables and other foods of plant origin, is protective, and so too are diets high in whole grain cereals.

Dietary risk factors for stomach cancer include inadequate intake of fresh fruits and vegetables, high salt intake, and consumption of smoked or cured meats or fish. The infectious bacterium *Helicobacter pylori* triggers excess cell proliferation within the stomach with chronic gastritis, and ulceration is also considered a risk factor for stomach cancer.

Early forms of stomach cancer are usually asymptomatic. The most common symptom is a mild pain in the upper abdomen, which is often confused as simple indigestion. Generalized and nonspecific symptoms include fatigue, loss of energy, and a decrease in appetite.

Like all forms of cancer, the definitive diagnosis of stomach cancer is done by taking a biopsy. CT or MRI scans provide information on size, location, and spread of the cancer.

Surgery is the most important treatment for stomach cancer. The extent of surgical removal of the stomach depends on the location of the tumor and extent of tissue involvement. Often a large part of the stomach or all of the stomach will need to be removed. Radiation therapy is especially important in cases where the tumor cannot be removed. The most commonly used chemotherapy agents for treating stomach cancer include 5-fluorouracil, folinic acid, etopside, adriamycin, methotrexate, cisplatin, or caboplatinum. See Figure 4–1►.

## Colorectal

Cancers of the colon and rectum are most common in Western societies where consumption of high-fat food, refined carbohydrates, and animal protein combined with low physical activity is common. In the United States an estimated 112,340 cases of colon cancer and 41,421 cases of rectal cancer occured in 2007.

Screening is necessary to detect colorectal cancer in its early states. Advanced forms of colorectal cancer may cause rectal bleeding, blood in the stool, a change in bowel habits, and pain in the lower abdomen. See Figure 4–2►. Colonoscopy enables visual inspection of the entire large bowel and recturm. The procedure is a safe and effective means of evaluating the large bowel. The technology for colonoscopy has evolved to provide a very clear image of the mucosa through a videocamera attached to the end of the scope. The camera connects to a computer, which can store and print color images selected during the procedure. Colonoscopy is especially useful in detecting small adenomas; however, the main advantage of colonoscopy is that it allows for identification and removal of cancerous lesions or polyps as well as for biopsy of suspect tissue.

The risk of colorectal cancer increases with age; more than 90% of cases are diagnosed in individuals age 50 years and older. Certain inherited genetic mutations, including familial

Figure 4–1 ► Stomach cancer. (Javier Domingo/Phototake NYC)

Figure 4–2 ► Radiograph of colon cancer. (ISM/Phototake NYC)

adenomatous polyposis and hereditary nonpolyposis colorectal cancer, are nonmodifiable risk factors for colorectal cancer. Modifiable risk factors include obesity, physical inactivity, smoking, heavy alcohol consumption, a diet high in red and processed meat, and inadequate intake of fruits and vegetables.

Surgery is a curative for colorectal cancers that have not spread. A permanent **colostomy**, or the creation of an abdominal opening for elimination of body waste, is rarely needed for colon cancer and is frequently required for rectal cancer. Chemotherapy alone or in combination with radiation therapy is used to treat invasive tumors prior to and after surgery. Chemotherapeutic agents used to treat colorectal cancer include oxaliplatin and 5-fluorouracil. Two new targeted therapies recently approved in the United States are Avastin, which blocks the growth of blood vessels to the tumor, and Erbitux, which blocks the effects of hormone-like factors that promote cancer growth.

## Liver

**Hepatocellular** carcinoma, or malignancy of the liver cells, accounts for 80% of all primary cancers in the liver. Liver cancer accounts for almost 4% of all cancers worldwide and affects men three times more frequently than women. The liver is the second most commonly involved organ in metastatic disease, after the lymph nodes.

In vitro studies have demonstrated the carcinogenic effects of hepatitis B virus and hepatitis C virus on **hepatocytes** or liver cells. Viral replication in infected cells and consequent immune response result in persistent inflammation that progresses toward chronic liver disease and malignant changes. In developing countries, dietary ingestion of toxins produced by mold is causally associated with hepatocellular carcinoma.

Common symptoms of hepatocellular carcinoma are abdominal pain, weight loss, fatigue, abdominal swelling, and **anorexia** or loss of appetite. Other signs include impaired liver function, **ascites** (accumulation of fluid in the abdominal cavity), **hepatomegaly** (enlarged liver), and **jaundice** (yellowish discoloration of the skin,

sclera, and bile). Liver cancer follows a rapid and progressive course, with only about a 10% survival at 5 years in the United States and lower in developing countries.

Most cases of liver cancer can be diagnosed by computed tomography (CT) and ultrasound. A definitive diagnosis depends on identification of cellular abnormalities obtained by a biopsy (Figure 4–3 ►).

The treatment of malignant tumors of the liver depends on the extent of disease and the underlying liver function. Surgical removal of the tumors with defined margins is the primary treatment for malignant liver neoplasms. Most hepatocellular cancers are not sensitive to chemotherapy. Radiation therapy can be used to control symptoms by shrinking the tumor. Liver transplantation is recommended when chemotherapy and radiation are ineffective.

## Female Reproductive Tract

*Cervical* Cervical cancer is the second most common cancer in women. The incidence and mortality have declined in the last 40 years in Western societies with the development of extensive screening programs.

Molecular and epidemiological studies have shown that certain human papillomavirus types (HPV) are central to the development of cervical cancer. High-risk sexual behavior, such as multiple sex partners, and early age at initiation of sexual activity potentially reflect the probability

**Figure 4–3** ► Cancer of the liver. (Dr. E. Walker/Science Photo Library/Photo Researchers, Inc.)

of infection with HPV and associated cervical cancer.

Precancerous changes in the cervix can be readily detected with the Pap test. Additional tests include a colposcopy (endoscopic examination of the cells of the cervix) and biopsy for a definitive diagnosis.

Moderate to severe precancerous changes to the cervix can be treated by killing the diseased tissue via freezing, or **cryosurgery**, or applying heat via **cautery** or **laser,** which vaporizes cells. If a larger area of the cervix needs to be removed, it is removed by a surgical procedure called a **cone biopsy.** Invasive cervical cancers are treated with radiation therapy and chemotherapy.

*Uterine* Cancer of the uterus or **endometrium** is the seventh most common cancer of women worldwide, with the highest incidence reported in the United States. Uterine cancer occurs in women of middle age and older, with a peak incidence in the late 50s and early 60s.

Endometrial cancer is linked to reproductive life, with a higher rate among women who have never been pregnant and women in late menopause. Oral estrogen therapy and prior removal of the ovaries also increase the risk for endometrial cancer. This disease is also associated with obesity, diabetes, and hypertension.

The most common sign of uterine cancer is **metrorragia**, or uterine bleeding, especially after menopause. Other signs of the disease are those linked to a mass in the abdomen such as **dysuria** (difficult urination), constipation, or bloating.

Enodovaginal echography and hysteroscopy are useful in identifying the tumor. Histological examination provides a more definitive diagnosis.

Precancerous lesions of the endometrium are treated by surgical removal of the uterus or **hysterectomy.** A total abdominal hysterectomy with removal of the ovaries is the definitive treatment for carcinoma of the uterus. Postsurgical radiation therapy is also recommended in patients at risk for relapse following surgery. In inoperable cases, pelvic radiation therapy may be the sole treatment.

*Ovarian* Cancer of the ovary may develop in one or both ovaries and may spread to other parts of the abdomen. Because the ovaries are situated deep within the pelvis, the early stages may cause no symptoms, so that ovarian cancer is frequently diagnosed in advanced stages of the disease. See Figure 4–4 ▸.

A family history is the single most important risk factor for ovarian cancer. Cancer of the ovary is influenced by hormones and reproductive factors, and the risk is greater among women with a prior history of breast cancer and no history of pregnancy. A history of pelvic inflammatory disease, polycystic ovary disease, and endometriosis has also been associated with increased risk.

The majority of patients with ovarian cancer usually present after the disease has spread outside the ovary. Symptoms include abdominal discomfort, bloating, abnormal vaginal bleeding, and gastrointestinal or urinary tract abnormalities.

Abdominal and vaginal ultrasound are used to detect the presence of an ovarian tumor; however, a definitive diagnosis requires surgical examination and a biopsy.

Surgery is often the first option for diagnosis via biopsy and treatment of ovarian cancer. Surgical treatment of the disease includes a total abdominal hysterectory with removal of the ovaries, appendectomy, and removal of pelvic lymph nodes. Chemotherapy agents used to treat advanced stages of ovarian cancer include

Tumor —

**Figure 4–4** ▸ Tumor on ovary.

cisplatin, paclitaxel, vincristine, actinomycin, bleomycin etopside, and cyclophamide in various cycles and duration. Despite treatment, the overall five-year survival rate for all stages of ovarian cancer ranges from 30% to 50%.

## Male Reproductive Tract

***Prostate***  Prostate cancer is the third most common cancer in men worldwide, with approximately 543,000 new cases each year. In the United States there are approximately 317,000 new cases per year. The incidence and the mortality increases with age and peaks around the seventh decade of life. Thus, approximately three-quarters of the cases occur in men age 65 years and older.

Age is the leading risk factor for prostate cancer. Dietary pattern studies suggest that a diet high in saturated fat is a significant risk factor, whereas ingestion of micronutrients such as vitamins A, D, E, selenium, lycopene, and calcium has a protective effect. The role of hormones in the development in prostate cancer has been suggested, though the exact role of hormones in prostate carcinogenesis is still not understood.

There are no symptoms that are absolutely specific to prostate cancer. The symptoms, including urinary hesitancy, frequency, urgency, dribbling, weak stream; blood in the urine; and pain in the lower abdomen resemble symptoms of a urinary tract infection or a benign growth of the prostate, also called **benign prostatic hypertrophy.**

Digital rectal examination is the simplest way to detect abnormalities of the prostate gland (Figure 4–5▶). A blood test for **prostate-specific antigen (PSA)** may support the diagnosis of prostate cancer. Ultrasound guided biopsy studies establish the dimensions of the tumor. Radiologic examinations such as CT scans and MRI are performed to help stage a diagnosed prostate cancer.

Surgery to remove the prostate is recommended for those with localized disease and a life expectancy greater than 10 years. Radiation therapy is recommended for men who are not suitable for surgery. Advanced disease is treated with radiation therapy and endocrine

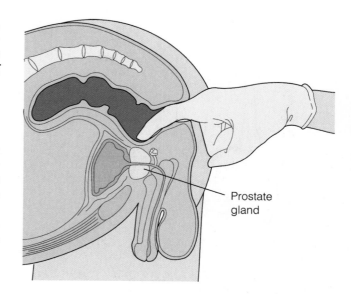

**Figure 4–5** ▶ Digital rectal examination to detect abnormalities of the prostate gland.

therapy. Endocrine therapy is aimed at reducing hormone levels that may continue to foster growth of the tumor.

***Cancer of the Testes***  Cancer of the testes accounts for 1.5% of all male cancers. Approximately 49,300 new cases are diagnosed each year. Cancer of the testes can occur at all ages, though the risk is greatest in men during the third and fourth decades of life.

The most common malignant tumors of the testes originate from germ cells. **Germ cells** are cells that have the potential to grow and develop into many different types of tissues. There are two types of germ cell tumors: **seminomas**, or cancer of sperm-producing cells, and **nonseminomas** cancers of embryomic cells. Seminoma are slow growing tumors and are sensitive to radiation therapy. See Figure 4–6▶.

Environmental causes of testicular cancer have not been established. There is an increased incidence of the disease in men with a history of undescended testicles and those with a family history testicular cancer. In utero exposure to exogenous estrogen may increase the

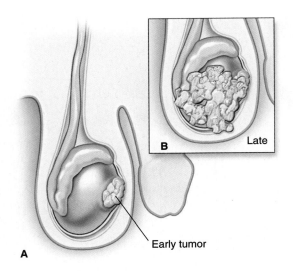

**A**

Early tumor

**B** Late

Figure 4–6 ► Early and late stage testicular tumors.

risk of undescended testes, also known as **cryptorchidism.**

Cancer of the testes is usually detected as a painless lump on the testicle. Rarely, the first noticeable symptoms of a nonseminomatous cancer are a lump in the neck, pain or discomfort in the back, or shortness of breath due to metastases in the lungs.

Current management of germ cell tumors includes surgical resection, radiation therapy, and chemotherapy. Approximately 80% of patients with advanced disease respond to all three treatments.

## Esophageal Cancer

Cancers of the esophagus are the sixth most frequent cancers worldwide. In Europe and in the United States, the annual mortality from esophageal cancer is up to five males and one female per 100,000 persons. In the United States, cancer of the esophagus is more common in people over the age of 60.

Consumption of tobacco and alcohol, associated with low intake of fresh fruits and vegetables, is causally associated with cancer of the esophagus. Greater than 90% of esophageal cancer is attributable to tobacco and alcohol,

with an additive risk among individuals who are exposed to both factors. Long-standing esophagitis due to reflux disease increases the risk of esophageal cancer.

Difficulty swallowing or pain with eating or drinking are the most noticeable symptoms. Unexplained weight loss, hoarseness of the voice, and bleeding from the throat may be associated with advanced disease.

Diagnosis of esophageal cancer requires microscopic examination of the diseased tissue, or biopsy. CT scan and endoscopic ultrasonography are useful in determining the extent of the tumor and whether there is spread to neighboring tissues. Barium dye x-rays provide information on how well the esophagus is functioning as well as the location of the tumor.

Primary treatment for local disease is surgical removal of the esophagus. Replacement of a prosthetic tube or a stent across the tumor **stenosis** (narrowing) may help restore swallowing in patients not suitable for surgery. Radiation therapy as well as multiple chemotherapy regiments have been used alone or combined with surgery, though these approaches are rarely curative. Despite the availability of treatment, the overall 5-year survival rate for esophageal cancer ranges from 10% to 20%.

## Bladder Cancer

Bladder cancer is the ninth most common cancer worldwide, with an estimated 330,000 new cases and 130,000 deaths per year. An estimated 67,160 new cases are expected to occur in the United States in 2007.

The most important risk factor for bladder cancer is cigarette smoking, which accounts for approximately 65% of male cases and 30% of female cases. Upon cessation of cigarette smoking, a substantial decrease in risk of bladder cancer is observed. Exposure to certain industrial chemicals, such as rubber, aromatic hydrocarbons, asbestos, and solvents used in paint and hairspray, is correlated with an increased risk. In certain endemic regions, infection with a worm, *Schistosoma haematobium*, is linked with up to a fivefold risk of bladder cancer.

The most common symptom of bladder cancer is **hematuria**, or blood in the urine. Pain is rarely associated with hematuria. Increased urinary frequency is also reported but is often mistaken for a less serious condition.

Surgery alone or in combination with radiation or chemotherapy is used to treat greater than 90% of cases. Localized tumors can be treated with immune therapy or chemotherapy administered directly into the bladder. For all diagnosed cases and stages combined, the 5-year survival rate of bladder cancer is 82%.

## Head and Neck Cancer

Cancer in the upper aerodigestive tract (which extends from the surface of the lips to the neck region), larynx, and pharynx comprise head and neck cancer. These cancers are among the eleventh most common worldwide, with 390,000 new cases of oral cancer, 65,000 new cases of pharyngeal cancer, and 160,000 cases of laryngeal cancer reported worldwide per year. The incidence rate is more than twice as high in men as women in the United States.

Smoking and excess alcohol consumption are the major risk factors for head and neck cancer. Smoking accounts for about 14% of laryngeal and oral/pharyngeal cancer cases in men and about 15% of cases in women worldwide. Tobacco smoking has also been found to be an important risk factor for nasopharyngeal cancer.

Symptoms of oral cancer include head or neck pain; bleeding; difficulty in opening the mouth, chewing, swallowing, and talking; and pain in the neck. Early disease is often painless and present as elevated, red mucosal patches or hardened ulcers or growths. With advanced disease, large masses with areas of **necrosis,** or death to surrounding tissue, may extend to the bone, muscle, and skin.

There are no general screening tests for head and neck cancers. Frequently these cancers are detected by dentists or primary care physicians as abnormal changes in oral tissue. Endoscopic examination to obtain a biopsy is useful for laryngeal and pharyngeal tumors.

Like many other forms of cancer, tumor resection is aimed at removing the tumor while preserving optimal tissue function. Radiation therapy along with surgery is a mainstay treatment for most head and neck cancers. Chemotherapy is applied for advanced stages of disease.

## Lymphoma

Lymphoma covers a heterogeneous group of neoplasms of lymphoid tissue. Lymphomas are categorized as either Hodgkin's disease or non-Hodgkin's lymphoma. Within each of these two categories are a range of diverse subtypes. There are around 287,000 new cases of non-Hodgkin's lymphoma and 62,000 new cases of Hodgkin's lymphoma diagnosed worldwide annually. An estimated 71,380 new cases of lymphoma will occur in the United States in 2007, including 8190 cases of Hodgkin's lymphoma and 63,190 cases of non-Hodgkin's lymphoma.

*Hodgkin's Disease*    Hodgkin's disease comprises approximately 23% of malignant lymphomas worldwide, and approximately 45% of cases can be attributed to Epstein-Barr virus (EBV). Hodgkin's disease is distinguished from non-Hodgkin's lymphoma by a particular type of cell termed **Reed-Sternberg cell.**

Hodgkin's disease most often occurs in young adults. The risk for Hodgkin's disease has been explained by infections with EBV, HIV, and chronic exposure to wood or wood products. The most common presenting symptom is a painless swelling of the lymph nodes in the neck, armpit, or groin. Other symptoms include fatigue, unexplained fever, night sweats, and indigestion in cases of gastric lymphoma.

Hodgkin's disease is often treated with chemotherapy with combinations of several different agents. Survival of Hodgkin's disease is related to the extent of disease at diagnosis; however, 5-year survival for all stages of the disease combined is estimated at 70% to 90%.

*Non-Hodgkin's Lymphoma*    Patients with HIV/AIDS or those who have received immune suppressive therapy are at a higher risk for developing non-Hodgkin's lymphoma. In addition to HIV, viral infections with HTLV1 and EBV are also associated with non-Hodgkin's lymphoma. Infection in the stomach with the bacterium *Helicobacter pylori* is linked with gastric lymphoma.

The most common presenting symptom of non-Hodgkin's lymphoma is painless swelling of the lymph nodes. Similar to Hodgkin's disease, nonspecific feelings of fatigue, night sweats, and fever are also reported. Accurate diagnosis requires microscopic evaluation of lymphoid tissue. X-rays, CT scans, MRI, bone marrow sampling, and lymphograms are useful in determining the extent of disease.

**Indolent** or slow growing lymphomas often present as advanced disease. Treatment with radiation and or chemotherapy can be administered as needed over a period of many years. The goal in treating advanced, slow growing lymphomas is to obtain a cure. This is accomplished with several doses and combinations of chemotherapeutic agents alone or in combination with radiation therapy. Recurrent lymphomas have been treated with bone marrow transplantation with some success.

## Leukemia

Leukemia, which causes massive proliferation of immature forms of white blood cells, occurs in more than 250,000 individuals worldwide each year. These cancers are further classified on the basis of malignancy involving either **lymphoid** (B cells or T cells in lymph tissue) or **myeloid** (bone marrow) cells and whether the disease is acute or chronic.

Leukemia is diagnosed 10 times more often in adults than in children, although it is often thought of as a childhood cancer. Symptoms include fatigue, paleness, weight loss, repeated infections, fever, bruising easily, and nosebleeds or other hemorrhages. These signs often appear suddenly in acute leukemia, whereas chronic leukemia can progress slowly with few symptoms.

Because the symptoms often resemble less serious conditions, leukemia is difficult to diagnose early. Blood tests and bone marrow biopsy provide definitive evidence for this disease.

Chemotherapy is the most effective method for treating leukemia. Supportive treatment with blood transfusions and antibiotics is needed to treat anemia and infections. Bone marrow transplantation from a matched donor is one form of therapy for late stages of this disease. Survival in leukemia depends on type,

ranging from a 5-year survival of 20% for those with acute myeloid leukemia to 74% for people with chronic lymphocytic leukemia.

## Pancreatic Cancer

Pancreatic cancer is a difficult disease to detect and treat. It is the fourteenth most common cancer worldwide, with approximately 216,000 new cases per year. In the United States, an estimated 33,370 deaths are expected to occur in 2007.

About 30% of cases of pancreatic cancer are attributed to smoking. Cigarette smokers develop this disease two to three times more often than nonsmokers. Diets low in fiber and high in consumption of red meat and fat are also associated with this disease.

The diagnosis of pancreatic cancer is rarely made during early stages of the disease. It is frequently diagnosed once patients present with clinical symptoms, including weight loss, nausea, diarrhea, weakness, jaundice, and upper abdominal pain.

Ultrasoundography is useful for initial diagnoses. CT scanning allows for clearer images of the head and tail of the pancreas as well as extent of involvement of surrounding tissues.

Currently, surgery offers patients the only chance for a cure. Palliative treatment is often needed for the treatment of jaundice and gastric obstructions. Simultaneous chemotherapy may provide a survival benefit. Survival from pancreatic cancer is poor, and the majority of pancreatic cancer patients die within one year of diagnosis.

## Melanoma

Melanoma is a malignant proliferation of pigment-producing cells or **melanocytes.** This disease occurs primarily in white-skinned individuals, with incidence rates more than 10 times higher in whites than in African Americans. Approximately 133,000 new cases are diagnosed annually worldwide, and approximately 59,940 persons are expected to be diagnosed in the United States in 2007.

The risk factors for melanoma vary by skin type; sensitivity to sunlight; extent of sun exposure; exposure to industrial chemicals such as

Figure 4–7 ► Malignant melanoma. (ISM/Phototake NYC)

coal tar, arsenic, and radium; and past history of skin, cancer. Melanomas can occur anywhere on the skin, though the majority of melanomas in men appear on the back, while in women the majority appear on the legs.

Early detection of skin cancer is possible by personal examination of the skin. Melanomas usually start as small, mole-like growths that increase in size and change in color (Figure 4–7►). A simple ABCD rule outlines the warning signs of the most common forms of melanoma: asymmetry, border irregularity, color, and diameter.

The diagnosis of a melanoma is made by a biopsy. If the lesion is found to be a melanoma, surgery is required to remove the lesion. Radiation therapy is used to treat recurrent disease or metastases. In general, melanomas are not very responsive to chemotherapy drugs. Biologi-

cal therapy with interferon-alpha and interleukin-2 produces treatment responses in some patients that last many years.

## Thyroid Cancer

Cancer of the thyroid gland is relatively rare, with an incidence of about 120,000 new cases worldwide annually. In general, thyroid cancer can occur at any age, including young adults and teens.

Radiation exposure, iodine deficiency, and radioactive iodine exposure are among known risk factors for thyroid cancer. This cancer is grows slowly and in many cases is cured by complete surgical removal of the thyroid gland.

Thyroid cancer commonly causes no obvious symptoms in its early stages. The vast majority of cancers become clinically palpable as thyroid nodules, although a minority of all thyroid nodules are malignant. Hoarseness, dyspepsia, and dysphagia may reflect local invasion to the larynx, trachea, or esophagus. A definitive diagnosis is achievable by biopsy.

## Kidney Cancer

The most common type of kidney cancer, renal carcinoma, occurs twice as frequently in men than in women. Renal carcinoma is the fifteenth most common cancer in the world and is most prevalent in developing countries.

Kidney cancer has consistently been found to be more common in cigarette smokers than in nonsmokers. An increased risk has been linked to obesity, especially in women. Leather tanners, shoe workers, and dry cleaning employees have an increased risk, as do workers exposed to asbestos.

# Prevention ✚PLUS!

### The ABCDs of Cancer

Perform skin examination regularly, and check for the ABCDs:

- A is for asymmetry; one-half of the mole does not match the other half.
- B is for border irregularity.
- C is for color; the pigmentation of the cancer is not uniform.
- D is for diameter greater than 6 millimeters, or approximately two-thirds of an inch.

Kidney cancer commonly causes no obvious symptoms in its early stages. Advanced disease symptoms include hematuria, flank pain, and a palpable kidney mass. Systemic symptoms of renal carcinoma result from overproduction of normal kidney proteins and hormones that cause hypertension, fevers, anemia, **erythrocytosis** (elevated number of red blood cells), abnormal liver function, and hypercalcemia (abnormally high calcium levels).

Urine tests are used as a screening tool to confirm the presence of blood cells in the urine. An intravenous pyelogram (IVP) is an x-ray in which a special dye is injected into a vein and x-ray pictures are taken as the dye passes through the kidneys. Ultrasound and CT scans are useful for evaluating the size, location, and spread of disease.

Surgery is the mainstay treatment for cancer of the kidney. Surgery can be curative for early disease and may help prevent further spread of disease when the disease has advanced. Renal cell carcinoma is responsive to treatments with immune modifiers such as interferon and interleukin-2 in combination with chemotherapy.

## Cancers of the Nervous System

The majority of adult tumors of the central nervous system are derived from **glial** cells, which are support cells in the nervous system. These cancers are rare and account for less than 2% of all malignancies worldwide. Brain tumors have two peaks of incidence. The first is in childhood, with a peak between three and twelve years of age. The second group is older adults, with a peak between 60 and 70 years of age.

Some brain tumors are associated with inherited cancer syndromes. The brain is also a frequent site of metastases from primary tumors that occur elsewhere in the body. Childhood brain tumors are thought to result from defects in cell cycle control mechanisms originating from fetal development. Rare cases of brain tumors are caused by therapeutic radiation. Children who have received preventative brain radiation for acute leukemia seem to have an increased risk of developing malignant gliomas.

The signs and symptoms largely depend on the location of the neoplasm and may include **paresis** or a slight paralysis, speech disturbances, and personality changes. Some patients have long histories of epileptic seizures. Large tumors can cause life-threatening pressures to build up in the central nervous system that may lead to unconsciousness and respiratory arrest. Headaches occur when the tumor infiltrates the **meninges** or membranes covering the brain.

CT scans of the brain will often show the position of a tumor, whether it is causing swelling around the brain, and whether it is blocking the flow of the cerebrospinal fluid. The MRI scan may provide additional information tumor location, size, and spread. An **EEG** or electrical brain activity recording device is useful for identifying seizure activity. If possible, a brain biopsy will provide a definitive diagnosis of the tumor type.

Surgical removal of the tumor usually involves a **craniotomy,** in which a flap of bone is temporarily removed. In some circumstances, the tumor may be surgically removed by use of a laser. Dexamthasome is a steroid medication that is very helpful in reducing swelling around brain tumors. Radiation therapy is often applied to the specific areas of the brain that are affected.

## Pediatric Cancer

Although uncommon, childhood cancer is the second leading cause of death in children. An estimated 10,400 new cases are expected to occur among children in the United States, aged 0 to 14 years, in 2007. The majority of childhood cancers are leukemia.

Like many adult forms of cancer, symptoms of early disease in children are often mistaken for less serious conditions. Common general symptoms include loss of energy, pallor, easy bruising, persistent pain, prolonged fever, frequent headaches, profuse vomiting, sudden changes in vision, and weight loss. See Table 4–5 ▶.

Childhood forms of cancer are treated by a combination of therapies, surgery, radiation, and chemotherapy. The number of treatment cycles as well as the agents used depends on the type and stage of cancer. Long-term survival from childhood cancer has improved, though many patients experience cancer treatment effects. Late effects of pediatric cancer treatment

## Table 4-5 ► Childhood Cancers

| Childhood Cancer | Childhood Cancer (%) | Disease Description | Disease Signs and Symptoms |
|---|---|---|---|
| Leukemia | 30 | Proliferation of abnormal white blood cells | Severe anemia, hemorrhages, slight enlargement of the lymph nodes or the spleen. Weakness, bone and joint pain, bleeding, and fever. |
| Brain, nervous system | 22.3 | Mostly medulloblastoma, which are undifferentiated primitive cells that appear on the cerebellum, brainstem, and spinal cord | Headache, nausea, vomiting, blurred or double vision, dizziness, and difficulty handling objects. |
| Neuroblastoma | 7.3 | Cancer of the sympathetic nervous system; consists of immature embryonic-like cells | Occurs most frequently in the mediastianal and retroperitoneal abdomen. Recognized by a lump or swelling on the abdomen. |
| Wilms' tumor | 5.6 | Malignant renal tumor that is composed of small spindle cells and cells that resemble embryonic glomerulii; often inherited as an autosomal dominant trait | May occur in one or both kidneys. Symptoms include swelling or palpable mass in the flank as well as moderate to severe pain. |
| Non-Hodgkin's lymphoma | 4.5 | Affects the lymph nodes but may spread to the bone marrow and other organs | May cause swelling of the lymph nodes of the neck, armpit, and groin. Fever and weakness may also be present. |
| Hodgkin's lymphoma | 3.5 | Cancer of the lymphoid tissue. Distinguished from non-Hodgkin's lymphoma by the presence of Reed-Sternberg cells. | Painless enlargement of the lymph nodes, spleen, or other immune tissue, fever, fatigue, night sweats |
| Rhabdomyosarcoma | 3.1 | A soft tissue sarcoma or tumor of red muscle. Occurs in the head, neck, genitourinary area, trunk, and extremities | Symptoms depend on the location of the tumor. The most common problem is pain in the area of the tumor. |
| Retinoblastoma | 2.8 | Eye cancer that occurs in children under the age of 4. May be familial form that is caused by autosomal dominant mutation of the retinoblastoma gene, which is a tumor suppressor gene | In familial cases the disease is usually bilateral, with multiple lesions within the eye. |
| Osteosarcoma | 2.4 | Occurs on the surface of bone and usually presents in adolescents | Most frequent site of occurence is in the long bones of the lower limbs. Osteosarcomas are associated with pain, tenderness, and inflammation to affected limb(s). Symptoms become persistent and worse with pain occuring at rest. |
| Ewing sarcoma | 1.4 | Develops prior to age 20 and occurs twice as frequently in males. Involves bone mostly in the extremities | Bone cancer often has no initial pain or symptoms. Advanced disease is associated with severe pain. |

Adapted from *Cancer Facts and Figures*, American Cancer Society, 2007.

include organ damage and malfunction, secondary cancers, and cognitive impairments.

## Cancer and Aging

More than 60% of all cancers in the United States occur in adults over the age of 65. With the expansion of the aging population, especially in the United States, the number of cancer survivors over the age of 65 is likely to continue to increase. Coupled with this cancer health risk, older adults are often living with chronic diseases of older adulthood and are likely to have concomitant health problems. These coexisting health conditions often affect prognosis and treatment outcomes in older adults.

The most common cancers of older adulthood are prostate, breast, colon, panaceas, bladder, stomach, and lung. Chronic illnesses that often accompany aging, such as heart problems, vision loss, decline in memory, hearing difficulties, decreased kidney function, and weight loss, may interfere with the older adult's ability to handle a stressful illness like cancer.

Cancer treatment in older adults is the same as in young and middle adults. The goals of cancer treatment in persons of all ages include curing the primary tumor, allowing the patient to live longer with good quality of life, reducing cancer symptoms, and maintaining functions of daily living. In older adulthood, unlike other stages in life, the availability of a caretaker to assist with the effects of treatment may be lacking. Often assistance is sought from children, extended family, and friends. Caregivers, along with the patient, experience emotional distress from the stress of cancer treatment and the inability to maintain a "normal" routine. Like their younger counterparts, older adults respond to cancer treatment, and with continued support can lead a fulfilling life.

## ▶ Cancer Screening, Early Diagnosis, and Prevention

**Cancer screening** refers to early testing in individuals with risk factors for cancer. For example, the Pap test is recommended for all females who have been sexually active, and a rectal examination is recommended in all males over the age of 50. The ideal screening test is one that can detect cancer in at an early stage. See Table 4–6▶.

**Early diagnosis** is the detection of cancer at an early stage. Early detection can occur as a result of appropriate screening test or through public education on warning signs of cancer. Early diagnosis, like screening, is especially important if the treatment of early forms of cancer produces better survival and treatment outcomes. See Box 4–1▶ for nonspecific warning signs of cancer.

**Prevention** of cancer can be achieved by removing known causes of cancer. For many, cancer prevention involves a lifestyle change or a change in behavior that is known to increase cancer risks.

---

### Box 4–1 ▶ Nonspecific Warning Signs of Cancer

- Change in bowel or bladder habits
- A sore that does not heal
- Unusual bleeding or discharge
- Thickening or lump in the breast or any other part of the body
- Indigestion or difficulty swallowing
- An obvious change in a wart or mole
- A nagging cough or hoarseness

*Source:* American Cancer Society, 2007.

---

### RESOURCES

American Cancer Society: www.cancer.org

World Health Organization: www.who.org

Centers for Disease Control and Prevention, Atlanta: www.cdc.gov

National Cancer Institute: www.cancer.gov/cancerinfo

## Table 4–6 ▶ American Cancer Society Recommendations for Early Detection of Cancer in Asymptomatic People

| Site | Recommendation |
|------|----------------|
| Breast | Annual mammography for women over 40<br>Annual breast exam<br>Monthly self-breast examination |
| Colon and rectum | Beginning at age 50:<br><br>• Fecal occult blood test every year or<br>• Flexible sigmoidoscopy every 5 years or<br>• Annual fecal occult blood test and flexible sigmoidoscopy every 5 years<br>• A double contrast barium enema every 5 to 10 years<br>• A colonoscopy every 10 years<br>• Combined testing every 5 years is preferred over annual tests; people at moderate or high risk should talk with doctor about a different testing schedule |
| Prostate | Prostate-specific antigen test and digital rectal exam should be offered annually beginning at age 50; men at risk should start testing at age 45 |
| Uterus | Cervix: All women who are sexually active or who are 18 and older should have an annual Pap test and pelvic exam<br>Endometrium: all women should be informed about the risks and symptoms of endometrial cancer |
| Cancer-related checkup | A cancer-related check up is recommended every 3 years for people aged 20 to 39 years and every year for people 40 and older; exam should include health counseling and, depending on a person's age, examinations for cancers of the thyroid, oral cavity, skin, lymph nodes, testes, ovaries, as well as for some nonmalignant diseases |

Adapted from the American Cancer Society, 2007.

# Prevention ✚PLUS!

## Guidelines on Nutrition and Physical Activity for Cancer Prevention

Eat a variety of healthful foods, with an emphasis on plant sources:

• Eat five or more servings of vegetables and fruit each day.
• Choose whole grains in preference to processed (refined) grains and sugars.
• Limit consumption of red meats, especially high fat and process meats.
• Choose foods that help maintain a healthful weight.

Adopt a physically active lifestyle:

• Adults: Engage in at least moderate activity for 30 minutes or more on 5 or more days of the week; 45 minutes or more of moderate to rigorous activity on 5 or more days per week may further enhance reductions in the risk of breast and colon cancer.
• Children and adolescents: Engage in at least 60 minutes per day of moderate to vigorous physical activity at least 5 days per week.

Maintain a healthful weight throughout life:

• Balance caloric intake with physical activity.
• Lose weight if currently overweight or obese.

If you drink alcoholic beverages, limit consumption.

# DISEASES AT A GLANCE
## Cancer

| DISEASE | ETIOLOGY | SIGNS AND SYMPTOMS |
|---|---|---|
| Lung cancer | | |
| Non–small cell lung cancer | Cigarette smoke, radon, industrial asbestos | Cough, wheezing, stridor, dysphagia, blood in sputum, chest pain, loss of appetitite |
| Small cell lung cancer | Cigarette smoke | Cough, wheezing, stridor, dysphagia, blood in sputum, chest pain, loss of appetitite |
| Breast cancer | Age, female gender, genetics, overweight and obesity, postmenopausal hormone replacement therapy, physical inactivity, consumption of alcohol | Palpable lump on the breast, abnormality detected on a mammogram, thickening, swelling, distortion, and tenderness of the breast, spontaneous discharge or ulceration of the nipples |
| Stomach cancer | Diet, inadequate intake of fresh fruits and vegetables, consumption of smoked or cured meats and fish, infection with the bacterium *Helicobacter pylori* | Mild pain in the upper abdomen, fatigue, loss of energy, decreased appetitite |
| Colorectal cancer | High consumption of fat, refined carbohydrates, and animal protein and low physical activity, genetics, including familial adenomatous polyposis and hereditary nonpolyposis | Blood in stool, change in bowel habits, pain in the lower abdomen |
| Liver cancer | | |
| Hepatocellular carcinoma | Viral hepatitis B and hepatitis C infections, ingestion of toxins | Abdominal pain, weight loss, abdominal swelling, ascites, hepatomegaly, jaundice |
| Female reproductive tract | | |
| Cervical cancer | Human papilloma virus infections, high-risk sexual behavior, early age at initiation of sexual activity | Usually asymptomatic |

| DIAGNOSIS | TREATMENT | PREVENTION | LIFESPAN |
|---|---|---|---|
| | | | |
| Chest x-ray, sputum analysis, bronchoscopy with a biopsy, PET scan | Surgery, radiation therapy, chemotherapy | Good health, good hygiene, do not smoke | Incidence increases from age 40 to 70 years |
| Chest x-ray, sputum analysis, bronchoscopy with a biopsy, pet scan | Surgery, radiation therapy, chemotherapy | Good health, good hygiene, do not smoke | Incidence increases from age 40 to 70 years |
| Mammography, breast ultrasound, biopsy | Surgery (lumpectomy or mastectomy), radiation therapy, chemotherapy, hormone therapy | Regular breast cancer screening, good health with physical activity | Risk increases after the age of 40 years |
| CT scan, MRI scan, biopsy | Surgery, radiation therapy, and chemotherapy | Healthy eating with fresh fruits and vegetables, prompt treatment for infections caused by *Helicobacter pylori* | Incidence increases in person over the age of 60 years |
| Colonoscopy with biopsy | Surgery, radiation therapy, chemotherapy | Healthy eating, including consumption of fresh fruits and vegetables, limiting consumption of animal protein, genetic screening, regular screening examinations | Occurs more commonly in individuals aged 50 years and older |
| | | | |
| CT scan, ultrasound, biopsy | Surgery, radiation therapy, chemotherapy | Prompt treatment for viral infections, healthy eating | More common in adults, rarely occurs in childhood |
| | | | |
| Pap test, colposcopy with biopsy | Precancerous changes are treated with cryosurgery or lazer | Practice safe sex, use condoms to prevent infections | Second most common cancer in women; all women are at risk |

# DISEASES AT A GLANCE

## Cancer (*continued*)

| DISEASE | ETIOLOGY | SIGNS AND SYMPTOMS |
|---|---|---|
| Uterine cancer | Oral estrogen therapy, no history of pregnancy, removal of the ovaries, history of obesity, diabetes, or hypertension | Metrorrragia after menopause, dysuria, constipation, bloating |
| Ovarian | Family history, prior history of breast cancer, no history of pregnancy, polycystic ovary disease, pelvic inflammatory disease, endometriosis | Abdominal discomfort, bloating, abnormal vaginal bleeding, gastrointestinal or urinary symptoms |
| Male reproductive tract | | |
| Prostate | Diet high in saturated fat, age | Urinary symptoms, including hesitancy, frequency, dribbling, poor urine stream, blood in the urine, pain in the lower abdomen |
| Cancer of the testes | History of undescended testes (cryptorchidism), family history of testicular cancer, prenatal exposure to exogenous estrogen | Painless lump on the testicle |
| Esophageal cancer | Tobacco smoke, or chewing tobacco, consumption of alcohol, history of esphgitis | Difficulty swallowing, pain with eating or drinking, weight loss, hoarseness of the voice |
| Bladder cancer | Cigarette smoke, exposure to industrial chemicals such as rubber, aromatic hydrocarbons, asbestos, and solvents, infections with *Schistosoma haematobium* | Hematuria, increased urinary frequency |
| Head and neck cancer | Tobacco smoking and excessive alcohol consumption | Oral pain, bleeding, difficulty opening the mouth, chewing, swallowing and talking, pain in the neck |

| DIAGNOSIS | TREATMENT | PREVENTION | LIFESPAN |
|---|---|---|---|
| Endovaginal echography, hysteroscopy, biopsy | Abdominal hysterectomy, radiation therapy | Healthy lifestyle, regular cancer screening exams | Occurs most commonly in women of middle age or older, with a peak incidence around 50 to 60 years |
| Abdominal or vaginal ultrasound, biopsy | Surgery, including a total abdominal hysterectomy, removal of the ovaries, appendectomy, removal of the pelvic lymph nodes, and chemotherapy | Healthy lifestyle, treatment of polycystic ovary disease and pelvic inflammatory disease, regular cancer screening checkups, especially in individuals with a prior family history of ovarian cancer | All women are at risk |
| Digital examinate, PSA test, ultrasound, biopsy | Surgery, radiation therapy, endocrine therapy | PSA screening tests for all men over the age of 50 years, or 45 years for men at risk | Incidence and mortality increases with age; most cases occur in men age 65 years or older |
| Biopsy, physical examination of the testicles | Surgery, radiation therapy, chemotherapy | Self-examination of testicle, annual cancer screening exam, surgical treatment of cryptorchidism | Can occur at all ages, risk is greatest in men during the third or fourth decades of life |
| Biopsy, endoscopic ultrasound | Surgery, radiation therapy, chemotherapy | Do not smoke or chew tobacco, avoid excessive consumption of alcohol, treatment of reflux disease to prevent esophagitis | More common in individuals over the age of 60 years |
| Ultrasound, biopsy | Surgery, radiation therapy, and chemotherapy | Do not smoke tobacco, avoid exposure to industrial chemicals | Occurs more frequently in adults over the age of 65 years |
| Endoscopic examination, biopsy | Surgery, radiation therapy, chemotherapy | Do not smoke tobacco, limit consumption of alcohol | Occurs more commonly in males aged 65 years or older |

# DISEASES AT A GLANCE

## Cancer (*continued*)

| DISEASE | ETIOLOGY | SIGNS AND SYMPTOMS |
|---|---|---|
| Lymphoma | | |
| Hodgkin's disease | Infection with Epstein-Barr virus, human immunodeficiency virus | Painless swelling of the lymph nodes in the neck, armpit, or groin |
| Non-Hodgkin's lymphoma | HIV/AIDS viral infections with HTLV1 and EBV | Painless swelling of the lymph nodes in the neck, armpit, or groin |
| Leukemia | Unknown | Fatigue, weight loss, repeated infections, fever, easy bruising, nosebleeds, hemorrhages |
| Pancreatic cancer | Tobacco smoke, diet low in fiber, high in consumption of red meat | Weight loss, nausea, diarrhea, weakness, jaundice, and upper abdominal pain |
| Melanoma | Fair skin, sensitivity to sunlight, exposure to industrial chemicals | Appearance of a mole-like growth that increases in size and changes in color |
| Thyroid cancer | Exposure to radiation, iodine deficiency, radioactive iodine exposure | Palpable thyroid nodule, hoarseness, dyspepsia, dysphagia |
| Kidney cancer | | |
| Renal carcinoma | Cigarette smoking, obesity, greater risk among dry cleaning workers, leather tanner and shoe workers, exposure to asbestos | Hematuria, lower back pain, palpable kidney mass, hypertension, fever, anemia or erythrocytosis |
| Wilms' tumor | Unknown | Swelling, palpable mass, moderate to severe pain |

| DIAGNOSIS | TREATMENT | PREVENTION | LIFESPAN |
|---|---|---|---|
| Microscopic examination of lymph tissue, presence of Reed-Sternberg cells, x-ray, CT scan, MRI, bone marrow sampling, and lymphograms | Chemotherapy, radiation, bone marrow transplantation | Treatment of Epstein-Barr virus, safe sex practices to prevent infection with human immunodeficiency virus | Often occurs in young adults |
| Microscopic examination of lymph tissue, x-ray, CT scan, MRI, bone marrow sampling, and lymphograms | Chemotherapy, radiation, bone marrow transplantation | Safe sex to prevent infection with HIV | Often occurs in young adults |
| Blood tests, bone marrow biopsy | Chemotherapy, bone marrow transplantation | Unknown | Diagnosed 10 times more often in adults, also occurs in children |
| Ultrasound, CT scanning, biopsy | Surgery, chemotherapy | Do not smoke tobacco | Common in individuals older than 65 years of age |
| Skin examination, biopsy | Surgery, radiation therapy | Use of sunscreen, avoidance exposure to sunlight in susceptible individuals | Can occur at any age |
| Physical examination, biopsy | Surgery, radiation therapy, chemotherapy | Eat salt fortified with iodine, regular examinations following high radiation exposure | Can occur at any age |
| Urine test, intravenous pyelogram, ultrasound, CT scan, biopsy | Surgery, radiation therapy, chemotherapy, immune modifiers | To not smoke, cancer physical exams for high risk individuals | Renal carcinoma occurs primarily in adults; Wilms' tumor occurs primarily in children |
| Urine test, intravenous pyelogram, ultrasound, CT scan, biopsy | Surgery, radiation therapy, chemotherapy, immune modifiers | Unknown | Pediatric cancer occurs between the ages of birth and 14 years |

# DISEASES AT A GLANCE
## Cancer (*continued*)

| DISEASE | ETIOLOGY | SIGNS AND SYMPTOMS |
| --- | --- | --- |
| Cancer of the central nervous system | | |
| Malignant glioma | Radiation therapy, prior history of leukemia | Paresis, speech disturbance, seizures, headaches |
| Meduloblastoma | Defects in cell cycle control originating in fetal development | Headache, nausea, vomiting, blurred vision, dizziness, difficulty handling objects |
| Cancer of the sympathetic nervous system | | |
| Neuroblastoma | Unknown | Lump or swelling of the abdomen |
| Sarcoma | | |
| Rhabdomyosarcoma | Unknown | Tumor of red muscle, pain in the area of the tumor |
| Osteosarcoma | Unknown | Bone pain |
| Ewing sarcoma | Unknown | Bone pain commonly felt in the extremities |

| DIAGNOSIS | TREATMENT | PREVENTION | LIFESPAN |
|---|---|---|---|
| | | | |
| CT scan, MRI, EEG, biopsy | Surgery, radiation therapy, chemotherapy, corticosteroid medication | Unknown | Incidence peaks between ages 60 and 70 years of age |
| CT scan, MRI, EEG, biopsy | Surgery, radiation therapy, chemotherapy, corticosteroid medication | Unknown | Incidence peaks between 3 and 12 years of age |
| CT scan, biospy | Surgery, radiation therapy, chemotherapy | Unknown | Pediatric cancer occurs between the ages of birth and 14 years |
| | | | |
| CT scan, biopsy | Surgery, chemotherapy, radiation therapy | Unknown | Pediatric cancer occurs prior to the age of 20 years |
| CT scan, biopsy | Surgery, chemotherapy, radiation therapy | Unknown | Pediatric cancer occurs prior to the age of 20 years |
| CT scan, biopsy | Surgery, chemotherapy, radiation therapy | Unknown | Pediatric cancer occurs prior to the age of 20 years |

# Interactive Exercises

## Cases for Critical Thinking

1. A 45-year-old male presents to his physician's office with a persistent productive cough. He has recently missed a week of work due to fever, weakness, and hoarseness. What diagnostic procedures should be used to rule out lung cancer? What type of historical information is needed to diagnose lung cancer?

2. A 30-year-old female has recently noticed a lump in her breast. She has never been pregnant, and she has noticed a discharge from her left nipple. Describe some of the risk factors and diagnostic tests for breast cancer. What are the most definitive tests for the diagnosis of breast cancer?

## Multiple Choice

1. Which of the following does not control cell growth?
   a. growth inhibitors       b. cell cycle proteins
   c. mutation                d. apoptosis

2. _____ are(is) responsible for repairing errors in DNA replication.
   a. oncogenes
   b. tumor suppressor gene
   c. DNA repair genes
   d. apoptosis

3. _____ is(are) the major cause of lung cancer worldwide.
   a. tobacco
   b. industrial chemicals
   c. radiation
   d. chronic infections

4. Inherited mutations, including familial adenomatous polyposis and hereditary nonpolypois, are nonmodifiable risk factors for _____ cancer.
   a. lung        b. liver
   c. stomach     d. colorectal

5. Molecular and epidemiological studies have linked the human papilloma virus to _____ cancer.
   a. breast      b. cervical
   c. uterine     d. ovarian

6. The most important risk factor for the development of prostate cancer is _____.
   a. diet high in saturated fat
   b. age (greater than 65 years)
   c. hormones
   d. hypertrophy of the prostate

7. Malignant tumors in the testes originate from _____ cells.
   a. seminoma    b. epithelial
   c. squamous    d. germ

8. The most important risk factor for bladder cancer is _____.
   a. human papillomavirus
   b. infection
   c. cigarette smoking
   d. exposure to environmental chemicals

9. Hodgkin's disease is distinguished from non-Hodgkins lymphoma by the presence of _____ cells.
   a. squamous      b. Reed-Sternberg
   c. epithelial    d. lymphoid

10. Leukemia is diagnosed _____ times more often in children than in adults.
    a. 2       b. 4
    c. 8       d. 10

## True or False

_____ 1. Lymphoma is characterized by massive proliferation of white blood cells in plasma.

_____ 2. The diagnosis of pancreatic cancer is rarely made during early stages of the disease.

_____ 3. Risk factors for the development of melanoma include sensitivity to sunlight, extent of sun exposure, and exposure to industrial chemicals.

_____ 4. Kidney cancer is more common in cigarette smokers than in nonsmokers.

_____ 5. Wilms' tumor is a malignant tumor that occurs in childhood.

_____ 6. Neuroblastoma is a central nervous system tumor.

_____ 7. Cancer is primarily a genetic disease.

_____ 8. A mutation is an inherited form of a normal gene.

_____ 9. Oncogenes normally regulate cell growth, differentiation, and cell death.

_____ 10. Exposure to asbestos increases the risk for mesothelioma.

## Fill-Ins

1. _____ is the most significant source of ultraviolet radiation.

2. Chronic infections with _____ and _____ viral infections have been linked to liver cancer.

3. Solid tumors can often be removed with _____.

4. The infectious bacterium _____ is a risk factor for stomach cancer.

5. _____ carcinoma accounts for more than 80% of all primary cancers in the liver.

6. Precancerous lesions on the cervix can be readily detected by the _____ test.

7. Neoplasms of lymphoid tissue are referred to as _____ .

8. A melanoma is a proliferation of _____ or pigment-producing cells.

9. Iodine deficiency is a risk factor for _____ cancer.

10. The majority of adult tumors in the central nervous system are derived from _____ cells.

## Labeling Exercise

Use the blank lines below to label the following photos.

1. _____

2. _____

3. _____

4. _____

# Multimedia Preview

Additional interactive resources and activities for this chapter can be found on the Companion Website. For videos, audio glossary, and review, access the accompanying DVD-ROM in this book.

## ▶ DVD-ROM Highlights

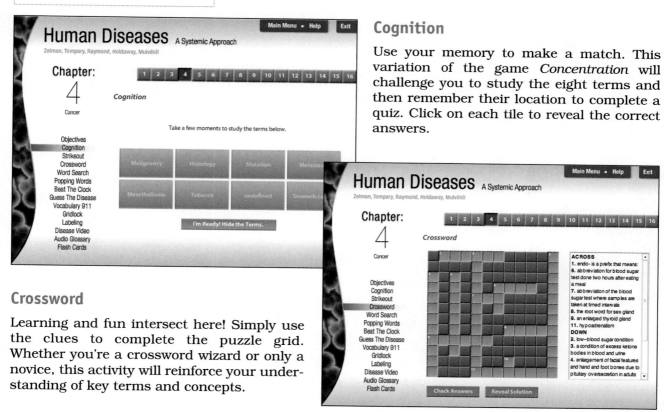

### Cognition

Use your memory to make a match. This variation of the game *Concentration* will challenge you to study the eight terms and then remember their location to complete a quiz. Click on each tile to reveal the correct answers.

### Crossword

Learning and fun intersect here! Simply use the clues to complete the puzzle grid. Whether you're a crossword wizard or only a novice, this activity will reinforce your understanding of key terms and concepts.

## ▶ Website Highlights—www.pearsonhighered.com/zelman

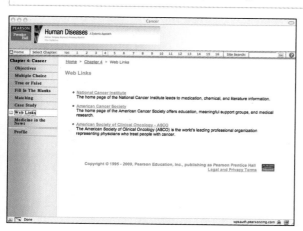

### Web Links

Take advantage of the free-access online study guide that accompanies your textbook. This online activity challenges you to visit selected web links where you can explore important issues to reinforce your understanding. By clicking on this URL you'll also access links to current news articles and an audio glossary.

# Heredity and Disease

CHAPTER

# 5

## Learning Objectives

After studying this chapter, you should be able to

- Describe DNA's unique composition and its role in heredity
- Describe mechanisms of transmission of hereditary diseases and give examples
- Explain genetic diseases based on abnormal chromosome construction
- Describe genetic diseases involving anomalies and numbers in the sex chromosomes
- Compare and contrast congenital diseases and hereditary disorders
- Discuss the concept of gene therapy

## Fact or Fiction?

Familial hypercholesterolemia, a disorder in which a person has very high blood cholesterol, can be inherited.

*Fact: Five types of hypercholesterolemia are known and all can be inherited; a common form is an autosomal dominant disorder.*

# Disease Chronicle

## Then and Now: Marfan Syndrome

Some say that President Abraham Lincoln had a hereditary disease called Marfan syndrome, which today affects 1 in 10,000 people. President Lincoln exhibited key traits associated with Marfan, including a tall stature with a slender skeleton, long fingers, and a long, narrow face. Marfan also causes an abnormally shaped chest, loose joints, and weak ligaments, which results in curvature of the spine. Weakened connective tissue in the walls of large arteries leads to aortic aneurysms. With aging, or in demanding situations, the heart and other organs fail.

In 1986, Flo Hyman, captain of the 1984 U.S. Olympic Volleyball team died of a ruptured aorta during a match in Japan at age 31; at age 29, Sergei Grinkov, an Olympic skating champion died in a similar fashion in 1995. Ronalda Pierce, a 6 foot, 5-inch basketball player for Florida State University apparently died of Marfan syndrome at age 19 in 2004. In 2007, Guy Ntang, a recruit basketball player for Wichita State University, died suddenly at age 19 in a pick-up basketball game. Could this genetic disease forecast a premature fate for some tall, lean athletes especially during strenuous activities?

# ▶ Introduction

**DNA**, which stands for **deoxyribonucleic acid**, is the blueprint for directing all cell activities and especially protein synthesis within the cell. DNA is a double helix similar in shape to a spiral staircase. It is made of four chemical bases, pairs of which form the "rungs" of the DNA molecule. All **genes** are made from segments of these four bases, arranged in different orders and in different lengths (Figure 5–1 ▶).

Within the nucleus of cells, the DNA is assembled into stranded units called **chromosomes**, which must be copied during cell division and distributed to the resulting daughter cells. DNA has the unique ability to replicate itself and code for its partner RNA (ribonucleic acid). The coordination of these two allies will direct the program for hereditary and metabolic activities. Within each primary sex organ (ovary or testis),"parent" sex cells contain 46 chromosomes and divide by a process called meiosis (Figure 5–2 ▶) to produce gametes (egg and sperm) that contain 23 chromosomes each. Egg and sperm unite during fertilization; therefore, each human cell contains 46 chromosomes in 23 pairs.

The chromosomes contain thousands of genes, each of which is responsible for the synthesis of a particular protein, an RNA molecule or DNA molecule. Forty-four of the chromosomes are called **autosomes**, and two are called the X and Y (or sex) chromosomes. A male has a combination of one X and one Y chromosome, and a female has two X chromosomes. The complete chromosomal composition of the nucleus is called the **karyotype** of the cell. The karyotype can be visualized by extracting the chromosomes from the nucleus and photographing them under a microscope. In this way, abnormalities in number or structure of the chromosomes can be detected (Figure 5–3 ▶).

In 1990, the U.S. Human Genome Project (HGP) began a 13-year effort coordinated by the U.S. Department of Energy and the National Institutes of Health. Project goals were to identify all of the approximate 30,000 genes in human DNA, determine the sequences of the 3 billion chemical base pairs that make up human DNA, and store this information in databases.

**Trillions of cells**

Each cell:
• 46 human chromosomes
• 2 meters of DNA
• 3 billion DNA subunits (the bases: A, T, C, G)
• 25,000 genes code for proteins that perform all life functions

DNA the molecule of life

Cell

Chromosomes

Protein

DNA

Gene

**Figure 5–1** ▶ Each cell nucleus throughout the body contains the genes, DNA, and chromosomes that make up the majority of an individual's genome.

The full DNA sequence was completed and published in April 2003. Upon publication of the majority of the genome in February 2001, Francis Collins, the director of the National Human Genome Research Institute, noted that the genome could be thought of in terms of a book with multiple uses. "It's a history book—a

**(3) Meiosis II**

**(2) Meiosis I**

**(1) Interphase**

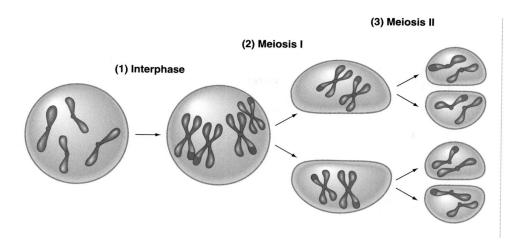

Figure 5–2 ▶ Meiosis involves two complete divisional operations forming four potential sex cells.

narrative of the journey of our species through time. It's a shop manual, with an incredibly detailed blueprint for building every human cell. And it's a transformative textbook of medicine, with insights that will give health-care providers immense new powers to treat, prevent, and cure diseases." Genes, chromosomes, and other causes for selected hereditary diseases have been located and are listed in the Diseases at a Glance table at the end of the chapter; a complete list can be found at www.ncbi.nlm.nih.gov.

The genes for a particular trait, such as eye color, hair color, and hair type, occupy a particular site on a chromosome. Each person has two sites or two copies of each gene, one copy from each parent. **Alleles** are alternative forms of a gene. If the pair of alleles is similar (hh, HH), the person is **homozygous** for that trait. If the alleles are different (Hh), one for dark and one for light hair, for example, the person is **heterozygous**. Some alleles always produce their trait when inherited and are said to be **dominant**. The result of the dominant allele is the same whether a person is homozygous or heterozygous. The allele for brown eyes, for example, is dominant to that for blue eyes. Other alleles are **recessive** and only manifest themselves when the person is homozygous for the trait. This combination is significant in many hereditary diseases.

Certain factors may cause a deviation from the basic principles of inheritance that have been described. Some alleles are codominant, so that when both are inherited, both traits are expressed. An example of codominant alleles is found in blood type AB. The allele for the A factor is inherited from one parent and that for the B factor from the other, but both alleles are expressed. At times, a dominant allele is not fully expressed, a condition known as *reduced penetrance*. Various factors modify the expression of genes, including other genes, environmental conditions, and gender. One example of a reduced penetrance trait is syndactyly, which results in varying degrees of webbing in fingers or

Figure 5–3 ▶ Human karyotype. (© Custom Medical Stock Photo)

toes. Polydactyly is another dominant trait that will be described later in the chapter.

## ▶ Transmission of Hereditary Diseases

Many of the diseases described throughout this book are called *hereditary* or *familial diseases.* Hereditary diseases or disorders are generally the result of metabolic breakdown caused by a lack of direction from a missing or compromised gene or chromosomal segment. Often the gene responsible for the production of a particular protein (e.g., enzyme or structural type) is missing or defective, and that interrupts the chain of events required to ensure proper metabolic activities. For example, hemochromatosis is rated as the most common genetic disorder in the United States, occurring in 1 in 200 to 400 people. This defect is a recessive trait and stems from the body's unusual ability to absorb extra iron.

Further explanation of the mechanism of transmission will now be explored. Some diseases are caused by inheriting a single autosomal dominant allele. One such defective gene causes Huntington's chorea, a disease described in Chapter 13, and another causes polydactyly, explained in the next section. Other diseases are caused by inherited autosomal recessive alleles. In this case, expression of the disease occurs only when that particular allele is inherited from each parent, making the person homozygous for that trait. Cystic fibrosis, described in Chapter 8, is such a disease. A third type of inheritance is sex-linked, in which the defective allele is located on the X chromosome. Red-green color blindness and hemophilia are examples of sex-linked inherited diseases and are explained later in this chapter.

### Autosomal Dominant

A defective dominant allele is usually transmitted from a parent who is heterozygous for the trait. If the other parent is normal for the particular condition, each child has a 50% chance of being affected and manifesting the genetic defect. This is illustrated in Figure 5–4▶. The disease appears in every generation, with males

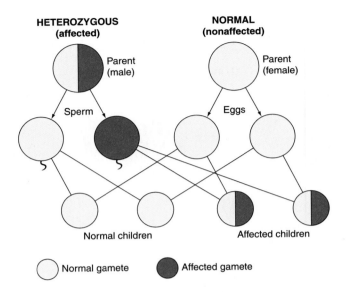

**Figure 5–4** ▶ Transmission of autosomal dominant disorders (50% chance for an affected child).

and females being equally affected. Exceptions to the rule are few.

**Polydactyly,** extra fingers or toes, is an example of an autosomal dominant disorder or it may occur on its own. A boy or girl inheriting the defective allele from either parent will have the abnormality. Polydactyly is apparent at birth but is not a major disorder and may be surgically corrected; however, it may occur in conjunction with other genetic disorders.

**Achondroplasia** is another disorder resulting from one defective dominant allele (Figure 5–5▶). In this disease, cartilage formation in the fetus is abnormal. Normally, the fetal skeleton first forms as cartilage and is gradually replaced by bone in a process known as ossification. In achondroplasia, the defective cartilage formation results in improper bone development and **achondroplastic dwarfism.** The long bones of the arms and legs are short, the trunk of the body is normal in size, the head is large, and the forehead is very prominent. The person has normal intelligence, develops sexually, and is muscular and agile.

**Marfan syndrome** results from the dysfunction of the gene that normally codes for the connective tissue protein fibrillin. Fibrillin is essential

Figure 5–5 ► A 12-year-old achondroplastic dwarf. (Note the disproportion of the limbs to the trunk, the curvature of the spine, and the prominent buttocks.)

for the maintenance of connective tissue in various organs, including tendons, heart valves, and blood vessels. Tendons and blood vessel walls with abnormal connective tissue become loose and cannot support normal body functions. Because connective tissue is widespread in the body, Marfan syndrome is a multisystemic disease affecting about 1 in 10,000 people. Blood exams support the diagnosis, by finding a lack of fibrillin. This protein deficiency causes skeletal changes, dilatation of the aorta, floppy heart valves, and ocular changes, including lens displacement, retinal detachment, and blindness.

Because there is no cure for Marfan syndrome, treatment is supportive. Annual visual exams plus echocardiograms (EKGs), and heart valve or vessel replacement are standard procedure. Usually the disease onset is by age 20,

and death is most often caused by heart failure or ruptured aortic aneurysm (vessel weakness).

**Familial hypercholesterolemia (FH)** affects 1 in 500 Americans and is a common cause of cardiovascular disease in this country. Frequently, familial hypercholesterolemia is caused by a mutation in the gene encoding the receptor for low-density lipoprotein (LDL). Blood screening confirms the increase of LDLs, which transport approximately 70% of the total blood cholesterol and are the principal carriers for the removal of cholesterol from the blood. The receptor deficiency in patients with familial hypercholesterolemia causes LDL cholesterol to be removed by a less efficient receptor-independent mechanism. Inefficient cholesterol removal results in hypercholesterolemia and the deposition of lipids in the arteries. This inefficiency results in accelerated atherosclerosis (plaque buildup) and increased incidence of coronary heart disease. In this case, the progression of familial hypercholesterolemia can be slowed by exercise, a low-fat diet, and drugs (statins) that block uptake of cholesterol in blood vessels.

Because this disease is actually caused by an **incomplete dominant** gene activity, it results in different outcomes. If the genes are both mutated in favor of hypercholesterol, then the person succumbs as a child. If one gene is normal and one mutated (heterozygous), then death would occur as a young adult.

## Autosomal Recessive

Autosomal recessive diseases manifest themselves only when a person is homozygous for the defective allele. Two parents who are both carriers of the recessive allele are themselves heterozygous for the trait but do not have the disease. Each of their children has a 25% chance of inheriting two recessive alleles and the disease. This potential probability is shown in Figure 5–6►. The chance for inheriting two recessive alleles increases in close intermarriage. Cystic fibrosis is an autosomal recessive disease affecting the respiratory and digestive systems and is discussed in Chapter 9.

**Phenylketonuria (PKU)** is an inborn error of metabolism caused by an autosomal recessive allele. Persons with PKU lack a specific enzyme

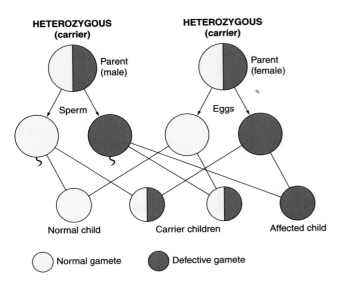

Figure 5–6 ▶ Transmission of recessive disorders (25% chance for an affected child).

that converts one amino acid, phenylalanine, to another, tyrosine. This mechanism is illustrated in Figure 5–7 ▶. As a result, high levels of phenylalanine and its derivatives build up in the blood and are toxic to the brain, interfering with normal brain development. PKU must be diagnosed

Figure 5–7 ▶ Enzyme block in phenylketonuria (PKU).

and treated very early or severe mental retardation results. Physical development proceeds normally, but the child is very light in color, somewhat similar to albinism. Production of the pigment melanin is impeded because of inadequate tyrosine, a result of the missing enzyme. The child may manifest disorders of the nervous system, such as a lack of balance, tremors, and hyperactivity, and may suffer convulsions. PKU frequency varies widely around the globe, but in the United States it occurs in about 1 in 10,000 people.

To prevent the serious mental retardation that accompanies PKU, newborn babies are screened by heel stick or Guthrie test for the defective gene or metabolic pathway. When the trait is found, a synthetic diet, such as Lofenalac, is prescribed that greatly reduces or eliminates phenylalanine. Good results have been achieved with this treatment. However, the diet is unpleasant, and controversy exists as to the length of time the diet must be maintained. Beginning treatment immediately and continuing during the earliest years of life seems to be the most critical factor in preventing mental retardation. Some soft drink and food labels alert consumers to the presence or lack of phenylalanine.

**Galactosemia** is another example of an inborn error of metabolism resulting from autosomal recessive inheritance. The person with this disease lacks the enzyme necessary to convert galactose, a sugar derived from lactose in milk, to glucose. Galactose accumulates in the blood and interferes with development of the brain, liver, and eyes. If untreated, mental retardation develops. The liver becomes enlarged and cirrhotic, and ascites fluid (see Chapter 9) accumulates in the abdominal cavity. Intestinal distress results in vomiting and diarrhea. Early diagnosis and treatment of galactosemia can prevent these problems, allowing development to proceed normally. Treatment consists of eliminating lactose from the diet or taking supplements like Lactaid to assist digestion and reduce symptoms. The occurrence is about 1 in 30,000 for the general population, and about 1 in 60,000 for Caucasians.

**Sickle cell anemia** is a severe anemia generally confined to the black population, who carry the sickle cell trait at a ratio of 1 per 12. Sickle cell anemia is an autosomal recessive disorder in which the hemoglobin (a protein molecule) is abnormal, resulting in deformed red blood cells. The improperly formed cells may become lodged in capillaries and block circulation, causing infarcts, pain, and necrosis (death of tissues). The sickle-shaped red blood cells rupture easily, and they are primarily removed from the circulation by the spleen. The depletion of red blood cells results in severe anemia.

The person with sickle cell anemia is homozygous, having inherited one altered allele from each parent. A person who is heterozygous has both normal and abnormal hemoglobin and possesses the **sickle cell trait**. The heterozygous person is mildly anemic, but the one defective allele provides an advantage because sickle cell trait confers increased resistance to malaria, which kills about 2 million persons per year, many of whom are children. See Chapter 7 for more information on this disease.

**Tay-Sachs** is an autosomal recessive condition that primarily affects families of Eastern Jewish origin; occurrence is approximately 1 in 3600 of the affected Ashkenazi (Jewish) community. Tay-Sachs is caused by the absence of the enzyme Hexosaminodase A (Hex-A). Without Hex-A, a lipid called GM2 ganglioside accumulates in cells, especially nerve cells of the brain. The result is progressive mental retardation and physical regression. Symptoms appear by 6 months of age when no new skills are learned, convulsions occur, and blindness develops. A cherry-red spot may be seen on each retina. Children usually die between 2 and 4 years of age. No cure exists, and treatment is aimed at relieving symptoms. Prevention may require genetic counseling and testing.

There are two tests available to determine if someone is a carrier of Tay-Sachs. The initial test uses an enzyme assay to measure the level of Hex-A in blood: a lower Hex-A quantity would indicate a carrier status, as carriers have less Hex-A than noncarriers. Next, a DNA-based carrier test looks for specific mutations in the gene that codes for Hex-A. Some carriers may not be identified by DNA analysis alone because not all known mutations in the Hex-A gene are detected by the test. Other mutations responsible for the disease have yet to be identified.

**Albinism** is an autosomal recessive disorder that is easily recognized. The skin and hair color are very white and do not darken with age. People with albinism have an increased risk for skin cancer and exhibit visual problems such as nearsightedness and abnormally high sensitivity to light. Even on cloudy days or overcast days, albinos may wear sunglasses, wide-brimmed hats, and full-length clothing or use umbrellas to reduce exposure. The occurrence for albinism is rare in the general population, but estimates as high as 1 out of 200 occur among the Hopi Indians of the American Southwest.

## Sex-Linked Inheritance

Diseases of sex-linked inheritance generally result from defective genes on the X chromosome, because the Y chromosome is small and carries very few genes. Because a male has only one X chromosome, if he inherits a defective recessive gene found on the X chromosome, that trait is expressed. A female may be heterozygous for the gene, having a defective recessive allele on one X chromosome but a normal allele on the other X. In that case, the female carries the disease, and she has a 50% chance of transmitting the allele to her sons and daughters. A male transmits the disease only to his daughters. His sons are unaffected, because the Y chromosome is normal and fathers contribute only the Y chromosome to males. This linkage is illustrated in Figure 5–8 ▶. Thus, the abnormalities of **sex-linked inheritance** tend to occur more frequently in males, but are transmitted by females. It is far less common for a female to inherit a sex-linked disease because she must inherit two defective X chromosomes. Duchenne's muscular dystrophy is an X-linked recessive disease that is discussed in Chapter 15.

*Color Blindness* Red-green color blindness, the inability to distinguish between certain colors, is a disorder of sex-linked inheritance. The defect that causes color blindness is apparently in certain specialized receptors of the retina called *cones*. Three types of receptors are stimulated by wavelengths of the primary colors: red, green, and blue. Impulses are then sent to the brain and interpreted. Diagnosis is made when the color-blind person is most frequently unable to

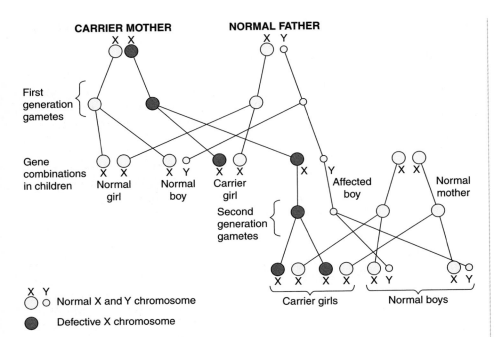

**Figure 5–8** ► Transmission of sex-linked disorders.

distinguish reds and greens. Corrective lenses are available that may offer some treatment for red-green color blindness. This condition is rare in women but occurs in about 1 out of 10 men.

*Hemophilia* People with hemophilia do not bleed more profusely or bleed faster than normal; they bleed for a longer period of time. Factor VIII, an intrinsic clotting factor, is usually inactive in cases of hemophilia. Diagnosis results from suspected bleeding episodes or family history. Beyond treatment with clotting factors (VIII) and blood transfusions, there have been significant advances in treating hemophilia in the last decade. A new genetically engineered clotting protein is now used for treatment of some types of hemophilia. Research is also underway to develop gene therapy for the disease. The therapy will replace the missing or deficient gene with one that has the instructions for producing the clotting factor. Gene therapy has been successful in treating mice with hemophilia B, and a procedure for it will be described near the end of this chapter.

*Fragile X Syndrome* **Fragile X syndrome** is a genetic condition associated with mental retardation. It is identified by thin, thread-like strands on the long arm of the X chromosome. This weakened area is more subject to breakage (thus the term *fragile* is used), and because this abnormality is associated with a sex chromosome, it is referred to as X-linked. Mothers are the carriers and their sons are at risk of being affected, whereas daughters are at risk of being carriers and sometimes are mildly affected. The prevalence of fragile X is approximately 1 in 1250 males (1 out of 2500 females), and the prevalence of carriers in the population is 1 in 600. Fragile X is the most commonly inherited cause of mental retardation known, accounting for up to 10% of the cases. Fragile X is diagnosed by DNA testing, and the gene responsible for fragile X has been identified as (FMR-1) for fragile X mental retardation gene.

About 80% of boys with fragile X have mental impairment ranging from severe retardation to low-normal intelligence. The majority of patients are mildly to moderately retarded. Men and boys with fragile X are usually socially engaging, but they have an unusual style of interacting. They tend to avoid direct eye contact during conversation, and hand-flapping or hand-biting is common. They may have an unusual speech pattern characterized by a fast and fluctuating rate of repetitions of sound, words, or phrases. They also may have a decreased attention span, hyperactivity, and motor delays. Girls are much less affected because they have two X chromosomes, and estimates are that about 30% with the condition have some degree of mental retardation. The physical features, including a long, narrow face and protruding ears, are much more subtle in females.

There is no cure for fragile X syndrome, but medical intervention can improve the problems related to attention and hyperactivity. A variety of medications can treat attention span, hyperactivity, and other behavior problems. In addition, speech and physical therapy as well as vocational training can be beneficial.

*Familial Diseases* Some diseases appear in families, but the means of inheritance is not understood. Examples of diseases with a higher incidence in certain families are epilepsy, diabetes, cardiovascular problems, allergies, and familial polyposis. The cause of these diseases does not seem to be a single gene but the effect of several genes working together, known as a **multifactorial** trait. In fact, some familial diseases may not be inherited at all but instead result from unique environmental conditions or behaviors that are shared by family members.

## ▶ Abnormal Chromosome Diseases

The hereditary diseases described to this point result from a defective gene. Abnormalities in the chromosomes, either in their number or structure, also cause disorders. At times, chromosomes fail to separate properly during cell division, causing one daughter cell to be deficient and one to have an extra chromosome. The loss of an autosomal chromosome is usually incompatible with life because each autosome contains a large number of essential genes. A fetus affected by this condition is generally spontaneously aborted. The loss of a sex chromosome or the presence of an extra one is

less serious, but many abnormalities accompany the condition.

### Down Syndrome

**Down syndrome** is an example of a disorder caused by the presence of an extra autosomal chromosome. Chromosome 21 is inherited in triplicate, a condition called **trisomy 21**. The extra chromosome results from a **nondisjunction**, or the failure of two chromosomes to separate as the gametes, either the egg or the sperm, are being formed. Therefore, when an egg or sperm with a double chromosome 21 is fused with its counterpart at the time of fertilization, a trisomy chromosome is formed. The incidence of Down syndrome is about 1 out of 800 and is higher among children born to mothers over age 35.

The Down syndrome child has a characteristic appearance (Figure 5–9 ▶). The eyes appear slanted because of an extra fold of skin at the upper, medial corner of the eye; the tongue is coarse and often protrudes; and the nose is short and flat. The child is usually of short

Figure 5–9 ▶ Boy with Down syndrome.

stature, and the sex organs are underdeveloped. A straight crease extends across the palm of the hand, and the little finger is often shorter than normal.

The life expectancy of a child with Down syndrome is relatively short because of complications that accompany the condition, such as congenital heart disease. In addition, there is a greater susceptibility to respiratory tract infections, including pneumonia, and a higher incidence of leukemia among those with Down syndrome.

The Down syndrome child is always mentally retarded to some degree. The excessive enzyme production from the extra genes may cause a toxic effect on the brain. The child can be taught simple tasks and is generally very affectionate. Today, compared to in years past, the Down syndrome individual may receive more exposure to special education and cooperative work opportunities.

## Cri Du Chat Syndrome

**Cri du chat syndrome**, or cat cry syndrome, is caused by a deletion of part of the short arm of chromosome 5. The occurrence for this trait is 1 out of 20,000 to 1 out of 50,000. Infants with cri du chat syndrome have an abnormally small head with a deficiency in cerebral brain tissue. Those who are born alive have a weak, catlike cry. The eyes are spaced far apart, and children with cri du chat syndrome exhibit mental retardation. Treatment is supportive until the infant dies, usually in the first 5 or 6 years. Parents may seek genetic counseling and request a karyotype test to determine if one or both parents have a rearranged chromosome 5.

## ▶ Sex Anomalies

## Turner Syndrome

One of the sex chromosomes is missing in **Turner syndrome**, resulting in a karyotype of 45, XO, indicating the presence of 45 chromosomes, with only one X chromosome. The person appears to be female, but the ovaries do not develop; thus, there is no ovulation or menstruation, and the person is sterile. In physical appearance, the

**Figure 5–10** ▶ Karyotype for Turner syndrome (45, XO). (Catherine G. Palmer, Indiana University)

mammary nipples are widely spaced, the breasts do not develop, and the person is short of stature and has a stocky build. Congenital heart disease, particularly coarctation of the aorta (described in Chapter 6), frequently accompanies Turner syndrome. Facial deformities are often present. Figure 5–10 ▶ shows a Turner syndrome karyotype. The occurrence for Turner syndrome is about 1 in 2000 live births.

## Klinefelter Syndrome

An extra sex chromosome is present in **Klinefelter syndrome**, resulting in a karyotype of 47, XXY, indicating the presence of 47 chromosomes, including two X and one Y chromosomes. A fairly simple chromosome check will reveal the condition. The occurrence is about 1 in 500 to 1 in 1000 males. This person appears to be a male but has small testes that fail to mature and that produce no sperm. At puberty, with the development of secondary sex characteristics, the breasts enlarge and female distribution of hair develops. There is little facial hair, and the general appearance is that of an immature young adult. The person is tall and slender (with abnormally long legs), is mentally deficient, and is sterile (Figure 5–11 ▶).

Figure 5–11 ▶ Karyotype for Klinefelter syndrome (47, XXY). (Catherine G. Palmer, Indiana University)

Some cases of pseudohermaphroditism result from excessive production of sex hormones from the adrenal cortex. An affected female develops male secondary sexual characteristics at a very early age. The external genitalia of pseudohermaphrodites are ambiguous, resembling that of both males and females.

## ▶ Genetic Counseling

A genetic counselor usually begins with a complete family history of both prospective parents. A complete, detailed family history is called a *pedigree*. Pedigrees are used to determine the pattern of inheritance of a genetic disease within a family. When the pedigree is complete, the genetic counselor can inform prospective parents of the possibility of having genetically abnormal offspring, and the parents can make an informed decision.

## Hermaphrodites

The number of true **hermaphrodites** who have both testes and ovaries is small. **Pseudohermaphrodites** do develop, and they have either testes or ovaries, usually nonfunctional, but the remainder of the anatomy is mixed. This condition is referred to as *sex reversal*, in which the chromosomal sex is different from the anatomic sex. Sex reversal occurs during fetal life. The sex glands are neutral during the first few weeks after conception, until the male gonads differentiate at about the sixth week under the influence of masculinizing hormone (testosterone). In the absence of an adequate amount of this hormone, ovaries develop, and the individual develops anatomically female but chromosomally male (XY).

## Diagnosis of Genetic Diseases

Early diagnosis is critical to prevention and treatment of genetic diseases. During **amniocentesis**, a small amount of amniotic fluid is withdrawn after the fourteenth week of pregnancy. Fetal cells in the amniotic fluid are removed, the chromosomes are examined, and the amniotic fluid is analyzed for biochemical abnormalities. Test results in amniocentesis are available approximately 2 weeks after the procedure. Amniocentesis can detect approximately 200 genetic diseases before birth.

Chorionic villi are projections of the membrane that surrounds the embryo in early pregnancy. **Chorionic villus sampling** involves removing cells from the villi through the cervix.

## Prevention ✚ PLUS!

### Spontaneous Mutation

With spontaneous mutation, genetic diseases may not be preventable (e.g., Queen Victoria and the royal family lineage of hemophilia). However, with pedigree and DNA analysis and proper immunizations, many genetic disorders can be prevented.

Samples may be taken between 8 and 10 weeks of pregnancy. The chromosomes of the cells obtained can be analyzed immediately. Chorionic villus sampling gives embryonic or fetal results (gender and chromosomal information) sooner within the pregnancy, allowing time for options, including termination of pregnancy or preparation for a child with special needs.

## Gene Therapy for Genetic Diseases

Gene therapy is a procedure that involves identification, manipulation, and transference of genetic segments into a host to replace defective genes and to perform desired genetic activities. The genetic material used is compatible with human DNA that may be cultured in a microbe and delivered in a viral package or by injection. This sophisticated procedure is also referred to as genetic engineering.

Gene therapy has certain risks, but with continued improvement in techniques the future appears brighter. So far, treatment for genetic diseases has progressed in three stages:

1. Donors supply deficient or defective proteins, because genes are responsible for making the necessary protein products required by all cells; in this case, the defective genes could be circumvented.
2. New DNA is made by recombinant manipulation (multiple contributors) to produce pure protein agents.
3. New/replacement genes are inserted into the proper (deficient or defective) location for corrective measures.

Gene therapy requires specific guidelines or protocols to be followed in order to qualify for clinical trials. Basically, clinical trials determine the future prospects of most new therapy agents. Development, funding, and resources are necessary to ensure a successful research project.

A common form of gene delivery for gene therapy is the use of "tamed" viruses in a procedure called a **vector.** The original virus is stripped of its deleterious impact and its shell is used as a biological vehicle to deliver the prescribed genetic material into the selected site.

Other applications use various physical and chemical means, such as microinjection with or without liposomes (fat bodies) to slip DNA, encased in fat, through the fat-soluble membrane. DNA is unable to penetrate or be absorbed through a cell membrane on its own.

A new approach for the future is called **picoarray gene synthesis,** which uses artificial genes synthesized on microchips; this advancement may pave the way for quicker and less costly genetic procedures. As stem cell research expands, so too will the new ways of treatment and prevention of many genetic conditions.

## ▶ Congenital Diseases

**Congenital diseases** are those appearing at birth or shortly after, but they are not caused by genetic or chromosomal abnormalities. Congenital defects usually result from some failure in development during the embryonic stage, or in the first 2 months of pregnancy. *Therefore, congenital diseases cannot be transmitted to offspring.* The systems chapters in Part II of this book provide further discussion of selected congenital conditions.

Various factors—inadequate oxygen, maternal infection, drugs, malnutrition, and radiation—can interfere with normal development. Rubella, or German measles, contracted by the mother during the first trimester of pregnancy can produce serious birth defects. The rubella virus can cross the placental barrier and affect the central nervous system of the embryo, causing mental retardation, blindness, and deafness. Cerebral palsy and hydrocephalus can develop as a result of a viral infection. Cerebral palsy and mental retardation may be the result of oxygen deprivation, such as when the umbilical cord gets squeezed or contorted and slows or shuts down blood flow to the fetus. Low oxygen may also be a factor in very high altitude environments.

Syphilis can be transmitted to a developing fetus and cause multiple anomalies: structural deformities, blindness, deafness, and paralysis. Children with congenital syphilis may become insane. Syphilitic infection of a fetus frequently results in spontaneous abortion or a stillbirth. A mother with syphilis should be treated for it before the fifth month of pregnancy to prevent fetal infection. A child born with syphilis should be treated immediately with penicillin, but considerable irreversible damage may have already occurred. Syphilis is discussed further in Chapter 11.

The tragic effect of the drug thalidomide, introduced in the 1950s and used in early pregnancy until 1962, alerted the public to the danger of harmful drugs for the developing embryo. Within the first two months of pregnancy, some babies who had been exposed to thalidomide before birth were born without limbs or had flipper-like appendages. The Food and Drug Administration (FDA) subsequently banned thalidomide and thus spared many parents the congenital outcome just described.

Many congenital defects result from improper development, such as failure of organ walls to form or close or failure of two parts to unite and fuse. The chambers and vessels of the heart are sites of such abnormalities, and congenital heart diseases are discussed in Chapter 6. Spina bifida is an improper union of the lateral ridges of the embryo to form the vertebral column, a primary example of a neural tube defect (NTD). Although the cause of NTD is unknown, folic acid intake prior to and through the first few weeks of pregnancy decreases the incidence of NTD. Since neural tube closure occurs at 28 days after conception and prior to the recognition of pregnancy by many women, NTD prevention is best achieved by adequate folic acid (0.4 mg per day) intake throughout the reproductive years. Spina bifida is further explained in Chapter 13.

Cleft lip and cleft palate comprise the fourth most common birth defect in the United States. One of 700 newborns is affected by cleft lip and/or cleft palate, which is a gap between the left and right halves of the lip or upper palate (roof of the mouth). In trisomy 13, about 60% to 80% of babies born have cleft lip and palate. The defects are due to failure of the two sides of the embryo to fuse during gestation and affect speech, respiration, feeding, and physical appearance. Clefts can be corrected with surgery.

A variety of types of congenital defects occur in the alimentary tract. The absence of a normal opening in an organ is called atresia. The lack of an opening from the esophagus to the stomach is esophageal atresia; it is frequently accompanied by an abnormal opening between the esophagus and the trachea.

Intestinal atresia is a complete obstruction of the intestine, resulting in vomiting, dehydration, scanty stool production, and distention of the abdomen. Another congenital obstruction of the intestinal tract is pyloric stenosis, in which the pyloric sphincter hypertrophies, closing the opening between the stomach and the beginning of the small intestine (duodenum). Symptoms include projectile vomiting, dehydration, constipation, and weight loss. Corrective surgery has been very effective in removing these congenital obstructions of the intestinal tract, just as it has been for congenital heart disease.

The bile ducts are blocked in biliary atresia, causing severe jaundice to develop. In biliary atresia, the liver and spleen become greatly enlarged. Excess bile buildup may cause jaundice and brain damage due to toxicity.

## Age-Related Diseases

The DNA blueprint foretells the future and the past. Some genetic diseases are noticed on the day of birth or shortly thereafter. Disease onset may start at birth, such as with PKU and galactosemia, or appear in a few months, as with Tay-Sachs. However, diseases such as hemochromatosis may appear from age 30 to 40, and Parkinson's disease often exhibits first noticeable symptoms in middle age.

### RESOURCES

The National Center for Biotechnology Information: www.ncbi.nlm.nih.gov

The National Library of Medicine: www.nlm.nih.gov

The National Marfan Foundation: www.marfan.org

National Human Genome Research Institute: www.nhgri.nih.gov

Medline Plus: www.medlineplus.gov

# DISEASES AT A GLANCE

## Heredity*

| DISEASE | ETIOLOGY | SIGNS AND SYMPTOMS | DIAGNOSIS |
|---|---|---|---|
| **Autosomal dominant inheritance** | | | |
| Achondroplasia | Chromosome 4, autosomal dominant, usually spontaneous | Short arms and legs, normal trunk, dwarfism, megalocephaly, lordosis; may depend on parent age | Present at birth, DNA tests before birth |
| Marfan syndrome | Chromosome 15, autosomal dominant | Skeletal malformations, long facial appearance, aortic aneurysm, scoliosis, hypermobile joints, ocular lens defects | Onset is age 20, detection of protein fibrillin on skin, culture DNA tests |
| Familial hypercholesterolemia | Incomplete autosomal dominant | Atherosclerosis, coronary artery disease | Onset at birth, high LDLs |
| **Autosomal recessive inheritance** | | | |
| Fragile X syndrome | Constricted segment on long arm of X, FMR1 gene mutation | Mental deficiency, large head, flat feet, prominent ears and forehead | DNA sequencing |
| Galactosemia | Autosomal recessive, lack enzyme for lactose digestion | Enlarged liver, ascites, vomiting, diarrhea, cataracts, mental retardedness, cerebral palsy | High blood galactose levels |
| Hemochromatosis | Autosomal recessive, more males | Early—abdominal pain, arthritis; Later—diabetes, liver damage | Blood test for excess serum ferritin-iron, DNA test for HFE mutation, liver biopsy |
| Parkinson disease; see Chapter 13 | Chromosome 4, or multifactorial | Mask/stoic face, twitching hands and arms, stiff gait, depression | Blood check for dopamine |

*Exceptions or additions may be found in many of these cases; some diseases are covered further in system chapters.

| TREATMENT | PREVENTION | LIFESPAN |
|---|---|---|
| Nothing definitive | Family history, genetic counseling | Because of appearance there may be some mental issues, but usually thrive well into adulthood |
| Depends on afflicted areas. Drugs to reduce aorta expansion (e.g., beta blocker) or bone surgery | None without family history, genetic screening; 1/3 are sporadic cases | May die early due to cardiovascular problems |
| Exercise, low-fat diet, statins | None, detect early as possible | Relatively normal life if heterozygous with medication, diet, and exercise; homozygous results in death as young adult |
| Special education, physical and occupational therapy | None, perhaps counseling if aware | Symptoms throughout life, primarily affects males because of only one X chromosome |
| Diet control, no lactose in food | Screened at birth | Normally do well with early diagnosis and controlled diet |
| Phlebotomy, blood donation | DNA test, genetic screening | Onset age 30–40, liver damage may be critical, continue blood transfusion throughout normal life expectancy |
| L-Dopa, steroids, antidepressants, electrostimulator (Chapter 13) | None | Normally appears at 40+ years and is progressive; requiring continued medication |

# DISEASES AT A GLANCE

## Heredity (*continued*)

| DISEASE | ETIOLOGY | SIGNS AND SYMPTOMS | DIAGNOSIS |
|---------|----------|--------------------|-----------|
| Phenylketonuria | Chromosome 12, autosomal recessive | Light skin tone, blue eye, mental retardation if not corrected | Blood and urine levels of phenylalanine |
| Tay-Sachs | Mutant Hex-A gene on chromosome 15 | Mental retardation, very dependent | Genetic blood screening |
| Change in chromosomal structure | | | |
|    Cri du chat | Part of chromosome 5 missing | Mental deficiency, petite, wide space between eyes, cat cry sound | At birth |
| Change in chromosomal number | | | |
|    Down syndrome | Extra chromosome 21 due to nondisjuntion | Mentally challenged, rounded face, protruding tongue, short stature | Observation, chromosomal screen |
|    Klinefelter syndrome | Extra X chromosome (47 total) | Tall and slender, long legs, sparse body hair, weak breast development, usually sterile, male | Genetic screen |
|    Turner syndrome | Missing X chromosome (45 total) | Short stature female, broad-flat breast, malformed elbows, sterile, hearing problems | May not be known until puberty, lack physical development |

| TREATMENT | PREVENTION | LIFESPAN |
|---|---|---|
| Restricted diet within day of birth | Enzyme assay, strict diet, along with family history | If untreated within 4 months, results in severe brain damage, mental retardation, and social abnormalities. With early detection and diet restriction, life is basically normal. |
| Genetic counseling | Genetic blood screening for parental traits, familyhistory | Die by age 3–4 |
| Supportive until death | None | Most die within first year (rarely live beyond 5–6 years) |
| Supportive, special education | Mother age under 35 | Usually die by midlife; if beyond age 45, tend to have Alzheimer's disease |
| Counseling, family supported | None, chance occurrence | Varies, may have rather normal life with strong support and live to midlife |
| May get growth hormone and other supplements | None, mostly miscarried and die in fetus stage | May live relatively normal life to age 50–55 |

# Interactive Exercises

## Cases for Critical Thinking

1. What is the reason that Turner and Klinefelter syndromes can occur as a result of nondisjunction in either the sperm or the egg but XYY can occur only as a result of nondisjunction in the sperm?

2. Marfan syndrome is an autosomal dominant disease. What is the probability that a child with a parent with Marfan syndrome will have Marfan syndrome?

3. If a mother is a carrier for the X-linked disease hemophilia A, what is the probability that her male child will have hemophilia A? Her female child?

4. A 36-year-old father of three with a new job thought stress had brought on abdominal pain and joint pain. He had noticed a darkening of his complexion and consulted a doctor, who found excess ferritin levels in his blood. What problem seems evident, and what treatment would help this individual?

## Multiple Choice

1. What do polydactyly and achondroplasia have in common?
   a. Both are autosomal recessive.
   b. Both are sex-linked.
   c. Both are congenital defects.
   d. Both are autosomal dominant traits.

2. Except for sperm and ova, how many chromosomes do human cells each have?
   a. 23          b. 46
   c. 96          d. 21

3. What combination of alleles manifest themselves only when the person is homozygous for the trait?
   a. recessive          b. dominant
   c. homozygous          d. heterozygous

4. Why do sex-linked diseases affect men more than women?
   a. Men have two X chromosomes.
   b. Men have two Y chromosomes.
   c. Men have one X chromosome.
   d. Men have no Y chromosome.

5. Color-blind people most frequently can't distinguish which colors?
   a. red and yellow          c. red and green
   b. green and blue          d. blue and yellow

6. What type of disorder is galactosemia?
   a. autosomal dominant
   b. autosomal recessive
   c. sex-linked
   d. congenital

7. If a female is a carrier of a sex-linked disease, what is the chance (in percent) of transmitting the allele to her children?
   a. 25          b. 50
   c. 75          d. 100

8. If both parents are carriers of an autosomal recessive disease, what is the chance (in percent) of each of their children getting the disease?
   a. 0          b. 25
   c. 50          d. 100

9. If alleles are different for a trait, what would be the genotype for that individual?
   a. homozygous          b. recessive
   c. heterozygous          d. dominant

10. Forty-four of our chromosomes (22 pairs) of the 46 total are called _____.
    a. sex chromosomes          b. genes
    c. autosomes          d. alleles

## True or False

_____ 1. DNA contains genetic information.

_____ 2. The incidence of Down syndrome increases with the mother's age.

_____ 3. Fragile X syndrome is found equally in men and women.

_____ 4. A patient with Turner syndrome has an extra sex chromosome.

_____ 5. Tay Sachs is an autosomal dominant disease.

_____ 6. Marfan syndrome is caused by an extra sex chromosome.

_____ 7. Albinism is a sex-linked disease.

_____ 8. Homozygous traits tend to be expressed generation.

_____ 9. If one parent is heterozygous for an autosomal dominant disease and the other parent is normal, a child has a 50% chance of getting the disease.

_____ 10. Fragile X syndrome is more demonstrative in girls than boys.

## Fill-Ins

1. _____ diseases are those appearing at birth or shortly after, but they are not caused by genetic or chromosomal abnormalities.

2. _____ have both functional testes and ovaries.

3. _____ alleles manifest themselves when the person is heterozygous for that trait.

4. _____ encode information for the synthesis of proteins.

5. _____ are alternative forms of a gene.

6. _____ is the condition of extra fingers or toes.

7. _____ is the failure of two chromosomes to separate as the gametes are being formed.

8. Sex cells contain _____ chromosomes.

9. A recessive genetic disease basically controlled by diet is _____.

10. Replacement of genetic material by recombinant application is called _____ _____.

# Multimedia Preview

Additional interactive resources and activities for this chapter can be found on the Companion Website. For videos, audio glossary, and review, access the accompanying DVD-ROM in this book.

## ▶ DVD-ROM Highlights

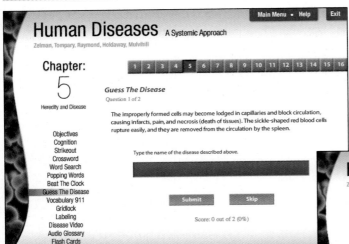

### Guess the Disease

Test your knowledge of human diseases! This fill-in-the-blank quiz provides instant feedback and allows you to check your score to see what you got right or wrong.

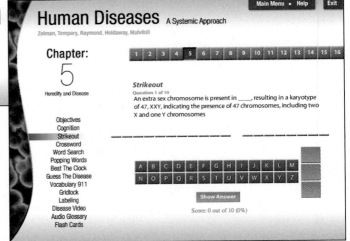

### Strikeout

Click on the alphabet tiles to fill in the empty squares in the word or phrase to complete the sentence. This game quizzes your vocabulary and spelling. But choose your letters carefully because three strikes means you're out!

## ▶ Website Highlights—www.pearsonhighered.com/zelman

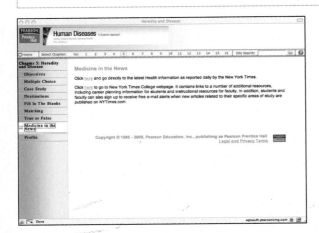

### Medicine in the News

Take advantage of the free-access online study guide that accompanies your textbook. You'll be able to stay current with a link to medical news articles updated daily by *The New York Times*. By clicking on this URL you'll also access a variety of quizzes with instant feedback and an audio glossary.

# Part II

# Diseases of the Systems

Part II presents diseases of the body's systems. Each chapter reviews the normal structure and function of a body system, and then discusses diseases associated with that system. Signs, symptoms, etiology, diagnosis, treatment, and prevention are described for each disease.

## Chapters

CHAPTER

6

# Diseases of the Cardiovascular System

## Learning Objectives

After studying this chapter, you should be able to

■ Describe the normal structure and function of the heart and blood vessels

■ Describe the key characteristics of the diseases of the arterial circulation and heart

■ Explain the association between arteriosclerosis and atherosclerosis

■ Identify the role of hyperlipidemia in atherosclerosis

■ Describe the etiology, signs, and risks associated with arterial hypertension

■ Compare and contrast pulmonary hypertension and arterial hypertension

■ Describe the role of varicose veins in peripheral vascular disease

■ Understand the risks associated with venous thrombosis

■ Differentiate between endocardial and myocardial diseases of the heart

■ Understand the distinguishing features of heart valve stenosis and heart valve regurgitation

■ Explain the different types of atrial and ventricular arrhythmias

■ Name the etiologies of shock

■ Describe normal fetal circulation

■ Describe the epidemiology, symptoms, etiology, diagnosis, and treatment of congenital heart abnormalities

■ Review and understand the differences between cyanotic and noncyanotic congenital heart disease

■ Review the risks and pathological changes associated with heart disease in older adults

## Fact or Fiction?

Aspirin therapy reduces the risk of myocardial infarction.

*Fact:* By minimizing platelet aggregation and clot formation, aspirin therapy reduces the risk of a myocardial infarction.

## Dr. Christiaan Barnard

Dr. Christiaan Barnard performed the first human heart transplant in 1967. In the Union of South Africa, Dr. Barnard performed this famous surgery on a 53-year-old dentist named Louis Washkansky. The dentist received the donated heart of a 25-year-old auto accident victim named Denise Davall. Although the surgery was a technical triumph and a beacon of hope for many with terminal heart disease, Washkansky died 18 days later from infection. Still risky today, heart transplants owe their successes to the generosity of Denise Davall, the courage of Louis Washkansky, and the brilliance of Dr. Barnard, who died of a heart attack in 2001.

# ▶ The Circulatory System

The main function of the circulatory system, which includes the heart and blood vessels, is transport. The circulatory system delivers oxygen and nutrients needed for metabolism to the tissues; carries waste products from cellular metabolism to the kidneys and other excretory organs for elimination; and circulates electrolytes and hormones needed to regulation various bodily functions. The circulatory system is divided into two parts: the systemic and the pulmonary circulation. The heart pumps blood, and the blood vessels serve as tubes through which blood flows. The arterial system carries blood from the heart to the tissues, and the veins carry it back to the heart.

## Structure and Function of the Heart

The heart is a hollow muscular organ located in the center of the chest. The heart consists of four chambers: a right and left atrium and a right and left ventricle. The chamber walls consist of cardiac muscle, known as **myocardium**, and their internal lining consists of a smooth, delicate membrane called the **endocardium**. The **pericardium**, a double-layered membrane, encloses the heart (Figure 6–1 ▶).

The right and left sides of the heart have an upper atrium that collects blood from the body and the lungs and a lower ventricle that ejects blood throughout the body and the lungs.

Valves between the atria and the ventricles, the atrioventricular (AV) valves, permit one-way blood flow from atria to ventricles. The **mitral valve** between the left atrium and left ventricle has two flaps called cusps that meet when the valve is closed. The **tricuspid valve** between the right atrium and right ventricle is named for its three cusps. Figure 6–2 ▶ shows these valves in the closed position.

The pulmonary semilunar valve permits one-way blood flow from the right ventricle to the pulmonary artery, while the aortic semilunar valve controls blood flow from the left ventricle to the aorta.

During every heart cycle, each heart chamber relaxes as it fills, and then contracts as it pumps

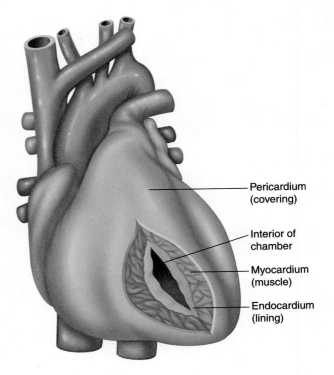

**Figure 6–1** ▶ Heart covering and layer of the heart.

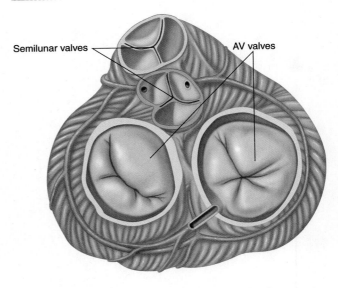

**Figure 6–2** ▶ Heart valves in closed position viewed from the top.

Superior vena cava
(from head and arms)

Aorta

Right
pulmonary
artery (to lung)

Left pulmonary artery
(to lung)

Pulmonary
semilunar valve

Right
pulmonary
veins (from
lung)

Left pulmonary veins
(from lung)

Right atrium

Left atrium

Tricuspid valve

Bicuspid (mitral) valve

Chordae tendineae

Aortic valve

Inferior vena cava
(from trunk and legs)

Left ventricle

Right ventricle

Figure 6–3 ▶ The blood flow through the heart.

blood. This filling period is the **diastole**, or the diastolic phase, while the contracting phase of each chamber is the **systole**, or systolic phase. The alternate contraction and relaxation of atria and ventricles comprises the **cardiac** cycle, which takes about 0.8 of a second. The flow of blood through the heart chambers, vessels, and lungs is reviewed in Figure 6–3 ▶.

Coronary arteries provide the heart muscle with a reliable blood supply. The left coronary artery begins at the aorta on the front of the heart and divides within an inch into the anterior interventricular coronary artery and the circumflex artery, which continues left around the back of the heart. The right coronary artery also branches from the front of the aorta and sends divisions to the right side and back of the heart (Figure 6–4 ▶).

Unlike skeletal muscle, cardiac muscle contracts continuously and rhythmically without conscious effort. A small patch of tissue, the **sinoatrial node** (SA node), acts as the pacemaker of the heart. The impulse for contraction initiates at the SA node spreads over the atria, and passes to the ventricles via conductive tissue called the AV node. The impulse continues along left and right bundle branches and terminates in the **Purkinje fibers**, which further branch throughout the ventricle walls. This conduction system is illustrated in Figure 6–5 ▶.

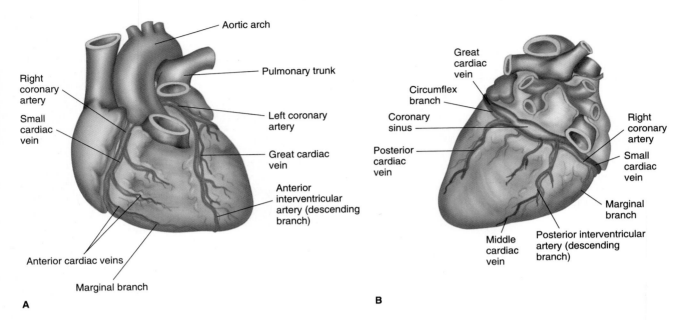

**Figure 6–4** ► Coronary arteries and major vessels.

Heart muscle does not depend on nerve stimulation for contraction, but it is influenced by the autonomic nervous system and hormones such as epinephrine. Two sets of nerves work antagonistically, one slowing the heart and the other accelerating it. The vagus nerve slows the heart rate during rest and sleep by means of a chemical it secretes, acetylcholine. The excitatory portion of the autonomic nervous system increases heart rate during periods of stress,

**Figure 6–5** ► Conducting system of the heart.

strenuous physical activity, and excitement. This excitation is brought about by the release of epinephrine and norepinephrine, which stimulate the heart's pacemaker.

Blood flows through two circulatory routes: the systemic circulation and the pulmonary circulation. The systemic circulation distributes oxygenated blood from the left ventricle, beginning at the **aorta** (large artery of the systemic arterial system) and continuing through arteries to all parts of the body, and returns deoxygenated blood by veins to the right atrium. The pulmonary circulation carries deoxygenated blood from the right ventricle, beginning at the pulmonary trunk and continuing through smaller arteries to the lungs to be oxygenated, and returns the blood through pulmonary veins to the left atrium. Partitions called the interatrial septum and interventricular septum separate oxygenated from deoxygenated blood in the atria and ventricles, respectively. See Figures 6–6▶ and 6–7▶.

Branches of the aorta carry blood to the head, upper extremities, chest, abdomen, pelvis, and lower extremities. These arteries continue to divide into smaller and smaller arteries, and eventually into vessels called **arterioles**, the smallest arteries. Arterioles lead into **capillaries**, the connecting links between arteries and veins. Capillaries deliver oxygen and nutrients to tissues.

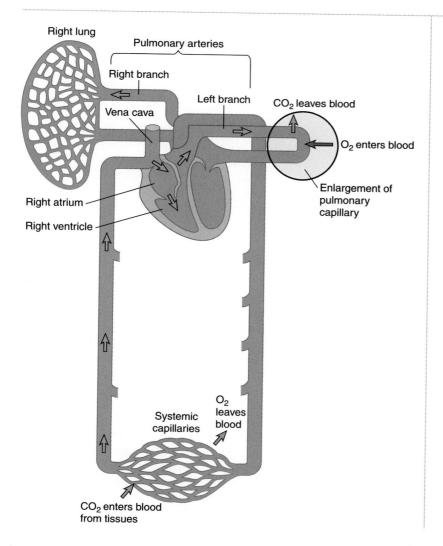

**Figure 6–6** ▶ Venous return to the heart and bloodflow to the lungs.

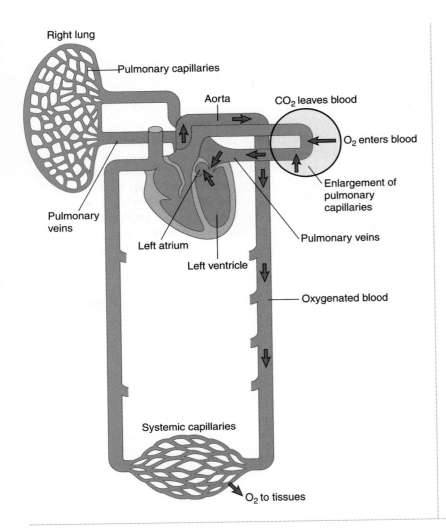

**Figure 6–7** ► Return of oxygenated blood to heart and entry into aorta (red = oxygenated blood, blue = deoxygenated blood).

Blood continues into **venules**, the smallest veins, and then into larger veins. Veins from the upper body empty blood into the superior vena cava, and veins of the lower body carry blood to the inferior vena cava. The superior and inferior **venae cavae** deliver systemic blood to the right atrium.

## Structure and Function of the Blood Vessels

The walls of arteries are muscular, thick, and strong, with considerable elastic tissue, and are lined with endothelium. Arterioles have a smaller diameter than arteries, with thinner walls consisting mostly of smooth muscle fibers arranged circularly and a lining consisting of endothelium. Arterioles can change their diameter by constricting or dilating, which alters blood flow to the tissues. Capillaries are minute vessels about ½ to 1 mm long with a lumen as wide as a red blood cell. Their wall consists only of a layer of endothelium. Vein walls are much thinner than companion arteries, but their lumens are considerably larger. With less muscle and elasticity in their walls, veins tend to collapse when empty. Veins, particularly those of the legs, contain valves that help return blood upward to the heart against gravity.

## ▶ Diagnostic Tests and Procedures for Cardiac Disorders

Many techniques for diagnosing and treating heart problems exist. **Auscultation**, listening through a stethoscope for abnormal sounds, and the electrocardiogram (ECG) provide valuable information regarding heart condition. The **electrocardiogram** is an electrical recording of heart action and aids in the diagnosis of coronary artery disease, myocardial infarction, valve disorders, and some congenital heart diseases. It is also useful in diagnosing arrhythmias and heart block. **Echocardiography** (ultrasound cardiography) is also a noninvasive procedure that utilizes high-frequency sound waves to examine the size, shape, and motion of heart structures. It gives a time-motion study of the heart, which permits direct recordings of heart valve movement, measurements of the heart chambers, and changes that occur in the heart chambers during the cardiac cycle. Color **Doppler echocardiography** explores blood-flow patterns and changes in velocity of blood flow within the heart and great vessels. It enables the cardiologist to evaluate valve stenosis or insufficiency.

An exercise tolerance test is used to diagnose coronary artery disease and other heart disorders. This test monitors the ECG and blood pressure during exercise. Problems that normally do not occur at rest are revealed.

**Cardiac catheterization** is a procedure in which a catheter is passed into the heart through blood vessels to sample the blood in each chamber for oxygen content and pressure. The findings can indicate valve disorders or abnormal shunting of blood and aid in determining cardiac output.

X-rays of the heart and great vessels, the aorta, and the pulmonary artery, in conjunction with **angiocardiography,** in which a contrast indicator (dye) is injected into the cardiovascular system, can detect blockage in vessels. **Coronary arteriography** employs a selective injection of contrast material into coronary arteries for a film recording of blood vessel action.

## ▶ Cardiovascular Disease

Cardiovascular disease includes a range of diseases that affect the heart and the blood vessels. Globally, mortality from cardiovascular disease is expected to increase to 19 million by 2020. Heart disease is the leading cause of death and a major cause of disability in the United States. Almost 700,000 people die of heart disease in the United States each year, about 29% of all U.S. deaths.

Disorders of blood flow and pressure and disorders of cardiac function are directly and indirectly responsible for many of the diseases that affect the pulmonary and systemic circulation. Disorders of blood flow and pressure include the diseases of the arterial circulation and the venous circulation. Disorders of cardiac function consist of diseases of the pericardium, coronary heart disease, myocardial and endocardial diseases, heart valve disease, cardiac conduction disturbance, heart failure, and heart disease in infants and children.

### Diseases of the Arterial Circulation

*Hyperlipidemia*   Hyperlipidemia is a general term used to describe an elevation of lipids or fats in the blood. Lipids include cholesterol, cholesterol esters, phospholipids, and triglycerides. Cholesterol is a soft waxy substance that forms cell membranes and various hormones. It is transported throughout the systemic circulation by transport proteins called **lipoproteins**.

**Low-density lipoprotein (LDL)** is the major cholesterol carrier in the blood. LDL transports cholesterol to the tissues of the body. LDL is also known as the "bad" cholesterol because accumulations of LDL form a **plaque** or thick hard deposit that narrows the arteries and impedes blood flow. **High-density lipoprotein (HDL)** carries about one-quarter to one-third of the cholesterol. Known as the "good" cholesterol, HDL carries cholesterol away from the arteries and to the liver, where it is eliminated from the body. **Triglycerides** are the form that fat exists in the human body. An increase in triglycerides is linked to coronary artery disease.

## Prevention ✚✚PLUS!

### Trans Fat

Americans obtain about 2% of their calories from trans fat—made when hydrogen is added to vegetable oil, a process called hydrogenation—twice the amount of American Heart Association recommendations. For example, if you eat 2000 total calories a day, your daily limit should be less than 2 grams (less than 20 of those calories) from trans fats.

*Hypercholesterolemia*  Hypercholesterolemia can be classified as primary, in which the hypercholesterolemia develops independent of other causes, and secondary, in which it is associated with other health problems or lifestyle.

Many types of primary cholesterolemia have a genetic basis. For example, the LDL receptor is deficient or defective in the autosomal dominant genetic disorder known as *familial hyperchloesterolemia.* Secondary causes of hypercholesterolemia include obesity and diabetes mellitus. High-calorie diets increase the production of LDL and cholesterol. Diets that are high in triglycerides and saturated fat increase cholesterol synthesis and suppress LDL receptor activity.

*Arteriosclerosis*  Arteriosclerosis and atherosclerosis are diseases of the arteries. Because these diseases significantly contribute to the development of many other diseases in the cardiovascular system, most notably heart disease, they are discussed first.

In **arteriosclerosis**, artery walls thicken and become hard and inflexible, partly due to calcium deposition. "Hardening of the arteries" aptly describes this condition, because affected arteries are unable to stretch and rebound in response to the pressure of blood as it is forced through them by contraction of the heart. As a result, arteriosclerosis leads to hypertension. The most common cause of arteriosclerosis is atherosclerosis (discussed next) in which fatty material accumulates within the walls of the artery (Figure 6–8 ▶).

*Atherosclerosis*  **Atheroslerosis,** or a hardening of the arteries, is a multifaceted disease that results from a number of insults that damage the vasculature. Hypercholesterolemia, smoking, hypertension, and diabetes are known risk factors that initiate the atherosclerotic process. The lesions associated with atherosclerosis are of three types: the fatty streak, the fibrous atheromatous plaque, and the complicated lesion.

A variety of tests are available to confirm the diagnosis of atherosclerosis. The electrocardiogram measures normal and abnormal electrical activity of the heart that may result from ather-

Figure 6–8 ▶ An artherosclerotic artery.

osclerotic disease. Coronary angiography is a test that is used to visualize the coronary arteries with the use of a contrast dye. A CT scan or computerized tomography scan sends x-rays through the body at various angles. The CT scan can directly visualize the heart arteries and measure the amount of calcium deposits in the arteries.

**Fatty streaks** are thin, flat discolorations in the vasculature that progressively enlarge and become thicker as they grow in length. Fatty streaks are present in children and increase in number until about the age of 20 years, and then they either remain static or regress.

The **fibrous atheromatous plaque** is the basic lesion of clinical atherosclerosis. It is characterized by the accumulation of intracellular and extracellular lipids and formation of scar tissue. The lesion begins as a whitish gray lesion thickening of the vessel intima (inner coat of the vessel) that contains a lipid core covered by a fibrous plaque. As the lesion increases in size, the artery may eventually occlude a vessel, causing a reduction of blood flow (Figure 6–9 ▶).

The more advanced or **complicated lesions** are characterized by hemorrhage, ulceration, and scar tissue deposits. **Thombosis**, or a clot within a blood vessel, is formed by turbulent blood flow in the region of the plaque and ulceration of the plaque.

Males and people with a history of cardiovascular disease have an increased risk for atherosclerosis. Modifiable risk factors such as hypercholesterolemia, high blood pressure, diabetes, obesity, physical inactivity, untreated or undertreated hypertension, and smoking can be controlled to reduce the risk for atherosclerosis.

Atherosclerosis is not usually associated with symptoms until the interior of the artery is extensively occluded. Symptoms depend on the location and the severity of the occluded artery. Occlusion of the coronary arteries may result in chest pain and shortness of breath. Blockage of the **carotid arteries** can reduce blood supply to the brain, causing a stroke. A hardening of the arteries in the legs, or **peripheral vascular disease**, leads to pain in the muscles of the leg; however, in severe cases ulceration or **gangrene** of the extremities may result.

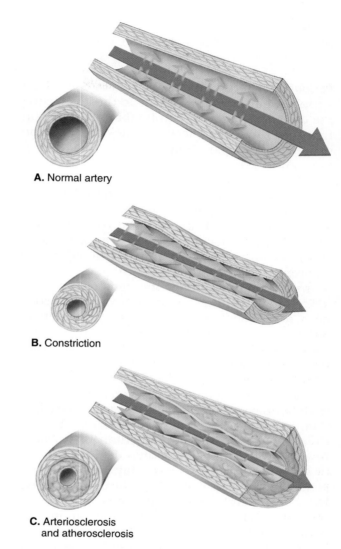

**A.** Normal artery

**B.** Constriction

**C.** Arteriosclerosis and atherosclerosis

**Figure 6–9** ▶ Blood vessels: (A) normal artery; (B) constriction; (C) arteriosclerosis and atherosclerosis.

Control of blood pressure, reduction of cholesterol, and lifestyle changes contribute significantly to the treatment and prevention of consequences that can result from atherosclerosis. Medications commonly prescribed in the treatment of atherosclerosis include antihypertensive and cholesterol-lowering medications. Numerous controlled clinical trials confirm the beneficial effects of controlling blood cholesterol levels. Treatment of hypertension reduces the potential for further injury and insult to the arteries.

***Peripheral Arterial Disease*** Diseases that affect peripheral arteries are similar to those affecting the coronary (heart) or carotid (brain) arteries in that they produce **ischemia**, or lack of blood and oxygen supply, pain, impaired function, infarction, and tissue necrosis. Atherosclerosis is an important cause of peripheral arterial disease. The most commonly affected arteries are the femoral (leg) or popliteal arteries. The disease is seen most commonly in men aged 70 to 80 years. The risk factors for this disease are the same as those for atherosclerosis, namely heredity and environmental risks.

Inspection of the limbs for signs of ischemia, such as subcutaneous atrophy, pallor, coolness, and absent pulses, provides a preliminary diagnosis. Doppler ultrasounography, ultrasound imaging, radionuclide imaging, and contrast angiography may also be used to confirm the diagnosis.

The primary symptom of chronic obstructive peripheral artery disease is **intermittent claudication**, or pain with walking. Other signs include a thinning of the skin and subcutaneous tissues of the lower leg. The foot may feel cool to the touch and a lower leg pulse may be faint or absent. When blood flow is significantly reduced, the oxygen and nutritional needs may not be met, and ischemic pain at rest, ulceration, and gangrene may result.

Treatment of peripheral vascular disease is aimed at prevention of further complications in the affected tissues. Walking slowly is usually encouraged because it increases circulation around the clots. Avoidance of injury is important because extremities affected by atherosclerosis are easily injured and slow to heal. Blood-thinning agents are used to prevent additional clots from forming. In severe cases, surgical bypass around the clot may be indicated. Removal of the clot may also be considered if the section of the diseased vessel is short.

***Raynaud's Disease*** **Raynaud's disease** is a functional disorder of the arteries caused by **vasospasms**, or intense spasms of the arteries and arterioles in the fingers and toes. Raynaud's disease usually occurs in healthy young women. It is often precipitated by exposure to cold or emotional stress and usually is limited to the fingers (Figure 6–10 ▶). The causes of vessel spasms are unknown, although hyperactivity of the sympathetic nervous system has been suggested.

Symptoms of vasospasm include changes in skin color from pallor to cyanosis accompanied by a sensation of cold, numbness, or tingling. The color changes are most noticeable in the tips of the fingers, later moving to the more distant parts of the fingers and hands. In severe progressive disease, the nails may become brittle, and the skin over the affected fingers may thicken. Deprivation of oxygen and nutrients in the affected area may give rise to arthritis, ulceration, or rarely gangrene of the fingers.

Treatment of Raynaud's disease is aimed at reducing triggers for the symptoms and protecting the hands from trauma. Abstinence from smoking, protection of the hands from cold, and avoidance of emotional stress are important. Medications that prevent vasospasm may be used in individuals with frequent symptoms.

***Aortic Aneurysm*** Aortic aneurysm refers to dilation of the aortic lumen. Aneurysms are usually described by their location, size, **morphology** (configuration and structure), and origin. The morphology of an aortic aneurysm is either **fusiform** or **saccular** (Figure 6–11 ▶). A **fusiform** aneurysm has a uniform shape, with symmetrical dilation that

**Figure 6–10** ▶ Raynaud's disease (Bart's Medical Library/ Phototake NYC).

**A**          **B**

Figure 6–11 ▶ Aneurysms: (A) saccular (Simon Fraser/RNC, Newcastle/Photo Researchers, Inc) and (B) fusiform (Zephyr/Photo Researchers, Inc.).

involves the circumference of the aortic wall. **Saccular** aneurysms, on the other hand, appear as an outpouching of only a portion of the aortic wall.

Ultrasound imaging, echocardiography, computed tomography (CT), and magnetic resonance imaging (MRI) scans are often used to diagnose and monitor the progression of an aneurysm.

Aneurysms usually occur in the abdomen below the kidneys (**abdominal aortic aneurysm**), or in the chest cavity (**thoracic aneurysm**). **Cerebral** or brain **aneurysm** is diagnosed less frequently. Regardless of location, the danger of an aneurysm is the tendency to increase in size and rupture, resulting in hemorrhage possibly in a vital organ such as the heart, brain, or abdomen.

Aortic aneurysms typically produce no symptoms and usually develop after age 50 and occur more frequently in men than women. Atherosclerosis is the most common cause of abdominal aneurysms. Other causes of aortic aneurysms include connective tissue diseases, infections, and conditions that cause inflammation of the vessels such as trauma or infections.

Depending on the size and rate of expansion, surgical repair of an aneurysm is at times indicated to prevent rupture. The diseased area of the vessel is removed and replaced with an artificial graft or segment of another blood vessel.

## Disorders of Arterial Pressure

*Arterial Hypertension*   Arterial blood pressure is a measure of the force of blood against the arterial walls. In healthy adults, the highest pressure, called the **systolic** pressure, is ideally less than 120 mm Hg, and the lowest pressure, called the **diastolic** pressure, is less than 80 mm Hg. Blood pressure normally varies throughout the day, increasing with activity and decreasing with rest (Table 6–1 ▶).

Hypertension is broadly defined as an arterial pressure greater than 140/90 mm Hg in adults on at least three consecutive measures. A blood pressure reading in the range of a systolic of

| Table 6–1 ▶ Adult Blood Pressure Guidelines | |
|---|---|
| Healthy (normal) | Below 120/80 mm Hg |
| Prehypertension | 120/80 to 139/89 mm Hg |
| Stage 1 hypertension | 140/90 to 159/99 mm Hg |
| Stage 2 hypertension | 160/100 mm Hg |

120 to 139 mm Hg or a diastolic of 80 to 89 mm Hg is classified as **pre-hypertension**.

Advancing age, sedentary lifestyle, excess weight, and excessive dietary salt and alcohol consumption are risk factors for the development of hypertension. Family history of hypertension and African American ancestry are also observed risk factors for developing high blood pressure. Pre-hypertension is associated with increased risk of progression to hypertension.

Hypertension is the most common cardiovascular disorder and affects about 20% of the adult population worldwide. It is considered one of the major risk factors for heart disease, stroke, and kidney disease (Table 6–2►). Due to the asymptomatic nature of hypertension, it remains untreated or undertreated in the majority of affected individuals.

Blood pressure measurements obtained by using a sphygmomanometer and stethoscope are important in the diagnosis and follow-up treatment for hypertension. The diagnosis of hypertension using this method is based on the average of at least two or more blood pressure readings taken on at least two separate physician office visits.

The etiology of hypertension is divided into two categories: primary and secondary hypertension. Primary hypertension is also called **essential** hypertension; this chronic increase in systolic and diastolic blood pressure occurs without evidence of other disease. Approximately 90% to 95% of hypertension is classified as primary or essential. In **secondary hypertension**, the elevation in blood pressure results from some other disease, such as kidney disease.

Primary hypertension typically does not cause symptoms. When symptoms do occur, they are usually related to the long-term effects of hypertension on the organ systems of the body, including the kidneys, heart, eyes, and blood vessels. Hypertension is a major risk factor for the development of atherosclerosis, cardiovascular disease (including heart failure), coronary artery disease, peripheral vascular disease, and cerebrovascular diseases and stroke.

Treatment of primary and secondary hypertension is aimed at reducing blood pressure to less than 140/90 mm Hg and preventing organ damage. For individuals with secondary hypertension, control of the disease causing the hypertension may often be curative. Lifestyle modifications such as weight loss, exercise, and reduction of salt intake enhance the effectiveness of medication therapy and help reduce further disease risks. The type of medication selected to treat hypertension depends on the stage of hypertension, age, other conditions, and patient-specific risk factors.

*Pulmonary Arterial Hypertension* Pulmonary arterial hypertension (PAH) is a condition of high blood pressure in the pulmonary artery. The average normal pressure in the pulmonary artery is about 14 mm Hg at rest. In PAH, pressures in the pulmonary artery are greater than 25 mm Hg at rest and greater than 30 mm Hg during exercise.

A number of tests are used to diagnose and assess the severity of PAH. Echocardiography provides information about the severity of the pulmonary hypertension, estimated pulmonary artery pressure, and potential causes. An electrocardiogram provides information on cardiac abnormalities. Pulmonary function tests, lung scans, and blood tests are useful for identifying secondary causes. Cardiac catherization provides a precise measure of the blood pressure in the pulmonary artery.

There are both idiopathic and secondary causes of PAH that cause three general changes in the pulmonary arteries: vasoconstriction, endothelial and/or smooth muscle proliferation,

| Table 6–2 ► Risk of Stroke and Heart Disease Increase with Increasing Blood Pressure | |
| --- | --- |
| **Blood Pressure (mm Hg)** | **Risk** |
| 115/75 | Normal |
| 135/85 | 2 times normal |
| 155/95 | 4 times normal |
| 175/105 | 8 times normal |

# Prevention ✚ PLUS!

### Sodium Intake

Most Americans consume more salt (sodium) than their bodies need. Heavy sodium consumption increases blood pressure in some people; a 25% to 35% reduction in salt intake can reduce the likelihood of heart attack or stroke. You can take action to reduce your blood pressure and decrease likelihood of stroke or heart attach in the following ways:

- Lose weight.
- Exercise.

- Limit alcohol consumption.
- Reduce fat intake and increase vegetable and fruit intake.
- Reduce dietary salt intake.

Weight loss is the single most effective nondrug method to reduce blood pressure.
Thirty to thirty-five minutes of exercise three times per week can decrease blood pressure, especially when combined with weight loss.
Alcohol raises blood pressure, even in the absence of hypertensive disease.
A diet high in vitamins and low in fats is associated with lower blood pressure.

Keep salt intake below 2400 mg per day, or less than 1 teaspoon (tsp) daily.

and intimal fibrosis and thrombosis of the pulmonary capillaries or arterioles. **Vasoconstriction** results in a narrowing of the walls of the arteries, which makes the lumen of arteries narrower. As the endothelial cells and smooth muscles proliferate, the walls of the pulmonary artery thicken. Scar tissues forms on the walls of the arteries, causing the lumen to narrow. Intimal fibrosis and thrombosis involves the formation of blood clots causing blockages.

PAH symptoms of pulmonary arterial hypertension include **dyspnea** (shortness of breath), fatigue, and **syncope** (loss of consciousness, or fainting). As the disease advances, the pumping ability of the heart weakens and symptoms occur at rest.

Without treatment, the prognosis of PAH is poor, with a median survival of less than three years. Patients with severe symptoms require aggressive treatment to remove the underlying cause, reduce symptoms and improve quality of life, slow endothelial proliferation and the development of further narrowing of the lumen, and increase the supply of blood and oxygen to the heart. Treatments include medications, oxygen therapy, and lung transplantation.

## Diseases of the Venous Circulation

*Venous Circulation of the Lower Extremities* The venous systems in the lower extremities consist of the superficial (saphenous) veins and the deep venous channels. Blood from the skin and the subcutaneous tissue accumulates in the superficial veins and then is transported into the deeper venous channels for return to the heart. Venous valves are located along the veins and prevent backflow of blood into the venous system. The leg muscles also assist in moving venous blood from the lower extremities to the heart.

*Varicose Veins* Varicose veins are dilated, distorted veins that usually develop in the superficial veins of the leg, such as the greater saphenous vein. The veins become swollen and painful and appear knotty under the skin. Varicose veins are caused by blood pooling within the veins because of decreased, stagnated blood flow (Figure 6–12▶).

Varicose veins can be an occupational hazard related to long periods of sitting or standing. Normally, the leg muscle movement moves blood up within the vein from one valve to the next. In the absence of this "milking action" of the muscles, the blood exerts pressure on the closed valves and thin walls of the veins. The veins dilate to the extent that the valves are no longer competent. The blood collects and becomes stagnant, and the veins become more swollen and painful.

Pregnancy or a tumor in the uterus can also cause varicose veins because pressure on veins causes resistance to blood flow. Heredity and obesity are also associated with varicose veins.

Complications of varicose veins include ulcers and infection, due to poor circulation, and hemorrhage, caused by weakened vein walls.

Figure 6–12 ► Development of varicose veins.

Figure 6–13 ► Spider veins (Courtesy of Jason L. Smith, MD).

Treatment depends on the severity of the symptoms. An elastic bandage or support hose may increase circulation and provide relief from discomfort. Symptoms can be relieved by walking, elevating the legs when seated, and losing weight. A surgical procedure called surgical vein stripping is very successful and involves removing the veins and tying off the remaining open ends. Collateral circulation tends to develop to compensate for the loss of the vein segment.

**Spider veins** are small, dense networks of veins that appear as red or blue discolorations on the skin. The cause of spider veins is unknown, though there appears to be a genetic link. Spider veins appear in both men and women, but more frequently in women. Female hormones may play a role in their development; puberty, birth control pills, pregnancy, or hormone replacement therapy may contribute to them. Spider veins can be treated with laser. The light heats and scars the tiny superficial veins, which closes them off to blood flow (Figure 6–13 ►). Another treatment is **compression sclerotherapy**, in which a strong saline solution is injected into

specific sites of the varicose veins. The irritation causes scarring of the inner lining and fuses the veins shut. The procedure is followed by uninterrupted compression for several weeks to prevent reentry of blood. A daily walking program during the recovery period is required to activate leg muscle venous pumps.

***Chronic Venous Insufficiency*** Chronic venous insufficiency (CVI) is a condition of poor venous blood return to the heart. The most common cause of chronic venous insufficiency is deep vein **thrombosis**, incompetence of the venous valves and muscles that aid in venous return.

Similar to other diseases, diagnostic screening consists of assessment of medical history, such as smoking, obesity, family history, pregnancy, and history of sedentary lifestyle. Additional tests include plethysmography studies and Doppler imaging studies. Outflow pleththysmography is a simple tourniquet procedure that requires placing and releasing a tourniquet on the lower extremities. Upon release of the tourniquet, the vein should return to baseline. Doppler imaging studies are used to assess venous flow and the presence of a thrombus.

Signs and symptoms associated with poor blood flow include tissue congestion, edema, necrosis or skin atrophy, and pain upon walking. In advanced disease, venous stasis ulcers may develop.

Risk factors for CVI include advancing age, family history of deep vein thrombosis, sedentary lifestyle, obesity, and smoking. The peak incidence of CVI occurs in women aged 40 to 49 years and men aged 70 to 79 years.

The treatment of CVI depends on the severity of the disease. Mild cases can be managed with controlled diet and exercise and the use of compression stockings. Compression stockings squeeze the leg and prevent excess blood from flowing backward. Surgical repair of the veins includes repairing the valves, bypassing the incompetent veins, and vein stripping (surgical procedure in which the diseased vein is removed). An incision is made below the vein, a flexible instrument is threaded up the vein, and the vein is grasped and removed.

*Venous Thrombosis* A clot, or **venous thrombosis**, can develop in the superficial or the deep veins of the lower extremities. Venous thrombosis is accompanied by an inflammatory response to the vessel wall that results from venous blood stasis, vessel wall injury, and increased blood coagulation

Risk factors for venous thrombosis include conditions that cause venous stasis, hypercoagulability, and vascular trauma. Older adults and postsurgical patients are at increased risk for venous thrombosis as immobilization results in decreased blood flow and venous pooling in the lower extremities.

Venous thrombosis is not associated with symptoms in about 50% of patients. Signs and symptoms of inflammation, such as pain, swelling, and deep muscle tenderness, are indications of venous thrombosis.

Early detection and prevention of venous thrombosis is vital to prevent potentially fatal complications such as **emboli**, or distant clots to vital organs such as the lung. Early ambulation after surgery or childbirth, exercising the legs, and use of compression stockings are measures that decrease the risk for thrombus formation. Blood thinners are beneficial for patients at high risk. Surgery is performed to remove the thrombus or embolism.

## Disorders of Cardiac Function

*Coronary Heart Disease* The coronary circulation supplies the heart with oxygen and nutrients to maintain cardiac function and thus supply the remainder of the body with blood. The body's metabolic needs change rapidly and widely, often requiring rapid adaptation of cardiac function and coronary blood flow. An imbalance in cardiac oxygen demand and supply can cause myocardial ischemia, cardiac contractile dysfunction, arrhythmias, infarction, and death.

A preliminary diagnosis of coronary heart disease requires a physical exam, patient medical history, and an electrocardiogram (EKG). A patient's medical history is used to identify hereditary and lifestyle risk factors for the disease. The EKG records the heart's electrical activity and can aid in identifying abnormalities in heart rate and rhythm as well as areas of damaged heart tissue. Additional diagnostic tests include echocardiograms, stress tests, nuclear imaging, and angiography.

Coronary heart disease (CHD) is a disease of reduced coronary blood flow most often due to atherosclerosis. More than 90% of persons with CHD have coronary atherosclerosis. Atherosclerosis can affect the major coronary arteries and their branches. Risk factor categories define major, emerging, and underlying conditions that influence the development of atherosclerotic CHD. See Table 6–3 ▶.

Coronary heart disease is the leading cause of death worldwide. Approximately 3.8 million men and 3.4 million women worldwide die each year from coronary heart disease. The aging world population will have major implications for CHD. By the year 2025, more than 60% of all CHD deaths will be among persons over 65 years of age and more than 40% among persons over 75 years of age.

Symptoms of CHD include chest pain, or **angina pectoris**, which is pain and pressure felt in the chest that results from ischemia; **palpitations**, or a sensation of a rapid pounding heartbeat; dizziness or fainting; weakness upon exertion or at rest; and shortness of breath. The most devastating sign of CHD is cardiac arrest or a heart attack, also known as a **myocardial infarction** (Figure 6–14 ▶). Crushing pain in the chest, shortness of breath, nausea, pallor, weakness, and faintness are among the symptoms of a myocardial infarction.

Treatment of CHD depends on the severity of the disease as well as patient risk factors that

### Table 6–3 ► Risk Factor Categories for Atherosclerotic Cardiovascular Disease

**Major Risk Factors**

- Cigarette smoking
- Elevated blood pressure
- Elevated LDL cholesterol
- Low HDL cholesterol
- Diabetes mellitus
- Metabolic syndrome

**Emerging Risk Factors**

- Prothrombotic state
- Proinflammatory state
- Insulin resistance

**Underlying Risk Factors**

- High-fat diet
- Obesity
- Physical inactivity
- Family history

*Source:* Adapted from S. M. Grundy (2007), "Cardiovascular and Metabolic Risk Factors: How Can We Improve Outcomes in the High-Risk-Patient." *The American Journal of Medicine*, 120(9A):S3–S9.

may contribute to additional morbidity and mortality. Medications used to treat CHD include blood pressure–lowering agents, blood thinners, diuretics (medication that increases excretion of water), nitrates such as nitroglycerin to stop chest pain, and lipid-lowering medication. Lifestyle changes, such as a healthy, low-salt diet and exercise, are important to prevent further progression of disease.

**Angioplasty** is a procedure used to open a partly occluded artery (Figure 6–15 ►). The procedure involves inserting a balloon-tipped catheter into the femoral artery, guiding it to the heart and into the narrowed coronary artery. The balloon is expanded to press against the vessel walls and open the lumen. A stent, which is a cylindrical wire mesh of stainless steel or other alloy, surrounds the balloon. Expansion of the balloon forces the mesh into the lining of the vessel, which physically holds the lumen open. Because the vessels commonly become occluded again (restenosis) within months or a year, stents are coated with drugs that prevent restenosis.

In cases of severe blockage of the coronary arteries, coronary artery bypass surgery may be

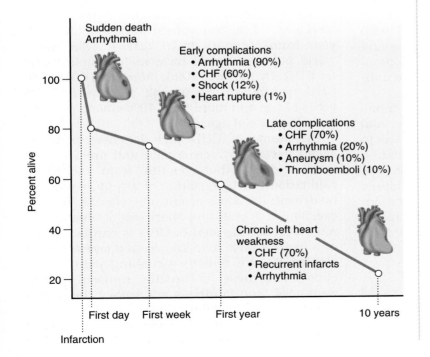

**Figure 6–14** ► Outcome of myocardial infarction. Forty percent of one-week survivors have late complications resulting in death. Ten-year survival is about 25%.

Figure 6–15 ► Angioplasty procedure. Note stent. (ISM/Phototake NYC)

needed. Coronary artery bypass surgery, also commonly called a CABG (cabbage) procedure, reroutes blood flow around the clogged arteries to improve blood flow and oxygen supply to the heart. A segment of a healthy blood vessel from another part of the body is attached or grafted from the aorta to the coronary artery below the blocked area. Depending on the number of blocked arteries, one or more grafts may be surgically placed. See Figure 6–16 ►.

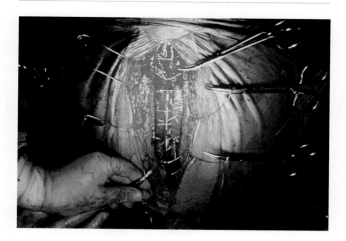

Figure 6–16 ► Bypass surgery of coronary blocked arteries. (Antonia Reeve/Photo Researchers, Inc.)

## Myocardial and Endocardial Diseases

*Myocarditis*  Myocarditis is an inflammatory disease of the heart muscle. Viruses such as the Coxsackie virus, adenovirus, and echovirus are the most common infecting viruses in the United States. Other potential etiologies include infections with the human immune deficiency virus and various bacterial infections.

Diagnosis of myocarditis can be suggested by clinical symptoms of the disease. An EKG recording provides evidence for conduction disturbances, and echocardiography may show an enlargement or inflammation of the heart muscle. Blood culture tests provide evidence for an infection. Elevations in certain heart muscle enzymes validate evidence for myocardial cell damage.

Myocarditis is often an asymptomatic condition. Patients usually have a history of viral illnesses, fever, chest pain that may feel like a heart attack, shortness of breath, and tachycardia, or a rapid heartbeat.

The goal for treatment of myocarditis is prevention of further myocardial damage through patient supportive measures. Bed rest and activity restriction help decrease myocardial work. Antibiotics may be prescribed in cases where an infectious organism has been identified.

*Cardiomyopathy*  **Cardiomyopathy** is a functional disease of the myocardium. There are three types of myocardial functional impairment: dilated, hypertrophic, and restrictive cardiomyopathy (Figure 6–17 ►). **Dilated cardiomyopathy** is the most common form and is characterized by dilation of the ventricle, contractile dysfunction, and symptoms of congestive heart failure. Ventricular hypertrophy is the dominant feature of **hypertrophic cardiomyopathy**. **Restrictive cardiomyopathy** is the least common form and is associated with reduced heart-filling pressures and endocardial scarring in the ventricle.

Dilated cardiomyopathy may result from infections, myocarditis, toxic agents, metabolic disorders, genetic disorders, and immune disorders. Often the cause is designated as **idiopathic dilated cardiomyopathy** as the etiology is unknown. The symptoms of dilated cardiomyopathy include dyspnea on exertion, orthopnea,

Figure 6–17 ▶ Cardiomyopathy.

weakness, fatigue, ascites, and peripheral edema. Treatment is aimed at relieving the symptoms with medications, rest, and surgical transplantation in severe cases.

Evidence for excessive ventricular growth is diagnostic for hypertrophic cardiomyopathy. Hypertrophic cardiomyopathy is a disease of young adulthood and is the most common cause of sudden cardiac death in the young. The etiology is often unknown, although genetic mutations are identified in a small number of cases. The treatment of hypertrophic cardiomyopathy includes medications and surgery. The goal of medication therapy is to decrease symptoms of the disorder and to prevent sudden cardiac death. Surgery consists of incision to the ventricular septum and removal of parts of the diseased tissue.

Restrictive cardiomyopathy is distinguished by restricted ventricular filling due to excessive rigidity of the ventricular walls. This condition is endemic in parts of Africa, India, South and Central America, and Asia. The most common cause is a condition called **amyloidosis**, a group of diseases in which one or more organ systems in the body accumulate deposits of abnormal proteins. Symptoms of restrictive cardiomyopathy include dyspnea, orthopnea, peripheral edema, ascites (accumulation of fluid in the abdomen), weakness, and fatigue.

## Diseases of the Endocardium

*Infective Endocarditis* **Infective endocarditis** is a microbial infection that affects the endocardial endothelium and the heart valves. It occurs in adults and children with predisposing conditions. Rheumatic heart disease, valvular disease, degenerative heart disease, congenital heart disease, and intravenous drug abuse increase the risk for endocarditis.

Many species of bacteria and fungi cause the majority of cases of infectious endocarditis. Acute forms of this disease involve the formation of nodules or **vegetations** that consist of the infectious organisms and cellular debris enmeshed in a fibrous clot. Typical lesions of endocarditis are shown in Figure 6–18▶. As fragments of the vegetations break apart, they enter the bloodstream to form emboli, which can travel to the brain, kidney, lung, or other vital organs, causing a variety of symptoms. The emboli can lodge in small blood vessels of the skin or other organs and cause the blood vessels to rupture.

Symptoms of infective endocarditis include fever, chills, a change in the sound or character of an existing heart murmur, and evidence for embolization of the vegetative lesions. A blood

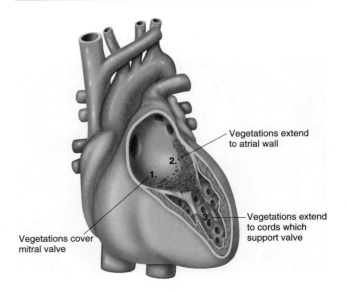

Vegetations extend to atrial wall

Vegetations cover mitral valve

Vegetations extend to cords which support valve

Figure 6–18 ▶ Bacterial endocarditis.

culture test provides a definitive diagnosis of the causative organism and directs antimicrobial treatment. Echocardiograms are useful to detect any underlying valve disease and vegetations.

Immediate and extensive antimicrobial treatment is necessary to eliminate the causative microorganism. Surgical interventions are indicated in cases where the heart is severely damaged by the infection.

***Rheumatic Heart Disease*** Rheumatic heart disease is a sequela of infection by group A hemolytic streptococci of skin, throat, or ear, although the organisms are no longer present when the disease presents itself. Approximately two weeks following the streptococcal infection, rheumatic fever develops, characterized by fever, inflamed and painful joints, and sometimes a rash.

Rheumatic fever is an **autoimmune disease** that results from a reaction between streptococcal antigens and the patient's own antibodies against them. All parts of the heart may be affected, frequently including the mitral valve. Blood clots deposit on the inflamed valves, forming nodular structures called vegetations along the edge of the cusps. The normally flexible cusps thicken and adhere to each other. Later, fibrous tissue develops, which has a tendency to contract.

If the adhesions of the cusps seriously narrow the valve opening, the mitral valve becomes stenotic. If sufficiently damaged, the cusps may not be able to meet properly, resulting in stenosis of the heart valves.

The incidence of rheumatic fever is highest among children and young adults. Prompt treatment of the streptococcal infection with antibiotics can prevent rheumatic fever and its complications.

## Valvular Heart Disease

Valves maintain unidirectional flow of blood through the heart. Valve disorders include stenosis and valvular insufficiency. **Stenosis** refers to a narrowing of the valves opening and failure of the valve to open normally. **Valvular insufficiency** or **regurgitation** refers to a valve that allows backward flow of blood within the heart. Stenotic valves produce distention of the heart chamber that empties blood through the diseased valve and impaired filling of the chamber that receives the blood. Incompetent valves produce distention and strain the chamber ejecting blood through the diseased valve.

***Mitral Stenosis*** In **mitral stenosis**, the mitral valve opening is narrow, and the cusps that form the valve, normally flexible flaps, become rigid and fuse together. A deep funnel shape develops, increasing resistance to blood flow from the left atrium to the left ventricle. As back-pressure develops in the left atrium, the left atrial wall hypertrophies. The right side of the heart is also affected (Figure 6–19▶). Pressure within the heart makes it difficult for the pulmonary veins to deliver blood to the right atrium, leading to increased pressure within veins. As the congestion builds in the veins, fluid from the blood leaks out into the tissue spaces, causing edema. Poor circulation causes cyanosis because an inadequate amount of oxygen is reaching the tissues. The backup of blood and congestion cause the heart to become exhausted and may lead to congestive heart failure. Another complication of a valve defect is the increased risk for a thrombus (blood clot) to form on the valve. If the thrombus becomes detached, it travels as an embolism and may occlude a blood vessel supplying the brain, kidney, or other vital organ.

The predominant cause of mitral stenosis is rheumatic fever, which can cause inflammation of the valve leaflets. The leaflets may further stick together and/or form rigid scar tissue. Rheumatic fever most often occurs in children aged 5 to 15 years; however, symptoms of mitral stenosis may not be seen for a number of years.

Stenotic valves may be widened to restore blood flow with valvuloplasty, a surgical technique similar to angioplasty. A complication of the surgery may be a leaky valve, in which case the valve may be surgically replaced with metal alloy or pig valve.

***Mitral Regurgitation*** In mitral insufficiency, also called mitral regurgitation, the valve is unable to close completely, which allows blood to leak into the atrium each time the ventricle contracts. As the volume of blood and pressure in the left atrium increases, blood pressure increases in other vessels, including the vessels leading from the lungs to the heart, resulting in lung

Superior vena cava

Pulmonary artery

Left atrial wall hypertrophies

Left atrium dilates

Left atrium

Stenotic mitral valve

Right atrium

Papillary muscles

Right atrium dilates

Inferior vena cava

Left ventricle

Right ventricle

Right ventricle dilates

**Figure 6–19** ► Effect of mitral valve stenosis on the heart.

congestion. The insufficiency is exacerbated by sclerosis and retraction of the valve cusps.

Another cause of regurgitation is the failure of specialized valve muscles in the ventricle, called papillary muscles. These muscles attach to the underside of the cusps by means of small cords (chordae tendinae) that normally prevent the cusps from flipping up into the atria when the ventricles contract. If the papillary muscles fail to contract, the cusps open upward toward the atria under the force of expelled ventricular blood. This failure is commonly called mitral valve prolapse (MVP).

Most individuals with MVP are asymptomatic and lead normal lives. Those who have moderate or more severe cases of MVP take antibiotics like amoxicillin to prevent bacteria from colonizing in the defective valves. If the prolapse becomes severe, it may be corrected with surgical reconstruction or replacement.

*Aortic Stenosis* **Aortic stenosis**, the narrowing of the valve leading into the aorta, occurs more often in men than in women and most frequently in men over 50 years old. It may result from

rheumatic fever, a congenital defect, or arteriosclerosis. Aortic stenosis is characterized by rigid cusps that adhere together and deposits of hard, calcified material, which give a warty appearance to the valve. Because the left ventricle pumps blood through this narrowed valve into the aorta, this chamber hypertrophies. Even with enlarged ventricles, inadequate blood flow to the brain persists and can cause **syncope** (fainting). This valve defect, like others, can be corrected surgically.

*Aortic Regurgitation* In aortic insufficiency, the valve does not close properly. With each relaxation of the left ventricle, blood flows back in from the aorta. Backflow of blood causes the ventricle to dilate, become exhausted, and eventually fail. This condition can result from inflammation within the heart, endocarditis, or a dilated aorta.

Symptoms of aortic regurgitation have a gradual onset. As the valve disease progresses, backflow of blood in the left ventricle increases, diastolic blood pressure falls, and the left ventricle enlarges. Most persons with aortic regurgitation remain asymptomatic for a number of years. The only sign for a number of years is a heart murmur. With advanced disease, symptoms of heart failure, such as dyspnea or shortness of breath on exertion and at rest, occur.

Valvular defects usually are detected through cardiac auscultation (heart sound) heard via a stethoscope. Diagnosis is confirmed by a number of tests, including echocardiography, cardiac catherization, or phonocardiogram. A phonocardiogram is a device that records heart sounds. An EKG tracing is usually collected simultaneously to correlate the sounds to ventricular and atrial contractions.

## Cardiac Conduction Disorders

*Cardiac Arrhythmias* Abnormal heart rhythms, or **arrhythmias**, develop from irregularity in impulse generation and impulse conduction. Electrical impulses from the heart's pacemakers stimulate contraction of the atria and the ventricles. Many forms of heart disease can disrupt the normal contraction and relaxation cycle of the atria and ventricles.

Cardiac arrhythmias are commonly divided into two categories: supraventricular and ventricular. The **supraventricular arrhythmias** include those that are generated by electrical abnormalities in the sinoatrial (SA) node, atria, atrioventricular node (AV) node, and junctional tissue in the heart. The **ventricular arrhythmias** include those that are generated in the ventricular conduction system and in the ventricle. Because the ventricles are the pumping chambers of the heart, ventricular arrhythmias are the most serious as they can be life threatening.

Disorders of cardiac rhythm can range from a sustained rapid heart rate of greater than 100 beats per minute, or **tachycardia,** to an abnormally slow heart rate of less than 50 beats per minute, or **bradycardia.** An interruption of the flow of impulses through the conduction system of the heart can lead to **heart block**. Heart block results when impulses are blocked, causing the atria and ventricle to contract independently of one another. The most serious effect of some forms of heart block is a slowing of the heart rate to the extent that circulation to vital organs such as the brain is blocked. An **ectopic pacemaker** is an excitable focus outside of the normally functioning pacemaker of the heart. Ec-

topic foci can cause additional beats (observed as premature contractions) or take over the normal pacemaker activity of the SA node.

Fibrillation is the result of disorganized current flow within the atria, called **atrial fibrillation**, or ventricle, called **ventricular fibrillation.** Fibrillation interrupts the normal contraction of the atria or the ventricles. In ventricular fibrillation, the ventricle quivers and does not contract and carry out effective coordinated contractions. Because no blood is pumped from the heart, ventricular fibrillation is a form of cardiac arrest. Immediate attempts at resuscitation must be made, or death will result.

Cardiac rhythm disturbances cause a wide variety of symptoms, including palpitations, **syncope** or lightheadedness, edema, or shortness of breath. The etiologies of arrhythmias are numerous and include a history of coronary heart disease, heart valve disease, myocardial infarction, hypertension, atherosclerosis, metabolic diseases, smoking, and drug abuse.

Medical therapy for the treatment of cardiac arrhythmias includes medications, electrocardioversion, and catheter ablation. Antiarrhythmic medications alter the physiological properties of the heart's conduction system. Electrocardioversion is accomplished using an external device or a surgically placed internal packemaker. A machine called an automated external defibrillator (AED) delivers electrical shocks and is used to re-establish normal heart rhythm (Figure 6–20▶). Defibrillators implanted under

Figure 6–20 ▶ Electrocardioverison paddles.

the skin of the shoulder resynchronize the heart on a daily basis, similarly to a pacemaker device. Catheter ablation is a nonsurgical procedure in which a catheter is inserted into the diseased area of the heart. A machine directs energy through the catheter to small areas of the heart that cause the abnormal heart rhythm. This energy severs the connecting pathway of the abnormal rhythm.

## ▶ Congestive Heart Failure

Congestive heart failure is a condition in which the heart cannot pump enough blood to meet the blood and oxygen needs of other body organs. It is a complication of most forms of heart disease, including coronary and peripheral atherosclerosis. There are nearly 23 million people living with heart failure worldwide. In the United States, approximately 550,000 new cases are diagnosed each year, and more than 287,000 people die each year from heart failure. Diagnostic methods for the diagnosis of heart failure include history and physical examination, laboratory studies, electrocardiography, chest radiography, and echocardiography. The patient history includes collecting information on symptoms related to shortness of breath, fatigue, and edema. A complete physical examination includes assessment of heart sounds, heart rate, and blood pressure; examination of the neck veins for congestion; and examination of the extremities for edema. Laboratory tests are used to diagnose anemia, blood disorders, or signs of liver congestions. Echocardiography is useful in assessing the anatomical and functional abnormalities of heart failure, and electrocardiographic studies are useful in diagnosing underlying disorders of cardiac conduction and rhythm. Chest x-rays provide information on the size and shape of the heart and surrounding vasculature. They can also be used to determine the severity of heart failure by revealing the presence of pulmonary edema.

The manifestations of heart failure depend on the extent of cardiac dysfunction, patient age, concurrent medical illnesses, and the extent and rate at which cardiac performance becomes impaired. The severity of impairment ranges from the mild, in which symptoms manifest clinically only during stress, to the most advanced form, in which the heart is unable to sustain life without external support. Mild symptoms of heart failure include ankle swelling and shortness of breath with exertion. Severe signs and symptoms include shortness of breath at rest, fatigue and limb weakness, neck vein swelling, rales (wet, crackly lung noises), pulmonary edema (fluid in the lungs), cyanosis, and abnormal heart sounds.

The goals of treatment for heart failure are aimed at relieving the symptoms, improving quality of life, and halting the progression of cardiac dysfunction. Treatment includes correction of the underlying causes, medications, restriction of salt and water intake, and modification of activities and lifestyle that are consistent with the functional limitations of the patient. Medication management of heart failure is complex and includes diuretics, medications that improve cardiac output, antihypertensives, antiarrhythmics, and medications that slow the heart rate and allow the heart muscle to relax and fill with blood. In severe cases, restriction of activity with bed rest often facilitates temporary improvement of heart function.

## ▶ Shock

Shock is a life-threatening condition in which blood pressure drops too low to sustain life. Any condition that reduces the heart's ability to pump effectively or decreases venous return can cause shock. This low blood pressure results in an inadequate blood supply to the cells of the body. The cells can be quickly and irreversibly damaged and die. Major causes of shock include cardiogenic, hypovelemic, anaphylactic, septic, and neurogenic shock. See Table 6–4 ▶ for types and etiology.

Untreated shock is usually fatal. The prognosis depends on the underlying cause, preexisting illnesses, the time between onset and diagnosis, and rapidity of response to therapy.

| Table 6–4 ▶ Types of Shock and Etiology | |
| --- | --- |
| **Type of Shock** | **Etiology** |
| Cardiogenic | Cardiac arrhythmias Myocardial infarction |
| Hypovelemic | Hemorrhage Trauma Surgery Extensive burns |
| Anaphylactic | Allergic reaction |
| Septic | Toxins released by a bacterial infection |
| Neurogenic | Damage to the central nervous system |

## ▶ Heart Disease in Infants and Children

### Fetal and Perinatal Circulation

Fetal circulation is anatomically different from postnatal circulation (Figure 6–21 ▶). Before birth, oxygenated blood flows through the placenta from the umbilical vein. The fetal lungs are entirely bypassed either by direct passage from the inferior vena cava to the right atrium through the foramen ovale to the left atrium, or from the right ventricle through the pulmonary artery through the ductus arteriosus to the aorta.

The umbilical vein connects to the fetal venous system, which returns blood to the fetal right atrium via the inferior vena cava. From the inferior vena cava, blood flows into the right atrium and then moves through the foramen ovale into the left atrium. It then passes into the left ventricle and is pumped into the ascending aorta to perfuse the heart and upper extremities. At the same time, venous blood from the heart

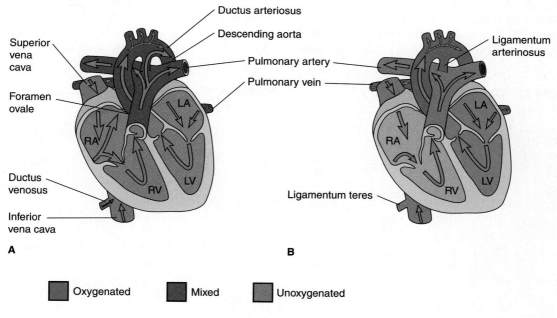

Figure 6–21 ▶ (A) Fetal circulation; (B) Postnatal circulation.

and upper extremities returns to the right side of the heart by way of the superior vena cava, moves into the right ventricle, and is pumped into the pulmonary artery. Blood that is ejected into the pulmonary artery gets diverted through the ductus arteriosus into the descending aorta. This blood perfuses the lower extremities.

When a baby takes its first breath after birth, the newly expanded lungs initiate a switch from placental to pulmonary oxygenation of the blood. Cord clamping and removal of the placental circulation cause an increase in left ventricular pressure. The decrease in right atrial pressure and decrease in left atrial pressure produce a closure of the foramen ovale. The newly expanded lungs favor the flow from the right heart via the pulmonary artery to the lungs as opposed to the ductus arteriosus. Closure of both the foramen ovale and the ductus arteriosus leads to the establishment of the postnatal circulation.

## Congenital Heart Disease

The embryological development of the heart is complex, and many errors can occur during development. Generic, environmental, and chromosomal changes may alter the development of the heart. Infants born to parents with a history of congenital heart disease are at a higher risk. Infants born with chromosomal abnormalities such as Down syndrome or Turner syndrome have an increased risk for congenital heart disease. Mater-

nal diabetes, congenital rubella, maternal alcoholism, and treatment with anticonvulsant drugs are also associated with congenital heart disease.

Approximately 8 babies of 1000 births have some form of a congenital heart disease. Due to advances in technology and early recognition of congenital heart disease, approximately 85% of infants born with congenital heart disease can be expected to survive into adulthood. Congenital defects can affect almost any of the cardiac structures or circulatory blood vessels.

Congenital heart disease is divided into etiologies that cause cyanosis, or blue babies, and those that do not cause cyanosis. For cyanosis to occur, deoxygenated blood must bypass the lungs and enter the systemic circulation.

## Cyanotic Heart Disease

***Tetrology of Fallot*** Tetrology of Fallot is one of the most serious of the congenital heart defects and consists of four abnormalities: (1) ventricular septal defect; (2) narrowing of the pulmonary outflow channel, including pulmonary valve stenosis, or a decrease in the size of the pulmonary trunk; (3) misplaced aorta that crosses the interventricular septum; and (4) hypertrophy of the right ventricle (Figure 6–22 ▸).

Maternal factors during pregnancy that are associated with tetrology of Fallot include a history of rubella, poor nutrition, overuse of alcohol, history of diabetes, and maternal age over

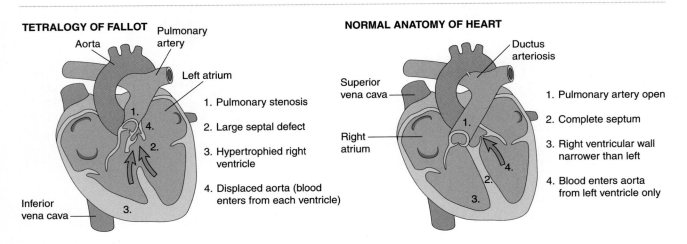

Figure 6–22 ▸ (A) Tetrology of Fallot; (B) normal anatomy.

40. Heredity may also play a role, as parents with a history of tetrology of Fallot have a greater risk of having a child with this disease. Children with genetic disorders such as Down syndrome often have congenital heart defects, including tetrology of Fallot.

Symptoms of this condition include difficulty feeding, failure to gain weight, poor development, cyanosis that becomes more pronounced during feeding, crying or defecation, fainting, sudden death, clubbing of the fingers, and squatting during episodes of cyanosis.

Surgical repair is often advised for all children born with this defect. More than one surgical procedure is required to increase blood flow to the lungs, patch the ventricular septal defect, open the narrowed pulmonary valve, and close any abnormal connections between the aortal and pulmonary artery.

### Transposition of the Great Arteries
In this condition, the aorta and the pulmonary artery connect to the wrong ventricle. The pulmonary artery is attached to the left ventricle, and the aorta is attached to the right ventricle; thus blood flow in the lungs and in the body occurs independently. Deoxygenated blood returns to the right heart and is pumped to the aorta, which pumps blood to the systemic circulation. The left heart receives blood from the lungs and then pumps the blood back to the lungs (Figure 6–23 ▶).

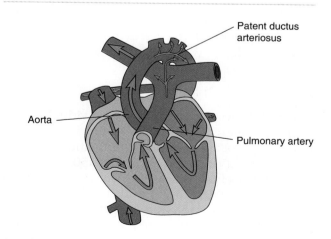

**Figure 6–23** ▶ Transposition of the great arteries

Symptoms include cyanosis, shortness of breath, poor feeding, and clubbing of the fingers. If diagnosed prior to birth, prostaglandins are administered to maintain a patent ductus arteriosus and allow mixing of oxygenated and deoxygenated blood to occur. Corrective surgery within the first two to three weeks of life is essential for long-term survival. An arterial switch procedure corrects both systemic and pulmonary blood flow.

## Non-Cyanotic Congenital Heart Disease

### Septal Defects
Septal defects may occur between the two atria, an atrial septal defect (ASD), or between the ventricles, a ventricular septal defect (VSD). Often these defects can be detected by the presence of a heart murmur on physical examination. In both conditions, blood in the right heart will be a mixture of deoxygenated blood and oxygenated blood that has traversed the left side of the heart (Figure 6–24 ▶).

Small ASDs may not cause any symptoms. Large atrial septal defects can lead to significant overload and enlargement of the right ventricle. Large ASDs require surgical repair.

A VSD causes increased blood flow to the lungs, which can eventually cause severe pulmonary hypertension. In the condition oxygenated blood is shunted from the left ventricle to the right ventricle, which contains deoxygenated blood. This results in increased pressures in the lungs. As pressure continues to build, the right ventricle shunts unoxygenated blood to the left ventricle, leading to cyanosis. Large VSDs required surgical correction.

### Patent Ductus Arteriosus
The ductus arteriosus serves as a fetal connection between the pulmonary artery and the aorta. In the fetal circulation, this allows blood to bypass the nonfunctional fetal lungs. At birth the ductus arteriosus normally closes. If the ductus remains open, blood intended for the body flows from the aorta to the lungs, overloading the pulmonary artery. Persistent increases in pulmonary arterial pressures can result in heart failure (Figure 6–25 ▶).

About 3000 infants are diagnosed with patent ductus arteriosus (PDA) each year in the United States. It is more common in premature infants but does occur in full-term infants. Premature

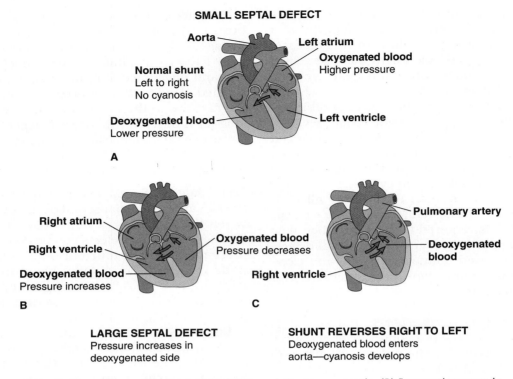

Figure 6–24 ► Effects of septal defects: (A) Normal shunt; no cyanosis; (B) Increased pressure in right ventricle; (C) Shunt reversal; cyanosis develops.

babies with PDA are more vulnerable to its effects. PDA is twice as common in girls as in boys.

A patent ductus can be treated medically with anti-inflammatory medications to close the PDA and antibiotics to prevent endocarditis. If medication therapy fails, a transcather device procedure or surgery may be performed to close the PDA.

***Coarctation of the Aorta*** Coarctation of the aorta is a congenital narrowing of the aorta that can occur anywhere along its length (Figure 6–26 ►). Most commonly it occurs near the ductus arteriosus. A severe coarcatation causes increases in resistance to the left ventricle and can eventually lead to heart failure.

Aortic coarcation occurs in approximately 1 out of 10,000 live births. It is often diagnosed in childhood, especially in cases where the narrowing is severe.

In severe cases symptoms are observed in infancy and include dizziness, shortness of breath, and cold legs. A harsh murmur heard on the back with the stethoscope along with x-ray scans, echocardiography, and doppler ultrasound provide a definitive diagnosis for this condition.

Surgery is often recommended to enlarge the narrowing of the aorta. The coarcatation of the aorta is surgically corrected by cutting the narrowed segment of the aorta and rejoining the healthy ends.

## Age-Related Disease

Worldwide, the population of individuals older than 65 years is projected to increase to 973 million (12%) by the year 2030 and comprise about 20% of the population in 2050.

Cardiovascular disease is the most frequent diagnosis in older adults and the leading cause of death in both men and women older than 65 years. Hypertension occurs in one-half to two-thirds of people over 65 years, and heart failure is the most frequently reported hospital dis-

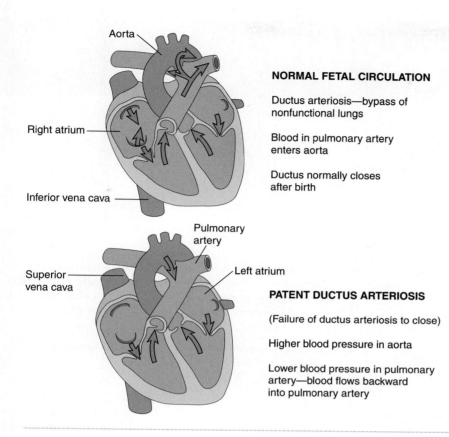

Figure 6–25 ► Patent ductus arteriosus.

Aorta

Right atrium

Inferior vena cava

**NORMAL FETAL CIRCULATION**

Ductus arteriosis—bypass of nonfunctional lungs

Blood in pulmonary artery enters aorta

Ductus normally closes after birth

Pulmonary artery

Superior vena cava

Left atrium

**PATENT DUCTUS ARTERIOSIS**

(Failure of ductus arteriosis to close)

Higher blood pressure in aorta

Lower blood pressure in pulmonary artery—blood flows backward into pulmonary artery

charge diagnosis among older adults in the United States.

Cardiovascular disease in older adults differs from that in younger persons. With age, systolic blood pressure and left ventricular mass progressively increase, and ventricular filling, heart rate and cardiac output, exercise capacity, and reflex responses of heart rate decrease. Cellular, enzymatic, and molecular changes in the arterial vessels lead to arterial dilation, thickening of the arterial intima, and vascular stiffness. With age, the cardiovascular system is less able to respond to increases in workload and stress; therefore, thresholds for symptoms of cardiovascular disease become more common with age.

Coarctation of aorta

Figure 6–26 ► Coarctation of the aorta.

## RESOURCES

Centers for Disease Control: www.cdc.gov

World Health Organization: www.who.int/en

American Heart Association: www.americanheart.org

National Institutes of Health: www.nhlbi.nih.gov. guidelines/cholesterol/atglance.htm

# DISEASES AT A GLANCE

## Cardiac System

| DISEASE | ETIOLOGY | SIGNS AND SYMPTOMS | DIAGNOSIS |
|---|---|---|---|
| Hypercholesterolemia | Genetic, lifestyle, obesity and diabetes, diet high in saturated fat | Elevated serum cholesterol | Blood test |
| Atherosclerosis | Genetic, lifestyle, obesity and diabetes, diet high in saturated fat | Occlusion of an artery. Symptoms depend on location of occlusion. | EKG, coronary angiography, blood tests, CT scan |
| Peripheral artery disease | Genetic, lifestyle, obesity and diabetes, diet high in saturated fat | Intermittent claudication, thinning of the skin of the lower leg, ulceration of the skin, gangrene can occur in advanced stages of this disease | Physical examination for ischemia, skin atrophy, pallor, absent pulses, Doppler ultrasounography |
| Raynaud's disease | Unknown | Changes in skin color from pallor to cyanosis, sensation of cold, numbness, or tingling | Physical examination |
| Aortic aneurysm | Atherosclerosis, connective tissue disease, infections, trauma, inflammation | Usually asymptomatic until rupture | Physical examination, ultrasound, echocardiography, CT scan, MRI |
| Arterial hypertension | Older age, sedentary lifestyle, overweight, excessive dietary salt intake, family history | Elevated blood pressure | Blood pressure measurement via sphygmomanometer |
| Pulmonary arterial hypertension | Etiology unknown in many cases, ventricular septal defect, patent ductus arteriosus | Asymptomatic | Echocardiography, pulmonary function test, lung scan, cardiac catherization |
| Varicose veins | Long periods of standing, pregnancy | Swollen veins of the legs, knotty appearance under the skin | Physical examination of the legs |
| Chronic venous insufficiency | Deep vein thrombosis, obesity, smoking, pregnancy, sedentary lifestyle | Tissue congestion, edema, necrosis or skin atrophy, pain with walking | Outflow plethysmography, Doppler imaging studies |

| TREATMENT | PREVENTION | LIFESPAN |
|---|---|---|
| Change in dietary habits, low-fat diet, cholesterol-lowering medication | Healthy lifestyle, diet and exercise, weight loss, low-fat diet | Can occur at any age |
| Weight loss, exercise, control blood pressure with antihypertensive, reduce cholesterol with cholesterol-lowering medication | Healthy lifestyle, diet and exercise, weight loss, low-fat diet | Occurs in adults, older adults |
| Weight loss, exercise, control blood pressure with antihypertensive, reduce cholesterol with cholesterol-lowering medication, | Healthy lifestyle, diet and exercise, weight loss, low-fat diet | Occurs in adults, older adults |
| Abstinence from cigarette smoking, protection of the hands from cold, medications that prevent vasospasm | Abstinence from cigarette smoking, protection of the hands from cold, medications that prevent vasospasm | Most often occurs in healthy young women |
| Surgery to repair aneurysm, control of blood pressure and atherosclerosis | Healthy lifestyle; control of hypertension, diabetes, and hypercholesterolemia | Usually develops after the age of 50 years |
| Blood pressure–lowering medication, diet, weight loss, and exercise | Healthy lifestyle with proper diet and exercise; control of diabetes, hypercholesterolemia, weight loss | Incidence of high blood pressure increases with age |
| Medications to lower pressure, oxygen, lung transplant | Unknown as etiology often unknown, surgical correction of ventricular septal defect and patent ductus arteriosus | Can occur at any age |
| Elastic bandages, support hose, walking, elevating the legs, surgical vein stripping, compression sclerotherapy | Weight loss, walking, elevation of the legs after long periods of standing | Occurs mostly in adults |
| Diet, exercise, compression stockings, surgical bypass procedure | Weight loss, control of atherosclerosis and hypercholesterolemia, diabetes, exercise, healthy eating | Peak incidence is between the ages of 40 to 49 years in women and 70 to 79 years in men |

# DISEASES AT A GLANCE

## Cardiac System (*continued*)

| DISEASE | ETIOLOGY | SIGNS AND SYMPTOMS | DIAGNOSIS |
|---------|----------|--------------------|-----------| 
| Venous thrombosis | Hypercoagulability, vascular trauma, surgery, immobilization | No symptoms in about 50% of individuals. Symptoms of inflammation such as pain, swelling, deep muscle tenderness | Doppler imaging, physical exam |
| Coronary heart disease | Atherosclerosis, high blood pressure, diabetes, obesity, inactivity | Angina pectoris, palpitations, myocardial infarction | Physical exam, EKG, stress test, nuclear imaging, angiography |
| Myocarditis | Coxackie virus, adenovirus, echovirus, HIV | Fever, chest pain, shortness of breath, tachycardia | Echocardiography, EKG, physical examination |
| Dilated cardiomyopathy | Infections, myocarditis, metabolic disorders, genetic disorders, immune disorders | Dyspnea, orthopnea, weakness, fatigue, ascites and peripheral edema | Echocardiography, EKG, physical examination |
| Hypertrophic (A) cardiomyopathy | Unknown | Excessive ventricular growth | Echocardiography, EKG, physical examination |
| Restrictive cardiomyopathy | Endemic in parts of Africa, India, south and central America, and Asia; amyloidosis | Dyspnea, orthopnea, peripheral edema, weakness, fatigue | Echocardiography, EKG, physical examination |
| Infective endocarditis | Rheumatic heart disease, valvular disease, degenerative heart disease, congenital heart disease, intravenous drug abuse, bacterial infections | Fever, chills, change in sound of an existing murmur, vegetative lesion on the heart valves | Blood cultures, echocardiography, EKG, body temperature, blood cultures to identify bacterium |
| Rheumatic heart disease | Infection with group A hemolytic streptococci | Fever, inflammation of the joints, rash | Blood cultures, EKG, echocardiography |

| TREATMENT | PREVENTION | LIFESPAN |
|---|---|---|
| Blood thinning medication, surgery to remove the thrombus | Early ambulation following surgery or childbirth, compression stockings | Can occur at any age, more common in adults and older adults |
| Angioplasty, coronary artery bypass surgery, blood pressure–lowering medication, blood thinners, diuretics, nitrates to stop chest pain, cholesterol-lowering medication, diet, exercise | Control of atherosclerosis; diet, exercise, weight loss if overweight or obese | Occurs in adults and older adults |
| Bed rest to prevent further myocardial damage, treatment of the viral infection | Unknown | Can occur at any age |
| Medications to treat symptoms, rest, heart transplant if severe | Unknown | Can occur at any age |
| Medications to treat symptoms and prevent sudden cardiac death | Unknown | Usually a disease of young adulthood. Most common cause of sudden cardiac death in the young |
| Medications to treat symptoms | Unknown | Can occur at any age |
| Antimicrobial therapy, surgery in severe cases to remove vegetations | Prompt treatment of bacterial infections, prophylactic antimicrobial therapy | Can occur at any age |
| Antimicrobial therapy | Prompt treatment of bacterial infections, prophylactic antimicrobial therapy | Incidence is highest among children and young adults |

# DISEASES AT A GLANCE

## Cardiac System (continued)

| DISEASE | ETIOLOGY | SIGNS AND SYMPTOMS | DIAGNOSIS |
|---|---|---|---|
| Valvular heart disease | | | |
| Mitral stenosis | Rheumatic fever | Increased pressure in the heart, congestion of the veins, cyanosis, congestive heart failure | EKG, echocardiography, phonocardiogram, cardiac catherization |
| Mitral regurgitation | Mitral valve prolapse | Usually no symptoms | EKG, echocardiography, phonocardiogram, cardiac catherization |
| Aortic stenosis | Rheumatic fever, congenital defect, arteriosclerosis | Hypertrophy of the left ventricle, calcified deposits on the valve | EKG, echocardiography, phonocardiogram, cardiac catherization |
| Aortic regurgitation | Endocarditis, dilated aorta | Dilation of the ventricle. Backflow of blood into the left ventricle, decreased diastolic pressure, symptoms of heart failure | EKG, Blood pressure check, echocardiography, phonocardiogram, cardiac catherization |
| Cardiac arrhythmias | | | |
| Supraventricular | Abnormalities in the SA node, AV node, and junctional tissue of the heart, myocardial infarction, hypertension, atherosclerosis, metabolic disease, smoking, and drug abuse | Tachycardia, bradycardia, heart block, syncope, edema, shortness of breath | EKG, blood pressure check, echocardiography, phonocardiogram, cardiac catherization |
| Ventricular | Generated by abnormalities in the ventricular conduction system and in the ventricle, myocardial infarction, hypertension, atherosclerosis, metabolic disease, smoking, and drug abuse | Tachycardia, bradycardia, heart block, syncope, edema, shortness of breath | EKG, blood pressure check, echocardiography, phonocardiogram, cardiac catherization |
| Congestive heart failure | Complication of most forms of heart disease | Shortness of breath, fatigue, edema | Physical examination, EKG, x-ray, echocardiography, blood pressure |

| TREATMENT | PREVENTION | LIFESPAN |
|---|---|---|
| Valvuloplasty, surgical valve replacement | Prompt treatment of bacterial infections, prophylactic antimicrobial therapy, treatment of cardiac symptoms | Can occur at any age |
| Surgery to replace valve | Prophylactic antimicrobial therapy prevents bacteria from colonizing defective valve | Can occur at any age |
| Surgery to replace valve | Prophylactic antimicrobial therapy prevents bacteria from colonizing defective valve | Occurs more frequently in men over 50 years of age than women |
| Surgery to replace valve | Unknown | Can occur at any age |
| Antiarrhythmic medications | Prevention of heart disease | Can occur at any age, most commonly occurs in adults and older adults as a consequence of heart disease |
| Antiarrhythmic medications | Prevention of heart disease | Can occur at any age, most commonly occurs in adults and older adults as a consequence of heart disease |
| Medication therapy includes diuretics, antihypertensive, antiarrhythmic medications, medications that improve cardiac output, bed rest | Treatment of underlying heart disease | Can occur at any age; most commonly occurs in adults and older adults |

# DISEASES AT A GLANCE

## Cardiac System (*continued*)

| DISEASE | ETIOLOGY | SIGNS AND SYMPTOMS | DIAGNOSIS |
|---|---|---|---|
| Shock | Heart disease, hemorrhage, trauma, surgery, allergic reaction, release of bacterial toxins, damage to the central nervous system | Drop in blood pressure too low to sustain life | Physical exam, medical history |
| Congenital heart disease | | | |
| Tetrology of Fallot | Maternal history of rubella, overuse of alcohol, maternal history of diabetes or poor prenatal nutrition. Infants born with Down syndrome | Difficulty feeding, failure to gain weight, poor development, cyanosis, fainting, sudden death | EKG, blood pressure check, echocardiography, phonocardiogram, cardiac catherization |
| Transposition of the great arteries | Unknown | Cyanosis, shortness of breath, poor feeding | EKG, blood pressure check, echocardiography, phonocardiogram, cardiac catherization |
| Septal defects | Unknown | Heart murmur, a vetriculoseptal defect causes increased blood flow to the lungs | EKG, blood pressure check, echocardiography, phonocardiogram, cardiac catherization |
| Patent ductus arteriosus | Unknown | Initially asymptomatic; increased pressure in the lungs can lead to pulmonary hypertension | EKG, blood pressure check, echocardiography, phonocardiogram, cardiac catherization |
| Coarctation of the aorta | Unknown | Increased pressure in the left ventricle, symptoms of heart failure in severe narrowing | EKG, blood pressure check, echocardiography, phonocardiogram, cardiac catherization, Doppler ultrasound |

| TREATMENT | PREVENTION | LIFESPAN |
|---|---|---|
| Rapid administration of fluids to increase blood pressure, medication to increase heart rate | Fluid replacement during surgery, prompt treatment of severe bacterial infections, prompt treatment of allergic reactions, blood transfusion in cases of severe blood loss | Can occur at any age |
| Corrective surgery | Unknown | Occurs in infants |
| Administration of prostaglandins at birth to maintain patent ductus arteriosus, until corrective surgery can be achieved | Unknown | Occurs in infants |
| Large defects require surgical correction | Unknown | Occurs in infants; small defects may persist unnoticed through adulthood |
| Antibiotics to prevent endocarditis, anti-inflammatory medication to close the patent ductus | Unknown | More common in premature infants |
| Surgical correction | Unknown | Diagnosed and corrected in infancy |

# Interactive Exercises

## Cases for Critical Thinking

1. The paramedics are called for a 59-year-old male who is experiencing severe chest pain while playing golf. What type(s) of heart or vascular disease should be considered in this patient?

2. A 65-year-old female reports to her physician with shortness of breath, feeling of faintness, dizziness, and productive cough, all of which have persisted over the past two months. Upon examination, the physician reports a blood pressure of 90/50 mm Hg, congestion in the lungs, and abnormal heart sounds. What type of heart diseases should be considered in this patient?

3. A 30-year-old obese female complains of pain with walking. The patient has a history of smoking cigarettes and is a "borderline diabetic." Explain the role of cardiovascular risk factors for cardiovascular diseases for this patient.

## Multiple Choice

1. Syncope is _____.
   a. hypertension
   b. shortness of breath
   c. lightheadedness
   d. fluid retention

2. Diastole is the _____.
   a. filling phase of the heart
   b. contracting phase of the heart
   c. alternation between relaxation and excitation of the heart
   d. impulse of the heart

3. The major cholesterol carrier in the blood is _____.
   a. HDL
   b. triglycerides
   c. blood
   d. LDL

4. Blockage of the _____ can reduce blood supply to the brain, causing a stroke.
   a. pulmonary artery
   b. carotid artery
   c. aorta
   d. coronary artery

5. The most common cause of an aortic aneurysm is _____.
   a. atherosclerosis
   b. hypertension
   c. enlarged artery
   d. embolism

6. A procedure involving insertion of a balloon-tipped catheter into the femoral artery to the heart is called a(n)_____.
   a. defibrillator
   b. angioplasty
   c. transcatheter procedure
   d. echocardiography

7. The mitral valve is located _____.
   a. between the right atrium and the right ventricle
   b. between the left atrium and the left ventricle
   c. in the atria
   d. in the ventricle

8. The pacemaker of the heart is the _____.
   a. atrioventricular valve
   b. His-Purkinje fibers
   c. ventricle
   d. sinoatrial node

9. An inflammatory disease of the heart muscle is _____.
   a. myocarditis
   b. pericardial disease
   c. cardiomyopathy
   d. coronary heart disease

10. Rheumatic heart disease is also known as a(n) _____ disease because it results from a reaction between bacterial antigens and the patient's antibodies.
    a. hemolytic
    b. vegetative
    c. autoimmune
    d. tricuspid valve

## True or False

_____ 1. Infants born with chromosomal abnormalities have a higher risk for congenital heart disease.

_____ 2. Salt and water restriction is one form of treatment for congestive heart failure.

_____ 3. An interruption of the flow of impulses through the conduction system is called bradycardia.

_____ 4. In ventricular fibrillation, the heart quivers and is able to maintain cardiac output.

_____ 5. In mitral valve stenosis, delivery of blood via the pulmonary veins to the right atrium is impaired.

_____ 6. Cardiomyopathy is a structural disease of the heart.

_____ 7. The most common cause of infective endocarditis is a bacterial infection.

_____ 8. The basic lesion of clinical atherosclerosis is a fatty streak.

_____ 9. Intact aortic aneurysms typically cause symptoms.

_____ 10. Hypertension is broadly defined as an arterial pressure greater than 120/80 mm Hg.

## Fill-Ins

1. The most common cause of chronic venous insufficiency is deep vein _____.

2. More than 90% of patients with coronary heart disease have _____.

3. _____ is associated with reduced heart-filling pressure and endocardial scarring.

4. _____ refers to a narrowing of the valves.

5. The predominant cause of mitral stenosis is _____.

6. Backflow of blood in aortic regurgitation causes the _____ to dilate.

7. An _____ is an excitable focus outside of the normally functioning pacemaker of the heart.

8. A machine called an _____ delivers electrical shocks and is used to re-establish normal heart rhythm.

9. Two forms of cyanotic congenital heart disease are _____ and _____.

10. The _____ arteries provide the heart muscle with blood and oxygen.

## Labeling Exercise

Use the blank lines below to label the following image.

1 _____

2 _____

3 _____

4 _____

5 _____

6 _____

7 _____

8 _____

9 _____

10 _____

11 _____

12 _____

13 _____

14 _____

15 _____

16 _____

# Multimedia Preview

Additional interactive resources and activities for this chapter can be found on the Companion Website. For videos, audio glossary, and review, access the accompanying DVD-ROM in this book.

## ▶ DVD-ROM Highlights

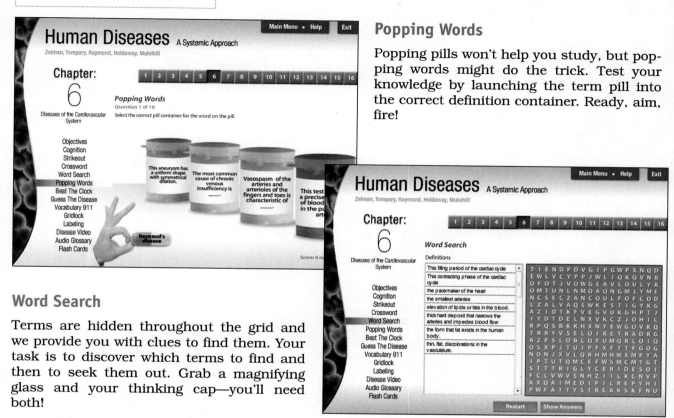

### Popping Words

Popping pills won't help you study, but popping words might do the trick. Test your knowledge by launching the term pill into the correct definition container. Ready, aim, fire!

### Word Search

Terms are hidden throughout the grid and we provide you with clues to find them. Your task is to discover which terms to find and then to seek them out. Grab a magnifying glass and your thinking cap—you'll need both!

## ▶ Website Highlights—www.pearsonhighered.com/zelman

### Labeling Exercise

Take advantage of the free-access online study guide that accompanies your textbook. You'll find a figure labeling quiz that corresponds to this chapter. By clicking on this URL you'll also access links to current news articles and an audio glossary.

CHAPTER

7

# Diseases of the Blood

## Learning Objectives

After studying this chapter, you should be able to

- Distinguish between formed elements and formed elements of the blood
- Delineate the function of red blood cells, white blood cells, and platelets
- Identify the etiology, signs and symptoms, diagnostic tests, and treatment for selected diseases of the blood

## Fact or Fiction?

Sickling of red blood cells results from inadequate oxygen saturation of red blood cells.

*Fact: In 1948, using the new technique of protein electrophoresis, Linus Pauling and Harvey Itano showed that abnormal hemoglobin, the oxygen-binding protein in red blood cells, was responsible for sickle cell disease. Under low-oxygen conditions, the abnormal hemoglobin causes red blood cells to sickle. Sickle cell disease was the first disorder linked to the presence of a specific abnormal protein.*

# Disease Chronicle

## Clinical Use of Leeches

The first clinical use of medicinal leeches (*Hirudo medicinalis*) occurred approximately 2500 years ago. This small invertebrate can produce a small bleeding wound that mimics venous circulation in an area of compromised blood flow. Upon biting a host, the leech releases important substances including an anticoagulant, a local vasodilator, and local anesthetic. These substances allow continued bleeding up to 10 hours after the animal has detached.

Today, medicinal leeches are used by plastic and reconstructive surgeons to restore venous circulation in regrafting procedures for amputated appendages such as fingers or toes. Severed blood vessels are often so damaged that they lack the ability to clear blood. Leeches apply enough suction to initiate blood flow when the patient's own blood supply isn't adequate. Research indicates that after about 3 to 5 days, new vessels in growth around flap margins develop sufficiently to restore effective venous drainage.

## ▶ Introduction

Blood is the medium for transporting oxygen, carbon dioxide, water, nutrients, proteins, and hormones where needed throughout the body and waste products to excretory organs of the body. The cellular components of the blood include the red blood cells, or erythrocytes, white blood cells, or leukocytes, and clotting cells, or platelets. These cells travel through the circulatory system suspended in the fluid portion of the blood called **plasma.**

### Red Blood Cells

**Erythrocytes**, or red blood cells (RBCs), make up about half of the blood's volume. Red blood cells are the most abundant cells in the human body. Erythrocytes normally number about 5 million/mm$^3$ in males and about 4.5 million/mm$^3$ in females.

Unlike other cells in the human body, red blood cells are biconcave sacs filled with an iron-rich oxygen carrying protein called hemoglobin. **Hemoglobin** is the most important component of red blood cells. It is composed of a protein called **globulin** and a **heme** molecule which binds to iron.

In the lungs, heme binds to oxygen in exchange for carbon dioxide. The oxygenated red blood cells are then transported to the body's tissues, where the hemoglobin releases the oxygen in exchange for carbon dioxide. The average life span of a red blood cell is 120 days. Old red blood cells are removed from the body by the liver and the spleen.

Erythrocytes are produced in the red marrow of the bones such as the vertebrae and the body of the sternum. The process of red blood cell formation, called **erythropoeisis,** is regulated by the hormone **erythropoietin.** Red blood cell synthesis begins with large nucleated stem cells that progress through many stages before emerging as mature red blood cells. In the process, hemoglobin accumulates within the cytoplasm and the nucleus disappears. Mature red blood cells emerge from the bone marrow as reticulocytes.

## ▶ Diagnostic Tests for Diseases of the Blood

Blood tests are diagnostic for systemic diseases as well as specific blood disorders. Blood analysis measures total blood counts (red blood cells, white blood cells, and platelets), hemoglobin, hematocrit, serum chemistry, and enzyme and hormone levels within the body. Differential blood analysis provides qualitative information such as size, shape, and ratio of one cell type to another.

A bone marrow smear is used to diagnose malignant blood disorders and increases or decreases in blood counts without any apparent cause. Bone marrow samples are obtained by needle aspiration of the bone marrow from the bone marrow cavity. Bone marrow analysis provides information on the function of the bone marrow and the qualitative characteristics of stem cells that give rise to all blood cells.

## ▶ Anemia

**Anemia** is a condition of reduced numbers of red blood cells. Potential causes, including hemorrhage, excessive destruction of red blood cells, nutritional deficiency, and chronic disease, decrease the number of red blood cells and oxygen delivery to the cells and tissues.

The clinical diagnosis of anemia requires a microscopic examination and analysis of red blood cells. A detailed medical history, including information on dietary habits, family history of anemia, and information regarding the patient's concurrent medical problems provides data for the potential etiology of the anemia.

The symptoms of anemia are due to tissue **hypoxia,** or lack of oxygen. Acute hemorrhages results in rapid appearance of symptoms and, if severe, many result in shock. Most patients develop anemia slowly and have few symptoms. Usual complains are fatigue, decreased tolerance for exercise, dyspnea, and palpitations. In physical examination, the major sign of anemia is pallor. Jaundice and enlargement of the spleen occurs with anemia caused by **hemolysis,** or red blood

# Prevention ✚PLUS!

## Anemia

For a half a billion women in developing countries worldwide, anemia is a lifelong burden that affects most of their infants and young children. Controlling anemia in these vulnerable groups could significantly reduce maternal and infant morbidity. It would also enhance intellectual and work capacity, thereby improving family, community, and national socioeconomic development.

Despite international efforts led by United Nations, the global prevalence of anemia has failed to decline. The reasons for this lack of improvement include the failure to identify the etiology of the anemia, underfunding, and poor health care with inadequate vitamin supplementation.

*Source:* From WHO, 2007, "Iron Deficiency Anemia, Assessment Prevention, and Control. A Guide for Programme Managers."

cell death. Cardiac signs of anemia include tachycardia, or rapid heartbeat, and heart murmurs.

## Iron Deficiency Anemia

Iron balance in the body is tightly controlled and designed to conserve iron for reutilization. There is no excretory pathway for iron, and the only means of iron loss from the body are blood loss and the loss of epidermal cells from the skin and the gut. Normally iron is replaced by sufficient dietary intake or from medicinal supplementation.

The amount of iron required in the diet to replace losses is approximately 1.0 to 1.4 mg of elemental iron per day. In the United States, the average iron intake in an adult male is 15 mg/d and 11 mg/d for females. Iron absorption takes place in the small intestine and is a carefully regulated process.

Iron deficiency anemia is the condition in which there is anemia with evidence of iron deficiency. The first stage in the development of iron deficiency anemia is a negative iron balance, in which the demands for iron exceed the body's ability to absorb iron from the diet. This stage can result from a number of physiological problems, including blood loss, pregnancy, rapid growth spurts in children and adolescents, and inadequate dietary intake. During pregnancy, the demands for red blood cell production by the fetus exceed the mother's ability to provide iron. During the first stage of iron deficiency, anemia may not be present.

The second stage of iron deficiency anemia occurs when the iron stores of the body become depleted. At this point the synthesis of hemoglo-

bin becomes impaired and a period of iron deficiency ensues. With progression of iron deficiency, the red blood cells lose their shape and appear as cigar- or pencil-shaped forms upon microscopic analysis on a peripheral blood smear (Figure 7–1 ▶).

Iron deficiency anemia is the leading cause of anemia worldwide. The prevalence of iron deficiency anemia is greatest among preschool children and adolescent and adult females. Approximately 52% of pregnant women in nondeveloped countries and approximately 23% of pregnant women in developed countries have iron deficiency anemia. The prevalence of iron

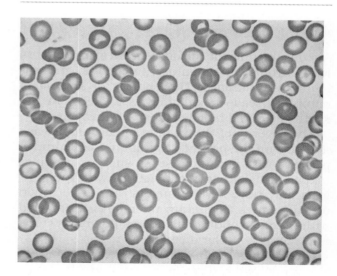

**Figure 7–1** ▶ Iron-deficient red blood cells. (Joaquin Carrillo Farga/Photo Researchers, Inc.)

deficiency anemia among preschool children ranges from 20% in developed countries to 39% in nondeveloped countries.

The most frequent cause of iron deficiency in men and postmenopausal women is gastrointestinal bleeding. In premenopausal women, iron deficiency occurs most frequently secondary to loss of iron with menstruation and during pregnancy. Dietary deficiency of iron most commonly seen in young children occurs when intake of iron does not keep pace with rapid growth and development.

Decreases in iron absorption occur with malabsorption syndromes and chronic disease. Iron absorption requires an intact gastrointestinal tract with healthy intestinal mucosal cells. Chronic disease, removal of the stomach, and bowel disorders limit the availability of iron.

Iron deficiency anemia is associated with weakness and fatigue. Mild to moderate iron deficiency can affect cognitive performance, behavior, and growth in preschool- and school-aged children. Iron deficiency during pregnancy increases overall infant mortality or death.

The treatment of choice for iron deficiency is oral iron supplementation. Injectable iron supplements are available for individuals with malabsorption or those who cannot tolerate oral supplements.

## Anemia of Chronic Disease

Anemia of chronic disease occurs in patients with chronic inflammatory, infectious, and autoimmune diseases. The etiology of anemia of chronic disease most often is a defect in the synthesis of red blood cells, or erythropoeisis.

The severity of the anemia of chronic disease depends on the primary condition. For example, patients with chronic disease such as rheumatoid arthritis or chronic infections with tuberculosis may have severe anemia due to depletion of iron stores. Moderate anemia is associated with cardiac conditions such as angina pectoris and exercise intolerance.

The anemia of chronic disease may resolve if the underlying disease is treated. In some cases, therapy with erythropoietin, a hormone secreted by the kidney that stimulates synthesis of red blood cells, will stimulate production of red blood cells.

## Anemia of Renal Disease

Chronic kidney or **renal failure** is associated with moderate to severe anemia; the level of anemia correlates with the severity of renal disease. This type of anemia is due to a failure to produce adequate amounts of erythropoietin and a reduction in red blood cell survival. Assessment of iron status provides information to distinguish the anemia of renal disease from iron deficiency anemia. Patients with anemia of renal disease usually have normal serum iron; however, individuals on chronic hemodialysis may develop iron deficiency from blood loss through the dialysis procedure.

## Megaloblastic Anemia

The megaloblastic anemias are disorders caused by impaired DNA synthesis. Megaloblastic red blood cells tend to be large and contain an increased ratio of RNA to DNA. The number of red blood cells produced is decreased by ineffective erythropoeisis. Most megaloblastic anemias are due to a deficiency in vitamin $B_{12}$ and/or folic acid.

## Vitamin $B_{12}$ Deficiency Anemia

Vitamin $B_{12}$ is a complex compound that cannot be synthesized by the human body and must be supplied by the diet. The minimum daily requirement for vitamin $B_{12}$ is about 2.5 micrograms. Normally about 2 micrograms of vitamin $B_{12}$ are stored in the liver and another 2 micrograms are stored elsewhere in the body. It would take approximately three to six years for a normal individual to become deficient in vitamin $B_{12}$ if absorption were to cease abruptly.

Vitamin $B_{12}$ deficiency anemia, or **pernicious anemia**, is caused by inadequate absorption or intake of vitamin $B_{12}$ or a deficiency in a protein called **intrinsic factor**. Intrinsic factor is produced in the stomach and is essential for the absorption of vitamin $B_{12}$ from the small intestine. Without vitamin $B_{12}$ and intrinsic factor, the membranes of immature red blood cells rupture easily within the chemical environment of the bloodstream. The result is fewer than normal red blood cells and consequently a reduced oxygen-carrying capacity.

Causes of pernicious anemia include inadequate diet, inadequate absorption, inadequate utilization, increased requirements, and increased excretion of vitamin $B_{12}$. Principal dietary sources of vitamin $B_{12}$ come from animal products. Strict vegetarians who restrict all animal products develop pernicious anemia unless they consume vitamin $B_{12}$ supplements. Abnormal bacterial growth in the small intestine and bowel disorders induce pathological changes that either impair absorption or enhance elimination of vitamin $B_{12}$. Removal of the stomach or the bowel impairs availability of intrinsic factor and limits absorption of vitamin $B_{12}$.

Symptoms of pernicious anemia include abdominal distress, such as nausea and vomiting, and burning of the tongue. Neurological disturbances include numbness, weakness, and yellow and blue color blindness.

Vitamin $B_{12}$ supplementation effectively reverses the effects of pernicious anemia. Because vitamin $B_{12}$ cannot be absorbed into the bloodstream, it must be replaced by injection. Vitamin $B_{12}$ supplementation is required for life for strict vegetarians and for those with chronic bowel disorders or individuals who have had their stomach or bowel partially or fully removed.

## Folic Acid Deficiency Anemia

Folic acid is synthesized by many different types of plants and bacteria. Fruits and vegetables constitute the primary dietary source of folic acid. The minimum daily requirement is normally about 50 micrograms, but this may be increased during periods of enhanced metabolic demand such as pregnancy.

Normal individuals have about 5 to 20 micrograms of folic acid in various body stores, half of which is in the liver. Folic acid deficiency can occur within months if dietary intake or intestinal absorption is decreased.

Folic acid deficiency anemia is common in the Western world, where consumption of raw fruits and vegetables is low. Inflammation of the bowel, as in Crohn's disease, and adverse effects of certain medications impair absorption of folic acid. Body stores of folic acid are small, and folic acid deficiency anemia occurs within a few months. Pregnant and lactating females, alcohol abusers, and individuals with kidney disease are especially susceptible to folic acid deficiency anemia due to increased metabolic demands.

Measurement of serum folic acid levels is conclusive for folic acid deficiency anemia. Oral folic acid supplementation is effective in replacing folic acid and meeting increased requirements for those with increased metabolic demands.

## Hemolytic Anemia

Red blood cells normally survive 90 to 120 days in the circulation. The lifespan of the red blood cells may be shortened by a number of disorders, often resulting in anemia if the body is not able to replenish the prematurely destroyed red blood cells.

Hemolytic anemia is a reduction in circulating red blood cells that is caused by pathological conditions that accelerate destruction of red blood cells. Inherited abnormalities such as hemoglobin defects, enzyme defects, and membrane defects impair intrinsic physical properties that are needed for optimal red blood cell survival. Infectious agents, certain medications, and immune disorders may also reduce red blood cell survival.

Significant red blood cell destruction produces symptoms similar to those of other anemias. Unlike other anemias, hemolytic anemia produces increased serum levels of **bilirubin** that result from the degradation of heme in destroyed red blood cells. Accumulation of bilirubin causes a jaundiced or yellow-orange appearance in the tissues, urine, and feces.

Treatment of hemolytic anemia depends on the underlying etiology. **Splenectomy**, or removal of the spleen, is recommended in cases of inherited causes of hemolytic anemia. Removal of the spleen decreases the risk of gallstones, hemolytic crises, and pathological changes to the bone marrow. Blood transfusions are recommended in cases of severe blood loss such as trauma. Infectious causes can be adequately treated with appropriate antibiotics and other supportive therapies. Similarly, immune disorders can be treated with various immune suppressive therapies. Offending medications are discontinued and rarely restarted in patients who develop hemolytic anemia.

## Hemoglobinopathies

Hemoglobin is critical for normal oxygen delivery to the tissues. **Hemoglobinopathies** are disorders affecting the structure, function, or production of hemoglobin. These conditions are usually inherited and vary in the severity of symptoms.

Hemoglobinopathies are mutations that result from the synthesis of abnormal hemoglobin. The most common hemoglobinopathies are sickle cell anemia and thalassemia.

*Sickle Cell Anemia*  **Sickle cell anemia** is a genetically transmitted disorder marked by severe hemolytic anemia, episodes of painful crisis, and increased susceptibility to infections. Approximately 10% of African Americans have the sickle cell trait or are heterozygous for the disorder. Those with the disease are homozygous or have inherited two genes (one from each parent).

In sickle cell disease, red blood cells contain an abnormal form of hemoglobin, or hemoglobin S. As the red blood cell deoxygenates, hemoglobin S forms cross-links with other hemoglobin S molecules, and long crystals develop. Crystals continue to form as oxygen is released, and the red cells assume a sickled shape.

Sickled red blood cells are inflexible and rigid and cause mechanical obstruction of small arterioles and capillaries, leading to pain and ischemia. Sickled cells are also more fragile than normal, leading to **hemolysis**. Patients with sickle cell disease suffer from hemolytic anemia. Tissue death secondary to ischemia causes painful crises that progress to organ failure with repeated occlusive episodes.

Sickle cell disease is diagnosed on the basis of symptoms and by microscopic examination of red blood cells. The diagnosis is usually established in childhood, and genetic counseling is recommended for parents.

Sickle cell anemia cannot be cured. Patients with sickle cell disease require continuous care. Treatment is aimed at preventing sickle cell crisis, controlling the anemia, and relieving painful symptoms. Painful crises are adequately managed with narcotic analgesics. Blood transfusions and fluid replacement expand blood volume and oxygen exchange needed for reperfusion of occluded vessels.

*Thalassemia*  **Thalassemia** is a group of inherited blood disorders in which there is deficient synthesis of one or more alpha or beta chains required for proper formation and optimal performance of the hemoglobin molecule. Several

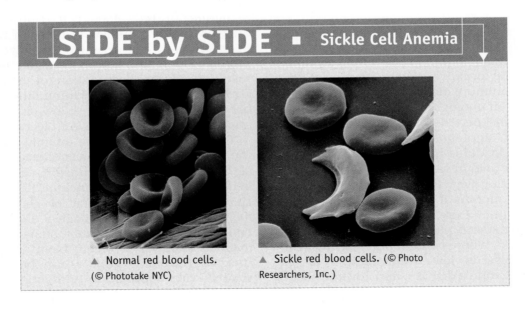

## SIDE by SIDE ■ Sickle Cell Anemia

▲ Normal red blood cells. (© Phototake NYC)

▲ Sickle red blood cells. (© Photo Researchers, Inc.)

different categories of thalassemia produce mild to severe symptoms.

Thalassemias are the most common genetic disorders in the world, affecting nearly 200 million people worldwide. About 14% of African Americans are silent carriers for alpha thalassemia. Beta thalassemia has a 10% to 15% incidence in persons of Mediterranean and Southeast Asia origin. The number of severe cases of thalassemia in the United States is about 1000 annually.

The most severe forms of thalassemia produce severe, life-threatening anemia, bone marrow hyperactivity, enlargement of the spleen, growth retardation, and bone deformities. Blood transfusions are required to sustain life, and life expectancy is reduced.

The diagnosis of most forms of thalassemia is readily made during childhood as children present with symptoms of severe anemia. The red blood cells in patients with thalassemia resemble red blood cells of severe iron deficiency anemia. Antenatal diagnosis of thalassemia syndromes is currently widely available through examination of fetal DNA obtained by amniocentesis or chorionic villus biopsy.

## Polycythemia Vera

Polycythmia describes a condition in which red blood cell mass is increased. This condition is categorized as relative or absolute. In relative polycythemia, the increase in red blood cell mass is due to a loss of plasma volume without a corresponding decrease in red blood cells. This may occur in cases of dehydration or excessive use of diuretics. Absolute polycythemia, also known as **polycythemia vera,** is a rise in red blood cell mass accompanied by an increase in white blood cells and platelets in the absence of a recognizable physiological stimulus.

Polycythemia vera is most commonly seen in men between the ages of 40 and 65 years. The etiology of this disease is unknown, although chromosomal abnormalities have been documented in some cases.

Signs and symptoms of this disease are due to increased viscosity of hemoglobin formed cells in the plasma. Uncontrolled growth of the blood cells can lead to neurologic symptoms such as dizziness, headaches, and visual disturbances. Hypertension accompanies increases in red blood cell mass. Because of the increased concentration of blood cells, patient may experience itching and pain in the fingers and toes. Thromboembolism with death may occur in severe undiagnosed cases of polycythemia vera.

Treatment of polycythemia vera is aimed at decreasing the thickness of the blood. This can be done by intravenously removing blood to reduce red blood cell volume. Chemotherapeutic agents may help suppress the production of all blood cells by the bone marrow. The symptoms of the disease can be managed with administration of pain medications, and antihistamines can help relieve the discomfort associated with itching.

## ▶ Disorders of Hemostasis

Disorders of hemostasis, commonly known as bleeding disorders, include a range of medical problems that lead to poor blood clotting and continuous bleeding. Bleeding disorders result from platelet dysfunction or deficiency, vitamin K deficiency, and clotting factor deficiencies. **Platelets** are blood elements produced in the bone marrow that are essential for blood clotting in response to immediate injury and for the mobilization of clotting factors. Clotting factors are formed in the liver and released in response to disuse injury and platelet fragments to form insoluble fibrin clots. Vitamin K is required for the synthesis of the prothrombin and thrombin clotting factors. Platelets, prothrombin, thrombin, vitamin K, and calcium are essential for **hemostasis**, or the arrest of bleeding.

## Thrombocytopenia

An abnormally small number of circulating platelets, or **thrombocytopenia**, result from conditions that either impair production, increase destruction, or cause sequestration of platelets. Thrombocytopenia is the most common bleeding problem among hospitalized patients.

Careful microscopic examination of the blood is essential in diagnosing thrombocytopenia. Bone marrow examination is useful for diagnosing impairments in the synthesis of platelets.

The production of platelets can be suppressed by malignant diseases or by destruction of the bone marrow most often secondary to cancer chemotherapies and radiation. Up to 30% of circulating platelets are normally contained in the spleen. Conditions that increase the size of the spleen cause increased trapping of platelets. Autoimmune disorders may increase platelet destruction or impair platelet function. Massive blood transfusions dilute circulating platelets and decrease platelet viability.

Regardless of cause, prolonged bleeding results from minor and major trauma. Spontaneous hemorrhages are often visible on the skin as small, flat, red spots called **petechiae**, or as larger purplish patches called **ecchymosis** (Figure 7–2 ▶). Spontaneous hemorrhages may also occur in the mucous membranes of the mouth and internal organs.

Thrombocytopenia can usually be corrected by treating the underlying cause. Preventative measures such as bed rest to avoid accidental trauma are highly recommended until platelet counts increase to acceptable levels. Platelet transfusions are reserved for severe thrombocytopenia or in cases of severe bleeding.

## Idiopathic Thrombocytopenic Purpura

Idiopathic thrombocytopenic purpura (ITP) is an autoimmune disorder resulting in excess destruction of platelets. ITP most commonly oc-curs as an acute problem in children less than five years of age following a viral infection. It is characterized by the sudden appearance of petechiae. Most children recover in a few weeks. In adults, this disorder is chronic and rarely follows an acute viral infection.

The diagnosis of ITP is based on the appearance of severe thrombocytopenia. In patients with a suspected immune disorder, analysis of the blood for the presence of antibodies or phagocytic cells is helpful.

The treatment of ITP depends on the age of the patient and the severity of the illness. Hemorrhage in patients with either acute or chronic ITP can usually be controlled by administration of corticosteroid medication. Removal of the spleen is reserved for patients who do not respond to medications or for those who are severely ill.

## Coagulation Defects

Blood clotting or coagulation is a complex process that involves many different plasma proteins in the control of bleeding. Coagulation involves forming of a blood clot, or a **thrombus**, that prevents further blood loss from damaged tissues, blood vessels, or organs.

Blood coagulation disorders can result from deficiencies or impairment of one or more of the clotting factors. Deficiencies can arise because

**A**

**B**

Figure 7–2 ▶ (A) Ecchymosis (Scott Camazine/Photo Researchers, Inc.) and (B) petechiae (© ISM/Phototake USA).

of defective synthesis, inherited disease, or increased breakdown of clotting factors.

***Impaired Synthesis of Coagulation Factors*** Certain coagulation factors are synthesized in the liver. In liver disease, synthesis of these clotting factors is reduced and bleeding may result. Coagulation factors VII, IX, X, and prothrombin require the presence of vitamin K for normal activity. In vitamin K deficiency, the liver produces an inactive form of the clotting factors. Vitamin K is a fat-soluble vitamin that is synthesized by intestinal bacteria; deficiencies occur when intestinal synthesis of vitamin K is interrupted or absorption of vitamin K is impaired. Vitamin K deficiency can occur in newborns before the development of intestinal flora required for the synthesis of vitamins occurs.

## ▶ Hereditary Disorders

The most common inherited bleeding disorders involve factor VIII, also known as hemophilia A and the von Willebrand Factor (vWF). According to the National Heart and Lung Institute, hemophilia A affects 1 in 5000 male live births and von Willebrand's disease may affect more than 1 in every 1000.

## Hemophilia A

Hemophilia A is an X-linked recessive disorder that primarily affects males. The severity of the disease depends on how the genetic defect affects the activity of the clotting factor. In mild to moderate forms of the disease, bleeding usually does not occur unless there is a local lesion or trauma such as surgery or dental procedures. Mild disorders may not be detected in childhood. In severe hemophilia, bleeding usually occurs in childhood and is spontaneous and severe, occurring up to several times per month.

Bleeding often occurs in the gastrointestinal tract and in the joints of the hip, knee, elbow, and ankle. The bleeding causes inflammation with acute pain and swelling. Without proper treatment, chronic bleeding and inflammation

cause joint fibrosis that can progress to major disability. Intracranial hemorrhage is an important cause of death in severe hemophilia.

Treatment of hemophilia involves replacement of factor VIII chronically, with additional doses administered during phases of acute bleeding. Patients with mild hemophilia A can sometimes be treated with a synthetic hormone called desmopressin. Desmopressin stimulates the release of the carrier for factor VIII, thus causing increases in blood concentration of factor VIII.

## Von Willebrand Disease

Von Willebrand disease is an inherited bleeding disorder that is most often diagnosed in adulthood. There are many forms of this disease that cause a defect in the adhesion of platelets. Because vWF carries factor VIII, its deficiency may also be accompanied by reduced levels of factor VIII, contributing to impaired clotting.

Mild symptoms of von Willebrand's disease include frequent bruises from minor bumps, frequent nosebleeds, extended bleeding following dental procedures, heavy menstrual bleeds, and heavy bleeding following surgery. In severe cases, life-threatening gastrointestinal or joint hemorrhage may resemble symptoms of hemophilia.

Mild forms of von Willebrand's disease are often diagnosed following a severe bleeding episode. Examination of the blood for antigens, vWF activity, and examination of the structure of the vWF provides information on the type of defect as well as the severity of the defects. Examination of the platelets provides information on how well the platelets are functioning.

Treatment of von Willebrand's disease includes medications and lifestyle changes to minimize trauma. Medications are used to increase the release of von Willebrand factor into the blood, replace von Willebrand factor, prevent the breakdown of clots, and control heavy menstrual bleeding in women.

## Disseminated Intravascular Coagulation

**Disseminated intravascular coagulation (DIC)** is a potentially life-threatening condition that involves destruction of the platelets and consumption of clotting factors. DIC occurs in a variety of disorders, such as sepsis or blood infection, endothelial damage as in states of shock, obstetrical complications associated with delivery of a child, and various neoplasms or cancer.

The pathogenesis of DIC involves the release of thrombin into the systemic circulation, causing systemic coagulation and suppression of normal physiological anticoagulation mechanisms. Extensive clotting produces diffuse tissue ischemia, organ damage, and depletion of platelets and clotting factors. The depletion of platelets and clotting factors, also known as **consumptive coagulopathy,** results in extensive bleeding.

The diagnosis of DIC is based on the presence of clinical signs of bleeding in a patient with a clinical condition known to be associated with DIC. Clinically DIC is usually diagnosed on the basis of the underlying disease, observed low platelet counts on a peripheral blood test, increases in bleeding times, and the presence of degradation products in the blood plasma.

Treatment of the underlying disorder is the cornerstone of therapy for DIC. Supportive medical treatments include platelet transfusions, administration of concentrates of coagulation inhibitors, and administration of an intravenous anticoagulant where appropriate.

## ▶ White Blood Cells

**Leukocytes**, or white blood cells, include **neutrophils**, **eosinophils**, **basophils**, **monocytes**, and **lymphocytes** (Figure 7–3▶). White blood cells are synthesized in the bone marrow from their respective stem cells. The primary function of leukocytes is to defend tissues against infections and foreign substances. Quantitative abnormalities, inherited acquired defects, and neoplastic alterations result in disease and disability.

### Disorders of White Blood Cells

*Neutropenia* A reduction of circulating neutrophils increases the risk for bacterial and fungal infections. Because neutrophils are responsible for most clinical findings during an acute infection, the classic signs of infection may be

Figure 7–3 ▶ Neutrophils or white blood cells. (Carolina Biological Supply Company/Phototake NYC)

diminished or absent in a severely neutropenic individual.

Neutropenia is a frequent complication of medication used for cancer chemotherapy or medications used for immune suppression. These medications suppress cellular proliferation within in the bone marrow. Infectious complications depend on the severity of neutropenia and are usually profound and severe in cancer patients.

Immune destruction of neutrophils occurs with rheumatoid arthritis or as a primary condition with unknown causes. Neutropenia may be either mild or severe, and infectious complications are variable. Chronic and severe cases require medical treatment with medications that increase neutrophil proliferation or medications that suppress immune function.

Patients with chronic neutropenia may experience chronic infections. Acute and severe neutropenia may be associated with fever, skin inflammation, liver abscesses, and septicemia, or infection in the blood.

Diagnosis of neutropenia is based on assessment of a complete blood count. Examination of the bone marrow is useful to diagnose bone marrow failure syndromes that may be causing the neutropenia.

The treatment of neutropenia depends on its cause and severity. Sometimes neutropenia may resolve without treatment. Those with mild neutropenia generally have no symptoms and may not need treatment. People with severe neutropenia are at risk for high fevers and severe infections. Hospitalization with isolation and intravenous antibiotic therapy is needed for the severely neutropenic patient.

Growth factors, called colony-stimulating factors, which stimulate the production of white blood cells, are especially helpful for patients who develop neutropenia secondary to cancer treatment. Corticosteroids may help if the neutropenia is caused by an autoimmune reaction.

## Abnormalities of Eosinophils

*Idiopathic Hypereosinophilic Syndrome*   The onset of **idiopathic hypereosinophilic syndrome** occurs between the ages of 20 and 50 years, and there is a strong male predominance. Persistent increases in blood eosinophils and associated involvement of the heart and nervous system are responsible for the most important clinical symptoms. Cardiac involvement produces congestive heart failure, valvular dysfunction, conduction defects, and myocarditis. Congestive heart failure is a frequent cause of death. Neurologic findings may include altered behavior and cognitive function, spasticity, and ataxia.

Prognosis for the idiopathic hypereosinophilic syndrome historically has been poor, with median survival of approximately one year. However, chemotherapy has recently been reported to produce 70% survival at 10 years.

*Eosinophilia-Myalgia Syndrome*   A recently described disorder, **eosinophilia-myalgia syndrome**, is a chronic, multisystem disease with a spectrum of clinical symptoms ranging from self-limited myalgias, or muscle pain, and fatigue to a progressive and potentially fatal illness characterized by skin changes, nervous system abnormalities, and pulmonary hypertension. Elevation of circulating levels of eosinophils is a universal feature of this disorder, and the illness has been related to ingestion of the dietary supplement L-tryptophan.

## Age-Related Diseases

Anemia is the most common blood disorder in persons greater than 75 years of age. The causes of anemia in older adults are blood loss and nutritional deficiencies, chronic illness, and chronic renal failure. Decreased physical performance, mental status changes, and an increase in mortality are among the consequences of untreated anemia in older adults. White blood cell disorders, platelet disorders, and immune deficiency are often due to malignant disease. Neutropenia, thrombocytopenia, and nutritional anemias develop secondary to the malignancy and cancer treatments.

## RESOURCES

National Institutes of Medicine: www.nlm.nih.gov/medlineplus/bloodandblooddisorders.html

Centers for Disease Control: www.cdc.gov/ncbddd/hbd/default.htm

World Health Organization: www.who.int/nutrition/publications/anaemia_iron_pub/en

National Heart, Lung, and Blood Institute: www.nhlbi.nih.gov/health/dci/Diseases/vwd/vwd_whatis.html

# DISEASES AT A GLANCE

## Blood

| DISEASE | ETIOLOGY | SIGNS AND SYMPTOMS | DIAGNOSIS |
|---------|----------|--------------------|-----------|
| Iron deficiency anemia | Iron loss | Fatigue, decreased exercise tolerance, shortness of breath | Blood test |
| Anemia of chronic disease and renal disease | Defect in erythropoiesis | Fatigue, decreased exercise tolerance, shortness of breath | Blood test, evidence for primary disease |
| Vitamin $B_{12}$ deficiency anemia | Impaired intake or absorption of vitamin $B_{12}$ | Abdominal distress, nausea, vomiting, and burning of the tongue | Blood test, health history |
| Folic acid deficiency anemia | Impaired intake, depletion of body stores | Fatigue, decreased exercise tolerance, shortness of breath | Blood test |
| Sickle cell anemia | Genetics: results in formation of abnormal hemoglobin | Pallor, fatigue, shortness of breath, painful sickle cell crisis | Genetic testing, blood test |
| Thalassemia | Genetics: results in formation of defective hemoglobin | Pallor, fatigue, shortness of breath | Genetic testing, blood test |
| Polycythemia vera | Idiopathic, unknown | Dizziness, headaches, and visual disturbances | Blood test |
| Idiopathic thrombocytopenic purpura | Viral infection in children Unknown in adults | Bleeding | Blood test |
| Hemophilia A | Genetic: results in deficiency of clotting factor VIII | Bleeding | Genetic test, blood test |

| TREATMENT | PREVENTION | LIFESPAN |
|---|---|---|
| Iron replacement | Iron fortified diet, iron replacement in high-risk individuals | Can occur at any age |
| Administration of injectable erythropoietin and iron | Treatment of the underlying disease | Can occur at any age |
| Replacement of vitamin $B_{12}$ | Treatment of underlying condition impairing vitamin $B_{12}$ absorption | Can occur at any age |
| Replacement of folic acid | Folic acid–fortified diet | Can occur at any age |
| Prevention of sickle cell crisis; supportive therapy during crisis; blood transfusion | Cannot prevent sickle cell disease | Diagnosed in childhood and persists throughout life |
| Supportive care; blood transfusion if anemia is severe; treatment of iron overload from frequent blood transfusions | Cannot prevent thalassemia | Diagnosed in childhood and persists throughout life |
| Chemotherapeutic agents, blood letting | Unknown | Can occur at any age |
| Corticosteroid medications, splenectomy | Unknown | Can occur at any age; more common in adulthood |
| Replacement of factor VIII | Cannot prevent hemophilia | Diagnosed in infancy and persists throughout life |

# DISEASES AT A GLANCE

## Blood (*continued*)

| DISEASE | ETIOLOGY | SIGNS AND SYMPTOMS | DIAGNOSIS |
|---------|----------|--------------------|-----------|
| Von Willebrand's disease | Genetic: results in decreased platelet adhesion | Bleeding | Genetic test, blood test |
| Disseminated intravascular coagulation | Sepsis, endothelial damage, shock | Bleeding | Blood test; clinical signs and symptoms in high-risk patients |
| Neutropenia | Medications, cancer, chemotherapy, immune disorders | Infection, fever, skin inflammation, and fever | Blood test |
| Idiopathic hypereosinophilic syndrome | Unknown | Cardiac symptoms can lead to congestive heart failure | Blood test |
| Eosiniphilia myalgias syndrome | Ingestion of contaminated L-tryptophan | Skin changes, nervous system abnormalities, pulmonary hypertension | Blood test |

| TREATMENT | PREVENTION | LIFESPAN |
|---|---|---|
| Desmopressin; lifestyle changes to prevent trauma and bleeding | Cannot prevent von Willebrand's disease | Can occur at any age |
| Supportive; treatment of the underlying condition; platelet transfusions | Cannot prevent this condition; difficult to predict when this will occur | Can occur at any age |
| Administration of medications to increase neutrophil count; antibiotics to prevent infections | Cannot prevent | Can occur at any age |
| Chemotherapy agents | Unknown | Can occur at any age |
| Discontinue use of the offending agent | Unknown as contaminants can be present without notice | Can occur at any age |

# Interactive Exercises

## Cases for Critical Thinking

1. E.T. is a 42-year-old female who has been "all tired out" for the past few months. The onset of her illness was poorly defined, and aside from a lack of energy she has no other complaints. She reported being easily winded or short of breath when climbing the stairs or walking for any prolonged distance. She told her doctor that she had recently experienced a slight weight loss following the loss of her mother. What diseases or conditions should be considered in this patient? What additional information do you need to make a correct diagnosis?

2. B.K. is a 65-year-old male admitted to the hospital for surgery. BK had been on blood thinners in the past for the treatment of a clotting disorder. He is fearful of going to the hospital, because last time he had a severe bleeding episode. What conditions should BK's doctors be concerned about? What are some of the symptoms and diagnostic tests that should be considered for this patient?

## Multiple Choice

1. The most important component of red blood cells is

   _____.

   a. vitamin $B_{12}$  b. folic acid
   c. erythropoietin  d. hemoglobin

2. In anemia of chronic disease and anemia of chronic renal failure, the defect in the synthesis of red blood cells is due to a lack of _____.

   a. erythropoeisis  b. iron
   c. hemoglobin  d. folic acid

3. Pernicious anemia is due to inadequate absorption of

   _____.

   a. vitamin $B_{12}$  b. folic acid
   c. erythropoietin  d. hemoglobin

4. The minimum daily requirement of folic acid is about

   _____ micrograms.

   a. 200  b. 150
   c. 100  d. 50

5. Disorders affecting the structure and function or production of hemoglobin are classified as _____.

   a. hemolytic anemia
   b. iron deficiency anemia
   c. hemoglobinopathy
   d. folic acid deficiency anemia

6. Deficient synthesis of one or more of the alpha or beta chains of the hemoglobin molecule is characteristic of

   _____.

   a. hemolytic anemia  b. thalassemia
   c. sickle cell anemia  d. iron deficiency

7. A disease of increased viscosity of the blood with associate neurological symptoms is known as

   _____.

   a. polycythemia vera
   b. disseminated intravascular coagulation
   c. sickle cell anemia
   d. thalassemia

8. _____ is an autoimmune disorder resulting in destruction of platelets.

   a. Disseminated intravascular coagulation
   b. Polycythemia vera
   c. Hemophilia A
   d. Idiopathic thrombocytopenic purpura

9. _____ is an X-linked recessive disorder that primarily affects males and results in a deficiency of clotting factor VIII.

   a. Disseminated intravascular coagulation
   b. Polycythemia vera
   c. Hemophilia A
   d. Idiopathic thrombocytopenic purpura

10. _____ is a reduction in circulating red blood cells that increases the risk for severe bacterial and fungal infections.

    a. Hemophilia  b. Neutropenia
    c. Thrombocytopenia  d. Coagulopathy

## True or False

_____ 1. Chemotherapy increases survival in patients with idiopathic hypereosinophilic syndrome.

_____ 2. Hemoglobin is the most important component of white blood cells.

_____ 3. The production of red blood cells is regulated by a kidney hormone, erythropoietin.

_____ 4. The symptoms of neutropenia are due to hypoxia.

_____ 5. The clinical diagnosis of blood disorders requires careful microscopic examination of blood in a peripheral blood smear.

_____ 6. Vitamin K is required for the synthesis of clotting factors.

_____ 7. Von Willebrand's disease is a hereditary deficiency of vitamin K.

_____ 8. The depletion of platelets in disseminated intravascular coagulation is also known as a consumptive coagulopathy.

_____ 9. Enlargement of the spleen occurs in anemia caused by hemolysis.

_____ 10. The amount of iron needed in the diet to replace losses is approximately 1.0 to 1.4 mg of elemental iron per day.

## Fill-Ins

1. White blood cells are called _____.

2. Mature red blood cells are called _____.

3. Sickle cell disease causes formation of _____ that forms cross links and sickling of red blood cells.

4. Thrombocytopenia is a disease in the circulating levels of _____.

5. The most severe, life-threatening forms of thalassemia are _____ and
_____.

6. The leading cause of anemia worldwide is _____.

7. Vitamin $B_{12}$ and folic acid deficiency anemia are also called _____.

8. Red blood cells normally survive in the circulation for about _____ days.

9. A rise in red blood cell mass accompanied by an increase in white blood cells and platelets is known as _____.

10. The pathogenesis of disseminated intravascular coagulation involves the release of _____ into the circulation, causing extensive coagulation followed by consumption of platelets and clotting factors.

## Labeling Exercise

Use the blank lines below to label the following photos.

1. _____

2. _____

# Multimedia Preview

Additional interactive resources and activities for this chapter can be found on the Companion Website. For videos, audio glossary, and review, access the accompanying DVD-ROM in this book.

## ▶ DVD-ROM Highlights

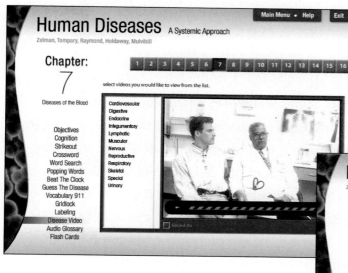

### Disease Investigation Videos

Become a human disease investigator! These videos explore the causes, signs, and symptoms of different diseases. By viewing concepts in moving, living color, you'll get a fuller picture of the pathologies presented in this chapter.

### Crossword

Learning and fun intersect here! Simply use the clues to complete the puzzle grid. Whether you're a crossword wizard or only a novice, this activity will reinforce your understanding of key terms and concepts.

## ▶ Website Highlights—www.pearsonhighered.com/zelman

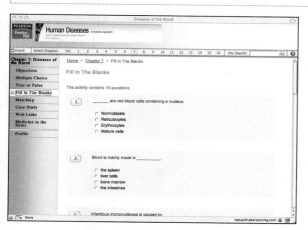

### Fill-in-the-Blanks Exercise

Take advantage of the free-access online study guide that accompanies your textbook. You'll find a fill-in-the-blank quiz that provides instant feedback and allows you to check your score to see what you got right or wrong. By clicking on this URL you'll also access links to current news articles and an audio glossary.

# Diseases of the Respiratory System

CHAPTER

8

## Learning Objectives

After studying this chapter, you should be able to

- Describe the normal structure and function of the respiratory organs
- Compare and contrast upper and lower respiratory tract infections
- Differentiate among influenza, the common cold, and allergies
- Compare acute bronchitis with chronic bronchitis
- Describe causes, symptoms, diagnosis, and treatments of sleep apnea
- Define COPD and name examples, causes, and treatments
- Discuss the causes and treatments of emphysema
- Describe the various forms of pneumonia and manifestations, causes, and treatments
- Explain pneumothorax and atelectasis in trauma, disease, and treatment
- Define pleurisy and describe primary causes, symptoms, and treatments
- Describe the signs, symptoms, diagnosis, treatment, and prevention of tuberculosis
- Understand the conditions and factors that bring challenges for future respiratory diseases

## Fact or Fiction?

Don't go out into the cold with wet hair or you might catch cold!

*Fiction: Viruses cause colds. However, sleeping in a draft, getting soaked in rain, or getting chilled can lower one's resistance to infection.*

# Disease Chronicle

## Respiratory Disease Old and New

**W**hat ancient respiratory disease is associated with disabling and causing death in the time of the pharaohs? The disease is tuberculosis (TB), caused by a resistive bacterium. Besides the lungs, tuberculosis may attack organs such as kidneys and the skeleton (bone). Travel and communications in the days of the pharaohs were very limited, and the spread of this dreaded disease could be restricted to isolated populations.

With the advent of the "wonder drugs" like penicillin in the 1940s, TB was considered beaten in the United States and developed countries. However, today TB kills an estimated 3 million people per year worldwide. This respiratory killer is considered a reemerging disease because it has not been stopped in endemic areas and now is advancing in countries with unstable governments lacking adequate health care. In addition, a more resistant strain of the bacterium that causes TB has emerged. Tuberculosis continues to be not only a major health threat, but the single most lethal bacterial pathogen in the world.

## ▶ Structure and Function of the Respiratory System

The primary function of the respiratory system is to obtain oxygen from the air and deliver it to the lungs for exchange with carbon dioxide and to the blood for distribution. In addition, respiratory structures in the nasal cavity filter, warm, and moisten inhaled air for entry into the lungs. Secondary functions of the respiratory system include coughing, sneezing, talking, and singing, none of which is required for oxygen delivery or carbon dioxide exchange.

Air enters the nasal cavity, or oral cavity, and passes back through the **pharynx**, or throat, and then down through the **larynx** to the **trachea**. Inferiorly the trachea branches into two primary **bronchi**, one going to each lung. The trachea and bronchi are continually kept open by ring structures called tracheal cartilages. The branching continues further into smaller and smaller tubules called **bronchioles**, which lack cartilaginous rings. The branching tubules resemble an inverted tree and are often referred to as the bronchial tree. The bronchioles terminate in the lungs as small air sacs called the **alveoli**. Figure 8–1 ▶ illustrates the respiratory system.

The alveoli are thin-walled sacs surrounded by blood capillaries and are the site of gaseous exchange (oxygen–carbon dioxide). With a moist surface, the alveoli tend to stick together, and

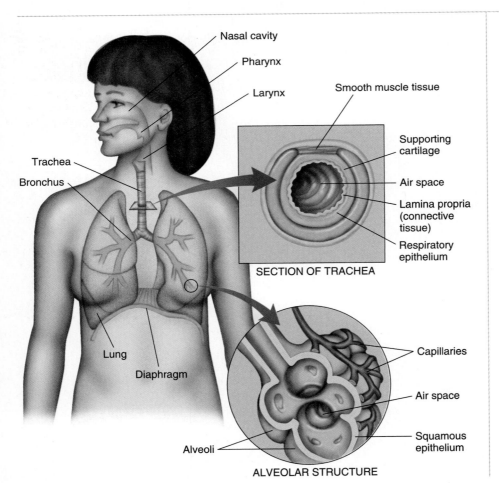

**Figure 8–1 ▶** The respiratory system.

Nasal cavity
Pharynx
Larynx
Smooth muscle tissue
Supporting cartilage
Air space
Lamina propria (connective tissue)
Respiratory epithelium

SECTION OF TRACHEA

Trachea
Bronchus

Lung
Diaphragm

Capillaries
Air space

Squamous epithelium

Alveoli

ALVEOLAR STRUCTURE

therefore an oily lubricant called **surfactant** bathes the inner surfaces to reduce the surface tension. Without the surfactant, the resistance to opening the balloon structures is felt in a distress situation like that found in premature newborns. Oxygen that is inspired, or inhaled, diffuses from the alveoli into the blood capillaries. The hemoglobin molecules of the red blood cells become saturated with oxygen. Carbon dioxide, a waste product of cellular metabolism, diffuses from the blood capillaries into the alveoli to be expired, or exhaled. This exchange of gases is illustrated in Figure 8–2 ►.

To deliver oxygen to the alveoli, air must be inspired into the lungs. The **diaphragm** and the muscles between the ribs called external intercostals are the main muscles of inspiration, or inhalation. Contraction of these muscles increases the volume of the chest cavity and decreases the pressure within the lungs, which allows air to rush in. When the same muscles relax, the volume of the chest cavity decreases, pressure within the lungs increases, and air is pushed out. Other muscles that assist exhalation include abdominal and in-ternal intercostal muscles, which are utilized during times of exertion, for example, running.

The lungs are encased by a double membrane consisting of two layers called **pleura**. One layer of this membrane covers the lungs, and the other lines the inner chest wall, or thoracic cavity. In between the pleura is the **pleural cavity**, which contains a small amount of fluid. This fluid lubricates the lung surfaces, reducing friction as the lungs expand and contract. The fluid also reduces surface tension, which helps keep the lungs expanded. The airtight space between the lungs and the chest wall has a pressure slightly less than the pressure within the lungs. This difference is called **intrapleural pressure**, which acts as a vacuum and prevents the lungs from collapsing.

The entire respiratory tract is lined with a mucous membrane, the **respiratory epithelium**. Numerous hair-like projections called **cilia** line the surface of this mucosa. The cilia exert a sweeping action, preventing dust and foreign particles from reaching the lungs. The breakdown of this mucous membrane paves the way for infection. The mucous membrane also protects the lungs by moistening and warming inhaled air starting in the nasal cavity.

Figure 8–2 ► Exchange of gases between lungs and blood. High concentration of $CO_2$ in blood capillary entering the lung diffuses into alveolus. High concentration of $O_2$ in alveolus diffuses into blood capillary leaving lung.

▶ **Common Symptoms of Respiratory Disease**

Respiratory diseases are common and many share similar signs and symptoms, including the following:

- Breathing irregularities, including **dyspnea** (labored breathing), **tachypnea** (rapid breathing), and wheezing
- Coughs—dry, productive (produces mucus), **hemoptysis** (coughing blood)
- Cyanosis (blue color in skin and nails)
- Fever
- Fatigue, due to labored breathing and less sleep
- Pain, especially sinuses, throat, and chest
- Sinus and nasal drainage
- Weakness of muscles and voice

## ▶ Diagnostic Procedures for Respiratory Diseases

The total lung volume for most individuals is about 6000 milliliters, or 6 liters. In order to have a baseline of pulmonary efficiency, the ventilation levels may be evaluated in two procedures. A vital capacity measurement is done using a spirometer. For this test, as much air as possible is drawn in and then expelled, with the volume expelled recorded. Normal vital capacity volumes range from about 2250 to 4500 milliliters. The vital capacity volume depends on age, gender, height, and general health. By comparing the spirometry test volume to a standard index volume, the test will demonstrate if the person is within normal range or deficient. This quick test will show lung conditions at the time and may well reflect current problems or some conditions from the past or chronic cases.

A second exam procedure is the one-second-forced-expiratory volume ($FEV_1$). This test reveals the maximum volume of air that can be expelled in one second of time. Any impedance of air flow within the tubule system within the bronchial tree, such as spasms, excess mucus, or tubule constriction, will tend to reduce the $FEV_1$.

**Oscillometry** is a newly developed test available to those as young as two years old. This test allows the patient to breathe normally (20 to 30 times per minute) and then it shoots sound waves into the air passageways and, depending on how the waves echo back, it measures the airway opening. Oscillometry helps the clinician distinguish patients who have persistently narrowed airways versus a confirmed diagnosis of asthma. Asthma patients are more at risk to develop damage to their lungs as they grow, and early diagnosis may allow these individuals a chance to improve their outcomes over the course of time.

Especially in chronic pulmonary deficiencies, arterial blood gases (ABGs) are used to analyze and evaluate gas levels of oxygen and carbon dioxide plus blood pH, which is a key indicator of respiratory function. Because of congestion, such as a thick respiratory membrane due to pneumonia or alveolar destruction and scar tissue from emphysema, less surface area is available for diffusing gases. ABGs normally show oxygen levels of 98% to 100%, while carbon dioxide levels are normally 35 to 45 mm Hg at rest. This procedure is somewhat invasive because it requires an arterial puncture to draw blood samples.

Sputum examination is helpful in the evaluation of pneumonia, TB, and malignancies. Gram-stained smears and cultures are useful in identifying causative organisms, determining proper antibiotic treatment, and diagnosing tuberculosis and fungal lung infections.

Several important imaging procedures include bronchoscopy, chest x-rays, and **fluoroscopy**, which permits visualization of the lungs and diaphragm during respiration. Computerized tomography, or CT scans, augment chest x-rays.

## ▶ Upper Respiratory Diseases

**Upper respiratory diseases** are typically infections, allergic reactions, or conditions like nasal polyps that occur within the head and inflame the sinuses, nose, and throat. Many upper respiratory diseases recur depending on current health status, immune sensitivity, and season.

### The Common Cold

The common cold is familiar to everyone. Why is it so common? More than 200 strains of viruses, including adenoviruses, rhinoviruses, and a type of paramyxovirus, are capable of causing colds. Unlike many other diseases, infection provides no immunity because so many strains of virus exist.

A relatively contagious disease, a cold is an acute inflammation of the mucous membrane lining the upper respiratory tract. The virus infection triggers swelling of the nasal mucous membrane and mucous secretion, causing nasal congestion. There is no cure for the common cold, but symptoms can be treated. Aspirin lowers fever, and antihistamines relieve nasal congestion. **Antitussives** control or suppress coughing. These agents may have opoid (e.g., codeine) or nonopoid components like benzonatate tessalon (or a combination), especially for severe cold symptoms (e.g., Robitussin A–C, usually in liquid (syrup) form). Occasionally, secondary infections of sinuses occur, and if they become bacterial, these infections may be treated with antibiotics (e.g., amoxicillin). Simple home remedies like hot soup and rest can be soothing.

## Sinusitis

In the United States, approximately one person in seven (33 to 37 million) has sinus problems, and the widespread nature of this illness costs more than 2.4 billion dollars per year, not counting surgical costs. The sinuses are air-filled spaces that reduce the weight of the skull and contribute resonance to the voice. The cavities are referred to as paranasal sinuses because they all are connected to, and drain their mucus secretions into, the nasal cavity. The sinuses are named for the skull bone in which

they are found: frontal, ethmoid, maxillary, and sphenoid.

In sinusitis, there is inflammation of the mucous membrane linings which causes pressure, pain, and often a headache. Children tend to have ethmoid sinus inflammation more commonly than do adults (Figure 8–3▶).

Sinusitis is caused by viruses, bacteria, and allergens. Environmental conditions such as changes in barometric pressure, airplane flights, swimming, and diving activities may precipitate sinusitis. Inflammation also may follow a tooth extraction or dental work. Nasal congestion may accompany the common cold and can reduce or block sinus drainage and thus cause sinusitis.

Sinusitis may be diagnosed using physical exam, patient history, x-ray, and endoscopic sinuscopy. Nasal discharge may be sent to the laboratory to confirm or rule out bacterial infections.

Over-the-counter drugs like decongestants and antihistamines (e.g., Sinade) are common, inexpensive measures for treating sinusitis. These agents cause swollen mucous membranes

**Figure 8–3** ▶ Paranasal sinuses are part of the upper respiratory system. From here, infections may spread via the nasopharynx to the middle ear or inferiorly to the bronchi.

to shrink. If pressure becomes chronic and painful, the sinuses may be drained with a sinus tap under local anesthesia.

Chronic sinusitis results in painful headaches, along with facial swelling, and requires a host of antibiotics, antihistamines, and steroid regiments. Some medications lose their effectiveness with increased frequency and may be inadequate to resolve the issue because of reinfection and deeper sinuses that are unable to be cleared properly. Some clinicians now use intravenous (IV) antibiotics in a two- to six-week trial in an attempt to avoid surgical measures. Home care procedures allow more flexibility for this IV treatment and an easier lifestyle accommodation. In other cases, a relatively new procedure, **balloon sinuplasty**, similar to angioplasty used for cardiac patients, is used to insert a balloon device into the natural sinus space and restore the normal drainage process. Both procedures are attempts to reduce the need for more elaborate surgical procedures that are more painful, expensive, and require more recovery time.

## Nasal Polyps

Nasal polyps are noncancerous growths within the nasal or sinus passageway. The exact cause of these growths is unknown. Certain chemicals found within these polyps may be the cause. Typically, nasal polyps form along with a sensitivity or allergic response to aspirin and some aspirin-like substitutes. Approximately 5% of the U. S. population is subject to these growths, although they are considered nonallergenic and do not demonstrate allergic responses. Individuals with asthma and chronic rhinitis (nasal inflammation) are susceptible, as are children with cystic fibrosis. Large polyps cause nasal drainage, interfere with smell capability, and occasionally may be linked to obstructive sleep apnea.

Treatment may include nasal sprays with cortisone-like drugs to control allergies, and surgery if the polyps are troublesome. However, even if surgery clears the passageway, it may not prevent the recurrence of the polyps.

## Snoring and Obstructive Sleep Apnea

Snoring is usually the production of exaggerated breathing sounds while sleeping caused by nasal congestion, postnasal drip, or inflamed sinuses. When the congested areas are cleared, the snoring sounds may be resolved. Heavy snoring on a more consistent basis is often a symptom that accompanies a more serious problem called **obstructive sleep apnea (OSA)**, the most common sleep disorder.

Interruption or hesitation of the normal breathing cycle during the sleep period is called **apnea**. The blood oxygen levels fall to a point that alerts the system to the need for a new breathing cycle with such a jolt that a snore results. Some individuals may actually wake themselves up or annoy a spouse or others in the immediate vicinity. On the surface, snoring individuals may appear to be getting a good, sound sleep when in fact they are not.

Sleep apnea is caused by various blockage areas within the air passageways (thus the name *obstructive sleep apnea*). The primary sites that are blocked are found within the nasal cavity, like deviated septum or nasal polyps; the base of the tongue; and soft tissue like the soft palate and enhanced uvula. Obstructive sleep apnea causes heavy, long, and loud snoring and snorting. Four or five episodes of sleep apnea per sleep hour significantly affect the quality of life, while 20 episodes per hour are severe. Extreme cases reach 100 to 500 apneic episodes in a single night. Without proper sleep, individuals awake tired and feel drowsy most of the day while functioning at a low capacity. It is estimated that in 75% of the cases, there is a decreased blood flow to the brain during these episodes. Therefore, the potential for cerebral stroke is increased, especially in moderate and severe apnea cases, which is another factor in seeking quick medical attention. Some studies dispute these findings, but most agree that obstructive sleep apnea is not a healthy situation, and corrective measures are warranted.

The incidence of sleep apnea is highest among middle-aged overweight males, but anyone may have this condition. Estimates are that 1 in 15, or about 6.62%, of the population have sleep apnea and about 70% of those or 4.37% have OSA, in the United States. Another 2% to 4% of Americans are considered to be undiagnosed suffers of this condition, which tends to worsen with age.

Those who are suspected of having OSA undergo a test known as a **polysomnography.** One test method is performed in a clinical setting to monitor brain waves, respiratory and auditory activities, and blood oxygen levels. Another test method allows the patient to be hooked up in an office and then take a computerized polysomnography program home to record happenings through the night; data are returned the next day.

Treatment depends on the cause or severity and ranges from behavioral therapy to mechanical or physical procedures (most common) or surgery. Issues with alcohol and tobacco may need to be addressed, and if being overweight is a problem, may suggest counseling and lifestyle changes. As little as a 10% decrease in weight may offer a 25% reduction in apnea episodes.

Mechanical or physical therapy tends to involve a mask placed over the nose to apply pressurized air into the nasal passages. Moderate and severe levels of obstructive sleep apnea are typically treated using a continuous positive airway pressure (C-PAP) device. This procedure keeps the airways open and clear of any minor obstructive material. Some machines have variable pressure mechanisms to adjust pressure during inhaling and exhaling (see Figure 8–4▶).

**Figure 8–4** ▶ Continuous positive airway pressure apparatus. (Custom Medical Stock Photo, Inc.)

The mask arrangement is somewhat uncomfortable, and about half of all patients eventually stop using the apparatus.

If sinuses or nasal cavities are misshaped or blocked, they need repair. Some patients find more relief with uvulo-palato-pharyngoplasty (UPPP), the trimming of the uvula (including laser treatment) to prevent blockage of the breathing passageway. The success rate using UPPP is about 50%, and it helps those who are not comfortable wearing a mask during the night. The most recent surgical procedure for snoring and sleep apnea is called radiofrequency (RF) procedure or **somnoplasty.** Using radio waves to shrink obstructive areas will allow the airways to remain open and snoring can be eliminated. Portions of the palate and tongue may be targets of tissue shrinkage.

When the soft palate has thickened, or drifts into the air passageway of the throat, a simple outpatient process known as the **pillar procedure** may be used. This technique inserts polyester implants into the palate in order to create scar tissue to contract and stiffen the palate, allowing the throat to remain open through the night. This unblocked area allows freedom of airflow that reduces or prevents snoring and addresses daytime sleepiness. If the palate is weak or drooping down into the pharynx passageway, even during relaxed periods, a **nasal valve procedure** may be used. In this procedure, a clip is anchored inside the nasal cavity and a thread is tied around the sagging section and pulled tight to secure an open passageway. Both of these procedures are performed on an outpatient basis and are relatively inexpensive.

Other control measures to consider when dealing with sleep apnea include avoiding or limiting alcohol indulgence, avoiding tranquilizers or sleeping pills, avoiding lying on the back, treating allergies or irritants promptly, and getting a full quota of sleep whenever possible.

## Hay Fever (Seasonal Allergic Rhinitis)

Hay fever, also called seasonal allergic rhinitis, is caused a by sensitivity to airborne allergens, especially pollens of ragweed and grasses.

Allergens trigger respiratory mucosa to secrete excessive mucus, causing a runny nose and congestion. Mucosal surfaces of the eyes react to the allergens, causing redness, tearing, and itching. Hay fever is the most prevalent chronic condition in patients under age 18 and affects about 1 in 6 Americans.

Because the release of histamine causes these signs and symptoms, treatment includes antihistamine medications. Antihistamines like diphenyldramine (Benedryl) or chlorpheniramine (Actified) are over-the-counter (OTC) medications. These medications do have side effects, including drowsiness, dizziness, or muscular weakness. Decongestants such as pseudoephedrine (Sinutab) may also be beneficial.

Many hay fever sufferers take allergy injections to **desensitize** them to pollen or other allergens. Desensitizing works by administering small doses of antigen and gradually increasing the dosage, allowing the person to produce antibodies against it. These antibodies can inactivate the pollen before it interacts with the nasal mucosa and thus prevent the hay fever reaction.

## Tonsillitis, Pharyngitis, Laryngitis

The tonsils, pharynx, and larynx can be irritated or infected with bacteria, viruses, or other pathogens. Infections of these tissues lead to difficulty swallowing and redness and pain in the throat (pharynx) area.

The palatine tonsils are masses of lymphatic tissue embedded into the lateral mucous membranes of the midsection of the throat (oropharynx). See Figure 8–5 ▶. When infected the tonsils may swell and become painful, making swallowing very difficult. If infections are severe and recurrent, the tonsils may be surgically removed (tonsillectomy). Surgery usually includes removal of the **adenoids** (pharyngeal tonsils) as well.

Pharyngitis, an inflammation of the pharynx, is characterized by pain in the throat. Foreign objects, hot liquids, or spicy foods may contribute to short-term pharyngitis. Breathing through the mouth due to nasal congestion

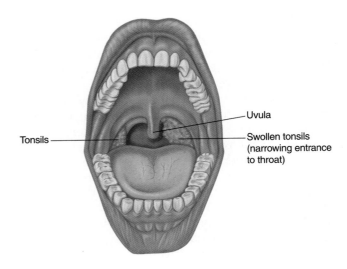

Tonsils

Uvula

Swollen tonsils (narrowing entrance to throat)

**Figure 8–5** ▶ Tonsils; normal and enlarged.

or falling asleep with an open mouth dries the throat and can cause temporary discomfort. Strep throat is caused by streptococci bacteria and is characterized by a red, purulent sore throat. A throat culture or a rapid immunological test can be performed in the healthcare provider's office to confirm the heavy presence of these causative agents in the throat. If throat cultures are inconclusive, blood tests will provide additional confirmation (or rejection) about the patient's status. Treatment includes antibiotics like Penicillin V or antitussive agents with codeine or without codeine, like Benylin.

Laryngitis, an inflammation of the larynx or voice box, is characterized by hoarseness or lost voice (**aphonia**). Bacteria, viruses, allergies, overuse of the voice, or exposure to caustic chemicals and smoke may cause a "lost voice." Antibiotics are used for bacterial infections. A viral infection called **croup** causes laryngitis especially in young children. Symptoms of the croup or other laryngitis forms can be alleviated by resting the voice, drinking fluids, and using steam inhalations. If symptoms do not improve rapidly, such as recurrent fever and continued lethargy, other respiratory conditions like pneumonia should be considered.

## Influenza

**Influenza** is a viral infection of the upper respiratory system. Many different strains of viruses cause influenza. Unfortunately, immunity for one strain does not protect against another strain.

The symptoms of flu are common and familiar. The onset is sudden, and within two days of exposure to the virus, symptoms develop, including chills, fever, cough, sore throat, runny nose, chest pain, muscle aches, and gastrointestinal disorders. The severity of flu cases varies from mild to severe, with pneumonia chief among the complications. The virus destroys the respiratory epithelial lining, and with the loss of this protection, the lungs become susceptible to a host of agents like *pneumococci*, *streptococci*, and *staphylococci*. All of these pathogens can cause pneumonia. Influenza is particularly serious in the elderly and chronically ill, as well as in young children.

No medication cures influenza. Treatments are symptomatic and include rest, fluids, and aspirin to reduce fever. Antibiotics are prescribed to treat secondary bacterial infections. Flu vaccines are available before the onset of the season, typically October and November, and are recommended for those considered at high risk. More recently, children have been advised to participate in the annual flu inoculation programs to reduce risk of sickness and hospitalization. Unfortunately, these flu inoculations do not give immunity for all strains of the influenza virus.

Allergy, influenza, and cold share some characteristics but actually are quite distinct (Table 8–1 ▶).

## ▶ Lower Respiratory Diseases

## Chronic Obstructive Pulmonary Disease

**Chronic obstructive pulmonary disease (COPD)** includes a number of diseases in which the exchange of respiratory gases is ineffective. COPD includes chronic bronchitis, chronic asthma, emphysema, cystic fibrosis, and pneumoconiosis.

*Bronchitis* **Bronchitis** is an inflammation of the bronchi that can be acute or chronic. The mucous membrane lining the bronchi becomes swollen and red, the typical inflammatory response. Irritants such as industrial fumes, automobile exhaust, viruses, and bacteria can cause acute bronchitis.

Acute bronchitis is most serious in small children, the chronically ill, and the elderly. The small bronchioles of children can become easily obstructed. The elderly or chronically ill are likely to have a secondary infection develop, such as pneumonia. Acute bronchitis is characterized by chest pains, **dyspnea**, cough, fever, and sometimes chills. The sputum may contain pus. Depending on the cause, antibiotics may be administered. Viruses do not respond to antibiotics, but vapors, sprays, and over-the-counter (OTC) cough medicines have been given for relief. However, as of the fall of 2007,

# Prevention ✚PLUS!

### Influenza Vaccination

Why do we hear about the influenza vaccine every year? Who should get the flu shot (vaccine)? Complications of influenza can be serious or fatal; on average influenza kills 36,000 Americans a year. Persons considered at risk should receive the vaccine, and that includes children (6 months to 18 years), those over age 50, the elderly, persons with chronic debilitating diseases or immune deficiencies, and healthcare workers. The vaccine formula is different every year because the virus strains are different. The viruses are capable of continual mutation; therefore, the immunity level an individual has in one year may not protect against a different strain that emerges the following year.

## Table 8–1 ▶ Comparison of Allergy, Cold, and Influenza

| Symptom/Sign | Allergy | Cold | Flu |
| --- | --- | --- | --- |
| Onset | Response to allergen | Slow | Fast |
| Duration | > Week | 1 week | 1–3 weeks |
| Season | Spring/summer | Fall/winter | Fall/winter |
| Fever | None | Rare, < 100°F | 102–104°F; lasts 3–4 days |
| Fatigue, weakness | Mild; varies | Quite mild | May last 2–3 weeks |
| Extreme exhaustion | Rare | Never | Early and prominent |
| General aches, pains | Varies | Slight | Usual; often severe |
| Headache | Usual | Rare | Prominent |
| Sneezing | Usual | Usual | Varies |
| Sore throat | Varies | Common | Varies |
| Stuffy nose | Common | Common | Varies |
| Nasal discharge | Clear | Yellow/greenish | Varies |
| Chest discomfort | Sometimes | Mild to moderate | Common; can be severe |
| Cough | None; dry | Yes | Yes; dry hacking |
| Vomit and/or diarrhea | Rare; varies | Rare | Common |

physicians advise children age 6 or less to avoid many cough medicines in favor of saline drip or humidifiers.

Chronic bronchitis is indicated by repeated attacks of acute bronchitis and coughing with sputum production lasting for at least 3 months for 2 consecutive years. It is more common in middle-aged men than in women. In the United States in 2002, approximately 4.4% or 1 in 22 showed signs of chronic bronchitis.

The symptoms of chronic bronchitis are the same as in acute bronchitis, but they persist. In chronic bronchitis, there is an excessive secretion of mucus from the mucous glands of the bronchial mucosa (lining). The mucous glands hypertrophy, and the mucosa itself is thickened and inflamed. The interference in the air passageway caused by the swelling and mucus reduces the person's ability to attain a proper blood oxygen level efficiently. **Hypoxia**, an insuf-

ficient oxygenation of the tissues, results. Poor drainage of the mucus sets the stage for bacterial infection. Parts of the respiratory tract can become necrotic, and fibrous scarring follows.

Chronic bronchitis may be a complication of another respiratory infection. It can result from long-term exposure to air pollutants or cigarette smoking. Respiratory diseases such as the flu or a common cold exacerbate chronic bronchitis. There is no cure for chronic bronchitis. However, the symptoms can be treated with antibiotics and moist vapors. Smoking cessation should be encouraged and clean air environments sought out at all times. When necessary, protective respiratory masks and respiratory therapy may be beneficial.

***Bronchial Asthma*** Following the common cold, asthma is one of the most common chronic conditions worldwide. The Greek derivation for *asthma* is "breathlessness or panting"; both features accurately describe a typical asthma attack. **Bronchial asthma** is the chronic inflammation of the bronchi and bronchioles that has ramifications throughout the lung tissue and denotes a location for the disease. Other types of asthma are known by virtue of timing, like nocturnal, or exercise induced or occupational by work environment.

The incidence of asthma has increased dramatically in the United States and worldwide since 1980 among all ages, gender, and ethnic groups, especially African Americans. As of 2002, approximately 30 million Americans of all ages had been diagnosed with this disease in their lifetime. The disease is increasing more aggressively in those under age 18, and it is calculated that 7% to 10% of children have asthma. Boys have a rate of asthma 30% to 50% higher than the rate for girls, although adult women have asthma about 7% more than do men. The cause of the rise in asthma cases has not been determined and may result from a complex set of factors dealing with environment, such as congested urban areas, processed foods, plus heredity and individual sensitivities.

Asthma kills 15 people daily in the United States, according to the American Lung Association. Bronchial asthma is characterized by hypersensitivity to various allergens, like dust, mold, pollen, animal dander, and various foods. In large urban areas even cockroach remains may act as a trigger for asthma attacks. Eighty percent of asthmatic children and 50% of adult asthmatics have allergies.

Constriction of smooth muscle in the walls of the bronchi and bronchioles narrows the lumen of the tubes. Recall the lack of cartilaginous rings in the bronchioles; this structural change allows spasms to occur. The spasm is caused by a sustained or intermittent contraction of the smooth musculature, making breathing, particularly expiration, very difficult. Figure 8–6 ▶ shows the narrowed bronchi resulting from muscular contraction. The mucous membrane becomes swollen with fluid, and that also narrows the lumen. Excessive secretion of mucus enhances the obstruction. A characteristic **wheezing** sound results from air passing

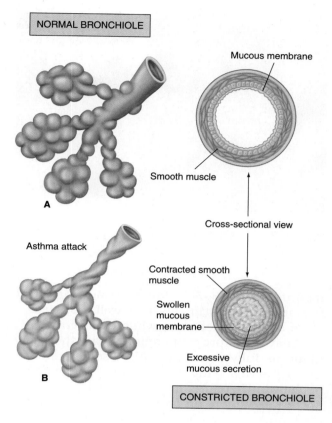

Figure 8–6 ▶ Normal bronchiole (A) and one constricted in asthma attack (B).

through the narrowed tubes. Stale air becomes trapped, which decreases the amount of fresh air that can enter the lungs.

Allergens typically trigger asthma symptoms because most asthma sufferers are prone to allergies. Nonallergenic causes include anxiety, overexertion, infection, bronchitis, and exposure to some aerosol sprays and perfumes. It is important to avoid the responsible allergens and other known triggers. Athletes should warm up before an event to prevent asthma responses caused by sudden overexertion. Asthma attacks tend to lead to fatigue, and a cough that continues to drain away vigor or vitality from an individual may progress to lung infection.

There is no definitive test for asthma, even though a simple instrument, the **spirometer**, can make a relative measurement in a rapid

Figure 8–7 ▶ Incentive spirometer.

manner (Figure 8–7▶). Children under age 4 are not able to perform this test well and need a more sophisticated test, while children ages 7 to 8 may not express or communicate their condition as fully as needed. Also, some tests are inconclusive if symptoms are absent at the time of testing. Therefore, in making their diagnosis, doctors rely more on family histories and thorough questioning about symptoms and allergen exposure.

The growing incidence of obesity has made asthma diagnosis more difficult. More children coming into healthcare facilities and getting diagnosed for asthma are found to be obese.

Therefore, when a child has a long-standing cough, shortness of breath, or wheezing, the parent and doctor should take particular notice.

Skin tests can show which allergens are responsible. Medication and allergy injections can reduce the incidence or severity of asthma attacks. Bronchodilators like proventil (Albuterol), ephedrine sprays, and **epinephrine** (adrenalin) applications are used to relieve an acute attack. Aerosol sprays delivered by a **nebulizer** are effective for acute attacks because they can emit a suspension of very small liquid droplets directly into the deeper bronchiole for immediate relief with little side effects. See Figure 8–8▶.

Inhaled glucocorticoids are mainly used for long-term prophylaxis of asthma, while oral glucocorticoids are used for short-term therapy of severe, acute asthma. Generally, oral medications are given at higher dosage and take longer to act; they are primarily used to help control or prevent attack onset.

Cortisone drugs may be used for prevention and to reduce inflammation, but long-term use is associated with negative side effects. All medications used in the treatment of asthma must be carefully controlled and administered under close supervision of the physician. Drugs are used to prevent asthmatic attacks or to terminate an acute attack. Antihistamines, although somewhat effective for hay fever, should not be used for asthma. A suggested natural remedy is omega-3-fatty acids from flax seeds and walnuts,

**A**

**B**

Figure 8–8 ▶ Nebulizer (A) and inhaler medication (B) delivery devices for asthma.

which tends to reduce inflammation; this may be combined occasionally with NSAID agents.

In the most severe form of asthma attack, called **status asthmaticus**, a **tracheotomy**, which is a surgical opening of the trachea, may be required. If not treated, status asthmaticus may end in respiratory failure and death.

There is no cure for asthma, although attacks may become less frequent or severe after age 18 and older. By learning the trigger for attacks and using proper medical aides, many patients do well to avoid asthma suffering. In older adults, asthma symptoms may return occasionally or be induced by medications and other respiratory ailments. Asthma attacks and symptoms may be caused by environmental occurrences like volcano dust or the particulates experienced by many survivors at ground zero in New York City on 9/11.

*Emphysema*  Emphysema is a disabling and debilitating disease caused by a restriction or obstruction resulting in the destruction of lung and vascular tissue. In emphysema, the alveolar walls break down, adjacent alveoli fuse, and the lungs lose their elasticity. Air cannot be adequately exhaled to allow oxygen to enter, and the lungs become filled with air that is high in carbon dioxide. Symptoms include a suffocating feeling and great distress due to the inability to breathe unimpeded (Figure 8–9 ▶). Intense pain accompanies the difficult breathing. To compensate for the reduced gas exchange, breathing becomes faster and deeper than normal. With the breakdown of alveolar walls, surrounding blood capillaries are damaged or lost, and this causes obstruction of the pulmonary artery. The large weak air sacs, formed by the fusion of the alveoli, tend to rupture. Air flows into the pleural cavity, the thin space between the lungs and the chest wall, causing a condition called a **pneumothorax**. Air in this space causes an increased intrapleural pressure and the lung is subject to collapse, called **atelectasis**.

The cause of emphysema is not known, but it is strongly associated with heavy cigarette smoking. An inherited form involves a genetic deficiency in alpha-1-antitrypsin, which leaves

**Figure 8–9** ▶ Typical appearance of emphysema patient. (Ray Kemp/911 Imaging)

the lungs susceptible to alveolar destruction. Other causes may include air pollution, long-term exposure to chemical irritants, and chronic bronchitis. In studies from the last 25 years, the prevalence of emphysema in the age 45–64 bracket is about 1.5% (or about 1 million), while in those over age 65 is about three times higher, at 4.5% (or about 3 million).

The most significant diagnostic test for emphysema uses a simple instrument, a **spirometer**, to measure the movement and volume of air in and out of the lungs. X-rays do not show emphysema in the early stages. Gradually, over time a physical exam reveals a chest wall permanently expanded, producing a characteristic "barrel" chest. A stethoscope placed on the chest detects abnormal respiratory sounds called **rales**. In addition, the right side of the heart becomes weak due to pulmonary resistance. Therefore, the blood is less saturated with oxygen (hypoxia) and that causes a blue-gray appearance of the skin called **cyanosis**.

Progression of the disease can be controlled by quitting smoking and avoiding polluted air containing smoke, fumes, irritating dust, and ozone, especially on days when the ozone level is high. Medications that clear mucus from the lungs help prevent infection. Emphysema cannot be cured, but some medications relieve difficult breathing. Physical therapy teaches the patient how to use more muscle groups for respiration from the abdomen and chest wall. Prognosis for emphysema depends on age, severity, and general health. Like other chronic conditions, this disease is manageable by close monitoring, for example, the activities of an athlete with emphysema or limitations found by mild exertion in the older patient.

*Cystic Fibrosis*  **Cystic fibrosis (CF)** is an inherited disease that affects the **exocrine glands** of the body, causing them to excessively secrete a viscous type of mucus which block gland ducts and prevents the glands from delivering their products. Exocrine glands are common glands that secrete mucus, wax, perspiration, and digestive enzymes.

The most serious manifestation of cystic fibrosis is in the respiratory system. The trachea and bronchi secrete thick mucus that accumulates and blocks the air passageway. Symptoms of cystic fibrosis are dyspnea, wheezing, persistent cough, and thick sputum. The abnormally thick mucosal surface increases susceptibility to recurrent bacterial infections. Bronchiectasis (weakened and dilated bronchial tubing) is a common complication of cystic fibrosis. Brochiectasis is not a disease but a sequela or residual effect of chronic inflammation and congestion. Lung collapse can result from the inability to inflate the lungs, and most deaths caused by CF involve younger adults and occur as a result of respiratory failure. Table 8–2 ► describes complications of cystic fibrosis.

Excessive mucus also blocks the ducts of the pancreas, preventing the release of digestive enzymes and resulting in weight loss and malnutrition. The lack of proper fat digestion results in a large, bulky, foul-smelling stool. In the pancreas, the secretory glands become dilated and develop into cysts containing thick mucus. Fibrous tissue then develops, which explains how cystic fibrosis gets its name.

Cystic fibrosis is recognized as a hereditary disease that first becomes manifested in young children. It is transmitted through a recessive gene carried by each parent (see Chapter 5). Before the disease was understood, the mortality rate of children was extremely high. Early diagnosis and treatment has greatly improved the prognosis and longevity.

In cystic fibrosis, the sweat glands excrete excessive perspiration and large amounts of salt, causing susceptibility to heat exhaustion. This increased excretion of salt in sweat is the basis for a "sweat test" that helps confirm cystic fibrosis.

Basic treatment includes pancreatic enzyme supplements that can be given with food. Antibiotic treatment reduces the incidence of respiratory tract infection, and regular respiratory

| Table 8–2 ► Complications of Cystic Fibrosis | |
|---|---|
| Malnutrition | Blockage of pancreatic duct prevents secretion of digestive enzymes and inability to digest and absorb nutrients |
| Dyspnea, lung collapse | Blocked airways, bronchiectasis (weakened airways) |
| Recurrent respiratory infections | Abnormal mucosal lining<br>Inability to clear thick mucus |
| Electrolyte imbalance | Abnormal salt excretion |

therapy relieves congestion in the respiratory tract.

*Pneumoconiosis* **Pneumoconiosis** is a COPD caused by dust particles that seem to infiltrate or embed into lung tissue. As a result of incomplete filtering by the normal action within the air passageways because of overload, the individual accumulates "grit" in the lungs, which causes shortness of breath, some wheezing, and low physical endurance. The dust usually is the result of industrial mining of coal and stone or milling of grains or environmental activity like asbestosis or volcanoes. Following respiratory testing by x-ray, spirometry, and exercise, individuals get some relief with bronchodilators to ease breathing and corticoid medications to reduce inflammation. Pneumoconiosis claims about 1100 victims per year in the United States.

## Pneumonia

**Pneumonia** is an acute inflammation of the lungs in which air spaces in the lungs become filled with an inflammatory exudate (fluid). Pneumonia can be caused by a variety of microorganisms, and it may affect different areas within the lungs. Aside from the infirmed or indigent and the vulnerable elderly, pneumonia typically runs in seasonal or cyclical patterns, somewhat like the flu.

Symptoms include dyspnea, fever, chest pain, and a productive cough. Listening to lung activity, a chest x-ray, and analysis of sputum can diagnose pneumonia and determine its cause.

*Lobar Pneumonia* **Lobar pneumonia** is inflammation of a section, often an entire lobe, of the lung. Lobar pneumonia is usually caused by the pneumococcus bacterium *Streptococcus pneumoniae.* Many people carry this bacterium in their respiratory passages, and it can infect the lungs under particular conditions or situations, like a weakened state (broken hip) or challenged immune system (Figure 8–10 ▶). Influenza, chronic bronchitis, and a weakened immune system increase the risk of developing lobar pneumonia.

Antibiotics like penicillin or amoxicillin are a common treatment.

*Bronchopneumonia* **Bronchopneumonia** is a form of pneumonia focused in small bronchi. Infection and inadvertent aspiration of gastric contents or vomit are common causes. Because many foci (sites) of infection develop in the various bronchi, the chest x-ray will show a diffuse pattern of inflammation. This type of pneumonia is more common in debilitated patients who are less mobile or bedridden from other diseases. Major factors that increase the risk for bronchopneumonia include

- Chronic bronchitis
- Measles or whooping cough
- Bronchiectasis
- Old age
- Cancer

*Primary Atypical Pneumonia* Also known as "walking pneumonia," **primary atypical pneumonia** is caused by a variety of pathogens, including viruses and atypical bacteria like *Mycoplasma pneumoniae.* Interstitial pneumonia, common in viral pneumonia, is a descriptive term denoting the diffuse pattern of the disease spread within the lungs on the x-ray. This disease is more common among adolescents and young adults due to crowded conditions in schools and contacts made by sharing of facilities and contaminated items. Initially, flu-like symptoms prevail, such as fatigue, fever, general weakness, headache, sore throat, and stomach and intestinal distress. This disease may not require a visit to a healthcare provider for otherwise healthy individuals who continue to go to school or work and keep up a basic routine. However, children and overstressed or more severely impacted individuals may suffer from pneumonia and other respiratory complications that require immediate attention to prevent hospitalization or home care. Advanced cases of pneumonia may be more common and serious for those with diabetes, cirrhosis, sickle cell disease, or cancer. Hospitalization may be required along with rest and a medication schedule to

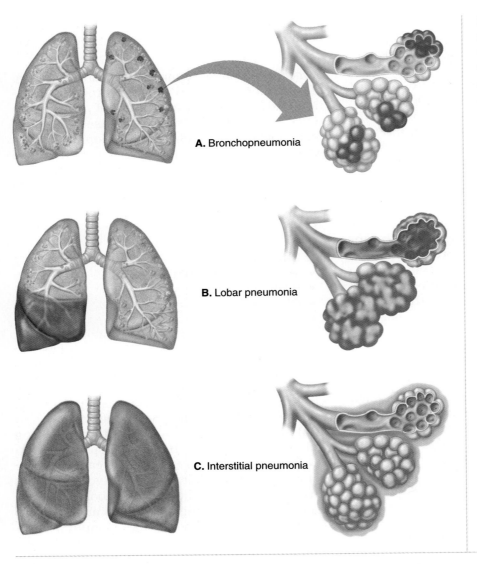

**A.** Bronchopneumonia

**B.** Lobar pneumonia

**C.** Interstitial pneumonia

**Figure 8–10** ▶ (A) Bronchopneumonia with localized pattern. (B) Lobar pneumonia with a diffuse pattern within the lung lobe. (C) Interstitial pneumonia is typically diffuse and bilateral.

treat and clear the lungs of the fluid buildup and congestion.

***Secondary Pneumonia*** Pneumonia can develop as a secondary disorder from other diseases that weaken the lungs or the body's immune system. Graft recipients and immunocompromised subjects, especially HIV/AIDS patients, are susceptible to pneumonia caused by unusual infectious agents like the fungi *Pneumocystis carini* and *Cryptococcus neoformans*. Postoperative patients, bedridden patients, and those with chronic respiratory illness may lack the ability to clear their lungs effectively and thus are at risk for developing pneumonia.

Perhaps the most dangerous **secondary pneumonia** is the one acquired as a complication of influenza. It was responsible for most of the estimated 20 million deaths worldwide in the influenza epidemic of 1918 to 1919. This devastating disease apparently started in the United States. It was carried to (and from) Europe by the huge influx of American troops and support personnel and always precipitated into double pneumonia (both lungs). Today, influenza still causes many cases of pneumonia; therefore, the flu vaccine is strongly recommended for persons at risk to prevent or reduce flu symptoms.

***Legionnaire's Disease*** This lung infection is caused by the bacterium *Legionella pneumophila.* The disease is predominately acquired by inhaling small droplets contaminated with the bacteria from large air conditioning cooling systems, humidifiers, hot tubs, and other equipment or environmental condition that produces contaminated aerosol water droplets. It is accompanied by flu-like symptoms, which sets it apart from other pneumonias, like lobar, and therefore suggests another atypical form of pneumonia. Because this is a serious and potentially fatal disease, it is important to differentiate it from other forms of pneumonia using sputum cultures and chest x-rays. The antibiotic erythromycin is the treatment of choice.

Residual effects of pneumonia, regardless of its form, occur in many victims and lead to long-term problems like fatigue, coughing, shortness of breath, and neuromuscular impairments. Complications from pneumonia range from lung abscesses to lung collapse and respiratory failure. In atypical forms of pneumonia, the symptoms may linger, as in "walking pneumonia" that may not be diagnosed or reported, or may be very severe, as with Legionnaires' disease. In general, pneumonia attacks over one million Americans per year and kills between 40,000 and 70,000 annually in the United States.

## Pleurisy (Pleuritis)

**Pleurisy** is an inflammation of the pleural membranes that occurs as a complication of various lung diseases, such as pneumonia or tuberculosis. It may also develop from an infection, trauma injury, or tumor formation. In addition to a cough, fever, and chills, pleurisy is ex-

tremely painful, with a sharp, stabbing pain accompanying each inspiration. The pain may stem from an excess or deficiency of pleural fluid, or from pus or blood in the pleural space. It is treated with antibiotics, heat applications, and bed rest.

## Pulmonary Tuberculosis

**Pulmonary tuberculosis (TB)** is a chronic infectious disease characterized by necrosis of vital lung tissue. Although TB most commonly attacks the respiratory system, it can secondarily attack, in similar fashion, other body systems as well (e.g., bone).

Tuberculosis is caused by the bacterium *Mycobacterium tuberculosis* and related bacteria. These bacteria are most commonly transmitted in contaminated sputum expelled in the coughs of infected persons, although tuberculosis can also be caused by contaminated milk from infected cattle. Expelled sputum may dry and settle in dust that can contain infective bacteria for a long time. Close quarters or contacts promote the spread of TB due to its contagious properties. Crowded campuses, cities, or airplanes are potential sites of tuberculosis exposure and outbreaks.

The inhaled bacteria infect the lungs and induce a chronic inflammatory response that leads to necrosis. The tissue in this site becomes soft and cheeselike, which is why it is described as a **caseous** lesion. The tissue heals with fibrosis and calcification, walling off the bacteria into pockets for months or many years. These lesions are called **tubercles**. During this period, a person may have no symptoms. A secondary infection occurs when the person is infected again or when the bacteria escape the walled-off lesions in the lungs. The bacteria may spread this way when resistance is reduced because of stress, infection, malnutrition, or immunodeficiency. During the secondary infection, leukocytes now recognize the bacteria and mount an attack that leads to greater necrosis and destruction of lung tissue. Necrotic tissue, blood, and bacteria may be coughed up. The bacteria may spread to other organs like the brain, kidney, and bones. Those in the secondary stage of the disease also lose weight and become cachectic (wasting away); this is the basis for the classic name for tuberculosis, *consumption.*

Screening for tuberculosis involves the Mantoux skin test, in which antigens from the bacteria are injected beneath the skin. If previously exposed to tuberculosis, the skin swells with slight elevation at the injection site. A positive skin test should be followed up with a sputum culture and a chest x-ray to determine if there is an active infection. Active infections are dangerous because they put others at risk for TB infection.

Antibiotics specially designed for *Mycobacterium* species include rifampin, isoniazid, and ethambutol. The drugs must be taken over an extended period of time, perhaps as long as 18 months, to ensure that the bacteria are killed or eliminated. This waxy coated bacterium is resilient and difficult to treat generally because it can be sealed in lung tissue (tubercles) or antibiotic resistant.

Tuberculosis is relatively uncommon in much of the United States, but its incidence has increased since the 1980s and 1990s. The evolution of antibiotic-resistant bacteria and the increased numbers of HIV-infected people, homeless people, and immigrants contribute to this increase (Table 8–3 ▶).

Worldwide, however, the incidence of tuberculosis is rising rapidly, especially in Asia, Russia, and parts of Africa. In fact, tuberculosis remains the largest cause of death due to infectious disease, killing 3000 people per day worldwide, and is a major cause of death among people infected with HIV. More than one-third of the world's population has been exposed to *Mycobacterium tuberculosis.*

## Thoracic Trauma and Pulmonary Distress

**Pneumothorax** literally suggests "air in chest." This condition involves the accumulation of air that escapes its normal entrapment within the lung, or outside air that enters from a breach in the chest wall (e.g., stab wound or gun shot). When the internal chest (intrapleural) pressure exceeds the internal lung pressure, then the lung will collapse, an event known as **atelectasis.** This term may also apply to lungs that fail to inflate in premature infants. Because these two events often occur together, they are considered to be the same thing.

Pneumothorax most commonly occurs in cases involving newborns that have a stiff or inflexible lung and results in **infant respiratory distress syndrome (IRDS).** Other cases involve ventilators or continuous positive airway pressure (CPAP) devices that may cause air to seep into the thorax. Acute atelectasis may compound the

| Table 8–3 ▶ Summary of Tuberculosis Increase in the United States | |
|---|---|
| **Primary Cause** | **Secondary/Support Causes for TB Spread** |
| Drug-resistant bacteria | More infections that cannot be treated with a single drug<br>More infections resistant to multiple drugs<br>Infections last longer and expose more people |
| Homeless/refugees/poverty | Reduced access to health care, screening, and treatment<br>Living conditions, malnutrition, and other infections increase susceptibility |
| Immigration | Infected immigrants from areas where the disease is endemic, prevalent, drug-resistant, and where there is little health care |
| HIV/AIDS | Reduced resistance and increased susceptibility to disease |

situation, and cause a reduced blood pressure because the relatively higher (internal) chest pressure slows blood flow to the heart. Therefore, with a circulatory deficiency, immediate medical attention is required. A needle and syringe are used to siphon air within the thorax to let the air pressure subside and allow the lung and chest membranes to adhere and reestablish their bond. A tube for ventilation may be left in place for a day or two to ensure complete adjustment.

If the internal pressure is slight or symptoms are not apparent, a healthcare provider may discover the problem when listening to each lung and noticing a lower sound quality to the air entering and leaving the lung on the side where the pneumothorax exists. Premature infants may receive a fiber optic examination that provides a transillumination effect and makes the defect more visible. In these cases the infant may be placed in an oxygen hood to assist breathing efforts.

Atelectasis may involve the whole lung or a partial lung that becomes airless or contracts. The primary reason the collapse comes about is an obstruction of a major bronchus. Blockage may be excess internal mucus forming a plug, a foreign object inadvertently inhaled, or a tumor or excessive fluid buildup in the pleural space. Accidental or acute atelectasis may result from a car accident involving chest compression or a fall onto a hard surface or object. Symptoms include shortness of breath, increased heart rate, and cyanotic appearance because the blood oxygen levels are low due to lack of respiratory function.

Diagnosis requires a physical exam and possibly a chest x-ray or CT scan: If obstruction is suspected, a bronchoscope may pinpoint the occluded site and assist removal. Antibiotics may be prescribed to reduce potential or anticipated infection that frequently develops in traumatized or inflamed tissues. If a chronic atelectasis situation ensues due to (slow) tumor development, residual excess fluid from unresolved pneumonia, or scarred areas, ventilation and antibiotics may be in order.

**Adult respiratory distress syndrome (ARDS)** may develop due to aspiration or inhalation of food or vomit material into the respiratory pathways. Heavy smoke from a burning structure or toxic fumes may scar the respiratory linings of the tubules and cause them to become less able to function. Oxygen assistance and respiratory therapy along with antibiotics and rest help resolve most cases. Chronic bronchitis or asthma symptoms may become considerations in advanced cases.

**Bronchogenic carcinoma** is the most common type of lung cancer, causing 28% of all cancer deaths worldwide, making it the leading cause of death from cancer among both men and women. *Bronchogenic* implies that the cancer originated in the bronchi of the lung versus another site. In addition to primary carcinoma of the lungs, the lungs are a frequent site of metastases from the breast, gastrointestinal (GI) tract, female reproductive system, and kidneys.

The great danger in bronchogenic carcinoma is blockage of the airway by the malignant tumor as it grows into the lumen of a bronchus, causing collapse of the affected part of the lung. Few symptoms or signs accompany early stage lung cancer, but symptoms of later stages include a persistent cough and hemoptysis. The blood in the sputum results from the erosion of blood vessels by the growing malignancy. Anorexia, weight loss, and weakness accompany the disease, caused partly by poor oxygenation of the blood. Other symptoms include difficulty in breathing caused by airway obstruction due to compression and body fluids such as mucus and blood. Because these symptoms develop late in the disease, when metastasis is likely to have occurred, immediate and aggressive treatment is in order. Prevention or early detection is preferred but not always achievable. At present, however, the average age for diagnosis is 60, and it is likely that many of these cancers began years earlier.

Approximately 80% of lung cancer is related to cigarette smoking, and it is 10 times more common in smokers than in nonsmokers. Other related causes include inhalation of carcinogens from second-hand smoke that kills 3000+ nonsmokers per year. Second-hand smoke increases the risk of developing lung cancer by 20% to 30%. Occupational hazards among

# SIDE by SIDE  ■  Lung Cancer

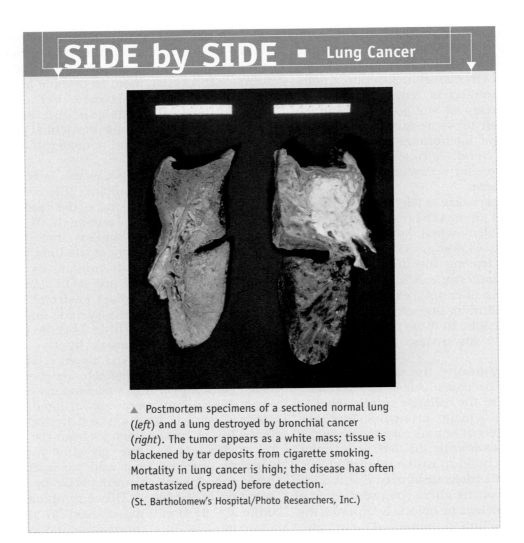

▲ Postmortem specimens of a sectioned normal lung (*left*) and a lung destroyed by bronchial cancer (*right*). The tumor appears as a white mass; tissue is blackened by tar deposits from cigarette smoking. Mortality in lung cancer is high; the disease has often metastasized (spread) before detection.

(St. Bartholomew's Hospital/Photo Researchers, Inc.)

workers also increase the probability of lung cancer due to a constant exposure to air pollution from exhaust gases and industrial fumes.

Diagnosis of lung cancer is made via x-ray, a biopsy of the tumor, detection of cancer cells in the sputum, or washings from the bronchoscopy examination. Coughing up blood is a major sign of lung cancer.

Treatment includes surgery that does not cure cancer but reduces a central source and mass, which allows other treatments to work. Where possible, radiation and/or chemotherapy are common approaches depending on the particular circumstance of tumor size, location, and general health.

## ▶ Age-Related Diseases

Because respiratory infections are generally highly contagious, they are common among infants and children. Historically, children have suffered a high mortality rate from diphtheria, pertussis, measles, and other contagious respiratory diseases. Vaccinations for these and other respiratory diseases have significantly reduced mortality in the United States. However, around the world where vaccines are unavailable, these diseases continue to kill many children.

The onset of asthma may be early or later in life, and while some cases of early-onset asthma may resolve, later-onset asthma generally tends to persist, but with less frequent attacks and at a reduced impact. Untreated sleep apnea tends to get worse with advancing years.

In the elderly, elastic tissue of the lungs deteriorates and reduces lung capacity in normal situations. This condition is exacerbated by weakening of respiratory muscles and arthritis in joints of the ribs and vertebrae. Prescribed exercises performed regularly can help maintain or improve lung capacity and benefit the cardiovascular system as well.

Some degree of emphysema occurs in many individuals age 50 to 70. On average, one square foot of the respiratory membrane is lost each year after age 30. Again, routine aerobic exercise or walking helps keep lungs in a healthier state.

The incidence of lung cancer increases with age. However, the cancer probably begins earlier in life, and this incidence reflects the relatively late age at diagnosis. Earlier treatment is crucial for a better life. Even with cancer, pneumonia will likely be the final disease and actual cause of death in the elderly who are weak and frail.

## RESOURCES

Centers for Disease Control and Prevention:
www.cdc.gov/nchs/fastats/asthma.htm
www.cdc.gov/tobacco/data_statistics/factsheets/
health_effects.htm

National Heart, Lung, and Blood Institute:
www.nhlbi.nih.gov

National Institutes of Health:
www.nlm.nih.gov/medlineplus

Stanford University:
www.stanford.edu/~dement/apnea.html

World Health Organization: www.who.org

# DISEASES AT A GLANCE

## Respiratory System

| DISEASE | ETIOLOGY | SIGNS AND SYMPTOMS | DIAGNOSIS |
|---------|----------|--------------------|-----------| 
| **Upper Respiratory** | | | |
| Pharyngitis | Bacteria, viruses, irritants | Red, sore throat; pus; dysphagia | Physical exam, throat culture |
| Tonsillitis | Bacteria, viruses, irritants | Sore throat, swollen tonsils, dysphagia | Physical exam, throat culture |
| Laryngitis | Bacteria, viruses, irritants | Sore throat, difficulty speaking | Physical exam |
| Common cold | Paramyxoviruses | Nasal congestion, cough, sore throat | Physical exam |
| Seasonal allergic rhinitis (hay fever) | Airborne allergens, pollens | Nasal and sinus congestion; watery, itchy eyes | Physical exam, allergy tests |
| Influenza | Viruses | Fever, headache, weakness, body aches | Physical exam |
| **Lower Respiratory** | | | |
| Asthma | Allergies, fumes, heavy exertion, roaches | Dyspnea, difficulty exhaling, wheezing | Spirometry, physical exam, family history |
| Bronchogenic carcinoma (lung cancer) | Smoking, fumes, air pollution | Obstruction of airways and associated complications, weight loss, weakness | Bronchoscopy, x-ray, CT scan, biopsy, sputum evaluation |
| Chronic bronchitis | Fumes, bacteria, viruses, smoking | Chest pains, dyspnea, chronic productive cough | Patient history, physical exam |
| Cystic fibrosis | Genetic, chromosome 7, recessive | Recurrent lung infections, dypsnea, coughing and lung obstruction, weight loss due to poor absorption of fats and vitamin D | Sweat test for excess salt |
| Emphysema | Cigarette smoking, fumes, genetic | Difficulty exhaling, cyanosis, fatigue, barrel chest, pneumonia as complication | Spirometry, physical exam |
| Pneumonia | Bacteria, viruses, fungi | Chest pain, fluid in lungs on x-ray, fever, productive cough | Chest x-ray, sputum analysis |
| Pulmonary tuberculosis | Mycobacterium | Primary may be asymptomatic, secondary with fever, weakness, weight loss/cachexia, cough producing blood, tissue, bacteria | Chest x-ray, skin test, sputum analysis |

| TREATMENT | PREVENTION | LIFESPAN |
|---|---|---|
| If bacterial, antibiotics | Maintain good health and hygiene; do not smoke or eat or drink spicy foods | Occurs at all ages |
| Antibiotics if bacterial infections | Maintain good health and hygiene; treat common cold | Typically in children, but also adults |
| Resting voice, steam inhalations, higher fluid intake | Maintain good health and hygiene; reduce voice usage | Occurs at any age |
| Antihistamines, aspirin | Reduce exposure, but difficult to prevent | Any and all ages |
| Antihistamines rhinitis (hay fever) | Reduce exposure, take medication as needed | Some are more susceptible |
| Bed rest, fluids, aspirin | Difficult especially in "flu" season, reduce exposure, vaccine for those with compromised health | Especially very young, compromised adolescents, elderly |
| Ephedrine sprays, epinephrine, cortisone-like drugs, allergy shots | With hereditary markers and/or environmental inducements may not be preventable. Do not smoke | Children, and middle age to older adults |
| Radiation, chemotherapy, surgery | Do not smoke, limit exposure in work environment if possible | Usually adults |
| Vapors, sprays, cough medicine; if bacterial, antibiotics | Avoid toxic areas or wear respiratory protection, do not smoke | Usually middle age to older adults |
| Respiratory therapy, antibiotics, pancreatic enzyme supplements | Basically set by heredity | At birth and throughout life |
| Elimination of inhaled irritants, mucus-thinning drugs | Do not smoke and limit exposure to aerial toxins. With genetic input, may not be preventable | Generally early to mid-adulthood, not curable |
| If bacterial, antibiotics | Uncertain, good health, try to avoid exposure (e.g., hospitals) | Any age; may kill the young and many older patients |
| Antibiotics like isoniazid and rifampin | Good health, but may not know of contagious source, thus unpreventable. Avoid known contact sources, reduce exposure to crowds | Any age, especially in areas of high exposure |

# Interactive Exercises

## Cases for Critical Thinking

1. A young man has chest pain, cough, difficulty breathing, and a fever. Obviously, these symptoms could be caused by a variety of diseases. What diagnostic procedures would be helpful in diagnosing the man's disease?

2. At age 62, Harry decided to retire from the grain mill where he had worked for 40 years. He was walking much slower and felt weaker even though he was walking less. He had enjoyed his smoke breaks and lunches with the guys, but now he had difficulty getting his breath, while his breathing rate had increased and his chest seemed inflated. What disease seems apparent here, and how may it be addressed?

3. Sara loved to run. She watched the track meets at school even as a first grader. An asthmatic, she occasionally had to use an inhaler, but she seemed determined to be an athlete. Should Sara be discouraged from pursuing her goal? Why or why not?

## Multiple Choice

1. What COPD is primarily caused by smoking, may have a genetic link, and has no cure?
   a. bronchitis
   b. diphtheria
   c. tuberculosis
   d. emphysema

2. Inflammation of bronchial membranes, destruction of cilia, and excess thick mucus production are characteristics of which disease?
   a. emphysema
   b. chronic bronchitis
   c. asthma
   d. tuberculosis

3. Which of the following diseases is typically NOT treated with antibiotics?
   a. pneumonia
   b. emphysema
   c. Legionnaire's disease
   d. pharyngitis

4. What disease was formerly known as "consumption"?
   a. pneumonia
   b. asthma
   c. tuberculosis
   d. lung cancer

5. What disease of the young or old may be triggered by allergies and emotions or heavy exercise?
   a. bronchitis
   b. sinusitis
   c. asthma
   d. pharyngitis

6. Which of the following tends to be caused by *streptococci*?
   a. pneumonia
   b. tuberculosis
   c. Legionnaires' disease
   d. influenza

7. A "barrel chest" is often indicative of what respiratory disease?
   a. pneumonia
   b. emphysema
   c. cancer
   d. bronchitis

8. Legionnaires' disease is caused by what condition or organism?
   a. fungi
   b. viruses
   c. low-humidity climates
   d. bacteria

9. What disease is characterized by a lack of alveolar surfactant that typically happens to premature infants?
   a. asthma
   b. infant respiratory distress syndrome (IRDS)
   c. TB
   d. pneumonia

10. Excess or deficient pulmonary fluid results in what painful disease?
    a. pulmonitis
    b. pneumonia
    c. pleurisy
    d. cystic fibrosis

## True or False

_____ 1. The flu can be prevented by vaccine.

_____ 2. The common cold is easily treated with antibiotics.

_____ 3. Laryngitis may be treated by removal of the tonsils.

_____ 4. The lungs are a common site for metastatic cancer.

_____ 5. Incidences of asthma and tuberculosis are declining because of new potent antibiotics.

_____ 6. Dyspnea is the coughing of blood.

_____ 7. Bronchiectasis is a collapse of lobes of the lung.

_____ 8. *Pneumothorax* simply means "air in the chest cavity."

_____ 9. *COPD* means "COntagious Pulmonary Disorder."

_____ 10. Pharyngitis is usually outgrown by age 15.

## Fill-Ins

1. The _____ test is used to screen for tuberculosis.

2. A lung collapse regardless of etiology is called _____.

3. The main cause of lung cancer is _____.

4. A simple breathing test for pulmonary functioning is _____.

5. The common cold, influenza, and atypical pneumonia are caused by _____.

6. Painful swelling of the membranes surrounding the lungs is called _____.

7. The most common form of pneumonia is _____.

8. Wheezing and difficulty in exhaling are symptoms of _____.

9. _____ is the newest treatment for snoring and sleep apnea.

10. Mucus secretion is thick and excessive in the inherited disease called _____.

## Labeling Exercise

Use the blank lines below to label the following images.

1 _____

2 _____

3 _____

4 _____

5 _____

6 _____

7 _____

8 _____

Additional interactive resources and activities for this chapter can be found on the Companion Website. For videos, audio glossary, and review, access the accompanying DVD-ROM in this book.

## ▶ DVD-ROM Highlights

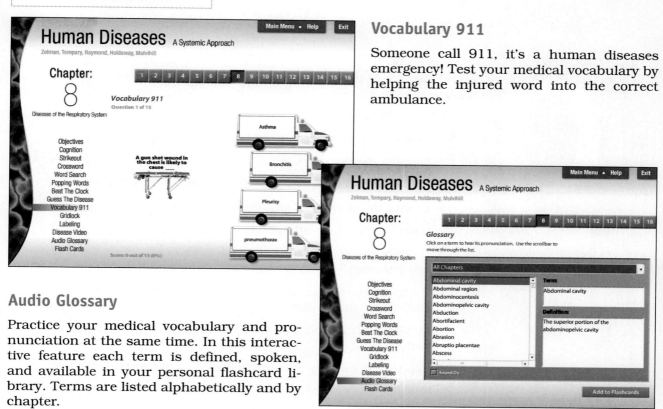

### Vocabulary 911

Someone call 911, it's a human diseases emergency! Test your medical vocabulary by helping the injured word into the correct ambulance.

### Audio Glossary

Practice your medical vocabulary and pronunciation at the same time. In this interactive feature each term is defined, spoken, and available in your personal flashcard library. Terms are listed alphabetically and by chapter.

## ▶ Website Highlights—www.pearsonhighered.com/zelman

### Labeling Exercise

Take advantage of the free-access online study guide that accompanies your textbook. You'll find a figure labeling quiz that corresponds to this chapter. By clicking on this URL you'll also access links to current news articles and an audio glossary.

CHAPTER

# 9

# Diseases of the Gastrointestinal System

## Learning Objectives

After studying this chapter, you should be able to

- Describe the normal structure and function of the digestive tract
- Describe the key characteristics of major diseases of the digestive tract
- Name the diagnostic tests for diseases of the digestive tract
- Explain the etiology of gastrointestinal diseases
- Describe the treatment options for diseases of the digestive tract
- Describe the normal structure and function of the liver, gallbladder, and pancreas
- Describe the key characteristics of major diseases of the liver, gallbladder, and pancreas
- Name the diagnostic tests for diseases of the liver, gallbladder, and pancreas
- Explain the etiology of liver, gallbladder, and pancreas diseases
- Describe the treatment options for diseases of the liver, gallbladder, and pancreas
- Describe age-related diseases of the digestive system

## Fact or Fiction?

Cancer of the colon or rectum is the second leading cause of cancer-related death in the United States.

*Fact:* The American Cancer Society estimates that each year 56,000 Americans will die of colorectal cancer, second only to lung cancer.

## Dysentery

**D**iseases of the digestive system include common ailments familiar to nearly everyone. Some are minor annoyances; others are serious, life-threatening diseases. The impact of digestive system diseases is undeniable. During the American Civil War, 81,360 soldiers died from dysentery, while 93,443 were killed in combat. Even today, 18,000 cases of bacillary dysentery occur annually in the United States. Despite modern medical diagnosis and treatment, cancer of the pancreas, colon, and liver remain deadly, and worldwide, dysentery remains a leading cause of death among children.

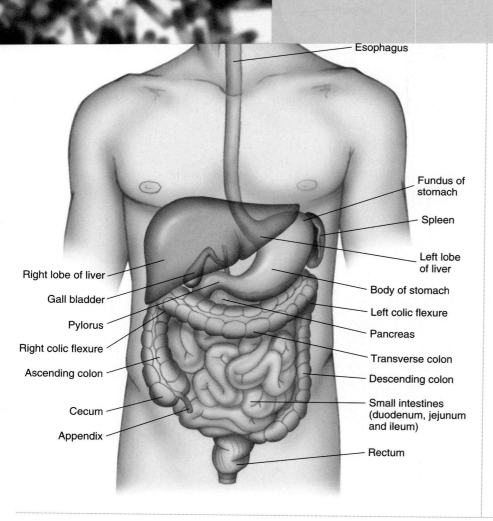

diaphragm and abdominal muscles; contraction of these muscles squeezes the stomach. The sphincter at the base of the esophagus is opened, and the gastric contents are **regurgitated**. A feeling of nausea often precedes vomiting. The cause of the nausea may be factors other than a gastric or intestinal irritant. Motion sickness produces this effect. A very unpleasant smell or sight can cause nausea with possible subsequent vomiting.

## ▶ The Gastrointestinal System

The digestive system consists of a digestive tract through which food passes and accessory organs that assist the digestive process. The digestive tract begins at the mouth and includes the pharynx, esophagus, stomach, small intestine, and large intestine. The accessory organs include the liver, gallbladder, and pancreas (Figure 9–1 ▶).

Digestion begins in the mouth with chewing, the mechanical breakdown of food. Salivation, the secretion of saliva, moistens the food and provides an enzyme for initial digestion of starch. The food is then swallowed and passes through the pharynx, or throat, and into the esophagus.

The moistened food moves down the esophagus to the stomach. A sphincter muscle at the juncture of the esophagus and stomach prevents regurgitation while digestion continues. The stomach secretes gastric juice that contains enzymes, biological catalysts that act on protein. Gastric juice also contains hydrochloric acid, which activates these enzymes. The acidic gastric contents would be irritating to the stomach lining if the lining were not protected by a thick covering of mucus. A great deal of moistening and mixing occurs within the stomach. The moistened, mixed, and acidic food is called chyme.

Chyme passes from the stomach into the small intestine through a sphincter muscle, the **pyloric sphincter.** This sphincter is closed until it

common bile duct. Bile is not an enzyme but an emulsifier, a substance that reduces large fat droplets into much smaller fat droplets, enabling the lipid enzymes to digest fat into small, absorbable units.

When digestion is complete, nutrients such as sugars and amino acids are absorbed into blood capillaries and lymph vessels in the intestinal wall. The inner surface of the small intestine is arranged to provide the greatest amount of surface area possible for digestion and absorption. This mucosal surface contains numerous fingerlike projections called villi, each of which contains capillaries and lymph vessels for absorption (Figure 9–2 ▶).

Material not digested passes into the large intestine, or colon. The first part of the colon is the cecum, to which the appendix, a fingerlike mass of lymphatic tissue, is attached. Water and minerals are absorbed from the large intestine, and the remaining matter is excreted as feces.

In this chapter, the diseases of each part of the digestive system are described. These include diseases of the mouth, esophagus, stomach, small and large intestines, pancreas, liver, and gallbladder.

## ▶ General Disorders of the Digestive Tract

General disorders of the digestive system, such as vomiting, diarrhea, constipation, and hemor-

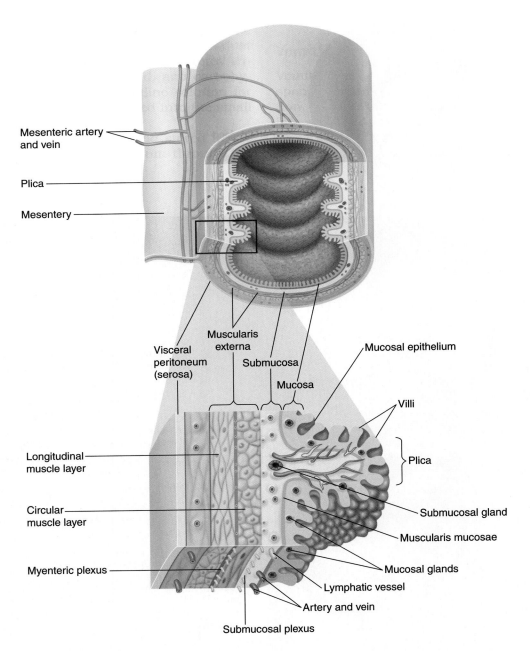

Figure 9–2 ▶ Mucosal surface of the small intestine.

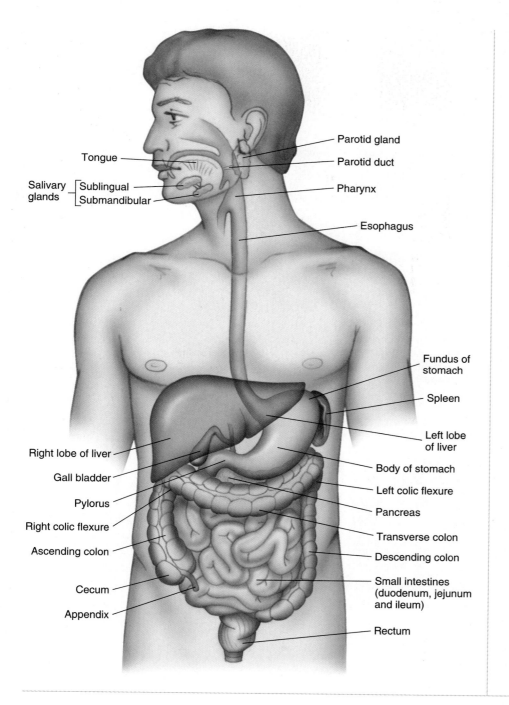

**Figure 9–1** ▶ The gastro-intestinal system.

Parotid gland

Parotid duct

Tongue

Pharynx

Salivary glands — Sublingual

Submandibular

Esophagus

Fundus of stomach

Spleen

Left lobe of liver

Right lobe of liver

Gall bladder

Body of stomach

Pylorus

Left colic flexure

Right colic flexure

Pancreas

Ascending colon

Transverse colon

Descending colon

Cecum

Small intestines (duodenum, jejunum and ileum)

Appendix

Rectum

diaphragm and abdominal muscles; contraction of these muscles squeezes the stomach. The sphincter at the base of the esophagus is opened, and the gastric contents are **regurgitated**. A feeling of nausea often precedes vomiting. The cause of the nausea may be factors other than a gastric or intestinal irritant. Motion sickness produces this effect. A very unpleasant smell or sight can cause nausea with possible subsequent vomiting.

Mesenteric artery and vein

Plica

Mesentery

Muscularis externa

Visceral peritoneum (serosa)

Submucosa

Mucosa

Mucosal epithelium

Villi

Plica

Longitudinal muscle layer

Circular muscle layer

Submucosal gland

Muscularis mucosae

Mucosal glands

Myenteric plexus

Lymphatic vessel

Artery and vein

Submucosal plexus

**Figure 9–2** ▶ Mucosal surface of the small intestine.

## Diarrhea

Diarrhea is the frequent passage of watery stools and results when the contents of the small intestine are rushed through the large intestine. It was stated earlier that the main function of the large intestine is to reabsorb water and minerals. In an episode of diarrhea, there is no time to reabsorb water because the smooth muscle in the walls of the intestine is so stimulated that peristalsis is intensified. Anxiety and stress can trigger this increased motility of the large intestine. Intestinal infections and food poisoning also can increase intestinal motility or impair water absorption by mucosal cells.

## Constipation

Constipation is the inability to eliminate feces from the colon and results when feces become hard and dry. Poor habits of elimination, dehydration, and low-fiber diets may cause constipation. Defecation should be allowed to occur when the defecation reflexes are strong; otherwise feces remain in the colon too long, excessive water reabsorption occurs, and the feces become dry, making elimination difficult. A diet containing adequate amounts of fiber aids elimination by providing bulk, which stimulates intestinal motility. Fiber is obtained from fresh fruits, vegetables, and cereals. This chapter will discuss several disorders and diseases of the digestive system that cause constipation.

## Hemorrhoids

Hemorrhoids are varicose veins in the lining of the rectum near the anus. Hemorrhoids may be internal or external. A physician can observe internal hemorrhoids with a **proctoscope**, a hollow tube with a lighted end. External hemorrhoids can be seen with a handheld mirror and appear blue because of decreased circulation; they can become red and tender if inflamed. Causes of hemorrhoids include heredity, poor dietary habits, inadequate fiber, overuse of laxatives, and lack of exercise. Straining to have a bowel movement can cause bleeding or cause the hemorrhoid to **prolapse**, or come through the anal

opening. Hemorrhoids frequently develop during pregnancy because of pressure from an enlarged uterus. Treatment includes adding fiber and water to the diet and stool softeners to reduce straining and subsequent inflammation. Medicated suppositories and anorectal creams relieve pain and reduce inflammation.

## ▶ Diseases of the Mouth

Complete coverage of diseases of the mouth is beyond the scope of this book. This chapter focuses instead on the major oral inflammatory diseases and neoplasms. Diseases of the mouth can adversely affect the ability to taste, chew, moisten, and swallow food.

### Oral Inflammation

Oral inflammation, or **stomatitis**, refers to a widespread inflammation of oral tissue. Depending on the cause, stomatitis may appear as patches, ulcers, redness, bleeding, or necrosis. Stomatitis can be caused by local infection of the mouth with bacteria, viruses, or fungi, or it may be a sign of a systemic infection.

Streptococci, spread in salivary and respiratory droplets, are a common cause of oral and throat bacterial infections, resulting in red, swollen mucosa. Bacteria also cause canker sores, small circular lesions with a red border. These painful lesions heal without scars after a week. *Neisseria gonorrhea*, the cause of the sexually transmitted disease gonorrhea, causes painful ulcerations in the mouth and throat. Also sexually transmitted, *Treponema pallidum* causes syphilis, which causes oral chancres and ulcerations. These bacterial infections are treated with antibiotics.

Herpes simplex is a common cause of oral virus infections. Transmitted by oral–genital contact, herpes simplex type 2 causes vesicles that rupture to form ulcers. These lesions can appear inside and outside the mouth. Herpes simplex type 1 can also be acquired from salivary droplets. Pain makes eating, drinking, and swallowing difficult. The symptoms typically subside within two weeks when the viruses move from the area to nerve tissue known as ganglia. The infection can be reactivated following stressful events or suppression of immune function. Treatment is aimed at reducing inflammation and pain with systemic anti-inflammatory and analgesic medications or topical anesthetics.

The fungus *Candida albicans* is present in the mouth in low levels normally, but can grow excessively in normal newborns and those with immune deficiencies or following long courses of antibiotic or corticosteroid treatment. The fungal overgrowth, called candidiasis or thrush, forms painless white patches that resemble cheese curds. Removing the white patches leaves a raw, damaged mucosal surface. Candidiasis of the esophagus causes throat pain and difficulty swallowing. Antibiotics and antiviral medications are not effective treatments for fungal infections (see Chapter 3). Oral candidiasis is treated with oral antifungal agents fluconazole, nystatin, or clotrimazole.

## Cancer of the Mouth

The most common form of oral cancer is squamous cell carcinoma. Most of these cancers appear on the floor of the mouth, tongue, and lower lip. An aggressive form of the cancer occurs on the upper lip. Mouth and throat cancer ranks eleventh among the leading causes of cancer death worldwide. While the causes remain unknown, it is clear that tobacco, smokeless tobacco, and alcohol use are major risk factors, and it appears that use of alcohol and tobacco in combination increases the risk. Treatment for lip and tongue cancer includes surgical removal. Radiation therapy may be used to treat local cancers on the floor of the mouth. See Chapter 4 for oral cancer specifics.

## ▶ Diseases of the Esophagus

The function of the esophagus is the controlled passage of food to the stomach. Esophageal disease manifests itself as **dysphagia**, or difficult or painful swallowing.

## Cancer of the Esophagus

Cancer of the esophagus occurs most commonly in men over 60 and is nearly always fatal. The disease ranks sixth among leading causes of cancer death worldwide but is most common in Japan, China, the Middle East, and parts of South Africa. Like mouth cancer, tobacco and alcohol use are major risk factors. The cancer narrows the esophageal lumen, causing the principal symptom, dysphagia. The obstruction causes vomiting, a bad taste in the mouth, and bad breath. Esophageal cancer is accompanied by weight loss because of the inability to eat. Diagnosis includes x-ray with barium swallow to study motility and functional defects. The cancer frequently metastasizes into adjacent organs, usually the lungs and liver, and to remote sites through the lymph vessels before it is detected. Because of early metastasis, the prognosis for esophageal cancer is poor. See Chapter 4 for further information on esophageal cancer.

## Esophageal Varices

Varicose veins that develop in the esophagus are called **esophageal varices**. Cirrhosis of the liver is the chief cause of esophageal varices. Cirrhosis impairs blood flow through the liver, which elevates pressure in the veins of the abdomen and elsewhere, including the esophagus. The increased venous pressure causes the esophageal veins to dilate and become knotty. The most serious danger in esophageal varices is hemorrhage. Bleeding esophageal varices require emergency treatment. Diagnosis usually requires endoscopy. Infusion of vasopressin may reduce bleeding, or bleeding can be stopped with pressure on the varices by inserting a Minnesota or Sengstaken-Blakemore tube. These are temporary measures: Surgical bypass of the portal vein to systemic circulation may reduce pressure in the veins and thus stop bleeding, but it will not repair liver damage and ultimately will not improve the prognosis.

## Esophagitis and GERD

**Esophagitis**, inflammation of the esophagus, causes burning chest pains, "heartburn," which can resemble the pain of heart disease. The pain may follow eating or drinking, and some vomiting of blood may occur. The most common trigger of esophagitis is a **reflux**, a backflow of the acid contents of the stomach. The condition is known as **gastroesophageal reflux disease** or **GERD**. GERD may be caused by an incompetent **cardiac sphincter**, which normally prevents stomach contents from ascending the esophagus. Other causes include hiatal hernia and medications that compromise the sphincter or induce excess acid secretion. The incidence of GERD increases with age, which suggests that age-related changes occur in the sphincter. Whatever the cause, regurgitated stomach acid irritates the lining of the esophagus and stimulates an inflammatory response. Diagnosis is based on history, signs, symptoms, as well as barium fluoroscopy, measure of esophageal pH, or endoscopy. Risk factors for GERD include old age, obesity, and pregnancy. Treatment includes a nonirritating diet, antacids, and acid-reducing medications. Frequent, small meals are recommended. Painful symptoms frequently occur at night while the body lies prone and relaxed; thus patients are advised to sleep with head elevated and to avoid eating 2 to 3 hours before sleeping. Alcohol is an irritant to the inflamed mucosal lining and should be avoided.

## Hiatal Hernia

A hernia is the protrusion of part of an organ through a muscular wall or body opening. A **hiatal hernia** is the protrusion of part of the stomach through the diaphragm at the point where the esophagus joins the stomach. The condition is caused by either a congenital defect in the diaphragm or by increased intraabdominal pressure associated with obesity. Figure 9–3► shows this condition. Indigestion and heartburn may occur after eating; shortness of breath may also occur. Diagnosis is based on a chest x-ray that may show air behind the heart, or a barium radiograph that can show a bulge at lower esophagus, or endoscopy to visualize the hernia and rule out cancer or varices. The aim of treatment is to reduce symptoms. The most effective treatment is cholinergic drugs,

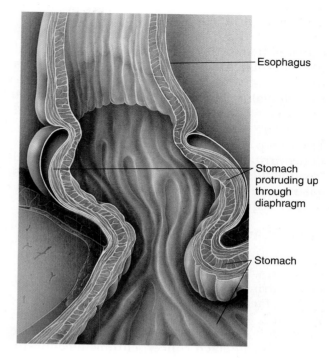

Esophagus

Stomach protruding up through diaphragm

Stomach

**Figure 9–3** ► Hiatal hernia. (© K. Somerville/Custom Medical Stock Photo)

which strengthen the cardiac sphincter and reduce reflux after eating. Patients should avoid irritants such as spicy foods and caffeine, should take frequent small meals, and, if obese, should lose weight. Surgery may be required to correct the structural defect, but hiatal hernias tend to recur following surgery.

## ► Diseases of the Stomach

The stomach is well adapted for storing and mixing food with acid and enzymes. Alterations in the stomach lining or malignancies can cause painful and sometimes serious disease.

### Gastritis

Acute **gastritis** is an inflammation of the stomach frequently accompanied by vomiting of blood. Acute gastritis is caused by irritants such as aspirin, excessive coffee, tobacco, alcohol, or infection. Acute alcoholism is a major cause of hemorrhagic gastritis. Chronic alcohol use stimulates acid secretion, which irritates the mucosa. **Gastroscopy** with biopsy is extremely valuable in diagnosing this disease. A camera may be attached to the gastroscope, and the entire inner stomach is photographed. Treatment includes avoiding the aforementioned irritants and treating infections. Medical treatment includes cimetidine, which blocks gastric secretion. If bleeding is involved, surgery may be required.

### Chronic Atrophic Gastritis

Chronic atrophic gastritis is a degenerative condition in which the stomach lining does not secrete intrinsic factor and hydrochloric acid. Intrinsic factor is required for absorption of vitamin $B_{12}$, and hydrochloric acid aids protein digestion. Chronic atrophic gastritis may be caused by stomach cancer, chronic alcoholism, or chronic exposure to certain irritants such as alcohol, aspirin, and certain foods. The term **atrophic** (wasting) suggests that little can be done to treat this disease. The underlying diseases or causes should be eliminated.

### Peptic Ulcers

Ulcers are lesions of any body surface where necrotic tissue forms as a result of inflammation and is sloughed off, leaving a hole. Ulcers of the stomach and small intestine are termed **peptic ulcers**. Ulcers of the stomach are called **gastric ulcers**, and those of the small intestine are called **duodenal ulcers**. Approximately 80% of peptic ulcers are duodenal ulcers and occur most frequently in men between ages 20 and 50. Figure 9–4▶ shows common sites of peptic ulcers.

Peptic ulcers have three main causes, including infection with **_Helicobacter pylori_**, use of nonsteroidal anti-inflammatory drugs, and an inherited disorder of acid hypersecretion. Because hydrochloric acid secretion is under nerve and hormonal control, stressful situations can trigger or exacerbate ulcers. Gastric contents contribute to ulcer formation in all cases. The ulcers are caused, in part, by pepsin, a proteolytic enzyme secreted by the stomach. Hydrochloric acid of the stomach and intestinal juice, including bile, which is regurgitated through the pyloric sphincter, also irritate the gastric mucosa. Irritated and inflamed mucous membrane may become necrotic, leaving a hole.

## SIDE by SIDE ■ Gastric Ulcer

▲ Normal mucosa showing openings of gastric glands.
(© C. Abrahams, M.D./Custom Medical Stock Photo)

▲ Superficial gastric ulcer in the stomach lining.

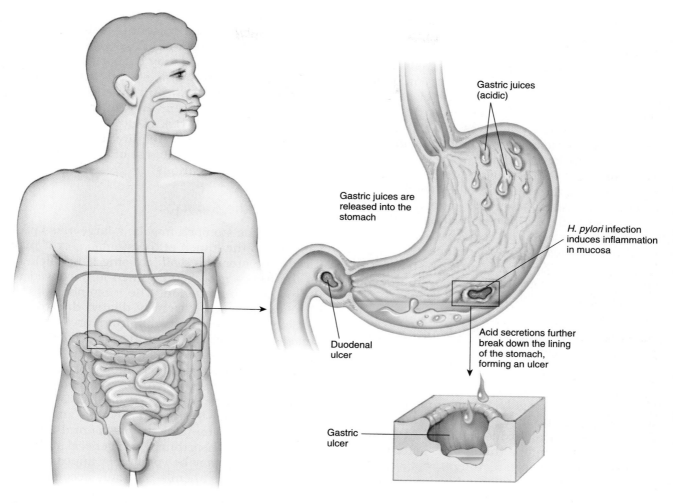

Gastric juices (acidic)

Gastric juices are released into the stomach

*H. pylori* infection induces inflammation in mucosa

Acid secretions further break down the lining of the stomach, forming an ulcer

Duodenal ulcer

Gastric ulcer

Figure 9–4 ► Peptic ulcer disease (PUD).

Heartburn and indigestion are frequently the first signs of an ulcer. The ulcer pain is caused by the action of hydrochloric acid on the exposed surface of the lesion. The muscular contractions of peristalsis also intensify the pain. Symptoms of gastric ulcer include nausea, vomiting, abdominal pain, and, occasionally, massive gastrointestinal bleeding.

A potential complication of any ulcer is hemorrhage; severe hemorrhage may lead to shock. It is possible for a large artery at the base of the ulcer to rupture as the lesion erodes deeper into underlying tissues. Bleeding from the ulcer may appear as **hematemesis** or bloody vomitus, or the

blood may appear in stools, where it gives the stools a dark, tarry appearance, referred to as **melena**. A serious ulcer complication is **perforation**. If an ulcer perforates—that is, breaks through the intestinal or gastric wall—there is sudden and intense abdominal pain. **Peritonitis**, inflammation of the lining of the abdominal cavity, usually results when the digestive contents enter the cavity, because this material contains numerous bacteria. Surgical repair of the perforation is required immediately. Obstruction of the gastrointestinal tract can result from an ulcer and the scar tissue surrounding it. Obstruction occurs most frequently in a narrow area of the stomach, near the pyloric sphincter. Ulcer pain can cause the sphincter to go into spasm, also resulting in obstruction.

Diagnosis is based on an upper gastrointestinal barium swallow, an x-ray, detection of blood in stools, blood tests to determine elevated levels of white blood cells, and gastric content analysis. The main objectives of treatment for peptic ulcer disease are to promote healing, prevent complications and recurrences, and provide pain relief. Acid reducers, such as omeprazole or ranitidine, are more effective for peptic ulcers than are antacids and mucosal barriers such as sucraflate. However, antibiotic therapy in combination with acid reducers is required to eradicate *H. pylori* and to reduce the rate of ulcer relapse. If the ulcer is stress or tension related, certain changes in lifestyle or approach to stress might be beneficial.

## Gastroenteritis and Food Poisoning

Gastroenteritis is an inflammation of the stomach and intestines. Symptoms include anorexia, nausea, vomiting, and diarrhea. The onset may be abrupt, with rapid loss of fluid and electrolytes. Possible causes are bacterial or viral infection, chemical toxins, lactose intolerance, or other food allergy, although the actual cause is not always clear. Treatment replaces fluid and nutritional requirements, including the lost salts. Antispasmodic medications can control the vomiting and diarrhea.

Food contaminated with human or animal feces may carry microorganisms that cause gastroenteritis and food poisoning. *Escherichia coli* is a normal inhabitant of human or animal intestines. Certain strains may cause disease, like traveler's diarrhea, or more serious diseases, like hemolytic uremic syndrome, in which toxins cause potentially fatal shutdown of the kidneys. To prevent infection, cook meat thoroughly and practice good hygiene in the kitchen.

One of the common forms of food poisoning is caused by the bacterium *Salmonella*. These bacteria invade the intestinal mucosa and cause sudden, colicky abdominal pain, nausea, vomiting, and sometimes bloody diarrhea and fever that begins approximately 6 to 48 hours after eating contaminated food and lasts up to

2 weeks. A stool culture can identify the bacteria. *Salmonella* food poisoning (salmonellosis) is associated with contaminated eggs and poultry, but most any food may harbor the bacteria. Treatment usually consists of replenishing water, electrolytes, and nutrients. Elderly individuals, young children, and immunocompromised people are at risk of developing serious infection, and they may require more intervention, including a short course of antibiotics and antidiarrheal medications.

## Cancer of the Stomach

Cancer of the stomach may be a large mass projecting into the lumen of the stomach, or it may invade the stomach wall, causing it to thicken. As the tumor grows, the lumen is narrowed to the point of obstruction. The remainder of the stomach becomes extremely dilated due to the blockage, and pain results from pressure on nerve endings. Infection frequently accompanies cancer, which causes additional pain. Because pain is not an early sign, carcinoma of the stomach may be very advanced before it is detected. It may even have spread to the liver and surrounding organs through the lymph and blood vessels. Early symptoms are vague and include loss of appetite, heartburn, and general stomach distress. Blood may be vomited or appear in the feces. Pernicious anemia generally accompanies cancer of the stomach, because the gastric mucosa fails to secrete intrinsic factor. The etiology of this malignancy is not known, but current research suggests an association with the consumption of preserved, salted, cured foods and a diet low in fresh fruits and vegetables. The incidence of stomach cancer in the United States has dropped dramatically over the past 30 years; it has become an uncommon disease and accounts for less than 1% of all cancers. Today the mortality rate for stomach cancer is about 6 per 100,000 men. Stomach cancer is the ninth leading cause of cancer death in men, and is more prevalent among men over age 40 than among women. Stomach cancer is not among the ten leading causes of cancer death among women.

Gastric analysis by means of a stomach tube demonstrates the absence of hydrochloric acid, or **achlorhydria**. Biopsy of any lesions seen through the gastroscope is an essential diagnostic procedure for carcinoma of the stomach.

*H. pylori* infection appears to increase the risk for stomach cancer, probably through its damaging effects on the mucosal cells. Good prognosis for this disease depends on early detection and treatment. See Chapter 4 for more information.

## ▶ Diseases of the Intestines

The small intestine is the site of most of the digestion and absorption that occurs in the digestive tract, while the large intestine absorbs remaining water and stores and concentrates the feces. Diseases in these areas may manifest themselves as diarrhea, constipation, changes in stool characteristics, or secondary diseases that arise as a result of poor nutrition.

### Appendicitis

Appendicitis is an acute and painful inflammation of the appendix. Appendicitis can occur at any age, but it is more common for males before puberty to age 25. The wormlike shape of the appendix and its location on the cecum make it a trap for fecal material, which contains bacteria, particularly *Escherichia coli.* Figure 9–5 ▶ illustrates this potential site of infection. Obstruction with fecal material and infections cause the appendix to become swollen, red, and covered with an inflammatory exudate. Because the swelling interferes with circulation to the appendix, it is possible for **gangrene** to develop.

The appendix then becomes green and black. The wall of the appendix can become thin and rupture, spilling fecal material into the peritoneal cavity, causing **peritonitis**. Before antibiotic treatment, peritonitis was almost always fatal. Rupture of the appendix tends to give relief from the pain, which is very misleading.

Diagnosis depends on physical exam. The pain of appendicitis is not always typical, but it often begins in the middle of the abdomen and shifts to the lower right quadrant. Patients may walk or lie bent over and draw the right leg up to the abdomen to seek pain relief. Other diagnostic signs and symptoms include nausea, vomiting, fever of between 99°F and 102°F, and elevated white blood cell count. Untreated appendicitis is fatal, and surgery must be performed before rupture occurs.

### Malabsorption Syndrome

The inability to absorb fat or some other substance from the small intestine is known as **malabsorption syndrome**. Signs and symptoms of malnutrition occur, including lack of energy and inability to maintain weight. Because fat cannot be absorbed from the intestine, it passes into the feces, and the result is unformed, fatty, pale stools that have a foul odor. The fat content causes the stools to float.

Although defective mucosal cells can cause the abnormal absorption, other diseases can result in secondary malabsorption syndrome. A diseased pancreas or blocked pancreatic duct deprives the small intestine of **lipase**. In the

Large intestine

Small intestine (ileum)

Ileocecal valve

Cecum

Opening into appendix

Appendix

Figure 9–5 ▶ Appendix attached to cecum into which the small intestine empties.

## Prevention ✚✚ PLUS!

### Bacteria, Coolers, and Food Poisoning

Refrigeration and freezing do not kill bacteria. The cold temperature inhibits their growth, which can resume at warmer temperatures. Bacteria can multiply rapidly; under optimum conditions, they may double their numbers every 30 minutes. A contaminated potato salad may be safe to eat right out of the refrigerator, but it may become the source of a serious infection if brought to a picnic and left to stand at air temperature for a couple of hours. In other words, it is a good idea to keep the potato salad in the cooler while you are playing softball at your next picnic!

absence of lipase, fat is not digested and cannot be absorbed. Inadequate bile secretion, due to liver disease or a blocked bile duct, also prevents lipid digestion and causes secondary malabsorption. One of the complications of the malabsorption syndrome is a bleeding tendency. Vitamin K, a fat-soluble vitamin that is essential to the blood-clotting mechanism, cannot be absorbed. Treatment for malabsorption syndrome depends on its cause, and diet is carefully controlled. Supplements are administered, such as the fat-soluble vitamins A, D, E, and K.

## Celiac Disease

Celiac disease is associated with gluten intolerance and is characterized by poor nutrient absorption. Signs and symptoms include recurrent diarrhea, gas, abdominal cramps, and systemic signs of malnutrition due to low caloric intake and poor absorption of vitamins. Onset is usually by age 1, when wheat products are first consumed. Celiac disease seems to be genetic, may involve immune dysfunction, affects twice as many females as males, and is more common among whites of European ancestry. Celiac disease affects about 2 million Americans, or 1 in 133 people. Celiac disease is diagnosed by the signs and symptoms as well as by biopsy of the small intestine, which reveals atrophy and flattening of intestinal villi. Treatment involves elimination of gluten from the diet, fluid replacement, and vitamin supplements.

## Diverticulitis

**Diverticula** are little pouches or sacs formed when the mucosal lining pushes through the underlying muscle layer of the intestinal wall. This condition is called **diverticulosis** and may

cause no harm in itself. **Diverticulitis** is an inflammation of the diverticula. Diverticulitis occurs when the sacs become impacted with fecal material and bacteria. The patient experiences low, cramplike pain, usually on the left side of the abdomen. As inflammation spreads, the lumen of the intestine narrows, an obstruction can develop, and abscesses frequently form. Diverticular disease is most prevalent in Western industrialized nations where fiber consumption is lowest. About 50% of older adults develop diverticulosis. Diverticular disease is diagnosed with a barium enema. Antibiotic therapy, together with a controlled diet, is usually effective. Figure 9–6 ► shows an example of diverticulitis.

## Regional Enteritis (Crohn's Disease)

**Regional enteritis** is an inflammatory disease of the intestine that most frequently affects the upper colon and sometimes the distal end of the ileum. Crohn's disease is most prevalent in adults ages 20 to 40, is two to three times more common among Jewish populations, and is least common in blacks. Possible causes include allergies, immune disorders, or stress, but the exact cause remains unknown. As inflammation progresses, the intestinal walls become thick and rigid. With thickening, the lumen narrows and a chronic obstruction develops. The pain of regional enteritis resembles that of appendicitis, occurring in the lower right quadrant of the abdomen, where a tender mass may be felt. Diarrhea alternating with constipation, and **melena** (dark stools containing blood pigments) are common. Severe diarrhea can cause an electrolyte imbalance because of the large amount of water and salt lost in the stools. **Anorexia**, nausea, and vomiting lead to weight loss. Periods of exacerba-

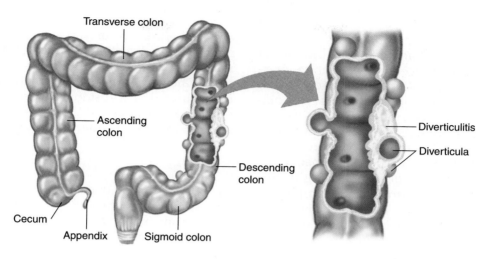

**Figure 9-6** ▶ Diverticulitis.

tion, remission, and relapse are common; during flare-ups, the inflammation can also manifest as rheumatoid arthritis. Severe cases entail a risk for hemorrhage or perforation. Crohn's disease is diagnosed by elevated levels of white blood cells; low levels of potassium, calcium, and magnesium; and by sigmoidoscopy or colonoscopy. Biopsy confirms the diagnosis. Crohn's disease is usually treated with anti-inflammatory medications such as corticosteroids and aminosalicylates, and with immunosuppressive agents such as azathioprine, sulfasalazine, and olsalazine. Surgery is performed to correct complications such as obstruction, perforation, or massive hemorrhage. Ileostomy is necessary if the large intestine has been severely damaged.

## Chronic Ulcerative Colitis

**Chronic ulcerative colitis** is a serious inflammation of the colon characterized by extensive ulceration of the colon and rectum. The incidence of ulcerative colitis remains unknown but may be as much as 100 per 100,000. Ulcerative colitis occurs primarily in young adults, especially women, and usually begins between ages 15 and 20. No known causes have been found; however, ulcerative colitis may be related to autoimmunity, *E. coli* infection, stress, or hypersensitivity to certain foods.

Typical symptoms include diarrhea with pus, blood, and mucus in the stools, and cramplike pain in the lower abdomen. Periods of remission and exacerbation are common in ulcerative colitis. Anemia often accompanies ulcerative colitis because of the chronic blood loss through the rectum. Increased risk for colon malignancy is associated with long-standing ulcerative colitis.

Diagnosis is based on colonoscopy and a barium x-ray in which the colon has a characteristic appearance; the normal pouchlike markings of the colon are lacking, and the colon appears straight and rigid, a "**pipestem colon.**"

Treatment is aimed at reducing symptoms, replacing nutrients, stopping blood loss, and preventing complications. The symptoms may be alleviated by reducing stress, eliminating foods found to trigger symptoms, and taking adrenal corticosteroids such as prednisone and hydrocortisone to control autoimmunity. If these treatments are not effective, surgery may be necessary, occasionally requiring a colostomy. A **colostomy** is an artificial opening in the abdominal wall with a segment of the large intestine attached. Fecal waste is evacuated through this opening and collected in a bag. A colostomy may be temporary or permanent depending on the nature of the colon surgery.

## Cancer of the Colon and Rectum

Cancer of the colon and rectum is a leading cause of death from cancer in the United States and is the fourth leading cause of cancer in the

United States. The incidence in men and women is roughly equal.

The symptoms vary according to the site of the malignancy. A change in bowel habits, diarrhea, or constipation is symptomatic. As the tumor grows, there may be abdominal discomfort and pressure. Blood often appears in the stools, and continuous blood loss from the malignant tumor causes anemia. The mass can partially or completely obstruct the **lumen** of the colon. As the tumor invades underlying tissue, the cancer cells spread through the lymph vessels and veins. Colorectal cancer is diagnosed with a digital rectal examination, sigmoidoscopy, colonoscopy, and biopsy.

Two diseases increase the risk for cancer of the colon: long-standing ulcerative colitis and familial polyposis of the colon. **Familial polyposis** is a hereditary disease in which numerous polyps develop in the intestinal tract. The polyps usually give no symptoms unless a malignancy develops. Another factor associated with risk for colon cancer is a diet high in red meat and low in food sources of fiber, such as vegetables, legumes, and whole-grain cereals.

Colorectal cancer grows slowly, tends to remain localized, and is thus potentially curable with early diagnosis. As in all cancers, early detection and treatment are essential to prevent its spread. Most malignancies of the large intestine are in the rectum or the sigmoid colon, which makes their detection and removal easier than malignant tumors in other areas of the digestive tract. Chemotherapy is used when the tumor has metastasized or if residual masses remain inoperable. (See Chapter 4.) If sections of the colon are removed, a colostomy may be necessary.

## Intestinal Obstructions

An obstruction can occur anywhere along the intestinal tract, preventing contents within the tract from moving forward. **Obstructions** are classed as **organic** when there is some material blockage, or as **paralytic**, in which case there is a decrease in **peristalsis**, preventing the propulsion of intestinal contents.

Tumors and hernias, both hiatal and inguinal, can cause organic obstructions. The intestine may be twisted on itself, a condition known as **volvulus** that may be unwound surgically (Figure 9–7 ▶). The intestine may be kinked, allowing nothing to pass. **Adhesions**, the linking of two surfaces normally separate, can distort the tract. Abdominal adhesions sometimes follow surgery, when fibrous connective tissue grows around the incision. Adhesions also develop as a result of inflammation. An-

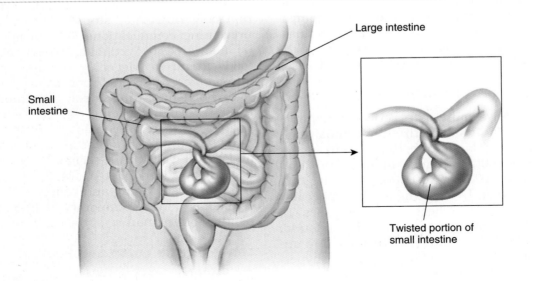

Large intestine

Small intestine

Twisted portion of small intestine

**Figure 9–7** ▶ Volvulus.

other type of organic obstruction is **intussu-sception**, in which a segment of intestine tele-scopes into the part forward to it. This occurs more often in children than in adults. Figure 9–8► shows various types of organic obstruc-tions. An acute organic obstruction causes se-vere pain. The abdomen is distended and vomit-ing occurs. There is complete constipation; not even gas, or **flatus**, is passed. Sometimes the ob-struction can be relieved by means of a suction tube, but frequently surgery is required. If the obstruction is a strangulated hernia, a protru-sion of intestine through the abdominal wall, surgery is required because the blood supply is cut off to the strangulated segment, and it can become gangrenous.

A paralytic obstruction can result from peri-tonitis. If a loop of small intestine is surrounded by pus from the infection, the smooth muscle of the intestinal wall cannot contract. Sphincters can go into spasm and fail to open as a result of intense pain.

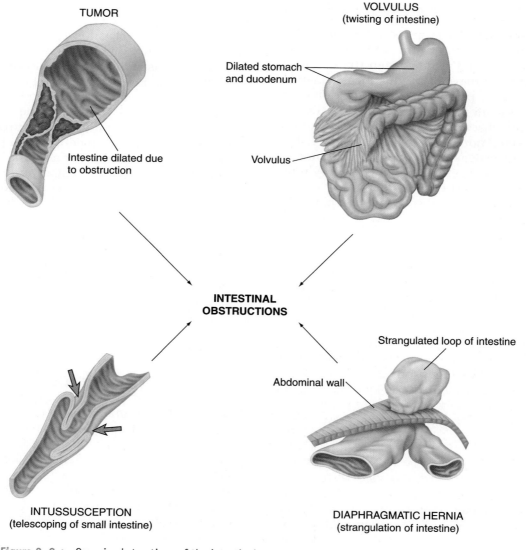

TUMOR

VOLVULUS
(twisting of intestine)

Dilated stomach
and duodenum

Intestine dilated due
to obstruction

Volvulus

INTESTINAL
OBSTRUCTIONS

Strangulated loop of intestine

Abdominal wall

INTUSSUSCEPTION
(telescoping of small intestine)

DIAPHRAGMATIC HERNIA
(strangulation of intestine)

Figure 9–8 ► Organic obstructions of the intestinal tract.

## Prevention ✚PLUS!

### Cancer Prevention through Detection

Early detection of colorectal cancer is the key to survival. Death rates are low for patients whose colorectal cancer is detected at an early localized stage; about 9% die within 5 years. Death rates are much higher, however, when the diagnosis occurs at an advanced stage; about 92% die within 5 years. Screening remains underused even though its benefits seem clear. Regular screening should be done for adults aged 50 years and over. This includes an annual fecal occult blood test, a flexible sigmoidoscopy every 5 years, and a colonoscopy every 10 years. These tests can identify precancerous polyps that can be removed, or they can detect cancer in the early localized stage, which can be treated before the cancer has a chance to spread.

## Spastic Colon (Irritable Bowel Syndrome)

**Irritable bowel syndrome** or **spastic colon** is relatively common, occurring in 20% of American adults and affecting more women than men. Irritable bowel is marked by diarrhea, constipation, abdominal pain, and gas. The difference between a spastic or **irritable colon** and the diseases already discussed is that the spastic colon has no lesion, no tumor, or ulceration. It is a functional disorder of motility, the movement of the colon. The pain is probably caused by muscle spasms in the wall of the intestine.

Abuse of laxatives and consumption of certain foods and beverages, particularly caffeine, alcohol, spicy foods, fatty foods, and concentrated orange juice, can irritate the bowel. Foods such as beans and cabbage, which contain carbohydrates fermented by colon bacteria, promote gas production and should be avoided. Laxatives should be avoided as well. Adding fiber to the diet helps prevent constipation. Emotional stress has an adverse effect on the digestive system, because the nerves of the autonomic nervous system affect digestion. If stressful situations can be alleviated, the colon will function more normally. Tension-relieving activities, sports, hobbies, or regular exercise may help.

## Dysentery

The terms *dysentery* and *diarrhea* are often incorrectly used interchangeably. Dysentery is an infectious disease; diarrhea is a symptom. **Dysentery** is an acute inflammation of the colon. The major symptom of dysentery is diarrhea containing pus, blood, and mucus accompanied by severe abdominal pain. Bacteria, parasitic worms, and other microorganisms can cause dysentery. The protozoan *Entamoeba histolytica*, which is transmitted in feces-contaminated food and water, causes amebiasis, also called amoebic dysentery. Amoebic dysentery is uncommon in the United States and is usually found among immigrants arriving from countries with poor water quality and sanitary procedures. American travelers acquire amoebic dysentery when drinking contaminated water abroad. *E. histolytica* invade the wall of the colon and cause numerous ulcerations, which account for the pus and blood in the stools. Bacillary dysentery is caused by various species of gram-negative bacteria in the genus *Shigella*. Antibiotics can be effective for bacillary dysentery, and amebicides are used for amoebic dysentery.

## ▶ Diseases Indicated by Stool Characteristics

Microscopic examination of stool may identify the cause of food poisoning, gastroenteritis, or dysentery. Other information can also be obtained from stool samples. Signs of several of the diseases discussed include blood in the stools. Blood appears differently, however, depending upon the site of bleeding.

If the blood in the stools is bright red, the bleeding originated from the distal end of the colon, the rectum. Streaks of red blood can indicate bleeding hemorrhoids. This symptom can also indicate cancer of the rectum. Dark blood

may appear in the stools, giving them a dark, tarry appearance, the condition of **melena**. This blood was altered as it passed through the digestive tract, so it originated from the stomach or duodenum. A bleeding ulcer or cancer of the stomach may be indicated by melena. Certain medications (those containing iron, for instance) can also give this tarry appearance to the stools. Blood may not be apparent to the naked eye, but a chemical test can show its presence. This is referred to as **occult blood**. It can indicate bleeding ulcers or a malignancy in the digestive tract.

If the stools are large and pale, appear greasy, and float on water, they contain fat. This is a symptom of malabsorption syndrome. It may also indicate a diseased liver, gallbladder, or pancreas. Diseases of these organs are discussed next.

## ▶ Functions of the Liver and the Gallbladder

The liver is located below the diaphragm, in the upper right quadrant of the abdominal region. The liver is the largest glandular organ of the body, and it is unique in that it has great powers of regeneration; it can replace damaged or diseased cells. Still, chronic liver disease may cause irreversible damage and loss of function.

The liver has a dual blood supply: It receives oxygenated blood from the hepatic artery and blood rich in nutrients from the portal vein. The blood reaching the liver through the portal vein comes from the stomach, intestines, spleen, and pancreas. Blood from the small intestines carries absorbed nutrients such as simple sugars and amino acids. One of the functions of the liver is to store any excess of these substances. The liver plays an important role in maintaining the proper level of glucose in the blood. It takes up excess glucose, storing it as **glycogen**. When the level of circulating glucose falls below normal, the liver converts glycogen into glucose, which is then released into the blood. The liver also stores iron and vitamins.

The liver synthesizes various proteins, including enzymes necessary for cellular activities. One means of evaluating liver function is to determine the level of these enzymes in the blood.

The liver also synthesizes plasma proteins. Albumin is the plasma protein that has a water-holding power within the blood vessels. If the albumin level is too low, plasma seeps out of the blood vessels and into the tissue spaces, causing edema. Other essential plasma proteins synthesized by the liver are those required for blood clotting: fibrinogen and prothrombin. If the liver is seriously diseased or injured and cannot make these proteins, hemorrhaging may occur.

The liver can detoxify various substances; that is, it can make poisonous substances harmless. Ammonia, which results from amino acid metabolism, is converted to urea by the liver. The urea then enters the bloodstream and is excreted by the kidneys. Certain drugs and chemicals are also detoxified by the liver. Specialized cells called **Kupffer cells** line the blood spaces within the liver. These cells engulf and digest bacteria and other foreign substances, thus cleansing the blood.

**Bile**, necessary for fat digestion, is secreted by the liver. Bile is an emulsifier, acting on fat in such a way that the lipid enzymes can digest it. The products of lipid digestion are then absorbed by the walls of the small intestine. In the absence of bile, the fat-soluble vitamins A, D, E, and K cannot be absorbed. Bile consists of water, bile salts, cholesterol, and bilirubin, which is a colored substance resulting from the breakdown of hemoglobin. It is bilirubin that gives bile its characteristic color of yellow or orange.

The gallbladder is a small, saclike structure on the underside of the liver. Bile is secreted continuously by the liver into the hepatic duct, which carries bile to the gallbladder for storage and concentration (Figure 9–9 ▶). The gallbladder releases the bile through the cystic duct to the common hepatic duct, which carries the bile to the duodenum. Release of bile is coordinated with the appearance of fats in the duodenum.

## ▶ Diseases of the Liver

Liver disease manifests itself when chronic damage to liver cells cannot be repaired. When fibrous tissue replaces liver cells, the normal functions of the liver become impaired.

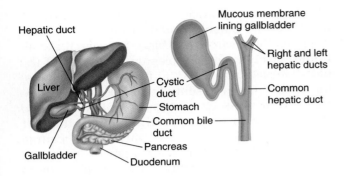

**Figure 9–9** ▶ Bile duct system of the liver and gallbladder.

## Jaundice

One sign frequently associated with liver disease is jaundice. **Jaundice**, or **icterus**, is a yellow or orange discoloration of the skin, tissues, and the whites of the eyes. It is caused by a build-up of bilirubin, a pigment that is normally secreted in the bile and removed from the body in the feces.

Jaundice has several causes. The normal flow of bile from the gallbladder to the duodenum may be obstructed by a tumor, a gallstone in the duct system, or a congenital defect. Because the bile cannot move forward, it leaks into the blood, with bilirubin coloring the plasma. When the blood reaches the kidneys, the bile appears in the urine, giving it a dark color. Because bile is unable to reach the duodenum, the stools are light in color. They are usually described as clay colored. Complications can result from this blockage to bile flow. Infection or inflammation of the gallbladder or bile ducts could occur. Lack of bile interferes with fat digestion and absorption, which means that the fat-soluble vitamins are not being absorbed. In the absence of vitamin K, bleeding tendencies may develop. The obstruction can also cause liver damage. Jaundice can also indicate liver disease, such as hepatitis or cirrhosis.

Hemolytic jaundice has an entirely different etiology. This type of jaundice accompanies the hemolytic anemias explained in Chapter 7. In these anemias, the red blood cells hemolyze, and an excess of bilirubin results from the breakdown of released hemoglobin. Abnormal discoloration follows.

## Viral Hepatitis

Hepatitis, or inflammation of the liver, is caused by a number of factors, including several viruses. Important causes are hepatitis virus A, hepatitis virus B, hepatitis virus C, and hepatitis virus D. Hepatitis E is uncommon in the United States.

Hepatitis virus A, formerly called *infectious hepatitis,* is the least serious form and can develop as an isolated case or in an epidemic. In the United States, as many as 30,000 people per year had hepatitis A infection until the vaccine was introduced, and since the 1990s this number has dropped dramatically. Still, in large crowded urban areas and in rural areas with poor sanitation, the rate of infection can exceed 20 per 100,000. The incubation period, the time from exposure to the development of symptoms, is from 2 to 6 weeks. The symptoms include anorexia, nausea, and mild fever. The urine becomes dark in color, and jaundice appears in some cases. On examination, the liver may be found to be enlarged and tender. Contaminated water or food is the usual source of the infection, which spreads under conditions of poor sanitation. The virus is excreted in the stools and urine, infecting soil and water. Hepatitis virus type A is usually mild in children; it is sometimes more severe in adults. Prognosis is usually good, with no permanent liver damage resulting. **Immunoglobulin** injections provide temporary protection against hepatitis virus type A for people exposed to it. A vaccine now in use has proven to be effective. Exposure to hepatitis A gives lifetime immunity.

Hepatitis virus B, formerly called *serum hepatitis,* is a more serious and common disease, affecting more than 60,000 Americans per year. In fact, 1.25 million American are chronically infected with hepatitis B, 25% of whom will die from cirrhosis. The symptoms are similar to those of hepatitis virus A but develop more slowly. The incubation period is long, lasting from 2 to 6 months. The severity of the disease varies greatly. Those with poor nutritional status, for example, will be more adversely affected by hepatitis. Occasionally, a **fulminating** form of hepatitis virus B develops, and it is fatal. This form has a sudden onset and progresses rapidly. Delirium is followed by a coma and death. Hepatitis virus B can be transmitted by donated blood or serum transfusions that contain the virus. It also is transmitted sexually and through contaminated needles or syringes used by drug addicts. Physical condition at the onset of the disease makes a difference in the seriousness of the infection. Blood and plasma are screened for hepatitis, but hospital personnel still must be well informed of the hazards that can lead to acquiring hepatitis. Precautions must be taken by nurses, laboratory technicians, dialysis workers, and blood bank personnel to prevent becoming infected. Vaccination provides immunity to the virus, and it should be administered to personnel who handle or come in close contact with blood or other bodily fluids (see Chapter 3).

Hepatitis C infections have declined in the United States to approximately 26,000 per year, somewhat fewer than hepatitis B, but hepatitis C remains the leading viral cause of chronic liver disease and cirrhosis and is now the most common reason for liver transplants. Because of the very high rates of infection seen in the 1980s, over 4 million Americans are infected today, 3.2 million of whom are chronically infected. The initial symptoms are nonspecific and similar to those of hepatitis A or B, but the disease persists for months, even years. About 20% of those infected develop cirrhosis, and a number of these cases can lead to end-stage liver disease. The virus is transmitted mostly through blood transfusions, although transmission has been traced to intravenous drug use, and epidemiologic studies show a risk associated with sexual contact with someone with hepatitis and with having had more than one sex partner in a year. Treatments of hepatitis C include interferon injections and oral ribavirin. Treatment for end-stage cirrhosis may include liver transplant.

Hepatitis D virus is described as a defective virus because it cannot reproduce in a cell unless the cell is also infected with hepatitis B. The resulting disease is more serious and more frequently progresses to chronic liver disease. Rates of hepatitis D are not known because surveillance is not systematically conducted; however, hepatitis D is quite uncommon but its transmission is known to be similar to that of hepatitis B.

Hepatitis E is very rare in the United States, but worldwide it is the leading cause of epidemics of infectious hepatitis. Major epidemics occur in Africa, Asia, and Mexico, where it is transmitted primarily through fecal-contaminated drinking water. Nearly every case in the United States occurs in travelers to areas where the disease is endemic. No effective treatment or vaccine exists. Fortunately, there is no evidence that type E progresses to chronic disease.

## Cirrhosis of the Liver

**Cirrhosis** is chronic destruction of liver cells and tissues with a nodular, bumpy regeneration. Cirrhosis is the twelfth leading cause if death in the United States, killing about 26,000 people each year. Alcoholic cirrhosis, the most common type of cirrhosis, is described in detail. This disease is also called portal, Laennec, or fatty nutritional cirrhosis (an accumulation of fat often develops within the liver). The exact effect of excessive alcohol on the liver is not known, but it may be related to the malnutrition that frequently accompanies chronic alcoholism, or the alcohol itself may be toxic. In the normal liver, there is a highly organized arrangement of cells, blood vessels, and bile ducts. A cirrhotic liver loses this organization and, as a result, the liver cannot function. Liver cells die and are replaced by fibrous connective tissue and scar tissue. This tissue has none of the liver cell functions. At first, the liver is generally enlarged due to regeneration but then becomes smaller as the fibrous connective tissue contracts. The surface acquires a nodular appearance. This is sometimes called a "hobnailed" liver.

In cirrhosis, circulation through the liver is impaired. As a result, high pressure builds in vessels of the abdomen and in other areas. The esophageal veins swell, forming esophageal varices. Abdominal organs like the spleen, pancreas, and stomach also swell. These organs and vessels may hemorrhage, causing hemorrhagic shock. Hemorrhage of vessels in the stomach or intestines may cause vomiting of blood, **hematemesis**. A characteristic symptom of cirrhosis is distention of the abdomen caused by

# SIDE by SIDE ■ Cirrhosis

▲ Normal human liver.

▲ Cirrhosis of the liver from chronic alcoholism.

the accumulation of fluid in the peritoneal cavity. This fluid is called **ascites** and develops as a result of liver failure. The pressure within the obstructed veins forces plasma into the abdominal cavity. This fluid often has to be drained. When the liver fails to produce adequate amounts of albumin, an albumin deficiency, **hypoalbuminemia**, develops and fluid leaks out of the blood vessels, causing edema. Because the necrotic cells of the cirrhotic patient fail to produce albumin, ascitic fluid develops, as does edema, particularly in the ankles and legs.

Blockage of the bile ducts, like that of the blood vessels, follows the disorganization of the liver. Bile accumulates in the blood, leading to

jaundice and, because bile is not secreted into the duodenum, stools are clay colored. The excess of bile, carried by the blood to the kidneys, imparts a dark color to urine.

Other signs are related to the fact that the diseased liver cannot perform its usual biochemical activities. Normally, the liver inactivates small amounts of female sex hormones secreted by the adrenal glands in both males and females. Estrogens then have no effect on the male, but the cirrhotic liver does not inactivate estrogens. They accumulate and have a feminizing effect on males. The breasts enlarge, a condition known as **gynecomastia**, and the palms of the hands become red because of the estrogen

## Prevention ✚ PLUS!

### Know Your Viruses

The more you know about how a virus is transmitted, the better prepared you can be to prevent infection. Hepatitis A is transmitted primarily through contaminated food and water. Workers in the food-service industry must use sanitary procedures when handling food, including the simple task of washing their hands. You can protect yourself at home by thoroughly cooking meat and seafood. Hepatitis B and C are transmitted through blood transfusions, contaminated needles and syringes, and sexual intercourse. Healthcare workers receive vaccination against hepatitis B, and blood is screened for contamination by hepatitis B and C.

level. Hair on the chest is lost, and a female-type distribution of hair develops. Atrophy of the testicles can also occur.

The damaged liver cells are unable to carry out their normal function of detoxification, so ammonia and other poisonous substances accumulate in the blood and affect the brain, causing various neurologic disorders. Confusion and disorientation, even to the point of stupor, and a characteristic tremor or shaking develop. This shaking is called "liver flap." Somnolence or abnormal sleepiness are symptoms of cirrhosis. **Hepatic coma** is a possible cause of death in cirrhosis.

Although chronic alcoholism is the leading cause of cirrhosis, other diseases can also cause cirrhosis. Severe chronic hepatitis, chronic inflammation of the bile ducts, and certain drugs and toxins can cause necrosis of the liver cells, which is the first step in the development of cirrhosis.

There is no effective treatment for cirrhosis. Liver damage can not be reversed, but further damage can be prevented by treating alcoholism or liver infections that are at the root of cirrhosis. Symptoms of cirrhosis may be treated. For example, edema is treated with diuretics and portal hypertension is remedied with beta blockers to reduce blood pressure. Liver transplant is the only way to restore liver function.

## Cancer of the Liver

**Hepatocarcinoma**, or cancer of the liver, is a primary malignancy of the liver that is rare but has a high mortality rate. While liver cancer comprises 1% of all cancers in the United States, it accounts for 6% and 2% of cancer deaths in men and women, respectively. Liver cancer is most prevalent in men over age 60, and the incidence increases with age. In Africa and parts of Asia, where there is a high incidence of hepatitis B infection, liver cancer comprises 10% to 50% of all cancers. Most cancer found in the liver is secondary, which means it results from metastasis from cancer in other organs, especially the colon, rectum, stomach, pancreas, esophagus, lung, or breast. Primary cancer of the liver is caused chiefly by viral hep-

atitis and cirrhosis. Other causes of liver cancer may include aflatoxin, a toxin from a mold that grows on peanuts and rice.

The symptoms of hepatocarcinoma vary according to the site of the tumor. If the tumor obstructs the portal vein, ascites develops in the abdominal cavity, as it does in cirrhosis. If the fluid contains blood, a malignancy is indicated. A tumor blocking the bile duct will cause jaundice. General symptoms may include loss of weight and an abdominal mass and pain in the upper right quadrant of the abdomen.

Diagnosis includes serum levels of enzymes that arise from diseased liver tissue, but correct diagnosis depends on needle biopsy or open biopsy. Prognosis for cancer of the liver is poor because usually the malignancy has developed elsewhere and has spread to the liver.

## ▶ Diseases of the Gallbladder

The gallbladder stores and concentrates bile. Gallbladder disease impairs the storage and delivery of bile to the duodenum.

## Gallstones (Cholelithiasis)

Gallstones are precipitated bile components in the gallbladder and bile ducts. Gallstones and gallbladder disorders (cholecystitis, discussed in the following subsection) are common, affecting about 1 million Americans per year. Gallstones affect twice as many women as men. The stones arise in the gallbladder when the bile composition changes or when gallbladder muscle activity reduces, as it may during pregnancy, use of oral contraceptives, diabetes mellitus, obesity, cirrhosis, and pancreatitis. The stones consist principally of cholesterol, bilirubin, and calcium when in excess. Gallstones, also called **biliary calculi**, may be present in the gallbladder and give no symptoms. There may be one gallstone present or several hundred, which can be large or small (Figure 9–10▶). Small stones, referred to as gravel, can enter the common bile duct and cause an obstruction with excruciating pain.

Figure 9–10 ► Gallbladder opening showing gallstones. (Martin Rotker/Phototake NYC)

Gallstones can be diagnosed and located by ultrasound and x-ray. The usual treatment for gallstones is surgical removal of the gallbladder, a **cholecystectomy**. The cystic duct is ligated and the common bile duct examined for stones. Occasionally, undetected cholesterol stones are retained in the common bile duct after surgery. Administering a solubilizing agent through a catheter into the bile duct may dissolve the remaining stones, preventing the necessity of repeated surgery.

## Cholecystitis

**Cholecystitis** is an inflammation of the gallbladder usually associated with gallstones (cholelithiasis). Acute cholecystitis is most common in middle age. The gallbladder becomes extremely swollen, causing pain under the right rib cage that radiates to the right shoulder. At this point, the gallbladder can usually be palpated. Chills and fever, nausea and vomiting, belching and indigestion are symptoms; in chronic cholecystitis these symptoms occur especially after eating fatty foods. The presence of fat in the duodenum stimulates the gallbladder to contract and release bile, and the contraction of the inflamed gallbladder causes pain. Prolonged inflammation causes the gallbladder to lose its ability to concentrate bile. The walls of the gallbladder may thicken, making it impossible for the gallbladder to contract properly. Serious complications can result from cholecystitis.

Lack of blood flow because of the obstruction brought about by the swelling can cause an infarction. With the death of the tissues, gangrene can set in. The acutely inflamed gallbladder, like an inflamed appendix, may rupture, causing peritonitis. A complication of chronic cholecystitis is that bile accumulates in the bile ducts of the liver. This causes necrosis and fibrosis of the liver cells lining the ducts. This is another form of cirrhosis, **biliary** (bile) **cirrhosis**.

## ► Structure and Function of the Pancreas

The pancreas is a fish-shaped organ extending across the abdomen behind the stomach. The head fits into the curve of the duodenum, where the pancreatic duct empties digestive enzymes from the pancreas. These enzymes include amylase, which breaks down carbohydrates; trypsin and chymotrypsin, which digest protein; and lipase, which breaks down lipid or fat.

Diseases of the pancreas severely interfere with digestion and absorption of nutrients. Also, a diseased pancreas may release enzymes that can damage the pancreas and surrounding tissues. Figure 9–11 ► shows the structure of the pancreas. Figure 9–12 ► shows the relationship between the pancreas and other digestive organs.

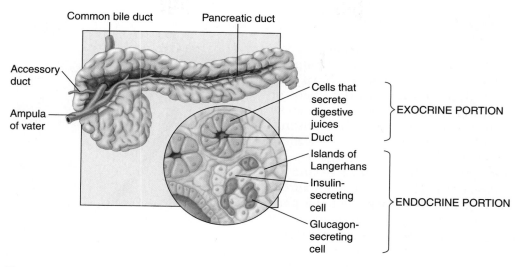

Figure 9–11 ► The pancreas: An endocrine and exocrine gland.

## ▶ Diseases of the Pancreas

### Pancreatitis

Acute **pancreatitis** is a serious, painful inflammation of the pancreas. Pancreatitis is more prevalent in women than in men and usually occurs after age 40. In men it is often associated with alcoholism or peptic ulcers. In women it is more commonly associated with gallbladder disease. The prognosis is good if pancreatitis is associated with gallbladder disease but is very poor if it is related to alcoholism. Pancreatitis

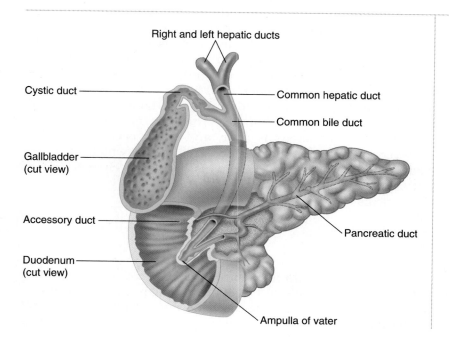

Figure 9–12 ► Relationship between the pancreas and the digestive system.

may be caused by local swelling, necrosis, hemorrhage, or trauma.

Severe, steady abdominal pain of sudden onset is the first symptom. The intense pain radiates to the back and resembles the sharp pain of a perforated ulcer. Drawing up the knees or assuming a sitting position may provide some relief. There may also be nausea and vomiting. Jaundice sometimes develops if the swelling blocks the common bile duct. If a large area of the pancreas is affected, both endocrine and digestive functions of the gland become impaired. In the absence of lipid enzymes from the pancreas, fat cannot be digested, resulting in greasy stools with a foul odor. Secondary malabsorption syndrome develops because fat that is not digested cannot be absorbed. In pancreatitis, the protein- and lipid-digesting enzymes become activated within the pancreas and begin to digest the organ itself. Severe necrosis and edema of the pancreas result. The digestion can extend into blood vessels, which causes severe internal bleeding and shock. When the condition becomes this severe, it is called acute hemorrhagic pancreatitis.

The most significant diagnostic procedures for pancreatitis are blood and urine tests for amylase. Treatment is aimed at maintaining circulation to the pancreas and surrounding tissues, maintaining blood and fluid volume, and reducing pain.

## Cancer of the Pancreas

Cancer of the pancreas, **adenocarcinoma**, has a high mortality rate. It occurs more frequently in males than in females, is most prevalent in men between age 35 and 70, and exhibits the highest prevalence in Israel, the United States, Sweden, and Canada. Pancreatic cancer is linked to cigarette smoking, high-protein and -fat diets, food additives, and exposure to industrial chemicals like beta-naphthalene, benzidine, and urea. Chronic alcohol abuse, chronic pancreatitis, and diabetes mellitus increase the risk of developing pancreatic cancer.

A malignancy in the head of the pancreas can block the common bile duct (Figure 9–13 ►), and symptoms are experienced earlier than those of cancer in the body or tail of the pan-

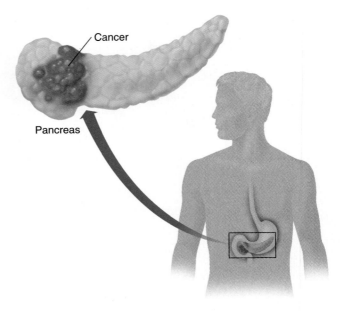

**Figure 9–13** ► Pancreatic cancer. A common site of pancreatic cancer is in the head of the pancreas within the pancreatic ducts.

creas, which can be very advanced before it is discovered. Obstruction of the bile duct causes jaundice and impairs digestion because the pancreatic enzymes and bile cannot enter the duodenum. This causes malabsorption of fat and clay-colored stools; sufficient nutrients and calories cannot be absorbed, and weight loss occurs. Great pain is experienced as the tumor grows, and the cancer usually metastasizes to the surrounding organs: the duodenum, stomach, and liver.

Diagnosis depends on laparoscopic biopsy and ultrasound. Prognosis for cancer of the pancreas is poor, and death occurs in a relatively short time. Treatment, which is rarely successful, includes surgery, chemotherapy, and radiation.

## ► Age-Related Diseases

Infants and young children are especially vulnerable to the effects of digestive system disorders and diseases because their growing and developing bodies require substantial fluids, calories, and nutrients. For example, unchecked vomiting and diarrhea can cause dehydration and malnutrition more easily in children than in adults. The digestive system functions fairly well in healthy elderly people, despite normal age-related changes like thinning mucosa and decreased muscle motility. However, some diseases occur with greater frequency with increasing age and thus significantly impact elderly populations.

## Mouth and Esophagus

Dental caries (cavities) are more prevalent in children than in adults. After adolescence, the incidence of caries reduces and the risk for gingivitis and periodontal disease increases. Periodontal disease and osteoporosis contribute to tooth loss in elderly people. The number of taste buds decrease, and together with decreased saliva secretion, this may lead to decreased appetite. Esophageal cancer incidence is highest in those over age 60. As stated earlier, this cancer is closely linked with the use of alcohol and tobacco.

## Gastrointestinal Tract

Infectious diarrheal diseases are the leading cause of death in children worldwide. Children cannot tolerate the loss of enormous amounts of water, electrolytes, and nutrients associated with diarrhea. Hiatal hernia is a common disorder in elderly people. Peptic ulcers are no more common in elderly than in middle-age people; however, the risk of hemorrhage is greater in old age. Colon cancer incidence increases after age 45, which emphasizes the importance of regular screening and early diagnosis. Diverticula are most common in elderly, and therefore the incidence of diverticulitis rises. Diarrhea poses a great risk of dehydration and malnutrition.

Therefore, gastrointestinal infections like food poisoning and dysentery can be serious diseases. Overall, the function of the intestines remains fairly normal, although intestinal motility is slightly decreased. Thus, changes in diet or new medications that affect intestinal motility can more easily lead to constipation or diarrhea.

## Liver and Gallbladder

Disorders are uncommon in children. In adulthood, liver function diminishes with increasing age, which results in the persistence of high blood levels of medications or toxins. In old age, levels of clotting factors decline, increasing the risk for hemorrhage. The incidence of cholelithiasis is highest in those over age 80.

## Pancreas

Disorders in children are uncommon, although insulin-dependent diabetes does have its onset in childhood. (See Chapter 12.) The incidence of pancreatic cancer peaks in the sixties and is most common among older men. Acute pancreatitis is common in the elderly. In younger people, acute pancreatitis is associated with alcoholism, while in the elderly acute pancreatitis is more likely due to gallstones that block the pancreatic duct.

## RESOURCES

American Cancer Society: www.cancer.org

American Gastroenterological Association: www.gastro.org

American Liver Society: www.liversociety.org

National Institute of Health, National Digestive Diseases Information Clearinghouse: digestive.niddk.nih.gov

# DISEASES AT A GLANCE

## Digestive System

| DISEASE | ETIOLOGY | SIGNS AND SYMPTOMS |
|---|---|---|
| Stomatitis | Bacteria, viruses, fungi | Redness, ulcers, patches, bleeding, depending on the cause |
| Cancer of the mouth | Use of tobacco products, especially in conjunction with consuming alcohol | Abnormal growths, sores, or lesions that don't heal |
| Cancer of the esophagus | Use of tobacco and alcohol | Dysphagia, vomiting, weight loss |
| Esophagitis | Acid reflux due to incompetent cardiac sphincter | Burning chest pain (heartburn), especially after eating or while lying down |
| Esophageal varices | Increased venous pressure; accompanies advanced cirrhosis | Dilated esophageal veins, hemorrhage |
| Hiatal hernia | Stomach protrudes through weakened diaphragm | Indigestion, heartburn following meals, acid reflux, and esophagitis |
| Gastritis | Aspirin, coffee, tobacco, alcohol, infection | Stomach pain, hematemesis |
| Chronic atrophic gastritis | Degeneration of stomach mucosa results in no HCl secretion and no intrinsic factor secretion | Gastritis, poor digestion and absorption of nutrients, weight loss |
| Peptic ulcer | Infection with *H. pylori* and erosion of mucosa by stomach acid | Upper abdominal pain, hemorrhage, blood in stool |
| Gastroenteritis | Food- and water-borne infection by bacteria, viruses, protozoa | Nausea, vomiting, diarrhea, abdominal discomfort or pain, and possibly fever, depending on the pathogen |

| DIAGNOSIS | TREATMENT | PREVENTION | LIFESPAN |
|---|---|---|---|
| Physical exam, immunodiagnostic tests, and pathogen culture | Antibiotics, antivirals, or antifungals, depending on the pathogen | Good oral hygiene; do not use antibiotics unnecessarily or incorrectly | More common in infants, young children, and older adults with weakened immune systems |
| Physical exam, biopsy | Surgical excision of tumor, radiation | Avoid tobacco products; use alcohol only in moderation | Occurs in adults; incidence increases with age |
| Endoscopy and esophageal washings | Surgery, radiation, chemotherapy | Avoid tobacco products; use alcohol only in moderation | Occurs in adults; incidence increases with age |
| Physical exam | Nonirritating diet, antacids, acid-reducing medications | Take small meals; avoid known irritants | Occurs in adults; incidence increases with age |
| Endoscopy, physical exam, history of alcoholism | Hemorrhage requires infusion of vasopressin or insertion of inflatable tube to compress veins; surgical bypass of portal veins to reduce intravenous pressure | Treat underlying alcoholism or liver disease | Occurs in adults; incidence increases with age |
| X-ray | Avoid irritating foods, eat frequent small meals, surgery to repair diaphragm | Avoid spicy food, caffeine; eat small meals | Occurs in adults; incidence increases with age |
| Gastroscopy | Avoid irritants, drink ice water, take antacid medications; surgery to control bleeding | Avoid known irritants | Occurs in adults; incidence increases with age |
| Analysis of stomach content reveals low levels of HCl and intrinsic factor | Avoid stomach irritants, take vitamin $B_{12}$ supplements | Avoid known irritants | Occurs in adults; incidence increases with age |
| Gastroscopy, gastric washings, barium x-ray | Antibiotics | Reduce stress | Occurs in adults; incidence increases with age |
| Stool culture, history | Fluid and electrolyte replacement; antidiarrheal medication; self-limiting in healthy people | Safe food handling, including correct storage, refrigeration, and thorough cooking as needed | Occurs at all ages; especially debilitating in young children and older adults |

# DISEASES AT A GLANCE

## Digestive System (*continued*)

| DISEASE | ETIOLOGY | SIGNS AND SYMPTOMS |
|---------|----------|--------------------|
| Cancer of the stomach | Idiopathic; associated with salted, cured foods and diet low in vegetables and fruit; associated with prior infections with *H. pylori* | Appetite loss, stomach discomfort, hematemesis, blood in stool, late-stage pain |
| Appendicitis | Obstruction with fecal material leads to infection, inflammation, and necrosis | Acute lower right quadrant abdominal pain, nausea, fever |
| Malabsorption syndrome | Congenitally abnormal intestinal mucosa or malabsorption secondary to diseases of pancreas or gallbladder | Malnutrition, failure to absorb fats and fat-soluble vitamins, failure to grow in children and weight loss in adults |
| Diverticulitis | Diverticula of colon become impacted with fecal material and infected or inflamed | Cramping and pain in lower abdomen |
| Regional enteritis (Crohn's disease) | Idiopathic; possible link to autoimmune disease | Lower right pain, diarrhea and constipation, emission and exacerbation, weight loss, melena |
| Chronic ulcerative colitis | Idiopathic; may be autoimmune, stress related, food allergy related | Diarrhea; pus, blood, mucus in stool; cramping in lower abdomen |
| Cancer of colon and rectum | Genetic; associated with familial polyposis and chronic ulcerative colitis | Change in bowel habits, diarrhea or constipation, blood in stool |
| Spastic colon/irritable bowel syndrome | Abuse of laxatives; irritating foods; stress | Diarrhea, pain, gas, constipation |
| Dysentery | Food- or water-borne intestinal infection by bacteria or protozoa | Abdominal pain, bloody diarrhea with pus and mucus |
| Viral hepatitis A (infectious hepatitis) | Food- or water-borne infection with hepatitis A virus | Anorexia, nausea, mild fever, jaundice, enlarged tender liver |

| DIAGNOSIS | TREATMENT | PREVENTION | LIFESPAN |
|---|---|---|---|
| Gastroscopy, biopsy, gastric fluid analysis (low HCl), barium x-ray | Surgery, chemotherapy | Reduce intake of salt and cured meat | Occurs in adults; incidence increases with age |
| Blood count, physical exam | Surgery | Maintain good bowel habits | Most prevalent puberty through 20s |
| Stool analysis and history | Manage diet and take vitamin supplements | Treat underlying diseases | Onset around age 1 as gluten introduced in solid meals |
| Endoscopy | Antibiotics, manage diet | Good bowel habits | Occurs in young adults; incidence increases with age |
| Stool analysis, endoscopy, patchy thickening of intestinal wall | Corticosteroids, occasionally surgery | None | Occurs in young adults; incidence increases with age |
| Stool analysis, endoscopy, diffuse thickening of colon (pipestem colon) | Corticosteroids, stress reduction, diet management, colostomy | Reduce stress | Occurs in young adults; incidence increases with age |
| Endoscopy, biopsy, barium x-ray, stool analysis | Surgery, radiation, chemotherapy | Regular screening to include endoscopy and biopsy if at risk | Occurs in adults; incidence increases with age |
| History and physical exam; no lesions present | Avoid caffeine, alcohol, spicy food, fat; increase fiber in diet; reduce stress | Avoid laxatives | Occurs in young adults; incidence increases with age |
| Stool culture and history | Antibiotics if bacterial and amebicides if caused by protozoa | Safe food and water handling | Occurs at all ages; especially debilitating for young children and older adults |
| Physical exam, stool analysis, immunodiagnostics | Immunoglobulin injections for exposures and infections | Vaccine; safe food and water handling | Occurs at all ages; especially debilitating for young children and older adults |

| DISEASE | ETIOLOGY | SIGNS AND SYMPTOMS |
| --- | --- | --- |
| Hepatitis B (serum hepatitis) | Blood-borne or sexually transmitted infection with hepatitis B virus | 2–6-month incubation period followed by anorexia, nausea, mild fever, jaundice, enlarged tender liver; may lead to chronic hepatitis and cirrhosis |
| Hepatitis C | Blood-borne or sexually transmitted infection with hepatitis C virus | Symptoms as for hepatitis A and hepatitis B following incubation period of months to decades; commonly results in cirrhosis and end-stage liver disease |
| Hepatitis D | Rare blood-borne or sexually transmitted co-infection with hepatitis D virus and hepatitis B virus | Same as for hepatitis B; more serious and frequently progresses to chronic liver diseases |
| Hepatitis E | Water-borne infection with hepatitis E virus rare in United States | As for hepatitis A |
| Cirrhosis | Alcohol-induced damage to liver; hepatitis | Jaundice, abdominal distension, ascites, bleeding tendencies, edema, malabsorption of fats, gynecosmastia, delerium tremens, hepatic coma |
| Cancer of the liver | Primary carcinoma is complication of cirrhosis; more common is secondary or metastatic | Bile duct obstruction, jaundice, impaired clotting, ascites, weight loss |
| Cholecystitis | Obstruction by infection/inflammation or by tumor | Upper right abdominal pain especially following a meal of fatty food; nausea, indigestion, belching |
| Cholelithiasis | Related to obesity; higher incidence in pregnancy and among women | None, or upper right abdominal pain especially following a meal |
| Pancreatitis | Idiopathic, commonly associated with excessive alcohol consumption or with gallstones | Acute, severe, sharp, radiating abdominal pain; risk of hemorrhage; jaundice; vomiting; malabsorption |
| Cancer of the pancreas | Linked to cigarette smoking, alcohol abuse, chemical carcinogens, chronic pancreatitis, diabetes mellitus | Malabsorption, jaundice, upper abdominal pain |

| DIAGNOSIS | TREATMENT | PREVENTION | LIFESPAN |
|---|---|---|---|
| Physical exam, stool analysis, immunodiagnostics | Immunoglobulin injections for exposures and infections, antiviral medications, vaccine for prevention | Vaccine | Occurs at all ages; especially debilitating for young children and older adults |
| Physical exam, stool analysis, immunodiagnostics | Ribavarin, interferon, liver transplant | Safe sex, avoid injection drug abuse | Occurs at all ages; especially debilitating for young children and older adults |
| Physical exam, stool analysis, immunodiagnostics | Immunoglobulin injections, antiviral | Safe sex, avoid injection drug abuse | Occurs at all ages; especially debilitating for young children and older adults |
| Physical exam, stool analysis, immunodiagnostics | No treatment, no vaccine | Safe food and water handling | Occurs at all ages; especially debilitating for young children and older adults |
| Patient history, physical exam, serum liver enzyme levels | No specific treatment; symptomatic treatment for edema and portal hypertension or bleeding; improved diet, liver transplant | Treat underlying alcoholism or liver disease | Occurs in adults |
| Ultrasound, CT scan, needle biopsy | Chemotherapy (prognosis poor) | None | Rare; occurs in adults and occasionally children |
| Ultrasound, CT scan, fecal fat test | Cholecystectomy | None | Occurs in young adults and prevalence increases with age |
| Ultrasound, CT scan, fecal fat test | Cholecystectomy, administration of solubilizing agent into bile duct | Reduce weight | Occurs in young adults and prevalence increases with age |
| Ultrasound, CT scan, serum pancreatic enzymes | No specific treatment; analgesics, fluid replacement, IV nutrients | Treat underlying alcoholism | Occurs in young adults and prevalence increases with age |
| Ultrasound, CT scan, needle biopsy | Chemotherapy (prognosis poor) | Stop tobacco use, alcohol abuse, treat underlying diabetes | Occurs in young adults and prevalence increases with age |

# Interactive Exercises

## Cases for Critical Thinking

1. A 45-year-old woman experiences frequent heartburn, difficulty swallowing, and sharp pains below her sternum. At night, she experiences gastric reflux, or a regurgitation of stomach acid into the esophagus, a condition that is extremely painful. What could produce these symptoms? What diagnostic procedures could be used? How should she be treated?

2. T. W. experiences sharp pain in his upper right abdomen after eating a high-fat meal. Also, he has noted that his feces are grayish white instead of brown. What disease is the likely cause of his symptoms? Explain why each of these symptoms occurs with this disease.

3. Explain how cirrhosis leads to each of these signs and symptoms: jaundice, malnutrition, hemorrhage, esophageal varices.

## Multiple Choice

1. Which of the following is a sign of gastritis?
   a. constipation
   b. inflammation of stomach mucosa
   c. achlorhydria
   d. diarrhea

2. Recurrent bloody diarrhea may be a symptom of
   _____.
   a. gastric ulcer        b. ulcerative colitis
   c. hiatal hernia        d. esophagitis

3. Which disease is characterized by the destruction of intestinal villi, leading to inability to absorb fats and other nutrients?
   a. ulcerative colitis
   b. celiac disease/malabsorption syndrome
   c. Crohn's disease
   d. peptic ulcer

4. Small pouches of the large intestine become inflamed during which disease?
   a. Crohn's disease      b. gastritis
   c. hemorrhoids          d. diverticulitis

5. Which statement about pancreatic cancer is FALSE?
   a. It is characterized by abdominal pain, weakness, weight loss.
   b. It has a higher incidence with age.
   c. Most cancers are diagnosed after the cancer has metastasized.
   d. The prognosis is good with an 85% cure rate.

6. Which statement about cirrhosis is FALSE?
   a. Irreversible degenerative changes occur in the liver.
   b. The normal liver tissue is replaced with fibrous scar tissue.
   c. It is most often caused by diabetes.
   d. It is associated with esophageal varices.

7. Acute pancreatitis is most closely associated with
   _____.
   a. hepatitis C virus infection
   b. chronic alcoholism
   c. bile duct obstruction
   d. complication of cirrhosis

8. Esophageal varices arise in which disease?
   a. cirrhosis            b. pancreatic cancer
   c. cholecystitis        d. cholelithiasis

9. Oral thrush is caused by _____.
   a. *Candida albicans*
   b. herpes simplex virus type 1
   c. *Treponema pallidum*
   d. *Streptococcus pyogenes* virus type 1

10. Pain in the upper right quadrant, especially after eating, could be a sign of _____.
    a. appendicitis         b. pancreatitis
    c. cholecystitis        d. colitis

## True or False

_____ 1. Hemorrhoids are caused by infection with *E. coli*.

_____ 2. Oral and esophageal cancers are linked to tobacco and alcohol use.

_____ 3. Drinking too much water causes diarrhea.

_____ 4. Dark stools are known as melena.

_____ 5. Neurologic disorders can accompany liver disease.

_____ 6. Hepatitis A is acquired through blood products.

_____ 7. Most cancer in the liver is primary liver cancer.

_____ 8. Gallstones are made of undigested food particles too large to pass.

_____ 9. There is no vaccine for hepatitis B.

_____ 10. Gastric ulcers are caused by infection with *Helicobacter pylori*.

## Fill-Ins

1. *Entamoeba histolytica* is the cause of _____ _____.

2. Thickened intestinal walls, leading to obstruction and abdominal pain, are found in _____ _____.

3. An abdominal _____ is protrusion of an organ through abdominal wall muscles.

4. An instrument called a(n) _____ is used to view the lining of the esophagus or other organs of the digestive tract.

5. Hepatitis type _____ is the major viral cause of cirrhosis.

6. Cholecystectomy is used to treat _____.

7. Biliary cirrhosis arises if there is obstruction of the _____ _____.

8. Accumulation of fluid in the abdomen is called _____.

9. Stomatitis refers to inflammation of the _____.

10. The primary function of the _____ _____ is to absorb water.

## Labeling Exercise

Use the blank lines on the right to label the following images.

1 _____

2 _____

3 _____

4 _____

5 _____

6 _____

7 _____

8 _____

9 _____

10 _____

11 _____

12 _____

13 _____

14 _____

15 _____

# Multimedia Preview

Additional interactive resources and activities for this chapter can be found on the Companion Website. For videos, audio glossary, and review, access the accompanying DVD-ROM in this book.

## ▶ DVD-ROM Highlights

### Labeling Exercise

A picture is worth a thousand words, but only if it's labeled correctly. Review pathology by clicking and dragging the terms that correlate to a figure from this chapter. The correct labels will lock into place beside the picture.

### Gridlock

Are you a *Jeopardy!* champ? Prove your quiz show smarts by clicking the tiles to answer the human diseases questions hidden beneath. Get them all right to clear the grid.

## ▶ Website Highlights—www.pearsonhighered.com/zelman

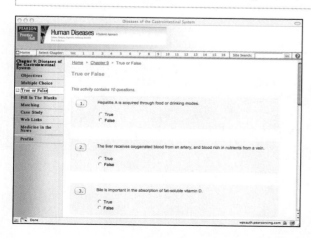

### True or False Quiz

Take advantage of the free-access online study guide that accompanies your textbook. You'll find a true or false quiz that provides instant feedback and allows you to check your score to see what you got right or wrong. By clicking on this URL you'll also access links to current news articles and an audio glossary.

CHAPTER

10

# Diseases of the Urinary System

## Learning Objectives

After studying this chapter, you should be able to

- Describe the primary functions of the major organs of the urinary system—the kidneys and the urinary bladder

- Identify the etiology, signs and symptoms, diagnostic tests, and treatment for selected diseases of the kidney

- Describe the etiology, signs and symptoms, diagnostic tests, and treatment of urinary tract infections (UTIs)

- Differentiate between ascending and descending modes of urinary tract infections

- Explain how urinary tract infections affect or dysfunctions affect other organ systems

- Distinguish among the various modes of kidney dialysis.

- Identify the etiology, signs and symptoms, and treatments of various types of kidney stones (renal calculi)

- Describe causes and treatments of inflammation within the urinary bladder and urethra

- Contrast neurogenic bladder with stress and other forms of urinary incontinence

- Recognize the etiology, signs and symptoms, and treatment for bladder cancer

- Describe age-related changes of the urinary system

## Fact or Fiction?

Renal calculi, or kidney stones, form only in the kidneys. They also form in the population equally throughout all regions of the United States.

*Fiction: Renal calculi may form anywhere within the urinary system, but they usually form in the renal pelvis or calyces of the kidney. Within the United States, there is an area considered the "stone belt." The southeastern region of the country tends to have a greater proportion of persons with renal calculi, but the exact cause is unknown.*

## Kidney Dialysis

In 1913, a pharmacologist at Johns Hopkins University named John Abel published an article about hemodialysis using animals. In the 1930s Dr. Willem Kolff, who at the time was struggling to develop an artificial kidney in the Netherlands, read the article and was curious about applying Abel's concepts to human dialysis. Even under the dark cloud of world war, Kolff and his associates managed to construct a dialyzer in 1943. However, progress was slow. The crude dialyzer failed to save the first 16 patients placed on it, and these patients suffered acute renal failure. In 1945, a woman in a uremic coma survived and lived seven more years and the future looked bright.

However, when Dr. Kolff moved to the United States following the war, he was not recognized or supported for his efforts. He struggled again for success. At Peter Bent Brigham Hospital in Boston, Kolff met George Thorn, who modified the dialyzer with a stainless steel container and later called it the Kolff-Brigham kidney. This new machine saved many American soldiers during the Korean War and paved the way for the first kidney transplant in 1954. Because machines were not thought to work as well over time as natural organs and puncture sites would be difficult to find after continual trauma, the dialyzer was not promoted.

Dr. Belding Scribner, from the University of Washington, formed a connection between an artery and a vein using plastic tubing and a shunt device with a new material called Teflon. By the 1960s, small portable units were made and hemodialysis could be performed at home. Dr. Kolff, however, is considered the father of dialysis, and he was instrumental in developing the heart-lung machine and the artificial heart. In the past 60 years, incredible advancements have been made in kidney treatments. Today, at age 93, Dr. Kolff is still inventing. Pioneers of the past like Drs. Kolff and Scribner continue to provide futures for so many in the present.

## ▶ Functions of the Kidney

The kidneys filter the blood, producing approximately 1 milliliter of urine per minute. In fact, between 20% and 25% of the body's blood volume is contained within the kidneys at any given time. As they filter the blood (plasma), the kidneys maintain water and **electrolyte balance**, and they maintain pH levels. The kidneys also produce hormones like erythropoietin, which stimulates red blood cell production, and renin, which elevates blood pressure.

### The Nephron

The functional unit of the kidney is the **nephron**. Approximately 1 million nephrons reside in each kidney. As blood passes through the nephrons, metabolic waste products are filtered from the blood plasma. At the same time, most of the water (99%) is reabsorbed along with nutrients such as glucose and amino acids. Extra water, unwanted ions, some drugs, and metabolic wastes are then excreted. The product at the end of the nephron is urine.

Each nephron consists of a pair of arterioles, a **glomerulus**, a glomerular capsule, a proximal convoluted tubule, a loop of Henle, and a distal convoluted tubule that leads to a collecting duct. The components of the nephron unit are shown in Figure 10–1 ▶.

### Formation of Urine

Blood in the renal arteries enters a tuft of capillaries called the glomerulus, which is situated inside the glomerular capsule. These capillary walls are very thin and porous, and the blood pressure within them is higher than the pressure in the surrounding capsule. When blood enters these capillaries, fluid filters into the glomerular capsule. This blood filtrate is equivalent to protein-free plasma. In a healthy nephron, neither protein nor red blood cells pass through the filter into the **glomerular capsule**.

In the proximal convoluted tubule, most of the nutrients and a large amount of water are reabsorbed and taken back into blood capillaries surrounding the tubules. Salts, particularly sodium and chloride, are selectively reabsorbed according to the body's needs. Eventually, about 99% of the water is also reabsorbed along with the salts.

The nitrogen-containing waste products of protein metabolism, **urea** and **creatinine**, pass on through the tubules to be excreted in the urine. Those substances that are in excess in the body fluids, such as hydrogen ions when the fluid is too acidic, are secreted into the distal tubules to be excreted.

**Aldosterone** and **antidiuretic hormone (ADH)** play very important roles in the regulation of salt and water reabsorption. These hormones are discussed in detail in Chapter 12.

Urine from all the collecting ducts eventually empties into the **renal pelvis**, the juncture between the kidneys and the **ureters**, and moves down the ureters to be stored in the urinary bladder. Following the signals given by the **micturition** process, the bladder empties urine into the urethra, which leads outside the body. Figure 10–2 ▶ illustrates the urinary system.

## ▶ Diagnostic Tests and Procedures

Pain, **dysuria** (painful urination), blood or pus in urine, or edema indicates kidney disease, but specific diagnostic tests are required to determine the nature of the disease. Edema is caused by the loss of protein from the blood; these blood proteins have a water-holding power within the blood vessels. With their depletion, fluid moves out of the capillaries and into the tissues, causing swelling or puffiness.

Significant information can be obtained by a simple diagnostic procedure, a urinalysis, in which a urine specimen is studied physically, chemically, and microscopically. Physical observation allows notation of urine color, pH, and specific gravity of a urine specimen. A centrifuged urine sample is examined microscopically for solids such as crystals, epithelial cells, or blood cells.

Chemical tests (e.g., Chemstrip) reveal the presence of abnormal substances such as protein (specifically albumin), glucose, and blood. Urine is normally yellow or amber, but hema-

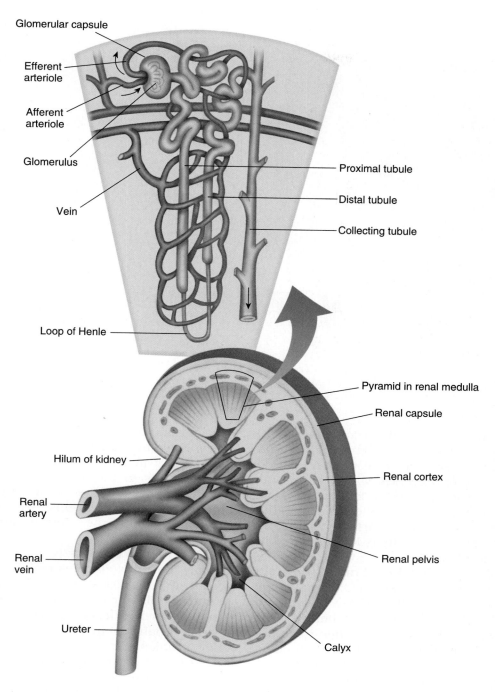

Figure 10–1 ▶ The kidney with an expanded view of the nephron.

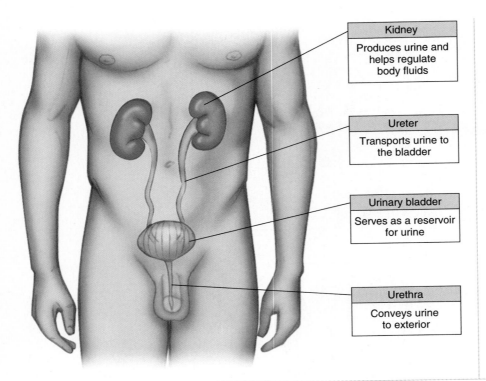

| Kidney |
|---|
| Produces urine and helps regulate body fluids |

| Ureter |
|---|
| Transports urine to the bladder |

| Urinary bladder |
|---|
| Serves as a reservoir for urine |

| Urethra |
|---|
| Conveys urine to exterior |

**Figure 10–2** ▶ The urinary system.

turia (blood in the urine) can darken the color to a reddish brown. The degree of color depends on the amount of water the urine contains. Urine is pale in the case of diabetics, whose water output is large. In long-standing kidney diseases, the ability of the tubules to concentrate the urine is lost. As a result, the urine is dilute and pale, and the specific gravity is low, as found in chronic glomerulonephritis.

The pH of urine has a broad range. The ability of the kidneys to excrete acidic or alkaline urine typically permits the kidney to regulate the pH of the blood within narrow limits. Urine specimens should be examined when fresh because they tend to become alkaline on standing due to bacterial contamination. Urine from a cystitis patient tends to be alkaline for the same reason.

Albuminuria indicates inflammation of the urinary tract, particularly of the glomeruli. The inflammation increases the permeability of blood vessels, allowing protein and albumin to enter the nephrons and appear in the urine.

This continual protein loss reduces the level of water "holding power" by the blood (plasma) and results in hypoproteinemia, leading to a loss of fluids to the surrounding tissues and causing edema. Clinitek 50 or Clinitek 100 microalbumin reagent strips are used on an overnight sample when determining hypoalbuminemia.

The presence of sugar (glucose) in the urine usually indicates diabetes mellitus. This is not a sign of a disease of the kidneys, but of the pancreas. Diabetes over an extended period of time adversely affects the kidneys (see Chapter 12). Diabetes insipidus is another endocrine problem due to the lack of ADH or reduced sensitivity of the kidney tubules to the hormone. In either case, the kidney loses its power to control water maintenance and the patient dehydrates due to copious water loss. Treatment involves ADH-type medication such as Pitressin (vasopressin) or Daipid (lypressin) that helps resolve the occurrence of dehydration.

Hematuria may be obvious to the naked eye or require microscopic determination. Hematuria is associated with many serious diseases of the urinary tract, including glomerulonephritis, kidney stones, tuberculosis, cystitis, and tumors. If the passage of urine is accompanied by pain, then a stone, an infection, or potentially tuberculosis would likely be the cause. Painless hematuria indicates the possibility of a malignant tumor in the urinary system.

Pyuria results from a suppurative inflammation caused by pyogenic bacteria that causes the urine to appear cloudy. Microscopic examination of the urine reveals numerous leukocytes. Diseases such as pyelonephritis, pyelitis, tuberculosis, and cystitis show pus in the urine.

Casts are shaped like cylindrical rods because they form within kidney tubules. These cast structures consist of coagulated protein, a substance not normally present in kidney tubules. Casts can include various kinds of blood cells as well as epithelial cells from the lining of the urinary tract, and they always indicate inflammation.

Microscopic examination determines the presence or absence of bacteria. Bacteria are found in tuberculosis of the kidney, pyelonephritis, and frequently in cystitis. For microscopic examinations, a urine sample may be removed from the bladder by catheterization to ensure that no external contamination occurs.

A cystoscopic examination enables the healthcare provider to view the inside of the bladder and urethra. The cystoscope is a long, lighted instrument resembling a narrow hollow tube. Tumors, stones, and inflammations may be identified with this device. Using an additional instrument, small tumors or polyps may be removed or biopsied. Stones in the bladder can be crushed or surgically removed.

The intravenous pyelogram (IVP) allows the visualization of the urinary system by means of contrast dyes injected into the veins followed by x-ray examination. When these dyes concentrate in the urinary system, it is possible to note tumors, obstructions, and other deformities. A kidney is viewed by renal ultrasound, and the whole urinary system is surveyed by computed tomography (CT) or kidney, ureter, bladder (KUB) exams.

## ▶ Diseases of the Kidney

### Glomerulonephritis

**Glomerulonephritis** is an inflammatory disease of the glomeruli. It is nonsuppurative; that is, no pus formation, and therefore no bacteria are found in the urine when examined microscopically during a urinalysis procedure. Glomerulonephritis is typically caused by an antigen-antibody reaction that occurs approximately 1 to 4 weeks following a skin (e.g., impetigo) or throat infection by a hemolytic streptococcus bacterium. Antigens from the streptococci and the defensive antibodies form complexes in the bloodstream that become trapped within the glomeruli, causing an inflammatory response. Numerous neutrophils crowd into the inflamed glomeruli, and blood flow to the nephrons is reduced. The impeded blood flow causes a reduction in the filtration rate and results in decreased urine formation. Many glomeruli degenerate, and the remaining glomeruli become extremely permeable, allowing albumin (plasma protein) and red blood cells to appear in the urine (Figure 10–3▶). Primary signs of glomerulonephritis include proteinuria, hematuria, edema, and hypertension.

Additional causes include other infective agents (e.g., viruses), parasites (malaria), vasculitis (inflamed blood vessels or lymph vessels), systemic lupus erythematosus (SLE), and Goodpasture syndrome, described later in this chapter.

Acute glomerulonephritis is most common in young children, but it can occur at any age and usually follows a streptococcal infection from a prior sore throat or skin inflammation (e.g., erysipelas). The symptoms include chills and fever, loss of appetite, and a general feeling of weakness. There may be edema, or puffiness, particularly in the face and ankles. A urinalysis shows **albuminuria**, the presence of the plasma protein albumin in the urine. **Hematuria**, blood in the urine, is also commonly found. **Casts**, which are the structural elements or molds of kidney tubules consisting of coagulated protein and blood, are present. The signs and symptoms of acute glomerulonephritis are presented in Figure 10–4▶.

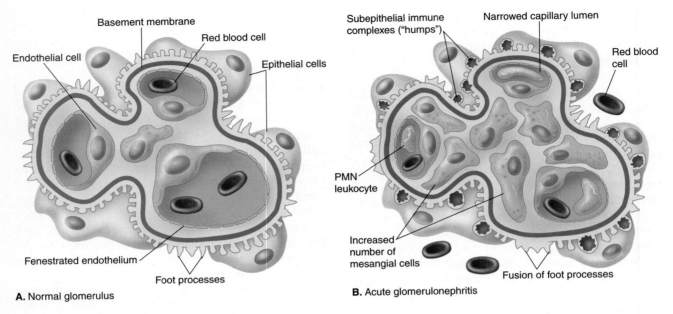

**A.** Normal glomerulus

**B.** Acute glomerulonephritis

Figure 10–3 ► Normal glomerulus and acute glomerulonephritis.

The prognosis for acute glomerulonephritis is good. Normal kidney function is generally restored following bed rest and dietary restrictions (e.g., reduced intake of salt). Medications used for treatment include diuretics, calcium channel blockers, and beta blockers.

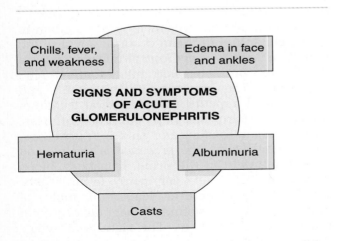

Figure 10–4 ► Signs and symptoms of acute glomerulonephritis.

Repeated attacks of acute glomerulonephritis can lead to weakened kidneys and a chronic condition.

## Chronic Glomerulonephritis

Chronic glomerulonephritis may persist for many years with periods of remission and relapse. Hypertension generally accompanies this disease. As more glomeruli are destroyed, blood filtration becomes increasingly impaired. Prevalence of glomerulonephritis is inconclusive, but the chronic cases are estimated at less than 1%.

Part of a urinalysis examination is a simple procedure using a **urinometer** to determine the extent of kidney function; this is known as a *specific gravity* (sp. gr.) measurement of a urine specimen. The sp. gr. measurement indicates the amount of dissolved substances or solid elements within a urine sample compared to distilled water. Distilled water has a specific gravity of 1.000, and the normal specific gravity of urine is about 1.015 to 1.025 within a broader overall range of 1.003–1.030. In advanced chronic glomerulonephritis, the specific gravity is low and fixed, indicating that the kidney tubules are unable to concentrate the urine. (See Appendix C for normal urine values.)

Urinalysis procedures basically require the visual observation of a urine sample, chemical tests (e.g., Chemstrip/Multistix) and microscopic evaluation.

Chronic glomerulonephritis causes the kidneys to shrink, as they gradually atrophy, and cease to function. **Uremia**, a buildup of metabolic toxins in the blood, results from kidney failure. Chief among these waste products is **urea**, a small, water-soluble nitrogenous molecule that easily penetrates red blood cells and causes their destruction (hemolysis). Therefore, uremia is often associated with gastrointestinal, neuromuscular, and cardiovascular insufficiencies.

Individuals suffering uremic toxicity experience nausea, headache, dizziness, and faint vision. Left unchecked, this condition may result in convulsions and coma. Dialysis treatment is quickly recommended to restore blood nitrogen and electrolyte balance, in order to reduce symptoms.

## Goodpasture Syndrome

Goodpasture syndrome (GPS) is a rarely occurring renal problem considered to be an autoimmune disease. The precise cause of Goodpasture syndrome is not known, although it may be triggered by viral agents attacking the respiratory system or by inhaling hydrocarbon solvents. Therefore, the lungs and kidneys may be stressed together or individually. It develops in days to weeks, and once the body attacks the agents mentioned above, or unknown causes, it tends to attack itself. The primary "glue" that the body uses for constructive support, a protein known as collagen, is somehow recognized as foreign and becomes the target of immune responses, somewhat similar to glomerulonephritis cases. Unfortunately, these autoantibodies are directed against the basement membranes of the glomerular capillaries; this disorder is also called *antiglomerular basement membrane glomerulonephritis*. In this case, the inflammatory disease results in scarring and fibrosis of the glomerular structure (see Figure 10–4).

These same autoantibodies (anti-GBM antibodies) are found in Goodpasture syndrome and must be removed in order to improve the functional unit.

Symptoms of GPS vary and include foamy urine, weakness, nausea, and vomiting. Signs include hematuria, **oliguria** (low urine production), and proteinuria. In addition, respiratory symptoms include hemoptysis, coughing, dypsnea, and chest pain. Diagnostics require physical exam, urinalysis, and more refined chemical tests.

Treatment requires cleansing the plasma of antibodies, and this is accomplished by plasmaphoresis. This process gleans out the causative agents and replaces lost plasma with donor plasma and/or fluids and protein. Dialysis may be required in progressive cases or when permanent kidney damage is moderate; in advanced cases, a kidney transplant is recommended.

Preventative steps are to avoid solvent-type fumes, many of which are aromatic (sweet smelling) and dangerous (e.g., glue sniffing). Use protective gear wherever industrial or commercial fumes are involved.

## Systemic Lupus Erythematosus or Lupus Nephritis

Lupus nephritis results when autoantibodies collect in the glomeruli which causes a major inflammation sufficient to create scars and reduce kidney functioning. Primary treatment involves two drugs in tandem; one to reduce inflammation, prednisolone, and one to suppress the immune system, cyclophosphamide or mycophenolate mofetil. Kidney function is vital, especially when the whole body is attacked by another (autoimmune) disease.

## IgA Nephropathy

In this disease, the immunoglobulin A (IgA) forms deposits in the glomeruli causing inflammation. The most common symptom is blood in the urine (hematuria), but it tends to go unnoticed and remain undetected for years. Even without exact numbers, IgA nephropathy is thought to be the most common cause of primary glomerulonephritis. This status, primary glomerulonephritis, excludes other causes like lupus or diabetes mellitus, which are systemic.

IgA nephropathy is more common in men and young people although it affects all age groups. Because it takes years to become recognized and cause complications, younger people seldom display symptoms. No treatment is recommended for mild cases with normal blood pressure and proteinuria levels, but elevated blood pressure requires medications like ACE inhibitors that seem to work quite well.

## Renal Failure

Ischemia (reduced blood flow), hemorrhage, poisons, and severe kidney disease may cause renal failure. In renal failure, the kidneys are unable to clear the blood of urea and creatinine, which are nitrogen-containing waste products of protein metabolism. These metabolic products are toxic if they accumulate in the blood. Uremia signifies the terminal stage of renal insufficiency.

The level of blood urea nitrogen, or BUN, reflects the degree of renal failure. Measurement of the glomerular filtration rate (GFR) also can assess the severity of renal disease or follow its progress. GFR is evaluated through tests designed to determine the ability of the kidney to clear the waste product creatinine. Serum creatinine level rises and creatinine clearance rate falls when the GFR is impaired. As may be expected, creatinine clearance levels decline in renal insufficiency and with aging. The test for creatinine is the most specific for kidney functioning and therefore a crucial diagnostic measurement.

*Acute Renal Failure*   Acute renal failure may develop suddenly but has a better prognosis than chronic renal failure. Acute renal failure is caused by various factors such as decreased blood flow to the kidneys resulting from surgical shock, including shock following an incompatible blood transfusion, or severe dehydration. Kidney disease, trauma, or poisons from toxic fumes or heavy metals can also cause acute renal failure.

Significant signs of acute renal failure are characterized by a sudden drop in urine volume, called **oliguria**, or complete cessation of urine production, called **anuria**. Symptoms include headache, gastrointestinal distress, and the odor of ammonia on the breath caused by accumulation in the blood of nitrogen-containing compounds. Of special concern is **hyperkalemia**. This elevated blood potassium causes muscle weakness and can slow the heart to the point of cardiac arrest. Treatment includes restoration of the blood volume to normal, with necessary electrolytes, restricted dietary fluid intake, and dialysis as needed.

*Chronic Renal Failure*   Chronic renal failure is life threatening and has a much poorer prognosis than acute renal failure. Chronic renal failure results from long-standing kidney disease such as chronic glomerulonephritis, hypertension, and **diabetic nephropathy (DN)**, a kidney disease resulting from diabetes mellitus.

Diabetic nephropathy, as in glomerulonephritis, is due to thickening of the glomerular apparatus that permits relatively high levels of protein (albumin) to escape into the urine. This glomerular change may be very slow, and routine urinalysis methods may not detect a small continual protein loss. Called microalbuminia, it requires a more comprehensive or sensitive test within the urinalysis procedure to detect protein. Unless other factors (e.g., hypertension, family history) indicate the need for a more reliable test, the albumin continually goes undetected. Early-stage diabetic nephropathy has no symptoms, but as the condition advances it becomes more noticeable and debilitating.

Diabetics are particularly at risk if blood glucose remains uncontrolled and high blood pressure is pronounced. A host of symptoms becomes apparent as diabetes nephropathy evolves over a 5- to 10-year span. These symptoms include fatigue, headache, generalized itching, frothy urine, frequent hiccups, and edema, particularly in the legs. A kidney biopsy is the confirming element of a diagnosis, and it helps determine the extent of the disease. However, if the protein loss is progressive or diabetic retinopathy is noted, the biopsy may be too risky.

Today DN is recognized as the most common cause of chronic kidney failure and end-stage renal disease (ESRD) in the United States.

Chronic renal failure responds to diuretic intervention until alternative measures are warranted, such as kidney dialysis or transplant. Drugs such as furosemide (Lasix) and torsemide (Demadex) will help reduce edema and hypertension as well, because hypertension is a medical priority. Either separately or in combination, angiotensin converting enzyme (ACE) inhibitors or angiotensin receptor blockers (ARBs) would be utilized. Additionally, controlling weight, blood lipids, and sugar levels and engaging in regular exercise are recommended. Common over-the-counter drugs like ibuprofen or aspirin tend to aggravate or weaken the kidney and are discouraged. As the condition worsens and ESRD develops, in which kidney function declines to less than 10% of normal, the option of choice is kidney transplant or kidney-pancreas transplant when available. Even with a successful transplant, continued diligence is necessary, such as dietary considerations for restricting salt and fluid intake and monitoring for anemia or infection.

The condition develops slowly, with urinary output dropping slowly over time. Metabolic wastes accumulate in the blood, with adverse effects on all body systems. For example, urea builds up to toxic levels, and some is converted to ammonia, which acts as an irritant in the gastrointestinal tract, producing nausea, vomiting, and diarrhea. Vision becomes dim, cognitive functions decrease, and convulsions or coma may ensue. Manifestations of chronic renal failure are summarized in Figure 10–5▶. These cases are now primarily considered end-stage kidney disease.

Renal failure is treated with kidney dialysis, a technique that removes toxic substances from the blood. Known as **hemodialysis**, blood is removed from the body, toxic substances are removed from the blood, and the blood is returned to the body (Figure 10–6▶). For hemodialysis, a patient typically must visit a clinic or hospital for dialysis and stay for 3 to 6 hours during the process. However, residential dialysis units are available that allow patients more convenient and private treatment. Small portable dialysis units have further reduced cost and have increased availability for treatment.

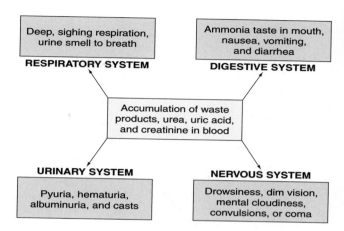

Figure 10–5 ▶ Manifestations of chronic renal failure.

In **peritoneal dialysis (PD)**, dialyzing fluid is introduced into the abdominal cavity, where the peritoneum (cavity lining) acts as a filter membrane. The fluid draws toxic materials out of capillaries surrounding the body cavity, and after a suitable amount of time, the peritoneal fluid is removed, along with its dissolved toxins. A bag may be attached externally to collect the fluid, permitting the patient to remain mobile and providing more freedom and flexibility during treatment. Dialysis may be required for years but may not be sufficient in advanced chronic renal failure.

Another alternative treatment for advanced kidney failure is kidney transplant. Advances in antirejection medications have reduced complications and allowed kidney transplants to prolong and save thousands of lives (Figure 10–7▶).

Prevention of ESRD requires early detection to halt chronic kidney failure, even though it may take many years (10–20) to develop. With advanced age, other ailments, or lack of attention, ESRD may not be preventable. Currently more than 400,000 Americans are on long-term dialysis and more than 20,000 have functioning kidney transplants.

## Pyelonephritis

**Pyelonephritis** is a suppurative urinary tract infection of the kidney and renal pelvis caused by pyogenic (pus-forming) bacteria, including *Escherichia coli, streptococci,* and *staphylococci.*

Figure 10–6 ► Continuous arteriovenous hemofiltration (CAVH).

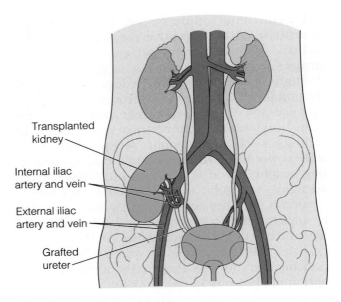

Figure 10–7 ► Placement of a transplanted kidney.

Obstruction of the urinary tract, such as a congenital defect, a kidney stone, or an enlarged prostate gland, slows urine flow and increases the risk for infection. The infection may originate in the bladder and ascends up into the kidneys, or it may originate in blood or lymph and descend to the kidneys as is found in tuberculosis. Figure 10–8► shows the possible routes of infection.

In pyelonephritis, abscesses form and rupture, draining pus into the renal pelvis and the urine. Pus in the urine is called **pyuria**, which causes a turbid or cloudy appearance in the urine sample, and may be detected during a **urinalysis procedure**. The abscesses can fuse, filling the entire kidney with pus. Left untreated, pyelonephritis may lead to renal failure and uremia. In less severe infections, healing occurs but scar tissue tends to form. Because fibrous scar tissue tends to contract, the kidney shrinks and becomes what is described as a granular contracted kidney.

Symptoms of pyelonephritis include chills, high fever, sudden back pain that spreads over the abdomen, **dysuria**, and hematuria. Microscopic examination of the urine reveals numerous pus cells and bacteria. Treatment includes antibiotics, such as aminoglycosides (Amikin) or sulfonamides (Bactrim, Septra), for the infection.

## Pyelitis

**Pyelitis** is an inflammation confined to the renal pelvis, the juncture between the ureter and the kidney. Pyelitis is caused by *E. coli* and other pyogenic bacteria. The bacteria may originate from a urinary bladder infection or the blood. Pyelitis occurs commonly in young children, particularly girls, because the **urethra** in females is much shorter than that of males. Microorganisms from fecal contamination can enter

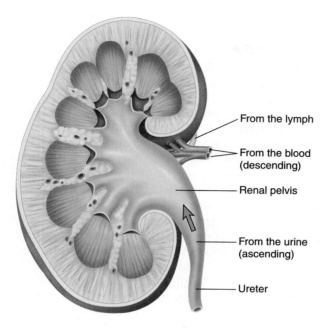

**Figure 10-8 ▶** Routes of infection for pyelonephritis.

From the outside and easily travel to the bladder. The infection can then spread up the ureter to the renal pelvis. Dysuria as well as increased frequency and urgency are common symptoms of pyelitis. A urinalysis exam will reveal numerous pus cells.

This disease responds well to treatment with antibiotics, as previously mentioned. Early diagnosis and treatment are important in preventing the spread of the infection into the kidney tissue, which leads to pyelonephritis.

## Renal Carcinoma

Kidney cancer, also called **hypernephroma**, causes enlargement of the kidney and destroys the organ. Renal carcinoma is a relatively rare type of kidney cancer, comprising only 3% of all adult cancers, but causes 85% of all kidney cancers. Two other types, *transitional cell carcinoma* and sarcoma, make up the remaining 15% of kidney cancers. The incidence of kidney cancer in men is twice that for women, and it normally occurs between ages 50 and 60.

Smokers are twice as likely as nonsmokers to develop kidney cancer.

The tumor may not manifest itself for several years. Painless hematuria eventually becomes the chief sign. When the tumor becomes large, an abdominal mass may be felt. This mass can then be detected on an x-ray as a tumor of the kidney. Metastasis to other organs often occurs before the presence of the kidney tumor is known. The malignancy frequently spreads to the lungs, liver, bones, and brain. Besides pain, typical signs include loss of appetite, weight loss, anemia, and an elevated white blood cell count (leucocytosis). Surgical removal (nephrectomy) is the best initial treatment.

A malignant tumor of the kidney pelvis that develops in children, usually diagnosed between ages 2 and 5, is **Wilms' tumor**, an adenosarcoma. A fast-growing tumor, it metastasizes through the blood and lymph vessels. Symptoms and signs include hematuria, pain, vomiting, and hypertension similar to symptoms of renal carcinoma in an adult. Diagnosis is done by an **IVP** and confirmed by kidney biopsy. In recent years, without metastasis, surgery and radiation (except stage 1) and chemotherapy treatment that may be intermittent, lasting 6 to 15 months, offer a good prognosis.

Wilms' tumor, found 1 in 10,000 individuals, has a genetic connection. It appears that at least three different genes influence the occurrence of this disease. The Wilms' tumor gene 1 (WT-1), whose actual function is unknown, seems to play an important role in embryonic development. When this particular gene is missing or mutated, congenital defects appear, and this abnormal tissue later becomes the site of cancer.

## Kidney Stones

Kidney stones, known as **urinary calculi**, predominantly form in the kidney. The prevalence of urinary calculi is approximately 10%, and by age 70, 5% to 15% of all U.S. citizens experience kidney stones. Men are four times more likely than women to produce renal calculi, with the first episodes occurring between ages 20 and 40.

Urinary calculi may be present and cause no symptoms, even when passed through the urinary tract, unless they are larger than a quarter-inch in diameter, in which case they become lodged in the ureter. The lodged stones cause intense pain that radiates from the kidney to the groin area. In addition to intense pain, other signs and symptoms include hematuria, nausea, vomiting, and diarrhea.

Kidney stones may cause urinary tract infections by blocking urine flow and permitting bacterial growth in the urinary tract. Conversely, a urinary tract infection that blocks urine flow can trigger kidney stone formation because of urine stasis in the renal pelvis. Calculi are formed when certain minerals in the urine form a precipitate; that is, come out of solution and grow in size. Bacteria in urine can serve as sites for calcium deposition. The resulting stones, if small enough, can be passed in the urine, but larger stones may require surgery or other treatment.

Four renal calculi formations are recognized. *Calcium stones* comprise 80% of all kidney stones and consist mainly of calcium salts, calcium oxalate, and calcium phosphate. Calcium excess often leads to stone formation. Hyperactive parathyroid glands can cause the excess of circulating calcium, promoting formation of urinary calculi. Therefore, the parathyroids may need to be controlled or surgically removed, especially with rapid recurrence of stones. No evidence suggests that "hard water" influences kidney stone formation. Men are four to five times more likely than women to form these stones. *Uric acid* stones comprise 10% of all stone formations and occur especially in men subject to gout. Colon surgery increases the risk for uric acid stones. When portions of the colon are removed, the urine becomes more acidic, which enhances the formation of uric acid stones. *Struvite* stones, also called infection stones, comprise nearly 10% of stone formations. Bacterial growth in these kidney stones produces ammonia, making the urine alkaline, which also triggers stone precipitation. When bacteria become encased in minerals, antibiotics are ineffective, and the stones tend to enlarge. A stone may become so large that it fills the renal pelvis completely, blocking the flow of urine, and requires surgical removal. A stone of this type, named for its shape, is the **staghorn calculus** illustrated in Figure 10–9►. A kidney containing numerous small calculi is also shown. Cysteine stones account for the remaining 1% of the renal calculi. These stones are aggregates of the amino acid cysteine, which does not dissolve easily in water. Cysteine stones result from a hereditary disorder in which the kidneys fail to reabsorb cysteine, which builds up in urine, precipitates, and eventually forms stones, more commonly in children.

Stones can also form in the urinary bladder. The presence of bladder stones causes urinary

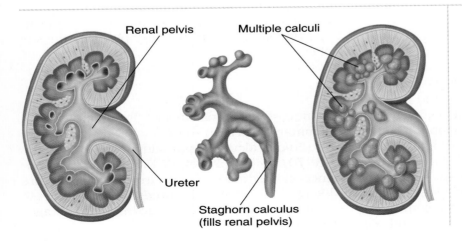

Renal pelvis    Multiple calculi

Ureter

Staghorn calculus
(fills renal pelvis)

**Figure 10–9** ► Urinary calculi.

# Prevention ✚ PLUS!

### Kidney Stones

To prevent kidney stones or their recurrence, it is recommended that urine output be increased. Drinking greater quantities of fluids, especially water, dilutes the urine and solubilizes the potential stones. Cranberries have been used for over 150 years to prevent urinary infection. Drinking the juice increases urine acidity, which reduces microbe growth and inhibits bacteria from adhering to the urinary bladder wall. Especially the unsweetened juice and even the capsule form seem to help prevent kidney stones.

tract infections because they frequently obstruct the flow of urine.

Diagnostic tools include CT, IVP, renal ultrasound/scan, and a KUB exam that consists of a single x-ray without dye to view the abdominopelvic region.

Urinary calculi may be treated with medication that partially dissolves the stone, permitting it to be passed in the urine. **Lithotripsy**, the crushing of kidney stones, is effective for the

20% of kidney stones that do not pass on their own. In lithotripsy, sonic vibrations are applied externally, and focused internally, to crush the stones. If performed while the patient is immersed in a tank of water, the procedure is called **hydrolithotripsy** (Figure 10–10▶). In this technique, the patient while partially submerged is subjected to the sonic waves that shatter the hard stones into sand-sized particles that can be eliminated within the urine

**A**

Beam focused on kidney stones

Reflector

Shock-wave generator

**B**

**Figure 10–10** ▶ Extracorporeal shock-wave lithotripsy. Acoustic shock waves generated by the shock-wave generator travel through soft tissue to shatter the renal stone into fragments, which are then eliminated in the urine. (A) A shock-wave generator that does not require water immersion. (B) An illustration of water immersion lithotripsy procedure.

stream. Recovery is rapid, but there may be some bruising, and the patient usually requires a maximum one-day hospital stay.

Recurrence of stones is not uncommon; after the first stone passes, 14% recur within the first year, about 35% recur within 5 years, and up to 52% recur within 10 years. To avoid or reduce recurrence, fluid intake should be increased to keep the urine dilute, and dietary calcium and protein should be reduced. Certain fruit juices (e.g., cranberry) are purported to benefit patients with calcium-forming stones.

## Hydronephrosis

As a result of urinary calculi, a congenital defect, a tumor, an enlarged prostate gland, or other obstruction of the renal pelvis, the kidney may become extremely dilated with pockets of urine (fluid). This condition is called **hydronephrosis**. The ureters dilate above the obstruction from the pressure of urine that is unable to pass and are referred to as **hydroureters**. Figure 10–11► shows this dilated condition. A physical cause for hydronephrosis is a **ureterocele**. In this case, the terminal portion of the ureter **prolapses**, or

Figure 10–12 ► Hydronephrosis. (Courtesy of Dr. David R. Duffell.)

slides into the urinary bladder. When detected, it can be corrected surgically.

Hematuria is generally present, and the degree of pain accompanying hydronephrosis depends on the nature of the blockage. If an infection develops because of the stagnation of urine, pyuria and fever occur (Figure 10–12►).

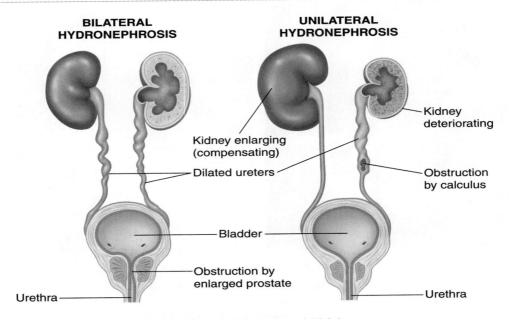

**BILATERAL HYDRONEPHROSIS**

**UNILATERAL HYDRONEPHROSIS**

Kidney enlarging (compensating)

Dilated ureters

Kidney deteriorating

Obstruction by calculus

Bladder

Obstruction by enlarged prostate

Urethra

Urethra

Figure 10–11 ► Hydronephrosis: bilateral (left), unilateral (right).

## Polycystic Kidney

Solitary renal cysts are relatively common, with sizes varying from a few millimeters to 15 mm (the latter may have little effect on kidney function). However, the polycystic kidney is a congenital defect, an error in development that usually involves both kidneys. An autosomal recessive gene causes polycystic kidney in children, while in adults it is caused by an autosomal dominant gene. Adult polycystic kidney disease affects 1 of every 500 to 1000 individuals.

The cysts are dilated kidney tubules that do not open into the renal pelvis as they should. Instead, the cysts enlarge, fuse, and usually become infected. As the cysts enlarge, they compress the surrounding kidney tissue. The accompanying Side by Side illustrates the polycystic kidney of an adult. By middle age, signs and symptoms appear, including pain, hematuria, polyuria, renal calculi, and hypertension. This disease may be diagnosed with a combination of a physical exam, a renal ultrasound or CT, or an IVP (see "Diagnostic Tests and Procedures").

No specific treatment is available. Renal failure eventually occurs, requiring dialysis or kidney transplant.

## ▶ Diseases of Urinary Bladder and Urethra

## Cystitis

**Cystitis** is an inflammation of the urinary bladder primarily caused by an infection. It is more common in women than in men because of women's shorter urethra. The chief cause is *E. coli*, which resides in the colon and can reach the urethra and ascend upward into the bladder. Cystitis can also develop following sexual intercourse if bacteria around the vaginal opening spread to the urinary opening. Occasionally, pressure from coughing or exertion squeezes the bladder, which pushes some urine into the urethra and then draws it back to the bladder. This action contaminates the normally sterile fluid within the urinary bladder.

The symptoms of cystitis are increased urinary frequency and urgency and a burning sensation during urination. Microscopic examination of the urine reveals bacteria, pus, casts, and leukocytes. Treatment depends on the type of bacteria and may include a type of penicillin, such as ampicillin or amoxicillin.

## SIDE by SIDE ▪ Polycystic Kidney

▲ Normal kidney. (© Logical Images/Custom Medical Stock Photo)

▲ Polycystic kidney. (Courtesy of the CDC/ Dr. Edwin P. Ewing, Jr., 1972)

# Urinary Incontinence (UI)

Very early in life, urinary incontinence is considered the norm, as it often is in the elderly years. Although adult incontinence is not a disease, it is abnormal and does require attention. Numbers range from 20 to 30 million sufferers in the United States. This involuntary (or unwanted) release of urine from the urinary bladder is an inconvenience and often an embarrassing problem for those individuals afflicted. Adults may alter their social and physical habits due to this problem.

For the infant, the inability to control micturition occurs because the nerves and muscles have not been coordinated to allow closure of the (voluntary) external urethral valve or sphincter. Automatic reflexive voiding of the urinary bladder occurs because the walls of the bladder expand, and the stretch receptors within the walls signal the internal valve to relax. Otherwise, until the bladder responds to the stretching, the collected urine is retained. A similar mechanism occurs in adults, but conscious efforts allow the voiding signals to be damped down and the external sphincter to remain closed. Urinary retention occurs when the bladder is unable to fully expel the contained urine in a timely fashion due to weak abdominal muscles or extraneous factors such as anesthesia (muscles need time to recover). Within the central nervous system, the pons, cerebral cortex, and spinal cord coordinate to inhibit micturition, or to allow it to occur. Once the timing is convenient and appropriate, urination proceeds.

A myriad of causes and treatments are found for UI. Obviously, UI is subject to various diseases, like infection or stroke, and heredity. Conditions such as childbirth, pregnancy, hysterectomy, and menopause may also be involved. A tumor or enlarged prostate that compresses the urethra, or a prostate surgery, may leave the male incontinent. UI may be inadvertently induced by medications that are used to control hypertension, antihistamines, muscle relaxants, and sleeping pills.

Whatever the primary cause, there are three basic forms of adult UI: (1) *overflow incontinence*, in which the bladder overfills and tends to dribble urine out the urethra; (2) *stress incontinence*, in which the urethral sphincter is weak or damaged and allows leakage upon coughing, sneezing, laughing, or increased abdominal pressure; and (3) *urge incontinence*, in which the muscular bladder wall has sudden uncontrolled contractions.

Depending on cause, severity, age, and other factors, UI is managed by methods ranging from the very simple to surgical. Wearing sanitary napkins, incontinence pads, or waterproof briefs may suffice initially or be preferred. Additional attention to voiding the bladder more often and extending the timing may help along with exercising the pelvic muscles and the urethral valves. These pelvic maneuvers are known as **Kegel** exercises and when performed several times each day may be sufficient to control some stress-type incontinence.

Collagen injections near the voluntary external sphincter may reduce the urethra passage sufficiently to prevent accidental urine release. Somewhat more invasive surgeries suspend the bladder to a greater degree to allow the bladder neck and urethra to form a better alignment and improve normal functioning. Overflow incontinence may be treated by voiding the bladder more frequently, on demand if possible, or if needed by medications like oxybutynin or tolterodine.

When the condition becomes chronic or causes pain or infection, a tubular catheter may be inserted up into the bladder via the urethra to insure voiding the bladder contents. Catheters are small-diameter flexible tubes made of "plastic" (polyvinyl chloride; PVC) or latex primarily inserted through the urethra into the bladder and range from 4 to 12 inches long per gender. A balloon device is at the inserted end and expanded once in place to prevent escape. Externally a retention bag is attached to the catheter and has a capacity of 0.5 L to 2 L depending on daily and overnight usage. It is important to empty the bag frequently (e.g., every 4 hours) and keep a fresh or cleansed container in place. For more mobility, the external retention bag may be strapped to the thigh, pelvic area, or calf position.

The catheter arrangement may be short term (a few days to 2 weeks) or long term (at least 2 years) depending on the circumstance. Long-term setups require a surgical procedure to tap directly into the bladder from the outside through the pelvic wall just superior to the symphysis pubis. Known as an **indwelling catheter**, these tubes are constructed of latex and may be coated with Teflon or silicone plus antibiotics if necessary.

Irritation by any tube in the bladder presents the potential for bladder infection (or beyond) and bladder stones. Therefore, an external catheter may be used such as a condom or penile sheath for men or a labial funnel-type device to adhere to the female external genitalia (or **vulva**). Either device is then attached to a tube that drains into a retention bag. Over time the type of catheter arrangement may change depending on situation or preference.

Incontinence that continues into the early juvenile years is called **enuresis**, or bedwetting. About 1 in 9 children has this UI, which is more common in boys by a margin of 2 to 3. Usually, it is outgrown within the first 11 years (72%) or by age 15 (99%).

Causes for enuresis, or **nocturia**, include lack of bladder growth or development, heredity (40%–70% of cases), heavy sleep, and a reduced level of ADH at night. Besides diapers or absorbent pads to prevent bedtime pools, the youngster may use a nasal spray (e.g., desmopressin acetate) that acts like ADH to prevent bedwetting. Some cases are better served through counseling, urination regiment, or bladder conditioning to reduce night-time urinating accidents.

## Neurogenic Bladder

A neurogenic bladder tends to result in urinary incontinence due to lack of nervous system control. Damage to the nerves supplying the bladder or a breakdown within the central nervous system (CNS) is the root cause of this problem. A common cause is a spinal cord injury from vehicular accident or other trauma. Physical dilemmas like herniated disks in the lumbar region or tumors compressing on the spinal cord and/or spinal nerves are highly probable causations. Metabolic disorders, especially diabetes, mental challenges like Alzheimer's disease, and other CNS dysfunctions like Parkinson's disease and multiple sclerosis (MS) tend to cause bladder impairment as well.

Symptoms vary with the severity or particular nerve(s) involved and the primary dysfunctional location. The bladder may spasm, fail to empty completely, or lack of the feeling of fullness or urgency, and thus the signal to evacuate may go undetected. Diagnosis is therefore difficult to ascertain. Beginning with an extensive patient history coupled with a full-scale neurological exam and a careful urological evaluation, a probable cause and prognosis may be set forth. The goal is to restore bladder function fully, and that may require a major neurological investigation. Urological treatments include indwelling catheters, hygiene training, and exercise. Lumbar disks may be repaired and drug treatments for CNS dysfunctions may assist the recovery. However, if nerve damage is severe or permanent, a neurogenic bladder will persist.

## Carcinoma of the Bladder

Certain industrial chemicals and cigarette smoking have been linked to carcinoma of the urinary bladder. Smokers generally have a risk 2 1/2 times higher of contracting bladder cancer than do nonsmokers. Bladder cancer accounts for 3.4% of all new cancers in men and 1.4% of all new cancer cases for women in the United States (2007). The tumor (or polyp) grows by sending fingerlike projections into the lumen of the bladder. Although these tumors can be seen with a **cystoscope** and removed, they tend to recur. A more invasive pattern of growth involves infiltration of the bladder wall, which cannot be surgically removed without destroying the bladder.

One treatment involves **fulguration**, an infusion of BCG solution (Bacillus Calmette Guerin), a weakened tuberculosis *bacillus* that coats the bladder's internal epithelial surface. This solution causes the inner lining to "peel off" and be replaced by new surface cells. This treatment lasts from months to years, depending on the status of the patient. If this procedure is not appropriate or is ineffective, then surgical removal of the cancer is required.

If the entire urinary bladder is surgically removed (radical cystectomy), an ileal conduit (see Figure 10–13 ▶) is likely constructed surgically to store and evacuate urine. See Chapter 4 for more information.

## Urethritis

Any part of the urinary tract can become inflamed, and the urethra is no exception. This tubular inflammation is called **urethritis**. In men, the cause may be a gonococcus or other bacteria, viruses, or noxious chemicals. A trauma caused by a "straddle" accident may cause irritation and damage to the urethra or stressful pressure (e.g., long-distance bicycle riding). Damage to nerves and blood vessels may occur at the same time, and this could cause testicular problems for the male. In women, urethritis frequently accompanies cystitis. An obstruction at the urinary opening may cause the inflammation in women. The symptoms of urethritis include a discharge of pus from the urethra, an itching sensation at the opening of the urethra, and a burning sensation during urination. Treatment includes antibiotics like amoxicillin for bacteria infections.

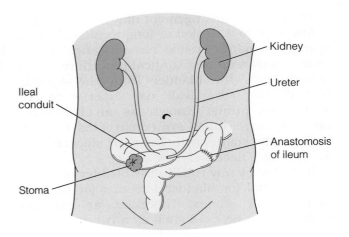

**Figure 10–13** ▶ Ileal conduit. A segment of ileum is separated from the small intestine and formed into a tubular pouch, with the open end brought to the skin surface to form a stoma. The ureters are connected to the pouch.

## ▶ Age-Related Diseases

Several changes accompany the aging urinary system. Basically there is less control over urination (the micturition reflex) because the urethral sphincter muscles lose tone, allowing urine to leak, and due to other factors mentioned earlier. Incontinence tends to be more common with aging, but some suggest that with more conscious effort, training, and some medical advice or attention (e.g., minor surgery) numbers of cases might be reduced or prevented by as much as 80%. Brain and spinal cord damage may lead to a weak micturition urination reflex.

Dehydration due to water loss via the aging kidneys is possible, because the total number of functioning nephrons declines with age, perhaps as much as 30% to 40% between ages 25 and 85, and the kidney loses sensitivity to ADH. The reduction of renin and therefore aldosterone activity causes a lack of salt and water retention, allowing more urine to be released by the kidney. Urinary retention occurs because bladders lose muscle tone and are unable to empty com-

pletely. Obstruction exacerbates urine retention and is common in men because of prostate enlargement. Urinary retention, in turn, increases the risk for urinary tract infections (UTIs). Cancer increases significantly past age 60 for the kidney, and at age 70 for bladder cancer.

## RESOURCES

National Kidney and Urologic Diseases Information Clearinghouse (NKUDIC): www.kidney.niddk.nih.gov

Renal Calculi: www.emedicine.com/emerg/topic499.htm

# DISEASES AT A GLANCE

## Urinary System

| DISEASE | ETIOLOGY | SIGNS AND SYMPTOMS |
|---|---|---|
| Kidney | | |
| Hydronephroma | Idiopathic, radiation | Painless hematuria, later pain, loss of appetite, weight loss, anemia, elevated white blood count |
| Wilms' tumor | Idiopathic, genetic (WT-1) chromosome II | In young children, signs and symptoms similar to hydronephroma in adults |
| Pyelonephritis | Pyogenic bacteria | Pyuria, chills, high fever, sudden back pain, dysuria, bematuria, eventual renal failure, uremia |
| Pyelitis | Pyogenic bacteria | Dysuria, frequency, urgency |
| Acute glomerulonephritis | Prior bacterial infection, antigen-antibody complex | Follow strep infection: chills, fever, loss of appetite, weakness, edema, albuminuria, hematuria, casts |
| Chronic glomerulonephritis | Hypertension and glomerular destruction | Remission and exacerbation of glomerulonephritis; may end with granular contracted kidneys and uremia; specific gravity low and fixed in advanced cases |
| Acute renal failure | Incompatible blood transfusion, severe dehydration | Sudden oliguria, may become anuria, headache, GI distress, odor of ammonia in breath, muscle weakness |
| Chronic renal failure | Hypertension, chronic glomerulonephritis, diabetic nephropathy | Slow development, urinary wastes increase in blood, nausea, vomiting, diarrhea, dim vision, central nervous system affected, convulsions, coma |
| Urinary calculi (kidney stones) | Hyperparathyroidism, excess calcium | No symptoms until they block ureter, then intense pain radiating to groin |

| DIAGNOSIS | TREATMENT | PREVENTION | LIFESPAN |
|---|---|---|---|
| X-ray | Surgery | Uncertain | Generally increased chance with aging |
| X-ray | Surgery, sometimes radiation | None | At birth and youngsters |
| Urinalysis, pus and blood in urine | Antibiotics | Depends on exposure and susceptibility | Especially in younger people, but older people too |
| Urinalysis, numerous pus cells in urine | Antibiotics | Same as above, good hygiene | Usually weaker immunity, age varies |
| Urinalysis, patient history | Antibiotics, steroids, immune suppression | As above or uncertain | Any age, often younger years |
| Urinalysis, urine specific gravity low, patient history | Antibiotics, steroids, immune suppression | Prevent negative kidney exposure, or uncertain | Tends to develop with prior infections; middle years + |
| Patient history, blood and urinalysis | Drugs, fluid control, antibiotics, dialysis | Uncertain | Any age |
| Patient history, urinalysis, blood analysis | Dialysis, kidney transplant | Implies prior kidney stress | More prevalent in elderly or caused by foreign substances (e.g., poison) |
| Patient history, blood and urinalysis, x-ray | Lithotripsy, surgery | Consider family history, prevent dehydration, diet | Usually 30s or 40s for initial onset |

# DISEASES AT A GLANCE

## Urinary System (*continued*)

| DISEASE | ETIOLOGY | SIGNS AND SYMPTOMS |
|---|---|---|
| Hydronephrosis | Renal obstruction, congenital defect | Pain, hematuria, pyuria, and fever if infection present |
| Polycystic kidney | Genetic | Hypertension, eventual renal failure, uremia |
| Carcinoma | Idiopathic, radiation, smoking | Early asymptomatic, hematuria may occur, later pelvic pain and frequent urination |
| Urinary Bladder | | |
| Cystitis | Usually bacteria infection | Urinary frequency, urgency, burning sensation during urination, blood in urine |
| Bladder cancer | Idiopathic, smoking, hazardous chemicals | Hematuria, dysuria, fatigue, anorexia |
| Urethritis | Microbial agents, viruses, some chemicals | Burning sensation during urination, itching, discharge; in females, accompanies cystitis |
| Incontinence | Neurological injury, aging | Involuntary loss of urine |

| DIAGNOSIS | TREATMENT | PREVENTION | LIFESPAN |
|---|---|---|---|
| Urinalysis, IVP cystoscopic exam | Relief of obstruction, surgery | Uncertain, depends on (e.g., obstruction due to enlarged prostate) | Varies; usually teens and beyond |
| Urinalysis, IVP cystoscopic exam | Kidney transplant | None | Recessive trait—child Dominant trait—adult |
| Cystoscopy | Surgery | Do not smoke, avoid radiation and other potential carcinogens | Chance increases with age |
| | | | |
| Microscopic exam of urine, may be diagnosed by patient's description of typical signs and symptoms | Antibiotics | Uncertain, good hygiene | In women any age; varies for men |
| Cystoscope, IVP, x-ray, CT | Fulguration, radiation, surgery | Uncertain; do not smoke, avoid radiation | Middle age and beyond |
| Microscopic exam of urine | Antibiotics | Uncertain, good hygiene | Higher incidence among females, any age |
| Patient history | Exercises for muscles of pelvic floor, antibiotics for infection | Varies; requires treatment | Newborn and elderly |

# Interactive Exercises

## Cases for Critical Thinking

1. Jane, a college sophomore, experienced painful urination and noticed blood in the urine. What can explain her symptoms and hematuria?

2. Britany, a thin fourth grader, experienced a significant weight gain within two weeks' time. Just before holiday break, she had a bad sore throat, but after a visit to the doctor, those symptoms subsided. Her abdomen was distended and she had edema of the extremities. She complained of abdominal discomfort and general aches. Urinalysis indicated proteinuria and hematuria. A follow-up blood screen found antibodies to streptococcal toxins. What may explain Britany's symptoms?

3. A mother of a 4-month-old infant, while giving a bath, noticed and palpated a mass on the right side of the child's abdomen. The child was irritable and somewhat lethargic. What might explain this mass, and what diagnostic techniques can help determine the nature of the disease?

4. A 52-year-old grandfather's urinalysis revealed blood (hematuria). The x-ray showed a renal mass on the right side. What is the probable cause for the hematuria, and what treatment would be recommended?

## Multiple Choice

1. Which of the following can cause chronic uremia?
   a. surgical shock
   b. severe dehydration
   c. complications of pregnancy
   d. diabetes mellitus

2. What is inflammation of the kidney tissue known as?
   a. pyelonephritis
   b. polycystic kidney
   c. hydronephrosis
   d. diabetic nephropathy

3. What is inflammation restricted to the renal pelvis called?
   a. pyelonephritis
   b. glomerulonephritis
   c. pyelitis
   d. congenital cystic kidney

4. Which disease or condition features a breath odor similar to the ammonia-like odor of urine?
   a. glomerulonephritis    b. pyelonephritis
   c. tuberculosis          d. uremia

5. Which of the following is TRUE about urinary tract infections?
   a. are more common in males
   b. usually exhibit dysuria, urgency, and frequency
   c. are commonly caused by a virus
   d. do not respond to antibiotics

6. Which form of kidney dialysis permits a patient to retain mobility?
   a. peritoneal dialysis    b. hemodialysis
   c. hemolysis              d. ileal shunt

7. The inability to control urination is called

   _____.

   a. micturition    b. incontinence
   c. anuria         d. nocturia

8. What dietary restriction helps to prevent uric acid calculi?
   a. protein
   b. dairy products
   c. pasta and citrus
   d. spinach, cabbage, and tomatoes

9. What primarily causes the edema associated with nephritic syndrome?
   a. hypertension
   b. hyperalbuminuria
   c. decreased plasma protein
   d. lower GFR

10. Which of the following includes a reduced sensitivity to ADH, incontinence, and increased urination frequency?
    a. overhydration    b. aging
    c. stress           d. excess nitrogen intake

## True or False

_____ 1. A sudden drop in urine volume indicates chronic renal failure.

_____ 2. Cystitis is often an ascending infection.

_____ 3. In acute uremia, fluid intake should be decreased.

_____ 4. Albuminuria leads to hypoproteinemia.

_____ 5. Painful and frequent urination accompanies tuberculosis of the bladder.

_____ 6. Bacteria are not found in acute glomerulonephritis.

_____ 7. Pyelonephritis is a suppurative disease.

_____ 8. The urinary bladder stores urine that may be reused.

_____ 9. Leukocytes in urine indicate anemia.

_____ 10. Calcium (oxalate, phosphate) is the most common form of renal calculus.

## Fill-Ins

1. _____ is pus in the urine.

2. _____ _____ is a kidney disease resulting from diabetes mellitus.

3. Urinary calculi, or _____ _____, may be present and cause no symptoms until they become lodged in the ureter.

4. _____, the external crushing of kidney stones, is now the preferable procedure to remove kidney stones, replacing the need for surgery.

5. _____ _____ is a congenital anomaly that usually involves both kidneys.

6. Scanty urine or _____ is low urine volume (or formation).

7. Loss of urine at night is called _____.

8. Struvite stones are associated with _____.

9. Adult polycystic kidney is a genetic disease caused specifically by an autosomal _____ gene.

10. An x-ray outline of the urinary system following an injection solution is the diagnostic technique called _____.

## Labeling Exercise

Use the blank lines below to label the following image.

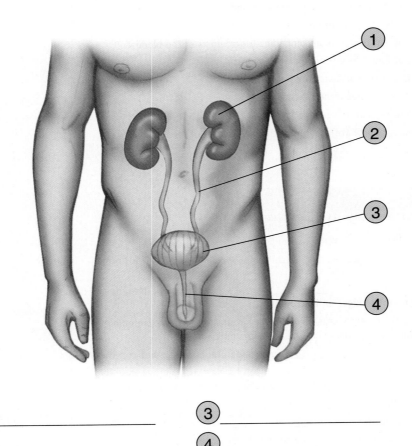

1 _____

2 _____

3 _____

4 _____

# Multimedia Preview

Additional interactive resources and activities for this chapter can be found on the Companion Website. For videos, audio glossary, and review, access the accompanying DVD-ROM in this book.

## ▶ DVD-ROM Highlights

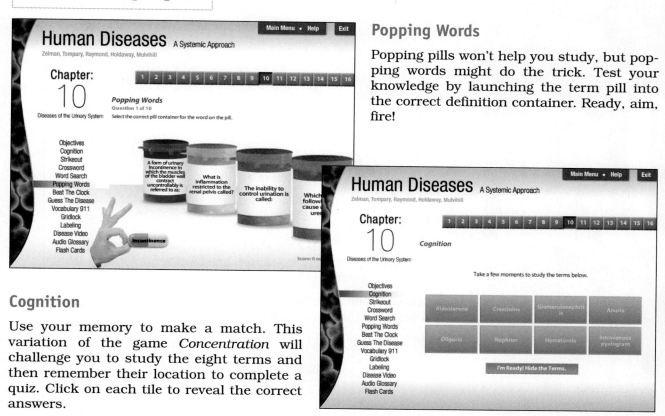

### Popping Words

Popping pills won't help you study, but popping words might do the trick. Test your knowledge by launching the term pill into the correct definition container. Ready, aim, fire!

### Cognition

Use your memory to make a match. This variation of the game *Concentration* will challenge you to study the eight terms and then remember their location to complete a quiz. Click on each tile to reveal the correct answers.

## ▶ Website Highlights—www.pearsonhighered.com/zelman

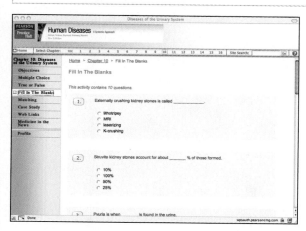

### Fill-in-the-Blanks Exercise

Take advantage of the free-access online study guide that accompanies your textbook. You'll find a fill-in-the-blank quiz that provides instant feedback and allows you to check your score to see what you got right or wrong. By clicking on this URL you'll also access links to current news articles and an audio glossary.

CHAPTER

# 11

# Diseases and Disorders of the Reproductive System

## Learning Objectives

After studying this chapter, you should be able to

- Identify diagnostic procedures used for conditions of the reproductive system
- Describe the normal structure and function of the reproductive system
- List signs and symptoms, causes, and treatments for diseases and disorders of the reproductive system
- Describe disorders of pregnancy
- List signs and symptoms, causes, and treatments for sexually transmitted infections
- List signs and symptoms, causes, and treatments for age-related diseases of the reproductive system

## Fact or Fiction?

All sexually transmitted infections (STIs) can be cured.

*Fiction: STIs caused by viruses cannot be cured. Medications can manage the signs and symptoms but cannot cure the infection.*

# Disease Chronicle

## Tuskegee Institute Experiment

In 1932, the U.S. Public Health Service, with the assistance of the Tuskegee Institute, recruited 600 African American men to participate in an experiment involving the effects of untreated syphilis. Of this group, 399 men had been diagnosed with syphilis but were never informed that they had syphilis or that their infection was sexually transmitted. Originally meant to last 6 to 9 months, the study instead lasted 40 years until the men died. When the story broke in 1972, Congress convened hearings about the Tuskegee study. The hearings resulted in the rewriting of the Department of Health, Education, and Welfare's regulations on the use of human subjects in scientific experiments. A $1.8 billion class-action suit was filed on behalf of the Tuskegee participants and their heirs. A settlement for $10 million was made out of court.

# ▶ Anatomy of the Female Reproductive System

The female reproductive system consists of the vagina, the uterus, the fallopian tubes, and the ovaries. The vagina is a tubular structure extending backward and upward to the cervix, the lowest part of the uterus. The expanded, upper portion of the uterus tapers down to form the narrow cervix, giving the organ a pear-shaped appearance. The uterine wall is very strong, comprised of smooth muscle and lined with a mucosal membrane, the endometrium, and is responsive to hormonal changes. Figures 11–1 ▶ and 11–2 ▶ show the female reproductive system.

The fallopian tubes extend laterally from each side of the uterus. The outer ends of the tubes are open to receive a released ovum. Fringelike projections at the outer ends, the **fimbriae**, propel the ova into the tube.

The ovaries, small, oval-shaped organs, are anchored near the open end of the fallopian tubes by ligaments. The ovaries contain hundreds of thousands of ova, which are present at birth. Surrounding each ovum is a single layer of cells, a **primary follicle**.

The external genitalia, the vulva, include the mons pubis, the labia majora and labia minora, the clitoris, and the vaginal opening. The urinary meatus is between the clitoris and the vaginal opening. The mons pubis, a pad of fat tissue over the pubic symphysis, becomes covered with hair at puberty. Extending back from the mons pubis to the anus are two pairs of folds, the labia majora and the labia minora. The clitoris, a tuft of erectile tissue similar to that of the penis, is located at the anterior junction of the minor lips. A membranous fold, the **hymen**, partly or completely closes the vaginal opening. Occasionally, this membrane is imperforate or abnormally closed and requires a minor surgical

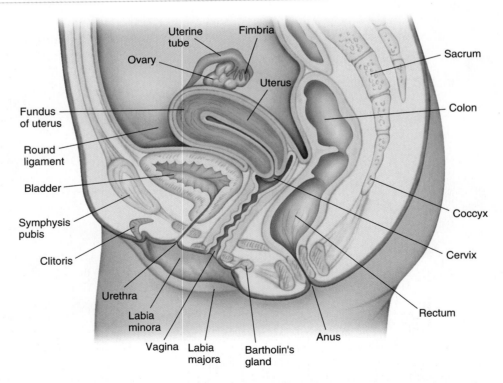

**Figure 11–1** ▶ Sagittal section of the female pelvis, showing organs of the reproductive system.

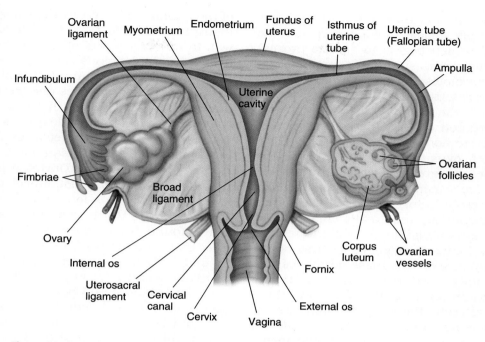

**Figure 11-2** ► The uterus, ovaries, and fallopian tubes.

procedure to open it. **Bartholin's glands**, a pair of mucus-secreting glands, are situated at the vaginal entrance. These glands produce a lubricating secretion during sexual intercourse.

The breasts, accessory organs of reproduction, consist of milk glands supported by connective tissue covered with fatty tissue and skin. Ducts of the milk glands converge at the nipple, which is surrounded by a darkly pigmented area, the areola. The breasts overlie the pectoral muscles of the chest.

## ► Physiology of the Female Reproductive System

The cyclic hormonal changes in the life of a woman prepare the uterus monthly for a possible pregnancy. The secretion of female hormones, estrogen and progesterone, is governed by two gonadotropic hormones—follicle-stimulating hormone (FSH) and luteinizing hormone (LH)—of the anterior pituitary gland, which is controlled by the hypothalamus of the brain. Failure of the ovary to secrete sex hormones or to ovulate may result from pituitary disease or disturbances in the central nervous system.

A woman's reproductive life begins with the onset of menstruation, the **menarche**, occurring generally between ages 10 and 15. The reproductive years terminate with the cessation of menstrual periods, menopause, which usually begins in the late 40s or early 50s. At the beginning of each monthly cycle, pituitary gonadotropic hormone stimulates ovarian follicles to develop. The stimulated follicles begin to grow and develop into **Graafian follicles**. One of these matures first and is released at the midpoint of the cycle, which is the process of ovulation.

As the follicles grow during the first half of the cycle, the ovary secretes **estrogen**, which is carried by the blood to the uterus. Estrogen stimulates the endometrium of the uterus to enter the proliferative phase, in which it thickens and becomes more vascular in preparation for pregnancy.

Once the ovum has been released from the ovary, the empty follicle is converted into the **corpus luteum**, which begins to secrete progesterone. Progesterone stimulates endometrial growth and promotes the storage of nutrients for nourishing a fertilized ovum. This is the secretory phase of the uterus.

If no fertilization occurs, the corpus luteum ceases to secrete hormones approximately 8 to 12 days after ovulation. At the end of the monthly cycle, the level of estrogen and progesterone drops, and menstruation, the sloughing of the endometrial lining, occurs. If pregnancy occurs, the corpus luteum greatly enlarges and continues to secrete high levels of progesterone. The placenta gradually assumes the role of the corpus luteum in secreting these hormones.

The placenta is formed from both maternal and embryonic tissue. Near the site of implantation in the uterus, the endometrium greatly thickens, becomes highly vascular, and develops large blood sinuses. An embryonic membrane, the chorion, develops fingerlike projections called villi, which dip into the maternal blood sinuses. This interdigitation of embryonic and maternal tissue constitutes the placenta. **Human chorionic gonadotropin hormone (HCG)** is secreted by the chorionic villi after implantation of the fertilized ovum in the uterus. Laboratory diagnosis of pregnancy is based on the presence of HCG in the mother's blood or urine.

The umbilical arteries extend into the chorionic villi, where carbon dioxide and waste are exchanged for oxygen and nutrients. Maternal and fetal bloods do not mix; the exchange of these substances is by diffusion across the blood vessel walls. Oxygen and nutrients return to the fetus through the umbilical vein.

## ▶ Diagnostic Procedures

Physical examination of the female reproductive system begins with a pelvic examination. Pelvic examination can detect certain cancers in their early stages, infections, and other reproductive system disorders. This exam includes inspection of the external genitalia, visual examination of the vagina and cervix through a speculum (an instrument used to spread and hold the vaginal wall in an open position), and palpation of the female internal organs by bimanual examination. During a bimanual examination, the healthcare provider places one hand on the abdomen and inserts fingers of the other hand into the vagina to feel the female organs between the two hands. A bimanual rectal examination allows palpation of the posterior aspect of the uterus and the rectum. During a pelvic examination, a sample for a Papanicolaou (Pap) test may be taken to look for changes in the cells of the cervix. CA 125 is a protein tumor marker that is found in greater concentrations in tumor cells than in other body cells and may be used for diagnosis of endometrial and ovarian cancer. In dilation and curettage (D&C), the cervix is widened (dilation) and part of the lining of the uterus is removed (curettage). D&C may be used in the diagnosis of endometrial cancer.

General visualization of the female reproductive system may be done using ultrasound or sonography and can aid the diagnosis of inflammatory diseases, uterine fibroid tumors, some cancers, **ectopic pregnancy**, and menstrual disorders. **Laparoscopy** is used to visualize the female reproductive organs; **colposcopy** is used to visualize the cervix; **hysteroscopy** is used to visualize the uterine lining. These visualization techniques can be used to diagnose inflammatory diseases, some cancers, menstrual disorders, and endometriosis. Mammography is an x-ray examination of breast tissue. If abnormalities or tumors are discovered, a biopsy may be performed.

Sexually transmitted infections are diagnosed by blood or urine cultures, DNA test, and antigen or antibody testing. Other laboratory tests that may be performed include urinalysis and hormone testing.

## ▶ Diseases of the Female Reproductive System

### Pelvic Inflammatory Disease (PID)

In PID, the pelvic reproductive organs become inflamed due to bacterial, viral, fungal, or parasitic invasion. The infection can ascend to the cervix (cervicitis), the endometrium (endometritis), fallopian tubes (salpingitis), and ovaries (oophoritis). The most common cause of PID is sexually transmitted infections, including gonorrhea and chlamydia.

The Centers for Disease Control (CDC) estimates that each year in the United States more than 1 million women experience an episode of acute PID. In the United States more than 150 women die annually from PID or its complications, and more than 100,000 women become infertile due to PID. A large proportion of the ectopic pregnancies that occur each year in the United States are due to the consequences of PID.

Because of vague symptoms, PID goes unrecognized by women and their healthcare providers about two-thirds of the time. Symptoms of PID vary from none to severe; the most common PID symptom is lower abdominal pain. Other signs and symptoms include fever, unusual vaginal discharge that may have a foul odor, painful intercourse, painful urination, and irregular menstrual bleeding.

PID can cause serious complications. Untreated bacterial infections can cause scar tissue formation. This scar tissue blocks or interrupts the normal movement of eggs into the uterus. If the fallopian tubes are totally blocked by scar tissue, sperm cannot fertilize an egg, and the woman becomes infertile. Infertility also can occur if the fallopian tubes are partially blocked or even slightly damaged. About one in eight women with PID becomes infertile, and if a woman has multiple episodes of PID, her chances of becoming infertile increase. In addition, a partially blocked or slightly damaged fallopian tube may cause a fertilized egg to remain in the fallopian tube. If this fertilized egg begins to grow in the tube as if it were in the uterus, it is called an ectopic pregnancy. An ectopic pregnancy can rupture the fallopian tube, causing severe pain, internal bleeding, and even death. Scarring in the fallopian tubes and other pelvic structures can also cause chronic pelvic pain that lasts for months or even years. Women with repeated episodes of PID are more likely to suffer infertility, ectopic pregnancy, or chronic pelvic pain.

A PID diagnosis is usually based on clinical findings. If symptoms such as lower abdominal pain are present, a physical examination is performed to determine the nature and location of the pain and check for fever, abnormal vaginal or cervical discharge, and for evidence of gonorrheal or chlamydial infection. Tests to identify the infection-causing organism (e.g., chlamydial or gonorrheal infection) or to distinguish between PID and other problems with similar symptoms may also be performed. A pelvic ultrasound can determine if the fallopian tubes are enlarged or an abscess is present. In some cases laparoscopy may be necessary to confirm the diagnosis.

Sexually transmitted infections (STIs) are the main preventable cause of PID. Women should take action to prevent STIs or get early treatment if they are infected. Treatment for PID includes antibiotics; however, antibiotic treatment does not reverse damage that has already occurred to the reproductive organs.

## Cervical Cancer

Cervical cancer is cancer of the cervix that begins in the lining of the cervix. **Carcinoma in situ** is the earliest stage of cervical cancer in which the underlying tissue has not yet been invaded. Some researchers estimate that carcinoma in situ is about four times more common than invasive cervical cancer. Progression from carcinoma in situ to an invasive malignancy may be slow. Ulceration then occurs, causing vaginal discharge and bleeding. The cancer spreads to surrounding organs: the vagina, bladder, rectum, and pelvic wall. The accompanying Side by Side shows a normal cervix and a cancerous cervix.

The American Cancer Society (ACS) estimates that in 2008 approximately 11,070 cases of invasive cervical cancer will be diagnosed and 3870 women will die from cervical cancer in the United States; approximately 550,000 women will be diagnosed with cervical cancer and 300,000 will die annually worldwide. Cervical cancer was once one of the most common causes of cancer death for American women; however, the death rate declined by 74% between 1955 and 1992 due to increased use of the Pap test (see Chapter 4). The HPV vaccine

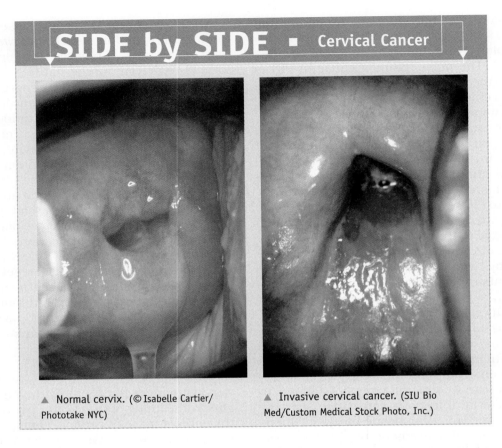

## SIDE by SIDE ■ Cervical Cancer

▲ Normal cervix. (© Isabelle Cartier/ Phototake NYC)

▲ Invasive cervical cancer. (SIU Bio Med/Custom Medical Stock Photo, Inc.)

Gardasil aims to further reduce the incidence of cervical cancer (see HPV and genital warts later in this chapter).

The most important risk factor for cervical cancer is infection by the **human papillomavirus (HPV)**. Women who smoke are about twice as likely as nonsmokers to get cervical cancer. Cervical cancer risk can be reduced by avoiding exposure to HPV and not smoking.

Cervical cancer can usually be diagnosed early through a Pap test. Between 60% and 80% of American women with newly diagnosed invasive cervical cancer had not had a Pap test in the past 5 years. The ACS recommends all women begin having a Pap test within 3 years of becoming sexually active or by age 21. For women under age 30, Pap tests should be done yearly (regular Pap test) or every 2 years (liquid-based Pap test). Beginning at age 30, if a woman has three normal Pap tests in a row, she can get a Pap test every 2 to 3 years or a Pap test every 3 years plus and HPV DNA test. The HPV DNA test is not used as a screening test for women under the age of 30 because HPV is very common and rarely causes cancer in those under 30.

Diagnosis of cervical cancer may include pelvic examination, Pap test, HPV DNA test, and colposcopy. Treatment may include surgery, radiation, and chemotherapy.

## Endometrial Cancer

In the United States, cancer of the endometrium is the most common cancer of the female reproductive organs. The ACS estimates that there will be 40,100 new cases of cancer of the body of the uterus diagnosed in the United States during 2008; most of these occur in the endometrium, and about 7470 women will die from cancers of the uterine body. Each year approximately 200,000 women will be diagnosed with endometrial cancer and 50,000 will die worldwide.

The cause of endometrial cancer is not known. Most endometrial cancers are hormone driven. A shift in the balance between estrogen and progesterone toward more estrogen increases a woman's risk for having endometrial cancer. Risk factors for endometrial cancer include total number of menstrual cycles, few pregnancies or infertility, estrogen therapy, polycystic ovarian syndrome, and obesity. The use of oral contraceptives, control of obesity and diabetes, and healthy diet and exercise can reduce the risk of endometrial cancer.

The malignant tumor may grow into the cavity of the uterus or invade the wall itself. Ulcerations develop, and erosion of blood vessels causes vaginal bleeding. Other signs and symptoms can include nonbloody vaginal discharge, pelvic pain, and weight loss. There are no early detection tests or exams that can find endometrial cancer early in asymptomatic women at average endometrial cancer risk. Diagnosis may include pelvic examination, CA 125 blood test, biopsy, hysteroscopy, and D&C. Surgery, radiation, chemotherapy, and hormone therapy are possible treatments.

## Fibroid Tumors of the Uterus

Benign tumors of the smooth muscle of the uterus, **leiomyomas** or fibroid tumors, are the most common tumors of the female reproductive system, with between 20% and 40% of women age 35 and older having fibroid tumors of significant size. Most women with fibroid tumors do not experience any symptoms, but signs and symptoms may include excessive vaginal bleeding, pelvic pressure, abdominal pain, abdominal enlargement, and pain during intercourse. Fibroids vary in size from a quarter of an inch to the size of a cantaloupe. The cause of fibroid tumors is unknown, although their growth is stimulated by estrogen. Uterine fibroids cannot be prevented. Diagnosis may include pelvic examination, ultrasound, sonography, and hysteroscopy. Treatment for fibroid tumors depends on severity of symptoms and childbearing plans. Birth control pills can decrease the bleeding caused by fibroids. Uterine artery embolization shrinks fibroids by cutting off their blood supply. Focused ultrasound surgery destroys fibroids using high-frequency sound waves. Endometrial ablation destroys the lining of the uterus and reduces the amount of bleeding during menstruation. Myomectomy is removal of the fibroid or fibroids that are causing symptoms. Hysterectomy may be necessary; one-third of hysterectomies performed in the United States are due to fibroids.

## Ovarian Cancer

The ovaries are a common site for cancer to develop (ovarian cancer ranks fifth as the cause of cancer death in women in the United States); however, their position deep in the pelvis makes early detection of the tumor difficult. The ACS estimates that about 21,650 new cases of ovarian cancer will be diagnosed in the United States in 2008, and 15,520 deaths will occur. Approximately 230,000 women are diagnosed with ovarian cancer and 140,000 die annually worldwide.

Extensive metastasis often occurs before there are noticeable symptoms, which include bloating, pelvic or abdominal pain, trouble eating or feeling full quickly, and changes in urinary urgency or frequency. The cause of ovarian cancer is not known. Risk factors include age; obesity; early menstruation; late menopause; not having children or having the first child after age 30; family history of ovarian, breast, or colorectal cancer; and a personal history of breast cancer. The use of oral contraceptives, tubal ligation, hysterectomy, child bearing, and breast feeding may reduce the risk of ovarian cancer.

Currently there is no screening test for ovarian cancer. Confirmation of the mass can be made by CT or MRI scan or ultrasound. Laparoscopy, biopsy, and CA 125 blood test may be performed. Treatment options include surgery, radiation, and chemotherapy.

## Breast Cancer

Breast cancer (also discussed in Chapter 4) is the second leading cause of cancer death in women, exceeded only by lung cancer. Women living in North America have the world's highest rate of breast cancer; annually approximately

1.3 million women will be diagnosed with breast cancer and 465,000 will die worldwide.

The most common sign of breast cancer is a lump or mass. Other possible signs and symptoms of breast cancer include swelling of all or part of the breast; skin irritation and dimpling; breast or nipple pain; nipple retraction; redness, scaliness, or thickening of the nipple or breast skin; a discharge other than breast milk; and a swelling of a lymph node in the armpit. Breast cancer spreads principally through the lymph system, and metastases are frequently found in the lungs, liver, brain, and bone. The cause of breast cancer is not known. Risk factors include gender, age, genetic risk factors, and family or personal history of breast cancer. Approximately 5% to 10% of breast cancer cases are thought to be hereditary. Women who inherit a BRCA1 or BRCA2 mutation have up to an 80% chance of developing breast cancer during their lifetime. A genetic screen for breast cancer is available. Breast cancer risk can be lowered by avoiding alcohol, exercising regularly, and maintaining a healthy body weight.

Regular screening and early diagnosis are critical to identify and treat breast cancer. Women are strongly urged to examine their breasts monthly for signs of cancer. Healthcare providers will examine breasts as part of routine gynecology exam. Mammography can detect small, early cancers, and the ACS recommends that women age 40 and older have a yearly mammogram. Ultrasound may be used to target specific areas of concern found on the mammogram. A biopsy of the suspected malignancy confirms the diagnosis or shows the tumor to be benign.

Treatment of breast cancer may include surgery, radiation, chemotherapy, targeted drug therapy, and hormone therapy. Lumpectomy removes only the breast lump and a surrounding margin of normal tissue. Partial (segmental) mastectomy or quadrantectomy removes more breast tissue than a lumpectomy. For a quad-

## Prevention ✚ PLUS!

### Self-Screening for Breast Cancer

Early detection of cancer is key to favorable outcomes. Women should perform monthly breast self-exams. The best time for a woman to examine her breasts is when the breasts are not tender or swollen.

#### HOW TO EXAMINE YOUR BREASTS

- Lie down and place your right arm behind your head.
- Use the finger pads of the three middle fingers on your left hand to feel for lumps in the right breast. Use overlapping dime-sized circular motions of the finger pads to feel the breast tissue.
- Use three different levels of pressure to feel all the breast tissue. Light pressure is needed to feel the tissue closest to the skin; medium pressure to feel a little deeper; and firm pressure to feel the tissue closest to the chest and ribs. A firm ridge in the lower curve of each breast is normal. Use each pressure level to feel the breast tissue before moving on to the next spot.
- Move around the breast in an up and down pattern starting at an imaginary line drawn straight down your side from the underarm and moving across the breast to the middle of the breastbone. Be sure to check the entire breast area, going down until you feel only ribs and up to the neck or collar bone.
- Repeat the exam on your left breast, using the finger pads of the right hand.
- While standing in front of a mirror with your hands pressing firmly down on your hips, look at your breasts for any changes of size, shape, contour, dimpling, or redness or scaliness of the nipple or breast skin.
- Examine each underarm while sitting up or standing and with your arm only slightly raised so you can easily feel in this area.

*Source:* American Cancer Society, "How to Examine Your Breasts," available at: www.cancer.org/docroot/CRI/content/ CRI_2_6x_How_to_perform_a_breast_self_exam_5.asp rantectomy, one-quarter of the breast is removed. For most women with stage I or II breast cancer, breast conservation therapy (lumpectomy/partial mastectomy plus radiation therapy) is as effective as mastectomy. However, breast conservation therapy is not an option for all women with breast cancer. Mastectomy involves removal of all of the breast tissue, sometimes along with other nearby tissues. In a simple or total mastectomy, the surgeon removes the entire breast, including the nipple, but does not remove underarm lymph nodes or muscle tissue from beneath the breast. Sometimes this is done for both breasts (a double mastectomy), especially when it is done as preventive surgery in women at very high risk for breast cancer. A modified radical mastectomy involves removing the entire breast and some of the axillary lymph nodes. This is the most common surgery for women with breast cancer who are having the whole breast removed. For some women with smaller tumors, one option may be a newer procedure known as a skin-sparing mastectomy, in which most of the skin over the breast (other than the nipple and areola) is left intact. Radical mastectomy is an extensive operation removing the entire breast, axillary lymph nodes, and the chest wall muscles under the breast. This surgery was once very common, but because of the disfigurement and side effects it causes and because modified radical mastectomy has been proven to be as effective as radical mastectomy, it is rarely done today.

▶ **Benign Conditions of the Breast**

Benign breast conditions are very common. Unlike breast cancer, benign breast conditions are not life threatening. Three types of benign breast conditions—**fibroadenomas,** breast cysts, and fibrocystic changes—are discussed.

## Fibroadenomas

Fibroadenomas are the most common benign tumor of the breast. Fibroadenomas are solid and firm and are usually painless. Fibroadenomas are most common in young women in their twenties and thirties, but they may occur at any age. The cause is unknown, and there are no known preventive measures. Diagnosis of fibroadenomas may include breast examination, mammogram, ultrasound, fine needle aspiration, and biopsy. They often stop growing or even shrink on their own without any treatment, and they may not require removal. Fibroadenoma surgery may involve removing a margin of surrounding breast tissue. However, scarring could occur that distorts the shape and texture of the breast, making future physical examinations and mammography more difficult to interpret.

## Breast Cysts

Breast cysts are tiny, fluid-filled sacs within the breast tissue. Cysts are oval or round, smooth and firm, and they move slightly when pressed. Breast cysts are common, especially in women over age 35. The cysts may vary in size during the menstrual cycle and may be tender. The cause of breast cysts is not known, and there are no known preventative measures. Diagnosis of breast cysts may include breast examination, mammogram, ultrasound, and fine needle aspiration. Cysts may resolve spontaneously or may need to be surgically removed.

## Fibrocystic Changes

Fibrocystic changes (FCCs) are characterized by breasts that are lumpy. FCCs primarily affect women ages 30 to 50. The cause of FCCs is not known, but estrogen and progesterone may play a role. FCCs are not preventable. FCCs may be diagnosed by breast examination, mammogram, ultrasound, and biopsy. For most women with FCCs and no symptoms, no treatment is needed. Women with mild discomfort may benefit from wearing a supportive bra or taking over-the-counter pain relievers.

▶ **Menstrual Disorders**

**Amenorrhea** is the absence of menstrual periods and is known as primary amenorrhea if menstruation fails to begin by age 16. Primary amenorrhea affects less than 1% of adolescent girls in the United States. Causes include chromosomal abnormalities, problems with the hypothalamus, pituitary disease, lack of reproductive organs, or structural abnormality of the vagina. The cessation of menstrual periods, for 3 to 6 months or more, once they have begun is termed secondary amenorrhea. Each year in the United States approximately 5% of menstruating women experience 3 months of secondary amenorrhea. Causes include pregnancy, contraceptives, breast feeding, stress, medication, chronic illness, hormone imbalance, low body weight, excessive exercise, thyroid disorders, pituitary tumor, uterine scarring, and premature menopause. Prevention of amenorrhea includes maintaining a sensible exercise program, maintaining a healthy weight, eating a healthy diet, avoiding excessive alcohol consumption, not smoking, and finding healthy outlets for stress. Diagnosis may include pregnancy test, pelvic examination, blood test to check hormone levels, and progestin challenge test. Treatment, if any, depends on the cause of amenorrhea and may include lifestyle changes related to weight, physical activity, or stress level; amenorrhea caused by thyroid or pituitary disorders may be treated with medications.

**Dysmenorrhea** is painful or difficult menses. The prevalence of dysmenorrhea is estimated to be between 45% and 95% among reproductive-aged women. Primary dysmenorrhea involves no physical abnormality and usually begins 6 months to a year after menstruation begins. Secondary dysmenorrhea involves an underlying physical cause, such as endometriosis or fibroid tumors. Symptoms of dysmenorrhea include cramping and dull to severe pelvic and lower back pain that may radiate to other areas. Prostaglandins are the cause of primary dysmenorrhea. Causes of secondary dysmenorrhea include PID, use of an intrauterine device (IUD), uterine fibroid tumors, and endometriosis. Prevention of dysmenorrhea includes avoiding risk factors for PID, obtaining early diagnosis and treatment of STIs, and not using an IUD. Diagnosis is made

based on pelvic examination, ultrasound, laparoscopy, and hysteroscopy. Treatment options include antibiotics, oral contraceptive therapy to regulate and decrease menstrual flow, nonsteroidal anti-inflammatory medications to reduce pain, and surgery to remove fibroid tumors.

**Menorrhagia** is excessive or prolonged bleeding during menstruation. Clinically, it is defined as total blood loss exceeding 80 mL per cycle or menses lasting longer than 7 days. Menorrhagia is one of the most common gynecologic complaints; gynecological surveys report that 30% of all premenopausal women perceive their menses to be excessive, and the World Health Organization (WHO) reports that 18 million women aged 30 to 55 years perceive their menstrual bleeding to be excessive. However, only 10% of these women experience blood loss severe enough to be defined clinically as menorrhagia. Nearly 30% of all hysterectomies performed in the United States are performed to alleviate heavy menstrual bleeding.

Causes of menorrhagia include hormonal imbalance, fibroid tumors, lack of ovulation, use of an IUD, pregnancy complications, medications (anti-inflammatory and anticoagulants), PID, thyroid disorders, endometriosis, and liver or kidney disease. Sometimes the cause of menorrhagia is unknown. Prevention of menorrhagia includes not using an IUD, avoiding risk factors for PID, and obtaining early diagnosis and treatment of STIs. Diagnosis may include pelvic examination, Pap test, blood tests, biopsy, and ultrasound. Treatment varies according to the cause of the disease and may include iron supplements, nonsteroidal anti-inflammatory drugs, oral contraceptives, and progesterone. Surgical treatment options include dilation and curettage, endometrial ablation or resection, and hysterectomy.

**Metrorrhagia** is bleeding between menstrual periods or extreme irregularity of the menstrual cycle. Metrorrhagia can be caused by a hormonal imbalance, endometriosis, infection, miscarriage, ectopic pregnancy, cancer, use of an IUD, thyroid disorders, diabetes, and blood-clotting disorders. Prevention of metrorrhagia includes early diagnosis, treatment of STIs, and not using an IUD. Diagnosis is based on record of menstrual cycle, pelvic examination, blood tests, hysteroscopy, x-ray, biopsy, and ultrasound. The treatment of metrorrhagia depends on the cause of the problem and may include hormone therapy, antibiotics, surgery, and other medications.

## Premenstrual Syndrome and Premenstrual Dysphoric Disorder

Premenstrual syndrome (PMS) is a group of symptoms that start one to two weeks before menstruation and cease with the onset of menses. Estimates of the percentage of women affected by PMS vary widely in the United States. According to the American College of Obstetricians and Gynecologists, at least 85% of menstruating women have at least one PMS symptom as part of their monthly cycle. Common PMS symptoms include breast swelling and tenderness, acne, bloating and weight gain, headache or joint pain, food cravings, irritability, mood swings, crying spells, fatigue, trouble sleeping, anxiety, and depression. The cause of PMS is not known, but hormonal changes trigger the symptoms. Prevention of PMS includes a high intake of calcium and vitamin D. Diagnosis is based on medical history, including symptoms, when symptoms occur, and how much the symptoms interfere with daily life. No single PMS treatment works for everyone. Over-the-counter pain relievers may help ease cramps, headaches, backaches, and breast tenderness. Contraceptives can be used to reduce PMS symptoms. Avoiding salt, caffeine, and alcohol; exercising; eating healthy foods; getting enough sleep; joining a support group; and managing stress may also help with symptoms of PMS.

For some women, the symptoms of PMS are severe enough to interfere with their lives. They have a type of PMS called premenstrual dysphoric disorder, or PMDD. PMDD affects 3% to 8% of menstruating women. There is evidence that the neurotransmitter serotonin plays a role in PMDD. Symptoms, which can be disabling, include feelings of sadness or despair, suicidal thoughts, feelings of tension or anxiety, panic attacks, mood swings, crying, lasting irritability or anger that affects other people, disinterest in daily activities and relationships, trouble thinking or focusing, tiredness or low energy, food cravings or binge eating, having trouble sleeping, and feeling out of control. Physical symptoms may include bloating, breast tenderness, headaches, and joint or muscle pain. The patient must have five or more of these symptoms to be diagnosed with PMDD. Prevention of PMDD includes getting plenty of exercise and rest, eating a well-balanced diet, and managing stress. In addition to the PMS treatments listed above, antidepressants that change serotonin levels in the brain have also been shown to help some women with PMDD.

## Endometriosis

**Endometriosis** is a condition in which endometrial tissue from the uterus becomes embedded outside the uterus. During menstruation, the tissue may be pushed through the fallopian tubes or carried by blood or lymph. The endometrial tissue can embed on the ovaries, the outer surface of the uterus, the bowels, or other abdominal organs and appears rarely on other body structures and organs. An estimated 5.5 million women in North America suffer from endometriosis.

The endometrial tissue by nature responds to hormonal changes even when outside the uterus. This tissue goes through proliferative and secretory phases, along with the sloughing with subsequent bleeding. The most common symptom of endometriosis is pelvic pain. Other symptoms can include diarrhea or constipation, abdominal bloating, menorrhagia, metrorrhagia, and fatigue. It is estimated that 30% to 40% of women with endometriosis are infertile. The etiology of endometriosis is unknown, and endometriosis cannot be prevented. The only certain means of diagnosing endometriosis is by seeing it with laparoscopy. Treatment of endometriosis may include pain relievers, hormone therapy, and surgery.

# ▶ Disorders of Pregnancy

## Ectopic Pregnancy

An ectopic pregnancy is a pregnancy in which the fertilized ovum implants in a tissue other than the uterus. Ectopic pregnancies are estimated to occur in 1 in every 40 to 1 in every 100 pregnancies. The most common site of an ectopic pregnancy is in the fallopian tubes. In rare cases, ectopic pregnancies can occur in the ovary, cervix, and stomach area. An ectopic pregnancy is usually caused by a condition that blocks or slows the movement of a fertilized egg through the fallopian tube to the uterus. Most cases are a result of scarring caused by a past infection in the fallopian tubes, surgery of the fallopian tubes, or a previous ectopic pregnancy. Up to 50% of women who have ectopic pregnancies have PID. Some ectopic pregnancies can be due to birth defects of the fallopian tubes, endometriosis, complications of a ruptured appendix, or scarring caused by previous pelvic surgery. Symptoms of ectopic pregnancy include lower abdominal or pelvic pain, mild cramping on one side of the pelvis, amenorrhea, metrorrhagia, breast tenderness, nausea, and low back pain. If the area of the abnormal pregnancy ruptures and bleeds, symptoms may get worse and may include severe, sharp, and sudden pain in the lower abdominal area; feeling faint or actually fainting; referred pain to the shoulder area; and internal bleeding due to a rupture, which may lead to shock. Shock is the first symptom of nearly 20% of ectopic pregnancies.

Most forms of ectopic pregnancy that occur outside the fallopian tubes are usually not preventable. Prevention of an ectopic pregnancy in the fallopian tube includes avoiding risk factors for PID and early diagnosis and treatment of STIs. Diagnosis of ectopic pregnancy is based on symptoms, pelvic examination, ultrasound, and measurement of HCG levels. Ectopic pregnancies cannot continue to term, so the pregnancy must be terminated. In cases in which a rupture will occur, the woman may be given a medication called methotrexate that allows the body to reabsorb the pregnancy. In the event of a rupture, a laparotomy is done to stop blood loss and terminate the pregnancy.

## Spontaneous Abortion or Miscarriage

A spontaneous abortion, commonly called a miscarriage, is loss of a fetus before the twentieth week of pregnancy. Most miscarriages result from a genetic abnormality of the fetus. Other possible causes of miscarriage include infection, physical problems in the mother, hormonal factors, immune responses, or serious systemic diseases of the mother like diabetes or thyroid disease. It is estimated that up to 50% of all fertilized eggs die and are spontaneously aborted, usually before the woman knows she is pregnant. Among known pregnancies, the rate of miscarriage is approximately 10% and usually occurs between the seventh and twelfth weeks of pregnancy. Possible signs and symptoms of spontaneous abortion include low back pain or abdominal pain that is dull, sharp, or cramping; vaginal bleeding; and tissue or clotlike material discharged from the vagina. About 20% of pregnant women have some vaginal bleeding during the first 3 months of pregnancy; approximately half of these women have a miscarriage. Very few miscarriages are preventable. Diagnosis of spontaneous abortion is based on pelvic examination and HCG levels. If all the pregnancy tissue does not naturally exit the body, medication or surgery may be used to help eliminate the remaining tissue.

## Preeclampsia

**Preeclampsia** is a disease that only occurs during pregnancy. Preeclampsia, pregnancy-induced hypertension (PIH), and toxemia are essentially interchangeable terms. Preeclampsia occurs in 5% to 10% of all pregnancies. Mild preeclampsia is characterized by high blood pressure and the presence of protein in the urine. Severe preeclampsia may also include headaches, blurred vision, inability to tolerate bright light, fatigue, nausea, vomiting, urinating small amounts, pain in the upper right abdomen, shortness of breath, and the tendency to bruise easily. The cause of preeclampsia in not known. Risk factors include family history of preeclampsia, being pregnant with twins, young maternal age, never having carried a pregnancy to term, and women who had high blood pressure, diabetes, or kidney disease prior to pregnancy. Prevention of preeclampsia includes maintaining a healthy weight before pregnancy and taking multivitamins. Diagnosis of preeclampsia is based on increased blood pressure and urine protein levels. If close enough to term, the baby will be delivered. However, if a woman has mild preeclampsia and is not close enough to term to be delivered, rest, frequent monitoring of blood pressure and urine, reduced salt intake, and increased water intake may be recommended. Severe preeclampsia may be treated with blood pressure medication.

## Gestational Diabetes Mellitus

Gestational diabetes is diabetes mellitus associated with pregnancy (diabetes mellitus is discussed in detail in Chapter 12). Approximately 4% to 6% of pregnancies in the United States are complicated by diabetes, of which 90% is gestational diabetes.

Increased metabolic demands during pregnancy require higher insulin levels, but certain normal, maternal, physiological changes during pregnancy can result in insufficient insulin levels, which, if uncorrected, result in diabetes. These changes include increased levels of estrogen and progesterone, which interfere with insulin action. In addition, the placenta normally inactivates insulin. The normal pregnancy-induced elevation of stress hormones, such as cortisol, epinephrine, and glucagon, raises blood glucose. Insulin requirements continue to rise as pregnancy approaches term. In a normal pregnancy, more insulin is secreted to compensate for these changes, but in some women, insulin levels remain low as blood glucose continues to rise.

Risk factors include a family history of type II diabetes, age, gestational diabetes in a previous pregnancy, a previous pregnancy which resulted in a child with a birth weight of 9 pounds or more, diagnosis of prediabetes, impaired glucose tolerance, or impaired fasting glucose.

Smoking doubles the risk of gestational diabetes. Women at risk for developing gestational diabetes should be screened early and monitored throughout their pregnancy. Signs and symptoms of gestational diabetes are similar to insulin-dependent diabetes mellitus (Chapter 12) but include maternal hypertension, polyhydroamnios (excessive amniotic fluid), excessive weight gain during the last 6 months of pregnancy, and a fetus large for gestational age. Prevention of gestational diabetes includes eating a healthy diet, maintaining a healthy weight, not gaining too much weight during pregnancy, engaging in exercise on a regular basis.

The prognosis for gestational diabetes is good if diagnosed and treated early. Diagnosis is made via a glucose tolerance test. Treatment consists of regular blood glucose monitoring, dietary control of blood glucose levels, weight control, and possibly insulin therapy. Untreated gestational diabetes mellitus entails many risks to mother and fetus. The fetus risks stillbirth, premature delivery, and high or low birth weight. Infants may experience severe hypoglycemia shortly after birth.

## ▶ Anatomy of the Male Reproductive System

The male reproductive system consists of a pair of testes that produce sperm and hormones, a system of tubules that convey sperm to the outside, and the penis, which transmits the sperm into the female tract. Accessory glands contribute to the formation of semen.

The testes are suspended in the scrotum, a saclike structure outside the body wall. The testes contain highly coiled tubules called the **seminiferous tubules**, which are the site of sperm development. When the sperm reach a certain maturity, they enter the **epididymis**, a coiled tube that lies along the outer wall of the testis. The epididymis leads into another duct, the **vas deferens**, which passes through the inguinal canal into the abdominal cavity.

Near the base of the urinary bladder, the vas deferens joins a duct of the **seminal vesicle**, an

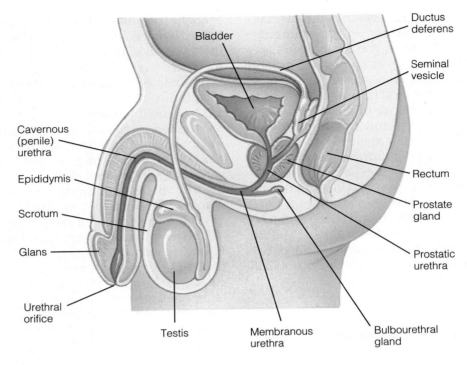

**Figure 11–3** ▶ The male reproductive system.

accessory gland, to form the ejaculatory duct. The ejaculatory ducts from each side penetrate the **prostate gland** to enter the urethra. Ducts of the prostate open into the first part of the male urethra. Another pair of glands, the **bulbour-ethral glands**, secrete into the urethra as it enters the penis. The male reproductive system is illustrated in Figure 11–3▶.

The penis contains erectile tissue composed of three cylindrical bodies filled with sinuses that become engorged with blood during sexual excitement. The urethra passes through one of these cylindrical bodies as it extends to the outside, and connective tissue supports the erectile structures. The distal, expanded end of the penis is the glans penis. A flap of loosely attached skin covering the glans, the prepuce or foreskin, is sometimes removed shortly after birth, a procedure called circumcision.

## ▶ Physiology of the Male Reproductive System

Spermatogenesis, the formation of sperm, begins in the male at puberty and continues through life. The development of sperm and the secretion of the male hormone, testosterone, are processes stimulated by gonadotropic hormones of the anterior pituitary gland. Maturation of sperm continues in the epididymis, where they acquire motility. Sperm are stored in both the epididymis and vas deferens, where they can live for several weeks. Once ejaculated, they live for 24 to 72 hours in the female reproductive tract.

The accessory glands produce a mucoid secretion, called semen, which nourishes and protects sperm. The seminal vesicles secrete an alkaline fluid that normally constitutes approximately 60% of the volume of semen. The alkaline nature of the seminal fluid helps to neutralize the acidic environment of the male urethra and female reproductive tract. Seminal fluid contains fructose to nourish the sperm and prostaglandins to stimulate uterine contractions and propel the sperm toward the fallopian tubes. The seminal vesicles release their secretions into the ejaculatory ducts at the same time that the vas deferens empty the sperm. The bulbourethral glands secrete an alkaline fluid into the urethra that neutralizes acidic urine in the urethra. At the same time, the bulbourethral glands secrete mucus that lubricates the urethra for easy passage of sperm. The prostate gland surrounds the upper portion of the urethra. The prostate gland secretes a milky fluid that contains citric acid to nourish the sperm and several protein-digesting enzymes such as PSA. Prostate secretions make up approximately 25% of the volume of semen.

Sexual stimulation of the male transmits impulses into the central nervous system, which initiates the male response. Erection of the penis is the first effect. Nerve impulses cause the dilation of penile arteries, allowing blood to flow under high pressure into the erectile tissue. The high pressure temporarily impedes the emptying of the penile veins and causes the penis to become hard, elongated, and erect.

Intense sexual stimulation causes peristaltic contractions in the walls of the epididymis and vas deferens, propelling sperm into the urethra. Semen typically contains between 50 and 150 million sperm. The seminal vesicles and prostate gland simultaneously release their secretions, which mix with the bulbourethral gland secretions and form the semen. Ejaculation of the semen, the culmination of the sexual act, occurs when contraction of this musculature increases pressure on the erectile tissue and the semen is expressed through the urethral opening.

## ▶ Diagnostic Procedures

Physical examination of the male reproductive system includes visual examination of the external genitalia. The testes are palpated to determine the presence of tumors. A digital rectal examination (DRE) allows the physician to palpate the prostate gland. PSA (prostate-specific antigen) is produced by cells of the prostate gland. The PSA test measures the level of PSA in the blood. Prostate cancer and benign prostatic hyperplasia can increase PSA levels. **Cytoscopy** is used to view the urethra and bladder. If abnormalities or tumors are discovered, a biopsy may be performed.

Sexually transmitted infections are diagnosed by blood or urine cultures, DNA test, and antigen or antibody testing. Others laboratory tests that may be performed include urinalysis and hormone testing.

## ▶ Diseases of the Male Reproductive System

### Prostatitis

**Prostatitis** is inflammation or infection of the prostate gland. According to the National Institutes of Health, prostatitis may account for up to 25% of all office visits for complaints involving the genital and urinary systems among young and middle-aged men. Prostatitis has been classified by the National Institutes of Health into four categories: Category 1 is acute bacterial prostatitis, category 2 is chronic bacterial prostatitis, category 3 includes the conditions previously known as nonbacterial prostatitis (prostatodynia and chronic pelvic pain syndrome), and category 4 asymptomatic inflammatory prostatitis. Approximately 5% to 10% of prostatitis cases are caused by bacterial infection.

The signs and symptoms vary depending on the category of prostatitis. Acute bacterial prostatistis usually comes on suddenly, and signs and symptoms may include fever and chills; flu-like symptoms; pain in the prostate gland, lower back, or groin; urinary problems, including increased urinary urgency and frequency, difficulty or pain when urinating, inability to completely empty the bladder, and blood-tinged urine; and painful ejaculation. The signs and symptoms of chronic bacterial prostatitis develop more slowly, usually aren't as severe as those of acute prostatitis, and tend to alternate with times when symptoms are worse. Signs and symptoms of chronic bacterial prostatitis include a frequent and urgent need to urinate, pain or burning sensation when urinating, pelvic pain, excessive urination during the night, pain in the lower back and genital area, difficulty starting urination or diminished urine flow, occasional blood in semen or urine, painful ejaculation, slight fever, and recurring bladder infections. The signs and symptoms of nonbacterial prostatitis are similar to those of chronic bacterial prostatitis, without fever.

Categories 1 and 2 prostatitis are caused by bacterial infections. The cause of categories 3 and 4 prostatitis is unknown. Prevention includes practicing good hygiene, maintaining adequate hydration, and seeking early treatment for infections. Diagnosis may include DRE and bacterial cultures of urine or prostate gland fluid. Pain relievers and several weeks of treatment with antibiotics are typically treatment for categories 1 and 2 prostatitis. Treatment for category 3 prostatitis may include alpha blockers to aid in urination, pain relievers, and muscle relaxants. Category 4 prostatitis is usually found during examination for another condition and may not require treatment.

## Epididymitis

**Epididymitis** is inflammation of the epididymis. Each year an estimated 1 in 1000 men suffer from epididymitis accounting for more than 600,000 medical visits per year in the United States. Signs and symptoms may include testicular swelling on one or both sides, scrotal pain ranging from mild to severe, tenderness in one or both testicles, tenderness in the groin, painful urination, painful intercourse or ejaculation, fever, penile discharge, and blood in the semen. A number of bacterial organisms can cause epididymitis, including gonorrhea and chlamydia. Other causes of epididymitis may include urinary infections spreading to the epididymis, anatomical abnormalities in the urinary tract, or catheter insertion. Prevention of epididymitis includes abstinence, monogamy, use of condoms and dental dams, and early

treatment for infections. Diagnosis may include physical examination, DRE, blood and urine tests, bacterial culture, ultrasound, and nuclear scan of the testicles. Antibiotics are the treatment for epididymitis.

## Orchitis

**Orchitis** is inflammation of the testes. The most common cause of orchitis is mumps; approximately 30% of male patients will develop orchitis during the course of the illness. Other causes of orchitis include bacterial infections or injury. The signs and symptoms of orchitis usually have an abrupt onset and may include testicular swelling on one or both sides, pain ranging from mild to severe, tenderness in one or both testicles, nausea and vomiting, fever, penile discharge, and prostate enlargement and tenderness. Prevention of orchitis includes vaccination against mumps, abstinence, monogamy, use of condoms and dental dams, and use of a protective cup over the genitals to guard against mechanical injury. Diagnosis may include physical examination, DRE, blood and urine tests, bacterial cultures, ultrasound, and nuclear imaging of the testicles. Treatment for viral orchitis is symptomatic and may include pain relievers, nonsteroidal anti-inflammatory drugs, bed rest, elevation, and application of cold packs to the scrotum. Bacterial orchitis is treated with antibiotics.

## Cryptorchidism

**Cyrptorchidism** is not a disease but a failure of the testes to descend from the abdominal cavity, where they develop during fetal life, to the scrotum. Approximately 3% of full-term male newborns have an undescended testicle at birth, and up to 30% of premature male newborns have at least one undescended testicle. Since the testicles typically descend late in fetal development, during the eighth month of gestation, the infant born before this time has a greater chance of having cyptorchidism. In over 50% of people being seen for cyrptorchidism, the testes descend by the third month, and by age one, 80% of all undescended testes have descended into the scrotum. Abnormal testicular development usually causes cryptorchidism. The affected testicles frequently have a short spermatic artery, poor blood supply, or both.

The major sign of cryptorchidism is not being able to feel one or both of the testicles in the scrotum. Cryptorchidism cannot be prevented. Diagnosis of cryptorchidism may involve palpating the scrotum and abdomen to locate the testicles while the patient is in the squatting position or in a warm bath and testing for testosterone and gonadotropin in the blood.

Cryptorchidism can cause other complications, including infertility and testicular cancer. It is reported that changes in an undescended testicle occur as early as 6 months of age, with the reported cancer rate in cryptorchidism at 22 times higher than in the general population. Treatment may include hormone therapy or surgery.

## Testicular Cancer

Testicular cancer is cancer in one or both testicles in young men. In about 90% of cases, men have a lump on a testicle that is painless but slightly uncomfortable, or they may notice testicular enlargement or swelling. Men with testicular cancer often report a sensation of heaviness or aching in the lower abdomen or scrotum.

The ACS estimates that about 8090 new cases of testicular cancer will be diagnosed during 2008 in the United States, and an estimated 380 men will die from the disease. Approximately 50,000 men annually will be diagnosed with testicular cancer and 9000 will die worldwide.

The cause of testicular cancer is not known. Risk factors include cryptorchidism (about 10% of testicular cancer cases occur in men with a history of cryptorchidism), a family history of testicular cancer age (90% of testicular cancer cases occur in men between the ages of 20 and 54), and race and ethnicity (the risk of testicular cancer among white men is about 5 to 10 times that of black men and more than twice that of Asian American men). The ACS recom-

mends a testicular examination as part of a general physical examination. Prevention of testicular cancer includes correcting cryptorchidism.

Diagnosis may include physical examination, ultrasound, and blood tests. Treatment may include surgery, radiation, and chemotherapy.

## ▶ Sexually Transmitted Infections

Sexually transmitted infections (STIs), also known as sexually transmitted diseases, are infections spread by sexual contact. Sexual contact includes unprotected oral, anal, or vaginal intercourse. STIs are caused by bacteria, viruses, and protozoans. The WHO estimates that more than 1 million new cases of sexually transmitted bacterial infections occur worldwide every day. The WHO also estimates that 80% to 90% of STIs occur in the developing world. The CDC estimates 19 million new STIs occur each year in the United States, almost half of them among people ages 15 to 24. The United States spends $14.1 billion in direct medical costs for STIs each year. Some STIs cause no or relatively minor symptoms, but undetected infections can have serious consequences, including infertility, PID, cervical cancer, and adverse pregnancy outcomes.

### HIV/AIDS

HIV/AIDS is covered in the discussion of immunity in Chapter 2.

### Gonorrhea

**Gonorrhea** is caused by the coccus bacterium *Neiserria gonorrhoeae*. Gonorrhea is transmitted through sexual contact and during childbirth. The CDC estimates that figure at more than 700,000 people in the United States get a gonorrheal infection each year; the WHO estimates that figure at more than 62 million people worldwide.

Although many men with gonorrhea are asymptomatic, some have some signs or symptoms that appear within two to five days after

## Prevention ✚PLUS!

### Preventing STIs

- **Don't have sex.**  The best way to prevent any STI is to practice abstinence, or not having vaginal, oral, or anal sex.
- **Be monogamous.**  Have a sexual relationship with one partner who has been tested negative for STIs.
- **Use condoms.**  Protect yourself with a condom EVERY time you have vaginal, anal, or oral sex. Condoms should be used for any type of sex with every partner. For vaginal sex, use a latex male condom or a female polyurethane condom. For anal sex, use a latex male condom. For oral sex, use a dental dam. A dental dam is a rubbery material that can be placed over the anus or the vagina before sexual contact.
- **Know that some methods of birth control, like birth control pills, shots, implants, or diaphragms, will not protect you from STIs.**  If you use one of these methods, be sure to also use a latex condom or dental dam correctly every time you have sex.
- **Talk with your sex partner(s) about STIs and using condoms.**  It's up to you to make sure you are protected. Remember, it's YOUR body!
- **Talk frankly with your healthcare provider and your sex partner(s) about any STIs you or your partner have or had.** Try not to be embarrassed.
- **Have regular pelvic exams.**  Ask your healthcare provider to test you for STIs.

*Source:* The National Women's Health Information Center, available at: www.4women.gov/FAQ/stdsgen.htm\#11

infection; signs and symptoms can take as long as 30 days to appear. Signs and symptoms include a burning sensation when urinating, or a white, yellow, or green discharge from the penis, and painful or swollen testicles. Most women who are infected with gonorrhea are asymptomatic. Even when a woman has symptoms, they can be so nonspecific as to be mistaken for a bladder or vaginal infection. The signs and symptoms in women include a painful or burning sensation when urinating, vaginal discharge, or vaginal bleeding between periods.

Untreated gonorrhea can cause serious and permanent health problems in both women and men. In women, gonorrhea is a common cause of PID. In men, gonorrhea can cause epididymitis, which can lead to infertility if left untreated. Gonorrheal infection in a newborn can cause blindness, joint infection, or a life-threatening blood infection. To prevent this infection, a drop of erythromycin is routinely placed in the eyes of newborn babies. Treatment of gonorrhea as soon as it is detected in pregnant women will reduce the risk of these complications.

Prevention of gonorrhea includes abstinence, monogamy, use of condoms and dental dams, and regular pelvic exams. Gonorrhea can be diagnosed by urine sample, bacterial culture, or Gram stain (Chapter 3). Gonorrhea is treated with antibiotics. Drug-resistant strains of gonorrhea are increasing in many areas of the world, including the United States, and successful treatment of gonorrhea is becoming more difficult.

## Syphilis

**Syphilis** is caused by the spirochete bacterium *Treponema pallidum*. Syphilis is transmitted through sexual contact, through direct contact with a syphilis **chancre**, and during childbirth. In 2006, 36,935 cases of syphilis were reported to the CDC. In the United States, men having sex with men account for 64% of syphilis cases. The WHO estimates that worldwide more than 12 million people annually are infected with syphilis.

The time between infection with syphilis and the appearance of symptoms can range from 10 to 90 days. The primary stage begins with the appearance of one or more chancres where *Treponema pallidum* entered the body (Figure 11–4 ▶). Chancres are a painless lesion that usually lasts 3 to 6 weeks and heals without treatment. If no treatment is administered, the

**Figure 11–4** ▶ Chancre of primary syphilis on the penis.

infection progresses to the secondary stage. Secondary syphilis is often marked by a skin rash that is characterized by brown sores about the size of a penny. The rash appears anywhere from 3 to 6 weeks after the chancre appears. While the rash may cover the whole body or appear only in a few areas, the palms of the hands and soles of the feet are almost always involved. Because active bacteria are present in these sores, any physical contact with the broken skin of an infected person may spread the infection at this stage. The rash usually heals within several weeks or months. Other signs and symptoms also may occur, such as mild fever, fatigue, headache, sore throat, as well as patchy hair loss and swollen lymph glands throughout the body. These signs and symptoms may be mild and, like the chancre of primary syphilis, will disappear without treatment. The signs and symptoms of secondary syphilis may come and go over the next one to two years.

If untreated, syphilis may lapse into a latent stage during which the disease is no longer contagious and no signs or symptoms are present. Many people who are not treated will suffer no further consequences of the disease. Approximately one-third of those who have secondary syphilis, however, go on to develop the complications of late, or tertiary, syphilis, in which the bacteria damage the heart, eyes, brain, nervous system, bones, joints, or almost any other part of the body. This stage can last for years, or even for decades. Late syphilis can result in

mental illness, blindness, other neurological problems, heart disease, and death.

Syphilis bacteria frequently invade the nervous system during the early stages of infection, and approximately 3% to 7% of persons with untreated syphilis develop neurosyphilis (syphilis that has reached the central nervous system). Some patients with neurosyphilis are asymptomatic; others may have headache, stiff neck, fever that results from an inflammation of the lining of the brain, and seizures. Patients whose blood vessels are affected may develop symptoms of stroke with resulting numbness, weakness, or visual complaints. In some instances, the time from infection to developing neurosyphilis may be up to 20 years.

It is likely that an untreated pregnant woman with active syphilis will pass the infection to her unborn child. About 25% of these pregnancies result in stillbirth or neonatal death. Between 40% and 70% of these pregnancies will yield a syphilis-infected infant. Some infants with congenital syphilis may have signs and symptoms at birth, but most develop symptoms between 2 weeks and 3 months later. These signs and symptoms may include skin sores, rashes, fever, weakened or hoarse crying sounds, swollen liver and spleen, jaundice, anemia, and various deformities.

Prevention of syphilis includes abstinence, monogamy, use of condoms and dental dams, and regular pelvic exams. Diagnosis of syphilis may include microscopic visualization of the bacterium from chancre scrapings. Laboratory tests may include antigen or antibody testing. Syphilis is treated with antibiotics; however, development of antibiotic-resistant strains is a serious threat. Treatment will kill the syphilis bacterium and prevent further damage, but it will not repair damage already done.

## Chlamydia

**Chlamydia** is caused by the coccus bacterium *Chlamydia trachomatis*. Chlamydia is the most frequently reported bacterial sexually transmitted infection in the United States. The CDC estimates that 2.8 million people in the United States are infected with chlamydia each year. Rates of bacterial STIs can vary by state. Table 11–1 ▶ shows the top ten states for each bacterial

**Table 11–1 ▶ Top Ten States Ranked by Rate (per 100,000) of Reported Bacterial STI Cases in 2006**

| Rank | Primary and Secondary Syphilis | Chlamydia | Gonorrhea |
|------|-------------------------------|-----------|-----------|
| 1 | Louisiana | Alaska | Mississippi |
| 2 | Alabama | Mississippi | South Carolina |
| 3 | Georgia | South Carolina | Louisiana |
| 4 | Nevada | New Mexico | Alabama |
| 5 | Maryland | Alabama | Georgia |
| 6 | California | Hawaii | North Carolina |
| 7 | Texas | Georgia | Delaware |
| 8 | Tennessee | Delaware | Missouri |
| 9 | New Mexico | Tennessee | Ohio |
| 10 | Florida | Illinois | Tennessee |

*Source:* CDC, STD 2006 Surveillance Report

STI. The WHO estimates that more than 92 million chlamydial infections occur worldwide each year. Chlamydia is transmitted by sexual contact and during childbirth. It is known as a "silent" disease because about three-quarters of infected women and about half of infected men are asymptomatic. If signs and symptoms do occur, they usually appear within 1 to 3 weeks after exposure. Women who have signs and symptoms may have an abnormal vaginal discharge, burning sensation when urinating, lower abdominal pain, low back pain, nausea, fever, pain during intercourse, or bleeding between menstrual periods. Men with signs or symptoms may have a penile discharge, burning sensation when urinating, and burning and itching around the urethral orifice.

In women, untreated infection can spread into the uterus or fallopian tubes and cause PID. This happens in up to 40% of women with untreated chlamydia. Complications among men are rare. Infection sometimes spreads to the epididymis, causing pain, fever, and infre-quently sterility. Rarely, genital chlamydial infection can cause arthritis that can be accompanied by skin lesions and inflammation of the eye and urethra known as Reiter's syndrome. In pregnant women, there is some evidence that untreated chlamydial infections can lead to premature delivery. Babies who are born to infected mothers can get chlamydial infections in their eyes and respiratory tracts. Chlamydia is a leading cause of early infant pneumonia and conjunctivitis in newborns. Prevention of chlamydia includes abstinence, monogamy, use of condoms and dental dams, and regular pelvic exams. Diagnosing chlamydia may include bacterial culture and antigen or antibody testing. Antibiotics are used to treat chlamydia.

## Trichomoniasis

**Trichomoniasis** is caused by the protozoan *Trichomonas vaginalis*. The CDC estimates that 7.4 million new cases occur each year in the United States. Trichomoniasis is transmitted by sexual contact. Most men with trichomoniasis are asymptomatic; however, some men may temporarily have urethritis, epididymitis, and prostatitis. Signs and symptoms usually appear in women within 5 to 28 days of exposure and may including a frothy, yellow-green vaginal discharge with a fishy odor, pain during intercourse and urination, and irritation and itching of the genital area.

Prevention of trichomoniasis includes abstinence, monogamy, use of condoms and dental dams, and regular pelvic exams. Diagnosis of trichmoniasis may include pelvic examination, microscopic visualization of the protozoan, protozoal culture, laboratory test, and pH test. Treatment of both partners with antiparasitic medication such as metronidazole is effective.

## Genital Herpes

**Genital herpes** is caused by the herpes simplex viruses type 1 (HSV-1) and type 2 (HSV-2). HSV-1 can cause genital herpes, but it more commonly causes infections of the mouth and lips, so-called fever blisters. Most genital herpes is caused by HSV-2. The CDC estimates that at least 45 million people age 12 and older, or one out of five adolescents and adults, have had a HSV-2 infection. Between the late 1970s and the early 1990s, the number of Americans with genital herpes infection increased by 30%. Genital HSV-2 infection is more common in women (approximately one out of four women) than in men (almost one out of five). This may be due to male-to-female transmission being more likely than female-to-male transmission.

Most people have no or minimal signs of HSV-1 or HSV-2 infection. Signs of HSV-1 and HSV-2 include one or more blisters on or around the genitals (Figure 11–5►). The blisters break, leaving ulcers or tender sores that may take up to 4 weeks to heal. Other signs and symptoms during the first herpes outbreak may include fever; itching, burning, or pain in the genital area; vaginal discharge; headache; muscle ache; pain during urination; and swollen lymph nodes. The herpes virus goes latent and can become active from time to time, causing an

**Figure 11–5** ► Genital herpes blisters as they appear on the labia. (© Visuals Unlimited)

outbreak of blisters. Over time these recurrences usually decrease in frequency. Active genital herpes has very serious consequences during pregnancy, causing spontaneous abortion or premature delivery and infection of the newborn.

HSV-2 may be diagnosed by physical exam and history, viral culture, and antibody testing. Prevention of HSV-1 and HSV-2 includes abstinence, monogamy, use of condoms and dental dams, and regular pelvic exams. There is no treatment that can cure herpes, but antiviral medications can shorten outbreaks and make them less severe. Taking antiviral medications on a regular basis may stop outbreaks from occurring and may decrease transmission of the virus.

## Human Papillomavirus and Genital Warts

Human papillomavirus (HPV) is one of the most common causes of STI in the world. According to the CDC, approximately 6.2 million new cases of sexually transmitted HPV infections occur every year in the United States. At least 20 million people in the United States are already infected with HPV. At least 50% of sexually active men and women acquire genital HPV infection at some point in their lives. By age 50, at least 80% of women will have acquired genital HPV infection. The WHO estimates the prevalence of genital HPV infection in the world to be 440 million.

More than 100 different types of HPV exist; approximately 30 types are sexually transmitted and are classified as either low risk or high risk. Low-risk types cause genital warts, while the high-risk types may lead to cancer. A person who is infected with HPV but has no signs or symptoms can still spread HPV to a sexual partner. One study sponsored by the National Institute of Allergy and Infectious Diseases reported that almost half of women infected with HPV had no obvious signs or symptoms. Most people who become infected with HPV will not have any signs or symptoms, and the immune system will clear the infection. Most women are diagnosed with HPV on the basis of abnormal Pap tests or an HPV DNA test.

**Genital warts** are the most easily recognized sign of genital HPV infection (Figure 11–6▶). However, many people have a genital HPV infec-tion without genital warts. Genital warts may appear within weeks after sexual contact with an infected partner, or they might not develop for several months. Genital warts are single or multiple growths or bumps that appear in the genital area and sometimes are cauliflower shaped. Warts can appear on the vulva, in or around the vagina or anus, on the cervix, and on the penis, scrotum, groin, or thigh. Genital warts are diagnosed by visual inspection and can be removed by medications, electrocautery (burning), cryosurgery (freezing), and laser surgery.

Prevention of HPV includes abstinence, monogamy, use of condoms and dental dams, and regular pelvic exams. There is no cure for HPV or genital warts. In June 2006, the Food and Drug Administration approved the Gardasil vaccine for females aged 9 to 26. Ideally, women should get the vaccine before they are sexually active. Gardasil is highly effective in preventing persistent infection with HPV types 16 and 18, two high-risk HPVs that cause 70 percent of cervical cancers, and types 6 and 11, which cause 90 percent of genital warts. Gardasil has not been proven to provide complete protection against persistent infection with other HPV types, some of which also can cause cervical cancer. Therefore, about 30% of cervical cancers and 10% of genital warts will not be prevented by the current vaccine.

**Figure 11–6** ▶ Genital warts. (Courtesy of the CDC/Dr. Wiesner, 1972)

## ▶ Female Age-Related Diseases

In older females, pubic hair thins and grays and the external reproductive genitalia acquire a wrinkled and sagging appearance due to a decrease in elasticity. Physical changes in the aging female include shrinking of internal reproductive organs, decrease in vaginal secretions and elasticity, and a decrease in breast tissue volume. The pH of vaginal secretions becomes more alkaline, making older women more susceptible to vaginal infections. Increased stimulation and lubrication may be necessary to facilitate sexual intercourse.

**Menopause**, the cessation of menstrual periods, is not a disease but is a physical change related to aging. Menopause usually takes place between 45 and 55 years of age. As a woman ages, the ovaries produce less estrogen and progesterone, causing cessation of ovulation and menstruation. Removal of the ovaries also causes menopause. Common physical signs and symptoms of menopause include hot flashes, night sweats, trouble sleeping, mood swings, trouble focusing, hair loss or thinning, facial hair growth, and vaginal dryness. Menopause is diagnosed by signs and symptoms, elevated FSH, and low estrogen. Hormone therapy may help with menopause signs and symptoms; however, each woman and her physician must weigh the benefits and risks of hormone therapy.

**Uterine prolapse** is the condition of the uterus dropping or protruding downward into the vagina. This condition results from trauma to the fascia, muscle, and pelvic ligaments during pregnancy and delivery, or atrophy of the pelvic floor muscles with age. The ligaments and muscles become so overstretched that they can no longer hold the uterus in place, so the uterus falls or sags downward. Symptoms include feelings of heaviness in the pelvic area, incontinence, and lower back pain. Diagnosis of uterine prolapse may include pelvic examination and fluoroscopy. Treatment consists of strengthening the pelvic floor muscles (Kegel exercises), inserting a pessary into the vagina to support the uterus, or surgery.

**Cystocele** is a downward displacement of the urinary bladder into the vagina. This condition results from trauma to the fascia, muscle, and pelvic ligaments during pregnancy and delivery, or atrophy of the pelvic floor muscles with age. Symptoms include pelvic pressure, urinary urgency and frequency, and incontinence. Diagnosis is made by pelvic examination. Treatment includes Kegel exercises, inserting a pessary into the vagina, or surgery.

A **rectocele** is the protrusion of the rectum into the posterior aspect of the vagina. This condition results from trauma to the fascia, muscle, and pelvic ligaments during pregnancy and delivery, or atrophy of the pelvic floor mus-

cles with age. Symptoms include discomfort, constipation, and fecal incontinence. Diagnosis is made by pelvic examination. Treatment includes surgical repair of the posterior wall of the vagina.

## ▶ Male Age-Related Diseases

In older males, pubic hair thins and grays and the external reproductive genitalia acquire a wrinkled and sagging appearance due to a decrease in elasticity. Testosterone levels decline gradually and the testes decrease in size. Sperm count is slightly reduced and prostate gland secretions are decreased. Increased stimulation may be necessary to achieve erection.

A common problem in older males is enlargement of the prostate gland, or **benign prostatic hyperplasia (BPH)**. BPH affects more than 50% of men over age 60 and as many as 90% of men over age 70. Signs and symptoms of BPH often come on gradually and may include a need to get up during the night and urinate, need to empty the bladder often during the day, difficulty starting urine flow, dribbling after urination ends, and decrease in size and strength of the urine stream. If the bladder cannot be fully emptied, residual urine provides a medium for bacterial infection, and cystitis develops. An imbalance of sex hormones frequently causes prostatic enlargement. The level of testosterone generally decreases with age, but estrogen from the adrenal cortex continues to be secreted, changing the ratio of the two. Diagnosis of BPH may include DRE, urine analysis, PSA blood test, ultrasound, urine flow study, cystoscopy, and x-ray.

Treatment may not be needed because the signs and symptoms of BPH clear up without treatment in as many as one-third of all mild cases. Since BPH can cause urinary tract infections, antibiotics may be given before treating the BPH. Medications can be used to relieve common symptoms of BPH. Other treatments may include destroying excess prostate tissue with microwaves or ultrasound and surgery. In the United States, 350,000 operations take place each year to relieve BPH symptoms.

## Prostate Cancer

Prostate cancer is the second leading cause of cancer death in American men, behind only lung cancer. Each year approximately 780,000 men will be diagnosed with prostate cancer and 250,000 will die worldwide. Prostate cancer is also discussed in Chapter 4.

The cause of prostate cancer is not known. Age is the strongest risk factor for prostate cancer; approximately two out of three prostate cancers are found in men over the age of 65. Other risk factors include race (prostate cancer is more common among African American men than among men of other races and occurs less often in Asian American and Hispanic/Latino men than in non-Hispanic whites), nationality (prostate cancer is most common in North America and northwestern Europe), and a family history of prostate cancer (having a father or brother with prostate cancer more than doubles a man's risk of developing this disease). The exact role of diet in prostate cancer is not clear, but studies have shown men who eat a lot of red meat or high-fat dairy products seem to have a greater risk of getting prostate cancer.

Signs and symptoms include dull pain in the lower pelvic area; urgency of urination; difficulty starting urination; pain during urination; weak urine flow and dribbling; intermittent urine flow; a sensation that the bladder does not empty; frequent urination at night; blood in the urine; painful ejaculation; general pain in the lower back, hips, and upper thighs; loss of appetite and weight; and persistent bone pain. Diagnosis is based on DRE, PSA blood test, and biopsy. The ACS believes that doctors should offer the PSA blood test and DRE yearly, beginning at age 50, to men who do not have any major medical problems and can be expected to live at least 10 more years. Men at high risk (African American men and men who have a close relative (father, brother, or son) who had prostate cancer before age 65) should begin testing at age 45.

Because prostate cancer often grows very slowly, some men (especially those who are older or who have other major health problems) may never need treatment for their cancer. An approach called "watchful waiting" may be suggested. This approach involves closely watching the cancer (DRE, PSA testing, and possible biopsy). Treatment of prostate cancer may include surgery, radiation, and hormone therapy.

**Erectile dysfunction (ED)**, also known as impotence, is the inability of the male to achieve and maintain an erection sufficient for sexual intercourse. ED is said to be primary if the man has never been able to complete intercourse successfully, and secondary if intercourse has been achieved successfully at least once. More than 18 million men in the United States age 20 and over suffer from ED. As men age, their risk for ED increases dramatically: 70% of men age 70 or over report erectile problems, compared with 5% of men age 20 to 40.

ED may be caused by psychological factors. The dilation of penile arteries that leads to engorgement of the erectile tissue of the penis and then erection is under the control of the autonomic nervous system, which is affected by stress, anxiety, and fear.

ED may also be physiologic in nature. Incidence of ED has a strong association with certain medical conditions. In a recent Johns Hopkins study, half of the study subjects with ED also had diabetes or a history of cardiovascular disease; of the subjects considered obese, 21% suffered from ED. There seems to also be an association between ED and lack of physical activity. Men who reported three or more hours of sedentary activity per day were approximately three times more likely to have ED than subjects who reported less than one hour of sedentary activity each day. Other possible physiologic causes of ED include surgical complications, urologic disorders, medications, premature ejaculation, drug abuse, and alcoholism.

Diagnosis of ED may include medical, sexual, and psychosocial history; physical examination; laboratory tests; and ultrasound. With correct treatment, ED can usually be overcome. Viagra, Levitra, and Cialis prevent the breakdown of nitric oxide, a chemical messenger that promotes relaxation and opening of the blood vessels that supply erectile tissue in the penis. Under the influence of nitric oxide, these vessels expand and stay dilated. Increased blood flow makes erectile tissue swell and compress the veins that carry blood out of the penis, resulting in a full erection. Lifestyle changes and therapy may also help improve ED.

## RESOURCES

American Cancer Society: www.cancer.org

Centers for Disease Control and Prevention: www.cdc.gov

The National Woman's Health Information Center: www.4women.gov

World Health Organization: www.who.org

## Reproductive System

| DISEASE OR DISORDER | ETIOLOGY | SIGNS AND SYMPTOMS |
| --- | --- | --- |
| Pelvic inflammatory disease | Infection | Lower abdominal pain, fever, unusual vaginal discharge that may have a foul odor, painful intercourse, painful urination, and irregular menstrual bleeding |
| Cervical cancer | Human papillomavirus | Vaginal discharge and bleeding |
| Endometrial cancer | Unknown | Vaginal bleeding, nonbloody vaginal discharge, pelvic pain, weight loss |
| Fibroid tumors of the uterus | Unknown | Asymptomatic or excessive vaginal bleeding, pelvic pressure, abdominal pain, abdominal enlargement, pain during intercourse |
| Ovarian cancer | Unknown | Bloating, pelvic or abdominal pain, trouble eating or feeling full quickly, changes in urinary urgency or frequency |
| Breast cancer | Unknown | Lump or mass, swelling of all or part of the breast, skin irritation and dimpling, breast or nipple pain, nipple retraction, redness, scaliness, or thickening of the nipple or breast skin, a discharge other than breast milk, swelling of a lymph node in the armpit |
| Breast cysts | Unknown | Tiny, fluid-filled sacs in breast tissue |
| Fibrocystic changes | Unknown | Lumpy breasts |
| Fibroadenoma | Unknown | Solid, firm tumor, usually painless |
| Amenorrhea | Primary—chromosomal abnormalities, problems with the hypothalamus, pituitary disease, lack of reproductive organs, or structural abnormality of the vagina Secondary—pregnancy, contraceptives, breast feeding, stress, medication, chronic illness, hormone imbalance, low body weight, excessive exercise, thyroid disorders, pituitary tumor, uterine scarring, premature menopause | No menstrual period |

| DIAGNOSIS | TREATMENT | PREVENTION/LIFESPAN |
|---|---|---|
| Physical examination, positive culture, ultrasound, laparoscopy | Antibiotics | Prevent STIs, early treatment of STIs |
| Pelvic examination, Pap test, HPV DNA test, colposcopy | Surgery, radiation, chemotherapy | Avoid exposure to HPV, Gardasil |
| Pelvic examination, CA 125 blood test, biopsy, hysteroscopy, D&C | Surgery, radiation, chemotherapy, and hormone therapy | Use of oral contraceptives, controlling obesity and diabetes, healthy diet, exercise |
| Pelvic examination, ultrasound, sonography, hysteroscopy | Uterine artery embolization, focused ultrasound surgery, endometrial ablation, birth control pills, myomectomy, hysterectomy | Not preventable |
| CT or MRI scan, ultrasound, laparoscopy, biopsy, CA 125 blood test | Surgery, radiation, chemotherapy | Use of oral contraceptives, tubal ligation, hysterectomy, having children, breast feeding |
| Breast exam, mammogram, ultrasound, biopsy | Surgery, radiation, chemotherapy, targeted therapy, hormone therapy | Avoiding alcohol, exercising regularly, maintaining a healthy body weight |
| Breast exam, mammogram, ultrasound, fine needle aspiration | None, surgery | Not preventable |
| Breast exam, mammogram, ultrasound, biopsy | None, supportive bra, OTC pain relievers | Not preventable |
| Breast exam, mammogram, ultrasound, fine needle aspiration, biopsy | None, surgery | Not preventable |
| Pregnancy test, pelvic examination, blood test to check hormone levels, progestin challenge test | If needed—lifestyle changes related to weight, physical activity or stress level, amenorrhea caused by thyroid or pituitary disorders may be treated with medications | Maintaining a sensible exercise program, maintaining a normal weight, eating a healthy diet, avoiding excessive alcohol consumption, not smoking, finding healthy outlets for stress |

| DISEASE OR DISORDER | ETIOLOGY | SIGNS AND SYMPTOMS |
| --- | --- | --- |
| Dysmenorrhea | Primary—prostaglands<br>Secondary—PID, use of an IUD, fibroid tumors, endometriosis | Cramping, dull to severe pelvic, lower back pain that may radiate to other areas |
| Menorrhagia | Hormonal imbalance, fibroid tumors, lack of ovulation, use of an IUD, pregnancy complications, medications (anti-inflammatory and anticoagulants), PID, thyroid disorders, endometriosis, liver or kidney disease, unknown | Excessive or prolonged bleeding during menstruation |
| Metrorrhagia | Hormonal imbalance, endometriosis, infection, miscarriage, ectopic pregnancy, cancer, IUD use, thyroid disorders, diabetes, blood-clotting disorders | Bleeding between menstrual periods, extreme irregularity of menstrual cycle |
| Premenstrual syndrome | Unknown but hormonal changes trigger the symptoms | Breast swelling and tenderness, acne, bloating and weight gain, headache or joint pain, food cravings, irritability, mood swings, crying spells, fatigue, trouble sleeping, anxiety, depression |
| Premenstrual dysphoric disorder | Unknown but hormonal changes trigger the symptoms | Feelings of sadness or despair, possibly suicidal thoughts, feelings of tension or anxiety, panic attacks, mood swings, crying, lasting irritability or anger that affects other people, disinterest in daily activities and relationships, trouble thinking or focusing, tiredness or low energy, food cravings or binge eating, having trouble sleeping, feeling out of control, physical symptoms, such as bloating, breast tenderness, headaches, joint or muscle pain |
| Endometriosis | Unknown | Pelvic pain, diarrhea or constipation, abdominal bloating, menorrhagia, metrorrhagia, fatigue |
| Ectopic pregnancy | PID, surgery of the fallopian tubes, previous ectopic pregnancy, birth defects of the fallopian tubes, endometriosis, complications of a ruptured appendix, scarring caused by previous pelvic surgery, or unknown | Lower abdominal or pelvic pain, mild cramping on one side of the pelvis, amenorrhea, metrorrhagia, breast tenderness, nausea, low back pain, severe, sharp, and sudden pain in the lower abdominal area, feeling faint or fainting, referred pain to the shoulder area, shock |
| Spontaneous abortion or miscarriage | Genetic abnormality of the fetus, infection, physical problems in the mother, hormonal factors, immune responses, diabetes, thyroid disease | Low back pain or abdominal pain that is dull, sharp, or cramping, vaginal bleeding, tissue or clotlike material discharged from the vagina |

| DIAGNOSIS | TREATMENT | PREVENTION/LIFESPAN |
|---|---|---|
| Pelvic examination, ultrasound, laparoscopy, hysteroscopy | Antibiotics, oral contraceptive therapy, non-steroidal anti-inflammatory medication, surgery | Not using an IUD, avoid risk factors for PID, early diagnosis and treatment of STIs |
| Pelvic examination, Pap test, blood tests, biopsy, ultrasound | Iron supplements, nonsteroidal anti-inflammatory drugs, oral contraceptives, progesterone, D&C, endometrial ablation or resection, hysterectomy | Not using an IUD, avoid risk factors for PID, early diagnosis and treatment of STIs |
| Record of menstrual cycle, pelvic examination, blood tests, hysteroscopy, x-ray, biopsy, ultrasound | Hormone therapy, antibiotics, surgery, medication | Not using an IUD |
| Symptoms, when symptoms occur, and how much the symptoms interfere with the patient's life | Over-the-counter pain relievers, avoiding salt, caffeine and alcohol, exercising, eating healthy foods, and getting enough sleep, support groups, stress management, contraceptives | High intake of calcium and vitamin D |
| Symptoms, when symptoms occur, and how much they interfere with the patient's life | PMS treatments plus antidepressants | Plenty of exercise and rest, eating a well-balanced diet, managing stress |
| Laparoscopy | Pain relievers, hormone therapy, surgery | Not preventable |
| Signs and symptoms, pelvic examination, ultrasound, measurement of HCG levels | Surgery, medication | In the fallopian tubes—avoid risk factors for PID, early diagnosis and treatment of STIs<br>Outside the fallopian tubes—usually not preventable |
| Pelvic examination, HCG levels | Medication, surgery | Not preventable |

| DISEASE OR DISORDER | ETIOLOGY | SIGNS AND SYMPTOMS |
|---|---|---|
| Preeclampsia | Unknown | Mild preeclampsia—high blood pressure, and the presence of protein in the urine<br>Severe preeclampsia—also includes headaches, blurred vision, inability to tolerate bright light, fatigue, nausea, vomiting, urinating small amounts, pain in the upper right abdomen, shortness of breath, and tendency to bruise easily |
| Gestational diabetes mellitus | Pregnancy | Maternal hypertension, polyhydroamnios, excessive weight gain during the last 6 months of pregnancy, a fetus large for gestational age |
| Prostatitis | Not always known; may be infection | Acute bacterial prostatits—fever and chills, flulike symptoms, pain in the prostate gland, lower back or groin, urinary problems, including increased urinary urgency and frequency, difficulty or pain when urinating, inability to completely empty the bladder, blood-tinged urine, painful ejaculation<br>Chronic bacterial prostatitis—frequent and urgent need to urinate, pain or burning sensation when urinating, pelvic pain, excessive urination during the night, pain in the lower back and genital area, difficulty starting urination or diminished urine flow, occasional blood in semen or urine, painful ejaculation, slight fever, recurring bladder infections<br>Nonbacterial prostatitis—similar to chronic bacterial without fever |
| Epididymitis | Infection, anatomical abnormalities in the urinary tract, catheter | Testicular swelling on one or both sides, scrotal pain ranging from mild to severe, tenderness in one or both testicles, tenderness in the groin, painful urination, painful intercourse or ejaculation, fever, penile discharge, blood in the semen |
| Orchitis | Infection, injury | Testicular swelling on one or both sides, pain ranging from mild to severe, tenderness in one or both testicles, nausea and vomiting, fever, penile discharge, prostate enlargement and tenderness |
| Cryptorchidism | Abnormal testicular development | Inability to feel one or both testicles |
| Testicular cancer | Unknown | Lump on a testicle that is often painless but slightly uncomfortable, testicular enlargement or swelling, sensation of heaviness or aching in the lower abdomen or scrotum |

| DIAGNOSIS | TREATMENT | PREVENTION/LIFESPAN |
|---|---|---|
| Blood pressure, urine protein levels | Delivery of the baby, rest, frequent monitoring of blood pressure and urine, limiting salt, drinking water, blood pressure medication | Healthy weight before pregnancy, taking multivitamins |
| Glucose tolerance test | Regular blood glucose monitoring, dietary control of blood glucose levels, weight control, insulin injections | Eating a healthy diet, maintaining a healthy weight, not gaining too much weight during pregnancy, regular exercise |
| DRE, bacterial cultures | Categories 1 & 2—pain relievers, antibiotics<br>Category 3—alpha blockers, pain relievers, muscle relaxants<br>Category 4—may not require treatment | Practice good hygiene, adequate hydration, seek early treatment for infections |
| Physical examination, DRE, blood and urine tests, bacterial culture, ultrasound, nuclear scan of the testicles | Antibiotics | Abstinence, monogamy, use of condoms and dental dams, early treatment for infections |
| Physical examination, DRE, blood and urine tests, bacterial cultures, ultrasound, nuclear imaging of the testicles | Pain relievers, nonsteroidal anti-inflammatory drugs, bed rest, elevation and applying cold packs to the scrotum, antibiotics | Vaccinating against mumps, abstinence, monogamy, use of condoms and dental dams, and wearing a protective cup over the genitals to guard against mechanical injury |
| Palpating the scrotum and abdomen, hormone testing | Hormone therapy, surgery | Not preventable |
| Physical examination, ultrasound, blood tests | Surgery, chemotherapy, radiation | Correcting cryptorchidism |

## Reproductive System (*continued*)

| DISEASE OR DISORDER | ETIOLOGY | SIGNS AND SYMPTOMS |
|---|---|---|
| Gonorrhea | *Neiserria gonorrhoeae* | Men—asymptomatic, burning sensation when urinating, or a white, yellow, or green discharge from the penis, painful or swollen testicles<br>Women—Asymptomatic, painful or burning sensation when urinating, increased vaginal discharge, or vaginal bleeding between periods |
| Syphilis | *Treponema pallidum* | Primary—chancre<br>Secondary—rash, mild fever, fatigue, headache, sore throat, as well as patchy hair loss, swollen lymph nodes throughout the body, illness, blindness<br>Neurosyphilis—asymptomatic others may have headache, stiff neck, fever that result from an inflammation of the lining of the brain, seizures, stroke symptoms<br>Congenital syphilis—skin sores, rashes, fever, weakened or hoarse crying sounds, swollen liver and spleen, jaundice, anemia, various deformities |
| Chlamydia | *Chlamydia trachomatis* | May be asymptomatic<br>Women—abnormal vaginal discharge, burning sensation when urinating, lower abdominal pain, low back pain, nausea, fever, pain during intercourse, bleeding between menstrual periods<br>Men—penile discharge, burning sensation when urinating, burning and itching around the urethral orifice |
| Trichomoniasis | *Trichomonas vaginalis* | Men—most are asymptomatic some have urethritis, epididymitis, prostatitis<br>Women—frothy, yellow-green vaginal discharge with a fishy odor, pain during intercourse and urination, irritation and itching of the genital area |
| Genital herpes | Herpes simplex type I and II | Blisters |
| Human papillomavirus and genital warts | Human papillomavirus | Asymptomatic, genital warts |

| DIAGNOSIS | TREATMENT | PREVENTION/LIFESPAN |
| --- | --- | --- |
| Urine sample, bacterial culture, Gram stain | Antibiotics | Abstinence, monogamy, use of condoms and dental dams, regular pelvic exams |
| Microscopic visualization, antigen and antibody testing | Antibiotics | Abstinence, monogamy, use of condoms and dental dams, regular pelvic exams |
| Bacterial culture, antigen or antibody testing | Antibiotics | Abstinence, monogamy, use of condoms and dental dams, regular pelvic exams |
| Pelvic examination, microscopic visualization, culture, laboratory and pH test | Antiparasitic medication | Abstinence, monogamy, use of condoms and dental dams, regular pelvic exams |
| Physical exam and history, culture, antibody testing | Antiviral medication | Abstinence, monogamy, use of condoms and dental dams, regular pelvic exams |
| Warts—physical examination HPV—abnormal Pap tests, HPV DNA test | Warts—medication, electrocautery, cryosurgery, laser surgery | Abstinence, monogamy, use of condoms and dental dams, and regular pelvic exams, Gardasil |

| DISEASE OR DISORDER | ETIOLOGY | SIGNS AND SYMPTOMS |
|---|---|---|
| Menopause | Aging | Hot flashes, night sweats, trouble sleeping, mood swings, trouble focusing, hair loss or thinning, facial hair growth, vaginal dryness |
| Uterine prolapse | Pregnancy, childbirth, aging | Feelings of heaviness in pelvic area, urinary stress, incontinence, lower back pain |
| Cystocele | Pregnancy, childbirth, aging | Pelvic pressure, urinary urgency and frequency, incontinence |
| Rectocele | Pregnancy, childbirth, aging | Discomfort, constipation, fecal incontinence |
| Benign prostate hyperplasia | Aging, hormone imbalance | Need to get up during the night and urinate, need to empty the bladder often during the day, difficulty starting urine flow, dribbling after urination ends, and decrease in size and strength of the urine stream |
| Prostate cancer | Unknown | Dull pain in the lower pelvic area, urgency of urination, difficulty starting urination, pain during urination, wek urine flow and dribbling, intermittent urine flow, a sensation the bladder does not empty, frequent urination at night, blood in the urine, painful ejaculation, general pain in the lower back, hips and upper thighs, loss of appetite and weight, persistent bone pain |
| Erectile dysfunction | Age, psychological, cardiovascular disease, diabetes, obesity, lack of physical activity, surgical complications, urologic disorders, medications, premature ejaculation, drug abuse, alcoholism | Inability to achieve and maintain an erection sufficient for sexual intercourse |

| DIAGNOSIS | TREATMENT | PREVENTION/LIFESPAN |
|---|---|---|
| Signs and symptoms, elevated FSH, low estrogen | Hormone therapy | Occurs with aging |
| Pelvic examination, fluoroscopy | Kegel exercises, pessary in the vagina, surgery | Occurs with aging |
| Pelvic examination | Kegel exercises, pessary in the vagina, surgery | Occurs with aging |
| Pelvic examination | Surgery | Occurs with aging |
| DRE, urine analysis, PSA blood test, ultrasound, urine flow study, cystoscopy, x-ray | May not be needed, antibiotics, medications, destroying excess prostate tissue with microwaves or ultrasound, surgery | Occurs with aging |
| DRE, PSA blood test, biopsy | Watchful waiting, surgery, radiation, hormone therapy | Occurs with aging |
| Medical, sexual, and psychosocial history, physical examination, laboratory tests, ultrasound | Medication, lifestyle changes, therapy | Occurs with aging |

# Interactive Exercises

## Cases for Critical Thinking

1. A young woman reports severe pelvic pain. Laproscopic examination found endometrial tissue on the uterine wall and ovaries. Name this disease. What is the cause? What treatments are available?

2. A 16-year-old, sexually active woman complains of a green, frothy, fishy-smelling vaginal discharge. What is the possible diagnosis? What test would you perform? What treatment is available?

3. A 63-year-old male says he gets up several times a night to urinate but has difficulty getting urination started. A DRE reveals an enlarged prostate gland. What are the possible diagnoses? What tests would you perform? What treatment is available?

4. A woman has been infected with genital herpes type II. Describe how she can reduce the risk of transmission of the infection to her sexual partner.

5. Why do many physicians sometimes recommend watchful waiting for prostate cancer?

6. When baby Christopher was born, the pediatrician discovered that his left testicle had not descended into the scrotum. Name this disease. What complications may arise? What treatments are available?

## Multiple Choice

1. Which is the most common tumor among females?
   a. ovarian cysts
   b. breast cancer
   c. uterine fibroids
   d. cervical cancer

2. Syphilis is caused by _____.
   a. human papillomavirus
   b. herpes virus
   c. *Trichomonas vaginalis*
   d. *Treponema pallidum*

3. Which statement is FALSE about syphilis?
   a. Primary syphilis chancres heal after a few weeks.
   b. A fetus can be infected and born with major physical and mental abnormalities.
   c. Syphilis is only transmitted by sexual contact.
   d. Secondary syphilis is characterized by a nonitching rash.

4. Which disease can lead to pelvic inflammatory disease?
   a. chlamydia
   b. cystitis
   c. prostatitis
   d. herpes

5. Excessive or prolonged bleeding during menstruation is known as _____.
   a. dysmenorrhea
   b. amenorrhea
   c. metrorrhagia
   d. menorrhagia

6. Protrusion of the rectum into the posterior aspect of the vagina is known as _____.
   a. uterine prolapse
   b. cystocele
   c. rectocele
   d. sepsis

7. Painful or difficult menses is _____.
   a. amenorrhea
   b. dysmenorrhea
   c. menorrhea
   d. metrorrhagia

8. Failure of the testes to descend from the abdominal cavity is _____.
   a. orchitis
   b. prostatitis
   c. cryptorchidism
   d. epididymitis

9. Fingerlike projections at the outer ends of the fallopian tubes are known as _____.
   a. hymen
   b. fimbriae
   c. Graafian follicles
   d. Bartholin's glands

10. Laboratory diagnosis of pregnancy is based on the presence of what hormone?
    a. progesterone
    b. estrogen
    c. human chorionic gonadotropin hormone
    d. luteinizing hormone

## True or False

_____ 1. Pelvic inflammatory disease can lead to infertility.

_____ 2. The Pap test detects endometriosis.

_____ 3. The most important risk factor for cervical cancer is infection by the human papillomavirus.

_____ 4. Herpes simplex type II virus causes syphilis.

_____ 5. Benign prostatic hyperplasia affects more than 50% of men over age 60.

_____ 6. Benign breast conditions are common.

_____ 7. Preeclampsia is a disease that occurs during pregnancy.

_____ 8. The only certain means of diagnosing endometriosis is laparoscopy.

_____ 9. The most common site for ectopic pregnancy is the ovary.

_____ 10. The cause of PMS is known.

## Fill-Ins

1. The site of sperm development is the _____.

2. _____ is inflammation of the testes.

3. The most frequently reported bacterial STI in the United States is _____.

4. The _____ surrounds the upper portion of the male urethra.

5. _____ is inflammation of the prostate gland.

6. _____ is an STI caused by a protozoan.

7. The herpes type _____ virus usually causes cold sores; the herpes type _____ virus causes genital herpes.

8. _____ is downward displacement of the urinary bladder into the vagina.

9. _____ is the cessation of menstrual periods.

10. _____ is the inability to achieve and maintain an erection sufficient for sexual intercourse.

## Labeling Exercise

Use the blank lines below to label the following image.

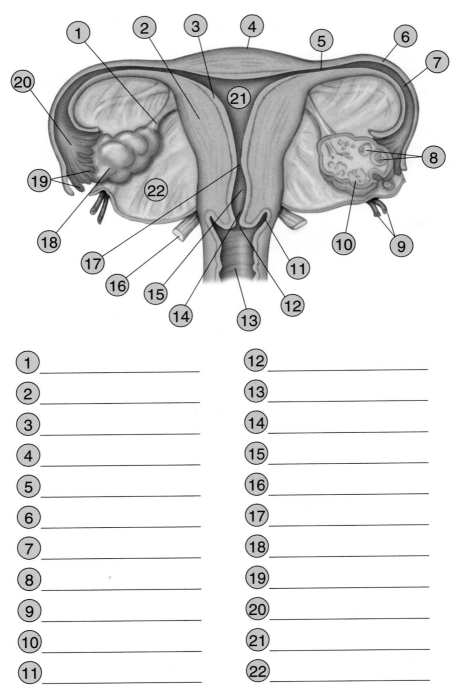

| | | | |
|---|---|---|---|
| 1 _____ | | 12 _____ | |
| 2 _____ | | 13 _____ | |
| 3 _____ | | 14 _____ | |
| 4 _____ | | 15 _____ | |
| 5 _____ | | 16 _____ | |
| 6 _____ | | 17 _____ | |
| 7 _____ | | 18 _____ | |
| 8 _____ | | 19 _____ | |
| 9 _____ | | 20 _____ | |
| 10 _____ | | 21 _____ | |
| 11 _____ | | 22 _____ | |

# Multimedia Preview

Additional interactive resources and activities for this chapter can be found on the Companion Website. For videos, audio glossary, and review, access the accompanying DVD-ROM in this book.

## ▶ DVD-ROM Highlights

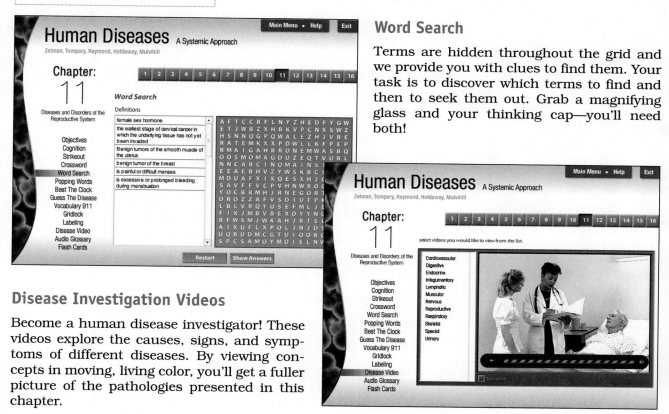

### Word Search

Terms are hidden throughout the grid and we provide you with clues to find them. Your task is to discover which terms to find and then to seek them out. Grab a magnifying glass and your thinking cap—you'll need both!

### Disease Investigation Videos

Become a human disease investigator! These videos explore the causes, signs, and symptoms of different diseases. By viewing concepts in moving, living color, you'll get a fuller picture of the pathologies presented in this chapter.

## ▶ Website Highlights—www.pearsonhighered.com/zelman

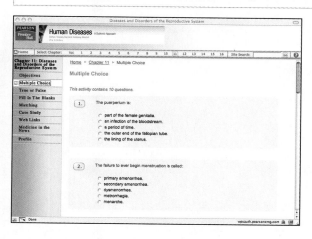

### Multiple Choice Quiz

Take advantage of the free-access online study guide that accompanies your textbook. You'll find a multiple-choice quiz that provides instant feedback and allows you to check your score to see what you got right or wrong. By clicking on this URL you'll also access links to current news articles and an audio glossary.

**CHAPTER**

# 12

# Diseases of the Endocrine System

## Learning Objectives

After studying this chapter, you should be able to

- Describe the functions of the endocrine glands
- Identify the hormones secreted from each endocrine gland and their normal functions
- Describe the consequences of hyposecretion and hypersecretion of endocrine hormones on various glands and organs
- Identify the endocrine functions of the pancreas
- Identify the etiology, signs and symptoms, diagnostic tests, and treatment for type 1 and type 2 diabetes
- Compare and contrast the consequences of type 1 and type 2 diabetes
- Describe the acute and chronic complications of diabetes
- Identify age-related changes in endocrine function

## Fact or Fiction?

The number of patients with type 2 diabetes is expected to increase dramatically and strain the healthcare system worldwide.

*Fact: The worldwide prevalence of DM has risen dramatically over the past two decades. The prevalence of type 2 DM is expected to rise more rapidly in the future because of increasing obesity and reduced activity levels. The number of diabetic patients will reach 300 million in 2025. More than 97% of these patients will have type 2 diabetes. The projected increase in the number of diabetic patients will strain the capabilities of healthcare providers worldwide. (International Diabetes Federation, 2001)*

# Disease Chronicle

## Diabetes

Ancient Hindu writings record distinctive signs of diabetes thousands of years ago: large volumes of urine, to which ants and flies were attracted; intense thirst; and a wasting of the body. No treatment or cure existed for this mysterious ailment, which killed children and whose complications crippled survivors. It was not until the late nineteenth century, when diabetes was observed in dogs whose pancreas had been removed experimentally, that the disease could be linked to a specific organ. The key component of the pancreas was eventually isolated and identified as the protein hormone insulin. Today, instead of treating patients with insulin extracted from dog pancreas, human insulin is synthesized using recombinant DNA technology. Early diagnosis, treatment, and effective management have lengthened and greatly improved the lives of diabetics. However, no cure for diabetes exists.

## ▶ Introduction

The endocrine system is responsible for the production, storage, and secretion of hormones, which are chemical messengers that regulate vital human functions. The major organs of the endocrine system include the pituitary, thyroid, and parathyroid glands; pancreatic islets; adrenal glands; and gonads (Figure 12–1 ▶). Endocrine glands communicate with other organs via complex networks involving the central and peripheral nervous system, hormones, **cytokines** (or regulators of immune response), and growth factors. Endocrine hormones affect many aspects of body functions, including growth, development, energy metabolism, muscle and fat distribution, sexual development, fluid and electrolyte balance, inflammation, and immune responses. Endocrine functions can be affected by anomalies in the primary gland responsible for producing a particular hormone, defects in circulating concentrations of stimulating hormones or releasing hormones, or anomalies in both the primary gland and the target or receiving organ. The result of endocrine abnormalities

**Figure 12–1** ▶ The endocrine glands.

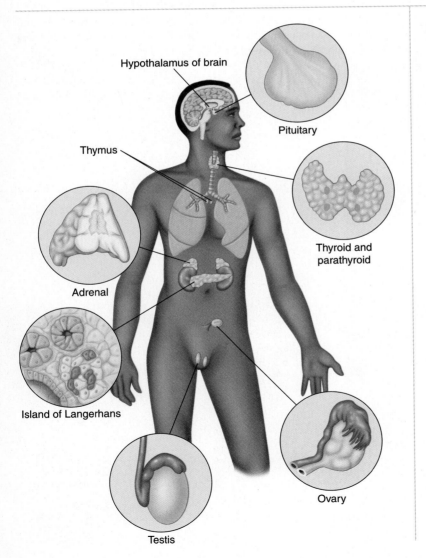

Hypothalamus of brain

Pituitary

Thymus

Thyroid and parathyroid

Adrenal

Island of Langerhans

Testis

Ovary

is either hypofunction or hyperfunction of a gland, hormone, or a target organ.

Impaired function of an endocrine gland can occur for a variety of reasons. Congenital defects can result in the absence of or impaired development of the endocrine gland or affect enzymes needed for hormone synthesis. The gland may be destroyed by **ischemia** or a disruption in blood flow, infection, inflammation, autoimmune diseases, or neoplastic growth. There may be a decline in function with age, or the gland may atrophy as the result of drug therapy or for unknown reasons. Some endocrine-deficient states are associated with receptor defect. Hormone receptors may be absent, receptor binding may be impaired, or cellular responsiveness to endocrine hormones may be impaired.

Hormones are released from endocrine glands into the bloodstream, where they affect activity in cells at distant sites. Some hormones affect the whole body, and others act only on target or distant organs. Most hormones are composed of proteins or chains of amino acids; others are steroids or fatty substances derived from cholesterol.

Most glandular activity is controlled by the pituitary, which is sometimes called the master gland. The pituitary itself is controlled by the hypothalamus.

The body is conservative and secretes hormones only as needed. For example, insulin is secreted when the blood sugar level rises. Another hormone, glucagon, works antagonistically to insulin and is released when the blood sugar level falls below normal. Hormones are potent chemicals, so their circulating levels must be carefully controlled. When the level of a hormone is adequate, its further release is stopped. This type of control is called a **negative-feedback** mechanism. Its importance becomes clearer as specific diseases of the endocrine system are considered.

Overactivity or underactivity of a gland is the malfunction that most commonly causes endocrine diseases. If a gland secretes an excessive amount of its hormone, it is hyperactive. This condition is sometimes caused by a hypertrophied gland or by a glandular tumor.

A gland that fails to secrete its hormone or secretes an inadequate amount is hypoactive. This condition may be caused by disease or tumor, or it may be caused by trauma, surgery, or radiation. A gland that has decreased in size and consequently is secreting inadequately is said to be atrophied. Each endocrine gland is discussed, with an emphasis on normal function and importance. The diseases caused by hypoactivity and hyperactivity of each gland are then explained.

## ▶ Structure and Function of the Pituitary Gland

The pituitary gland is a pea-sized organ located at the base of the brain. The gland has an anterior lobe called the **adenohypophysis** and a posterior lobe called the **neurohypophysis**. A stalk called the **infundibulum** connects the pituitary gland to the floor of the hypothalamus. The pituitary gland is regulated by the hypothalamus and feedback-control mechanisms in relation to blood concentrations of circulating hormones (Figure 12–2▶).

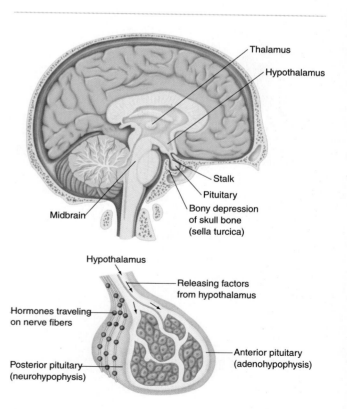

Figure 12–2 ▶ The pituitary gland.

The anterior pituitary produces six major hormones: prolactin, growth hormone, adrenocorticotropic hormone (ACTH), luteinizing hormone (LH), follicle stimulating hormone (FSH), and thyroid stimulating hormone. Each of these pituitary hormones elicits a response in target organs (Figure 12–3▶). The hormones of the posterior pituitary or neurohypophysis are produced in the hypothalamus. The neurohypophysis stores and releases two important hormones: antidiuretic hormone (ADH), also known as vasopressin, and oxytocin. Vasopressin stimulates the elevation of blood pressure by regulating the reabsorption of water in the kidney tubules. The target organ of oxytocin is the smooth muscle of the uterus, where it stimulates uterine contractions, and the mammary glands, where it stimulates milk letdown.

Table 12–1▶ lists the hormones of pituitary gland, target organs, and primary effects.

## ▶ Hormones of the Anterior Pituitary

### Growth Hormone

Growth hormone (GH; also called somatotropin) affects all parts of the body by promoting growth and development of the tissues. Before puberty, it stimulates the growth of long bones, increasing the child's height. Soft tissues—organs such as the liver, heart, and kidneys—also increase in size and develop under the influence of growth hormone. After adolescence, growth hormone is secreted in lesser amounts but continues to function in promoting tissue replacement and repair.

Growth hormone secretion is controlled by complex interactions between the hypothalamus and peripheral organs. Growth hormone releasing hormone is a hypothalamic hormone that stimulates growth hormone synthesis and release. Somatotropin release inhibiting factor (SRIF) is also synthesized in the hypothalamus and inhibits growth hormone secretion. Peripheral hormones that regulate growth hormone include insulin-like growth factors, glucocorticoids, and estrogen. Insulin-like growth factors and glucocoridoids feed back to the hypothalamus to inhibit growth hormone, whereas estrogen induces growth hormone release.

### Thyroid Stimulating Hormone

The thyroid gland regulates metabolism, the rate at which the body produces and uses energy. The anterior pituitary controls secretion of thyroid hormone by the thyroid gland. The pituitary hormone that stimulates the thyroid gland is thyroid stimulating hormone (TSH; also called thyrotropin). In the absence of TSH, the thyroid gland stops functioning.

### Adrenocorticotropic Hormone

The anterior pituitary also regulates the adrenal glands. The adrenal glands have an inner part, the adrenal medulla, and an outer portion, the

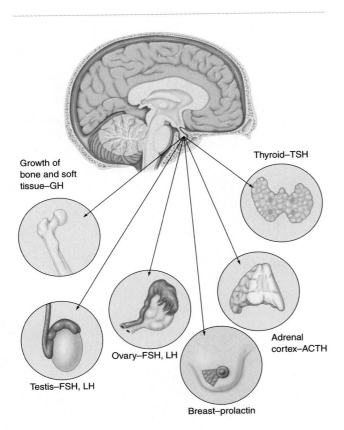

**Figure 12–3** ▶ Anterior pituitary and its target organs.

| Table 12–1 ▶ | Hormones of Pituitary Gland, Target Organs, and Primary Effects | |
| --- | --- | --- |
| **Hormone** | **Target Organ** | **Physiological Effects** |
| **Anterior Lobe** | | |
| Follicle stimulating hormone (FSH) | Ovary | In females: stimulates the growth of graffian follicles of the ovary and secretion of estradiol |
| | Testes | In males: stimulates the epithelium of the seminiferous tubules and subsequent spermatogenesis |
| Leutinizing hormone (LH) | Corpus luteum | In females: stimulates the production of the corpus luteum from the follicle; stimulates production of progesterone by the ovaries |
| | Interstitial cells of the testes | In males: stimulates production of testosterone |
| Prolactin | Female mammary gland | Stimulates milk production after birth |
| Growth hormone (somatotropin) | All body tissues | Increases the synthesis of protein and promotes the growth of bone and tissues |
| Adrenocorticotropic hormone (ACTH) | Adrenal cortex, skin, liver, and mammary gland | Stimulates the production of corticosteriods; increases metabolism and glycogen storage in the liver; responsible for darkening of the skin and nails |
| Thyroid stimulating hormone | Thyroid gland | Stimulates the production of the thyroid hormone |
| **Posterior Lobe** | | |
| Vasopressin or antidiuretic hormone (ADH) | Smooth muscle of the arterioles and the kidney tubules | Constricts blood vessels, increases blood pressure; stimulates reabsorption of water by the kidney |
| Oxytocin | Uterus and the mammary glands | Stimulates contration of the uterus; secrtion of milk or "milk letdown" by the mammary glands |

adrenal cortex. The cortex is controlled by the anterior pituitary. The adrenal cortex is stimulated by the anterior pituitary hormone, **adrenocorticotropic hormone (ACTH)**.

## Gonadotropins

The anterior pituitary regulates sexual development and function by means of hormones known as the **gonadotropins**. These are not sex hormones, but they affect the sex organs, the gonads. They are follicle stimulating hormone (FSH), luteinizing hormone (LH), and prolactin.

These gonadotropins regulate the menstrual cycle and secretion of male and female hormones.

## ▶ Diagnostic Procedures for Endocrine Diseases

Indications of pituitary hyperactivity or hypoactivity can be confirmed by serum assays. Growth hormone (GH) levels can detect hyperpituitarism (gigantism and/or acromegaly) and hypopituitarism (dwarfism). Thyroid stimulating hormone (TSH) assay is useful in confirming primary hypothyroidism or hyperthyroidism. Activity of the posterior pituitary can be evaluated by the water deprivation and vasopressin test. A urine specimen is taken after controlled water deprivation, and a blood sample is drawn. Dilute urine and high osmotic pressure in the blood indicate that water is not being absorbed by the kidney tubules. If vasopressin injection corrects the massive polyuria, diabetes insipidus is confirmed.

Diseases of the thyroid gland are diagnosed on the basis of the levels of the serum thyroid hormones, **tri-iodothyronine (T₃)** and **thyroxine (T₄)** and by the serum level of TSH. An elevated TSH indicates low $T_4$ function. A low TSH indicates an excess of $T_4$ caused by a functioning adenoma or carcinoma. A thyroid scan provides visualization of the thyroid gland after administration of radioactive iodine. It is usually recommended after discovery of a mass, an enlarged gland, or an asymmetric goiter. Thyroid ultrasonography evaluates characteristics of thyroid nodules and distinguishes between solid or cystic masses in the gland.

Diagnostic tests for parathyroid gland activity measure parathyroid hormone and calcium levels in the blood and can detect hyperparathyroidism.

Adrenal gland activity can be evaluated by the level of plasma cortisol from the adrenal cortex. Abnormal levels indicate hypersecretion (Cushing's syndrome) or hyposecretion (Addison's disease). Urine tests measure steroid level and detect hyperactivity of the gland.

A fasting blood glucose test helps detect diabetes mellitus and evaluate the clinical status of diabetic patients. An oral glucose tolerance test challenges the ability of the pancreas to secrete insulin in response to large doses of glucose. A glycated hemoglobin test, also called "hemoglobin A1c," is an important blood test that is used to determine how well diabetes is controlled. The test provides an average of blood glucose measurements over a 6- to 12-week period and is used in conjunction with a patient's home blood glucose monitoring devices.

## ▶ Diseases of the Anterior Pituitary

### Anterior Pituitary Insufficiency

Inherited disorders, malignant tumors, inadequate secretion of hormones, inflammation, and vascular changes of the pituitary gland can result in hypofunction or insufficiency of the pituitary gland. The manifestations of hypopituitarsim depend on which hormones are lost and the extent of the hormone deficiency. Growth hormone deficiency causes growth disorders in children and leads to abnormal body composition in adults. FSH and LH deficiency causes menstrual disorders, infertility, and decreased sexual function in women, and loss of secondary sexual characteristics in males. TSH deficiency causes growth retardation in children and features of hypothyroidism in both adults and children. ACTH deficiency leads to decreased production adrenal cortical hormones.

### Pituitary Dwarfism

Pituitary dwarfism results from a growth hormone deficiency. Growth retardation may become evident in infancy and persists throughout childhood. The child's growth curve, which is usually plotted on a standardized growth chart, may range from flat, indicating no growth, to shallow, indicating minimal growth. Normal puberty may or may not occur, depending on the degree to which the pituitary gland can produce sufficient hormone levels other than growth hormone.

There are approximately 7000 to 10,000 cases of pituitary dwarfism in the United States. Many cases are due to a tumor known as a craniopharyngioma. A rare form of this disease may be caused by an inherited autosomal recessive gene. Similar to pituitary insufficiency, pituitary dwarfism may also be associated with deficiencies in all pituitary hormones.

Symptoms of this disorder include slowed growth before the age of 5 years, absent or delayed sexual development, and short stature and height for age. Confirmation of the diagnosis is made by evaluation of blood pituitary hormone levels. Hand x-rays help determine bone age, and cranial x-rays are useful for identifying any abnormalities of the skull that may contribute to this condition. MRI scans provide detailed images of the pituitary and the hypothalamus.

Replacement therapy with injections of growth hormone is currently used to treat children with pituitary dwarfism who have isolated growth hormone deficiency. In cases of pituitary insufficiency, other associated hormone deficits should be corrected, especially glucocorticoids, thyroid hormone, and sex steroids. Treatment regimens that mimic physiologic hormone production allow for maintenance of satisfactory growth and metabolic homeostasis.

## Adult Growth Hormone Deficiency

**Adult growth hormone deficiency (AGHD)** is a rare condition that is usually caused by damage to the pituitary gland or the hypothalamus. Adults at risk for AGHD are those with a history of pituitary surgery, a previous tumor of the pituitary or hypothalamus, history of radiation to the head, and previously documented growth hormone deficiency in childhood.

Clinical features of AGHD include changes to body composition such as increased body fat, reduced exercise capacity, impaired heart function, reduced muscle mass, abnormal lipid profile, and atherosclerosis. Patients usually experience decreased energy and drive and a decreased ability to concentrate.

Radiographic imaging studies are used to diagnose masses or structural damage to the pituitary gland. Blood serum hormone concentrations of growth hormones are suppressed, and concomitant gonadotropin, thyroid hormone, and ACTH deficits may be present.

Replacement of growth hormone in AGHD is associated with body composition changes such as increased muscle mass and lower body fat. Women generally require higher doses of synthetic growth hormone than men.

## Hyperpituitarism

***Gigantism*** Gigantism is a rare condition of growth hormone excess that occurs during childhood. Prior to closure of the epiphyseal growth plate, excess growth hormone stimulates excessive linear growth. The most common cause of this disorder is a benign tumor of the pituitary gland.

The appearance of gigantism is usually dramatic, as all growth parameters are affected and accelerated linear growth occurs. Facial features may thicken, and the hands and feet may be disproportionately large.

Treatment of gigantism depends on the etiology of growth hormone excess. In cases of well-defined tumors, surgical resection may be curative. Radiation therapy may be used in conjunction with surgery or in cases where surgery is not possible. Medications that reduce growth hormone secretion are also used for cases where surgery is not possible.

***Acromegaly*** Acromegaly is a condition that results from excess growth hormone secretion after growth plate fusion has occurred. Worldwide, acromegaly occurs at a rate of 2.4 to 4 cases per one million. The mean age at the time of diagnosis is between 40 and 45 years.

The most common cause of acromegaly is a pituitary tumor. Other etiologies are excess release of growth hormone releasing hormone caused by hypothalamic tumors, or excess growth hormone releasing hormone secretion by nonendocrine malignant tumors.

Acromegaly has an insidious onset, and symptoms are usually present for a number of years before a diagnosis is made. The disease is characterized by weight gain, growth of the soft tissues, and enlargement of the small bones of the hands, feet, face, and skull. Prominent facial features include development of a bulbous nose, a protruding jaw, and slanted forehead, and changes in bite with difficulty chewing. Bony changes to the spine lead to **kyphosis**, or hunchback. Bone overgrowth eventually results in degenerative arthritis to the hip, knees, and spine.

The metabolic effects of acromegaly are numerous and life threatening. Excess growth hormone stimulates release of free fatty acid from fat tissue. Glucose intolerance and diabetes mellitus ensues, with changes in carbohydrate metabolism.

The treatment for acromegaly focuses on correcting metabolic abnormalities, improving adverse clinical features, and correcting the underlying cause. Surgical resection of tumors of the pituitary or hypothalamus is the treatment of choice. Medications that decrease growth hormone secretion may be administered prior to surgery or in cases where surgery is not possible to shrink the tumor. Radiation is also used to shrink the tumor and is used when medication therapy fails and in cases where surgery is not an option.

## ▶ Hypofunction of the Posterior Pituitary

### Diabetes Insipidus

Decreased secretion or action of ADH results in the syndrome of diabetes insipidus. The leading symptom of diabetes insipidus is the production of abnormally large amounts of urine, or **polyuria.** The polyuria produces symptoms of urinary frequency, disturbed sleep due to bed-wetting, and daytime fatigue. Excessive urination is accompanied by extreme thirst and a corresponding increase in fluid intake, or **polydipsia.**

The most common cause of diabetes insipidus is destruction of the neurohypophysis due to unknown causes. Diabetes insipidus can also occur when ADH levels are normal. This condition, nephrogenic diabetes insipidus, involves a defect in the kidney tubule that interferes with the reabsorption of water. The kidney fails to concentrate urine in response to the instructions of ADH. Figure 12–4▶ illustrates the normal action of the antidiuretic hormone; Figure 12–5▶ illustrates the effects of ADH deficiency.

The diagnosis of diabetes insipidus is based on the patient's history, physical examination, and results of urine tests. An MRI of the pituitary gland or the hypothalamus assists in identifying the etiological basis of the diabetes insipidus.

Treatment of diabetes insipidus is aimed at removing the primary cause and treating the symptoms to prevent dehydration. Central dia-

**Figure 12–4** ▶ Normal action of antidiuretic hormone.

**Hypothalamus**

**Sensors of osmotic pressure (blood concentration)**

**No ADH and no reabsorption of water from distal convoluted tubules or collecting ducts**

**Blood**

**Diseased or nonfunctioning posterior pituitary**

**Distal convoluted tubule**

$H_2O$

**Collecting duct**

$Na^+$
$Na^+$
$Na^+$

$Na^+$
$Na^+$

**Copious volume of dilute urine**

Figure 12–5 ► Effect of antidiuretic hormone deficiency.

betes insipidus may be controlled with vaso-pressin. Vasopressin is administered as either a nasal spray or tablets. Vasopressin is ineffective for nephrogenic diabetes insipidus. Treatment of nephrogenic diabetes insipidus requires compensatory fluid intake with effort to correct the underlying etiology.

## ► Structure and Function of the Thyroid Gland

The activity of the thyroid gland affects the whole body. It regulates the metabolic rate, the rate at which calories are used. The thyroid gland, through its hormone **thyroxine**, governs cellular oxygen consumption and thus energy and heat production. The more oxygen that is used, the more calories are metabolized ("burned up"). Thyroxine assures that enough body heat is produced to maintain normal temperature even in a cold environment.

## Structure of the Thyroid Gland

The thyroid gland is located in the neck region, one lobe on either side of the trachea. A connecting strip, or isthmus, anterior to the trachea connects the two lobes. The thyroid gland lies just below the Adam's apple, the protrusion formed by part of the larynx (Figure 12–6 ►). Internally, the thyroid gland consists of follicles, or microscopic sacs. Within these protein-containing follicles, the thyroid hormones thyroxin and tri-iodothyronine are stored. Thin-walled capillaries run between the follicles in a position ideal for receiving the thyroid hormones.

## Function of the Thyroid Gland

The thyroid gland synthesizes, stores, and releases thyroid hormones, which contain iodine. Most of the iodide ions of the body are taken into the thyroid gland by a mechanism called the iodide trap. Iodine combines with an amino acid, and the thyroid hormones are formed.

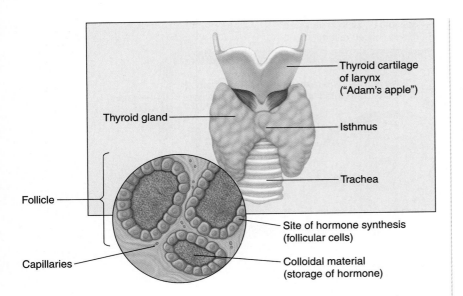

**Figure 12–6** ► The thyroid gland.

The hormones are stored in the thyroid gland until needed and then released into the blood capillaries. Tests to determine the activity of the thyroid gland are based on tri-iodothyronine ($T_3$) and thyroxine ($T_4$) levels in the plasma. In the $T_3$ and $T_4$ tests, a sample of the patient's serum is incubated with radioactive thyroid hormones and resin. The resin absorbs the hormones that are not bound to the blood proteins. Radioactivity counts of the serum and resin are made, and the percentage of thyroid hormones absorbed by the resin is calculated. A low percentage of absorption indicates a poorly functioning thyroid gland. A high percentage of absorption indicates hyperactivity. In the latter case, the patient's own thyroid hormones have saturated the plasma proteins, and the excess radioactive hormones are absorbed by the resin.

## Effects of Thyroid Hormones

Although there is more than one thyroid hormone, for clarity the thyroid hormones are referred to here as thyroxine, or $T_4$, the hormone that is secreted in the largest quantity. Thyroxine stimulates cellular metabolism by increasing the rate of oxygen use with subsequent energy and heat production.

Secretion of thyroxine leads to a compensatory increase in cardiac output. Faster cellular metabolism increases the cell's demand for oxygen, so more oxygen must be circulated to the cells. Nutrients are converted to energy in the presence of oxygen, and the waste products of metabolism, including carbon dioxide, are formed. These must be carried away from the cells. The circulatory system can meet these needs by increasing blood flow to the cells. Increased blood flow is obtained by greater cardiac output, or more heart activity.

As cellular metabolism increases, respiration increases. The greater need for oxygen and a corresponding accumulation of carbon dioxide stimulate the respiratory center of the brain. Stimulation of the respiratory center results in a faster rate and greater depth of breathing.

Thyroxine increases body temperature. Heat is produced through cellular metabolism, and thyroxine stimulates this process. In a cold environment, thyroxine secretion increases to assure adequate body heat. If excessive body heat is produced, it is dissipated in two ways. Blood vessels of the skin dilate, increasing blood flow at the body surface and giving the body a flushed appearance. As the blood flows through the skin's blood vessels, excess heat escapes. The body is also cooled by the perspiration mechanism. Body temperature is controlled by a regulatory center in the brain.

Thyroxine also has a stimulatory effect on the gastrointestinal system. It increases the secretion of digestive juices and the movement of material through the digestive tract. Absorption of carbohydrates from the intestine is also increased under the influence of thyroxine, assuring adequate fuel for cellular metabolism. The effects of thyroxin are illustrated in Figure 12–7 ▶. Many symptoms of thyroid diseases can be related to the effects of inadequate or excessive thyroxine secretion.

## Control of Circulating Thyroxine Level

The anterior pituitary gland stimulates the thyroid by releasing TSH. The thyroid, in turn, releases thyroxine, which circulates in the blood to all cells and tissues. When the level of circulating thyroxine is high, the anterior pituitary is inhibited and stops releasing TSH. This is an example of a negative-feedback mechanism. An adequate level of thyroxine prevents further synthesis of the hormone. When the level of thyroxine falls, the anterior pituitary is released from the inhibition and once again sends out TSH. This feedback mechanism is shown in Figure 12–8 ▶.

At times, this control mechanism fails, constituting one basis for a thyroid disease. The

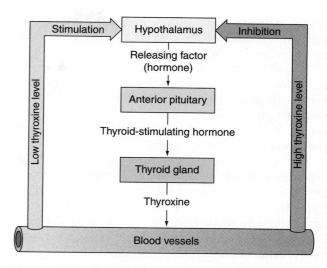

Figure 12–8 ▶ Control of thyroxine secretion through negative feedback.

thyroid gland also functions abnormally if the body's iodine supply is inadequate, if the gland is overstimulated or understimulated by the anterior pituitary, or if the thyroid gland itself becomes diseased. Some of these conditions are discussed in the following section.

## ▶ Diseases of the Thyroid Gland

### Hypothyroidism

Hypothyroid, or thyroid hormone deficiency, may affect almost all body functions. The severity of hypothyroidism ranges from mild and unrecognized symptoms to striking symptoms such as mental status changes, extreme and prolonged fatigue, weight gain, swelling or complaints of cold in the hands and feet, menstrual irregularities, muscle aches, and hair thinning.

The etiology of hypothyroid disease may be due to a primary disease in the thyroid gland or a lack of pituitary TSH. Primary hypothyroidism is the most common form of this condition and is generally caused by autoimmune disease, use of radioactive iodine, destruction or removal of the thyroid gland, dietary iodide deficiency, overtreatment with thyroid medications, and medical treatment for bipolar disorder with the

Figure 12–7 ▶ Effects of thyroxine.

drug lithium. Secondary hypothyroidism is caused by inadequate secretion of TSH caused by a disease of the pituitary gland.

Hypothyroid disease occurs more frequently in women. The average annual rate of autoimmune hypothyroidism is up to 4 per 1000 women, and 1 per 1000 men. The average age at onset of hypothyroid is around 60 years, and the prevalence continues to increase with age.

The most severe form of hypothyroidism is **myxedema coma. Myxedema** is a medical emergency with a high mortality rate. It is caused by hypothyroidism, but is usually precipitated by an acute illness or trauma. Physical signs may include severe hypotension, unresponsiveness, **bradycardia** (slow heart rate), shallow and slow breathing, convulsions, extremely low body temperature, and decreased oxygen delivery to vital organs such as the brain.

Thyroid hormone replacement therapy is often required for the duration of the patient's life. Regular blood tests to measure circulating levels of thyroxine are required to regulate the dose of thyroid replacement medication. Treatment of myxedema requires hospitalization and intensive administration of intravenous fluids, intravenous administration of thyroid hormone, warming, mechanical ventilation, and cardiac support.

## Congenital Hypothyroidism

Hypothyroid of the newborn, also known as cretinism, is most often the result of **hypoplasia** (underdevelopment), **aplasia** (absence), and failure of the thyroid gland to migrate to its normal anatomical position. Maternal factors such as excessive iodine intake and ingestion of antithyroid medications during pregnancy can cause hypothyroidism in both the mother and the fetus.

Most newborns with congenital hypothyroidism generally appear normal at birth and gain weight normally for the first three to four months of life. Symptoms that follow include physical and mental sluggishness, constipation, poor muscle tone, umbilical hernia and a protruding abdomen, hypothermia, bradycardia, and growth retardation. Physical growth retardation includes short stature, preservation of infantile facial features, and delayed dental eruption. Severe impairment of intellectual development with retardation of brain development is a severe consequence of untreated congenital hypothyroidism.

Congenital hypothyroidism is diagnosed by neonatal screening techniques usually within the first 10 days of birth. Adequate treatment with thyroid hormone supplementation started as soon as possible improves the prognosis of intellectual development and function later in life.

## Hyperthyroidism

Hyperthyroidism is a hypermetabolic condition of thyroid hormone excess. The symptoms of hyperthyroid range from mild increases in metabolic rate to severe hyperactivity. The term **thyrotoxicosis** refers to the clinical manifestations and etiologies associated with excess systemic thyroid hormone.

**Graves' disease** is the most common etiology of thyrotoxicosis. It is an autoimmune disease that is more common in women than in men. The onset of Graves' disease is between the ages of 20 and 40 years, and it is often associated with other autoimmune diseases, such as diabetes mellitus. Thyrotoxicosis is also caused by high levels of hormones secreted during pregnancy, pituitary tumors with excess secretion of TSH, and ingestion of excessive amounts of thyroid hormone medication.

Symptoms of thyrotoxicosis include nervousness, restlessness, heat intolerance, increased sweating, fatigue, weakness, muscle cramps, and weight loss. Women frequently report menstrual irregularities. Cardiac manifestations of thyrotoxicosis include a rapid pounding heart beat, cardiac arrhythmias, and heart failure, especially in older individuals with long-standing mild hyperthyroidism.

Treatment of hyperthyroid disease depends on the severity, etiology, and presence of complications. The goal of treatment is to bring the metabolic rate to normal with minimal complications. Medications, radioactive iodine, and surgery are used to treat hyperthyroidism. Drugs that inhibit the formation of thyroid hormone are administered until thyroid function returns to normal. If thyroid levels cannot be maintained, radiation or surgery may be performed. Medications that control heart rate and blood pressure are administered to prevent complications of thyrotoxicosis.

## Thyroiditis

**Thyroiditis**, or swelling of the thyroid gland, is associated with viral or bacterial infections, autoimmune disease, and aging. **Subacute thyroiditis** affects younger females and is usually associated with a viral infection. **Hashimoto's thyroiditis** is an autoimmune disease characterized by infiltration of leukocyte and progressive destruction of the thyroid gland.

Subacute thyroiditis commonly occurs in younger women and may or may not be associated with hyperthyroidism. Symptoms of pain, swelling, and thyroid tenderness last weeks or months and then disappear. Symptomatic management includes the use of anti-inflammatory and pain medications, observation, and treatment for severe symptoms of hyperthyroid.

Hashimoto's thyroiditis, or a firm enlargement or **goiter** of the thyroid gland, most often occurs in women around 40 to 50 years of age (Figure 12–9▶). The goiter is painless, although local symptoms may develop due to compression of the esophagus, trachea, neck veins, or laryngeal nerves. The goiter disrupts the function of the thyroid gland. Treatment of

**Figure 12–9** ▶ Thyroid goiter. (Newscom)

Hashimoto's thyroiditis is directed toward relief of compression symptoms by surgical removal of the goiter. Thyroid hormone supplementation is used if hypothyroid develops.

## ▶ Structure and Function of the Adrenal Glands

The adrenal glands are located on top of each kidney. Each of the glands consists of two distinct parts: an outer part (the adrenal cortex) and an inner section (the adrenal medulla). The cortex and medulla secrete different hormones. The adrenal cortex is stimulated by ACTH from the anterior pituitary gland. The adrenal glands are shown in Figure 12–10▶.

The adrenal cortex secretes many steroid hormones, which can be classified into three groups. One group, the **mineralocorticoids**, regulates salt balance. The principal hormone of this group is aldosterone. **Aldosterone** causes sodium retention and potassium secretion by the kidneys. Another group, the **glucocorticoids**, helps regulate carbohydrate, lipid, and protein metabolism. The principal hormone of this group is **cortisol** or **hydrocortisone**. The third group of hormones is sex hormones: **androgens**, the male hormones, and **estrogens**, the female hormones.

The adrenal medulla secretes **epinephrine** and **norepinephrine**. These hormones are secreted in stress situations when additional energy and strength are needed. Epinephrine causes vasodilatation and increases heart rate, blood pressure, and respiration. Norepinephrine brings about general vasoconstriction. Together, epinephrine and norepinephrine help shunt blood to vital organs when required.

Hyperactivity of the adrenal cortex is usually caused by hyperplasia (enlargement of the glands), a tumor. Hyperactivity may also result from overstimulation by the anterior pituitary gland.

Hypoactivity of the adrenal cortex sometimes results from a destructive disease, such as tuberculosis. Some steroid hormones can cause the adrenal glands to atrophy by interfering with the normal control mechanism for corticosteroid release.

**Figure 12–10** ► The adrenal glands.

## ► Diseases of the Adrenal Cortex

### Hypoadrenalism

**Primary adrenal insufficiency,** or **Addison's disease,** was first described in 1855 when Thomas Addison described symptoms associated with destruction of the adrenal glands. Addison's disease can result from any disease process that damages the entire adrenal cortex; however, approximately 75% to 80% of all cases are due to an autoimmune process. Other common causes of adrenal insufficiency include infectious diseases such as tuberculosis, fungal disease, opportunistic infections associated with AIDS, certain cancers, and hemorrhage of the

adrenal gland secondary to anticoagulation medication.

The prevalence of Addison's disease is rare, occurring in approximately 1 in every 1000 people in the United States. It is more common in females, with a female to male ration of 2 : 1, and is usually diagnosed in the third to fifth decades of life.

The lack of cortisol, aldosterone, and adrenal androgens contribute to the symptoms of Addison's disease. Weight loss, fatigue, and anorexia occur with a deficiency in cortisol. The most distinctive sign is hyperpigmentation found in non-sun-exposed areas of the body such as the gingival and in the creases of the palms of the hands. Gastrointestinal symptoms include anorexia or loss of appetite, abdominal discomfort, vomiting, and diarrhea. Fluid loss from these symptoms may contribute to low blood pressure or hypotension. Hypotension is often associated with dizziness, lack of blood sodium, and **syncope**, or fainting.

Diagnostic tests for Addison's disease include a 24-hour urine test for cortisol or blood tests for serum cortisol level. An ACTH stimulation test measures adrenal gland response to an intravenous dose of ACTH. An abnormal response to ACTH stimulation establishes adrenal insufficiency.

Addison's disease can result in a life-threatening condition known as acute adrenal insufficiency. It may occur in patients with chronic adrenal insufficiency in the setting of another acute illness such as infections, trauma, or severe physical stress such as surgery. Symptoms develop rapidly and include nausea, vomiting, abdominal pain, and severe hypotension. Death can result from shock and cardiovascular collapse. Immediate rehydration with salt solution along with intravenous glucocoricoid replacement are essential to prevent death.

The treatment of chronic adrenal insufficiency includes life-long replacement of both glucorticoids and mineralocorticoids. During stress, patients may require additional medica-tion as these patients are not able to increase endogenous cortisol production.

## Hyperadrenalism

Hyperadrenalism, or Cushing's syndrome, refers to the manifestations of excessive corticosteroids. The prevalence of Cushing's syndrome is approximately 1 in every 500,000 people in the United States. The etiology of Cushing's syndrome is most often due to benign pituitary adenomas causing hypersecretion of ACTH with excess stimulation of the adrenal glands. Other causes include nonpituitary neoplasm, such as small cell lung carcinoma that produce excessive amounts of ACTH, and adrenal tumors that cause excessive secretion of cortisol.

Excess cortisol secretion results in a number of metabolic abnormalities, including hyperglycemia, hyperlipidemia, fluid retention, weight gain, weakness, fatigue, and hypertension. Clinical signs of cortisol excess include central obesity, "moon face," fat accumulation behind the shoulders (also known as a buffalo hump), impaired wound healing, loss of elastic tissues, thinning of the skin, and emotional distress, including depression and psychosis (Figure 12–11 ▶). Untreated Cushing's syndrome

**A**          **B**

**Figure 12–11** ▶ A patient with Cushing's syndrome (A) before and (B) after receiving treatment. (Sharmyn McGraw)

can produce serious morbidity and even death. The patient may suffer from complications of hypertension or diabetes or from susceptibility to infections.

Laboratory test for Cushing's syndrome include blood tests for diabetes, electrolyte abnormalities, and signs of infection. Urine tests provide evidence for diabetes and excess cortisol. Radiographic tests, including MRI and CT scans, provide evidence for pituitary tumors or other tumors in the chest or abdomen that may be the source of excess ACTH.

The goal of treatment for Cushing's syndrome is to correct hypersecretion of adrenal hormones. Removal of pituitary tumors is accomplished through microsurgery or radiation therapy. Medications are administered to treat symptoms of diabetes, hypertension, hyperlipidemia, psychosis, and depression. Medications that block the synthesis of corticosteroids are useful in patients for whom surgery is not appropriate.

## ▶ Diseases of the Adrenal Medulla

### Pheochromocytoma

Pheochromocytoma is a rare epinephrine- and norepinephrine-producing tumor that occurs equally in men and women in the fourth and fifth decades of life. Most pheochromocytomas (85% to 90%) are located in the adrenal medulla.

Excess release of epinephrine and norepinephrine is responsible for the signs and symptoms of this disease. The most common clinical sign is hypertension. Headache, excessive sweating, and palpitations are the most common symptoms. Some patients may also suffer from anxiety, constipation, low energy level, and exhaustion.

Pheochromocytomas are diagnosed by biochemical evidence in both blood and urine of overproduction of epinephrine and norepinephrine. Imaging studies such as CT or MRI scan are essential for detection and localization of this tumor.

Surgery provides an effective cure by removing the tumor. Medication therapy is used to stabilize blood pressure and to treat associated symptoms. Often various combinations of medications are necessary to stabilize the patient's blood pressure.

## ▶ Structure and Function of the Parathyroids

### Structure of the Parathyroids

The parathyroids are four tiny glands located on the posterior side of the thyroid gland. Before the function of the parathyroid glands was understood, they were sometimes removed with a thyroidectomy. The hormone secreted by the parathyroids is **parathormone**, also called parathyroid hormone (Figure 12–12▶).

### Function of the Parathyroids

The parathyroid glands are extremely important in regulating the level of circulating calcium and phosphate. Ninety-nine percent of the body's calcium is in bone, but the remaining 1% has many important functions. Calcium is essential to the blood-clotting mechanism. It increases the tone of heart muscle and plays a significant role in muscle contraction.

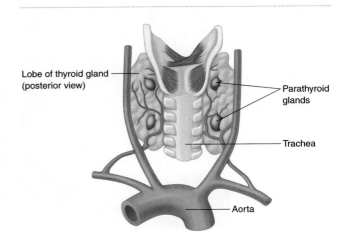

Lobe of thyroid gland (posterior view)

Parathyroid glands

Trachea

Aorta

**Figure 12–12** ▶ Parathyroid glands.

There is a constant exchange of calcium and phosphate between bone and the blood. Two kinds of cells are at work within bone: **osteoblasts**, which form bone tissue, and **osteoclasts**, which resorb salts out of bone, dissolving them. These salts are then released into the blood. The balance between these two processes, osteoblastic and osteoclastic, is governed by the parathyroid hormone.

When the blood calcium level falls, parathormone is secreted. The hormone acts at three distinct sites to raise the blood level of calcium to normal. Parathormone increases the amount of calcium that is absorbed out of the digestive tract by interaction with ingested vitamin D. It prevents a loss of calcium through the kidneys and releases calcium from bones by stimulating osteoclastic activity. When the proper level of circulating calcium is restored, parathormone is no longer released. An excess or a deficiency of calcium can have disastrous results. These conditions are usually the result of hyperactivity or hypoactivity of the parathyroid glands.

## ▶ Diseases of the Parathyroid Gland

### Hyperparathyroidism

Hyperparathyroidism, or excessive secretion of parathyroid hormone, is often caused by benign parathyroid tumors. The size of the tumor often correlates with the amount of parathyroid hormone secreted into the blood. Hyperparathyroidism occurs most frequently in persons over the age of 50 years and is more common in women than in men.

Excessive parathormone raises the level of circulating calcium above normal, a condition called **hypercalcemia**. Much of the calcium comes from bone resorption mediated by parathormone. As the calcium level rises, the phosphate level falls.

With the loss of calcium, the bones are weakened. They tend to bend, become deformed, and fracture spontaneously. Giant cell tumors and cysts of the bone sometimes develop. Excessive

calcium causes formation of kidney stones because calcium forms insoluble compounds. Calcium deposited within the walls of the blood vessels makes them hard. Calcium may also be found in the stomach and lungs.

Hyperparathyroidism, with its concurrent excess of calcium, causes generalized symptoms. There may be pain in the bones that is sometimes confused with arthritis. The nervous system is depressed, and muscles lose their tone and weaken. Heart muscle is affected, and the pulse slows. Symptoms include gastrointestinal disturbances, abdominal pain, vomiting, and constipation. These symptoms result from deposits of calcium in the mucosa of the gastrointestinal tract. Deposits of calcium sometimes form in the eye, causing irritation and excessive tearing. Hyperparathyroidism usually results from a tumor. If the tumor is removed, parathormone secretion returns to normal, and the level of circulating calcium is again properly controlled. See Box 12–1 ▶ for complications of hyperparathyroidism.

The most common laboratory findings in patients with hyperparathyroidism are elevated levels of blood serum calcium and excessive loss of phosphate in the urine. Imaging studies are used to locate the parathyroid tumor(s) and to guide surgical resection.

Medical treatment of hyperparathyroidism is aimed at lowering serum calcium level. This is accomplished through medication and intravenous hydration therapy. Medications called biphosphanates are potent inhibitors of bone resorption and can temporarily treat the hypercalcemia. Surgical resection is recommended for patients with severe chronic and recurrent symptoms.

### Box 12–1 ▶ Complications of Hyperparathyroidism: Hypercalcemia

- Kidney stone formation
- Calcification of blood vessel walls
- Calcification of organ walls
- Spontaneous fractures

## Hypoparathyroidism

Hypoparathyroidism is mostly a transient condition that commonly occurs in patients following surgical resection of the thyroid gland. Parathyroid deficiency can also be the result of damage from heavy metals such as copper or iron, or it can result from immune disorders and infections.

The principal manifestation of hypoparathyroidism is **tetany**, a sustained muscular contraction. In hypoparathyroidism, the muscles of the hands and feet contract in a characteristic fashion. The typical tetanic contraction of the hand is seen in Figure 12–13▸. Symptoms of chronic disease include lethargy, personality changes, anxiety, blurred vision and trembling of the limbs.

Common laboratory findings include low serum calcium, high serum phosphate levels, and low urine calcium. Imaging studies may show excessive calcification of bone and increased bone mineral density.

Acute hypoparathyroid tetany is a medical emergency that occurs after surgery and requires immediate treatment. Emergency replacement of calcium, magnesium, and vitamin D is used to maintain blood calcium in the appropriate range.

## ▸ Endocrine Function of the Pancreas

The pancreas is a long organ that lies across the middle of the abdominal cavity, below the stomach. It is divided into a head, body, and tail, with the head nearest to the duodenum and the opening of the **pancreatic duct**. (See page 221 in Chapter 9.) The pancreas carries out two types of functions: exocrine and endocrine. Most of the pancreas is devoted to exocrine secretion of digestive enzymes; the cells providing the endocrine function of the pancreas make up a smaller part. The endocrine functions of the pancreas consist of synthesis, storage, and release of two hormones, insulin and glucagon.

**Insulin** is secreted by certain cells of the pancreas called **beta cells**, located in patches of tissue named the islets of Langerhans or **pancreatic islets**. **Glucagon** is secreted by the **alpha cells** of the islets. Insulin and glucagon work antagonistically to each other. Insulin lowers the level of blood glucose, and glucagon elevates it. The combined effect of these hormones maintains the normal level of blood glucose.

Insulin is secreted when the blood glucose level rises. Insulin facilitates the entry of glucose into the cells, where it is primarily stored as glycogen and metabolized for energy. Glucose enters primarily skeletal muscle cells and fat cells.

As glucose enters cells and is converted to glycogen by the liver, the level of blood glucose falls. The normal level of glucose in the blood is about 90 mg/100 mL (or 90 mg/dL) of blood. This is also expressed as 90 mg percent.

When the level of blood glucose falls below normal, glucagon is released. Glucagon circulates to the liver and stimulates the release of glucose from its stored form, glycogen. This raises the level of blood glucose to normal. The control of glucose is illustrated in Figure 12–14▸.

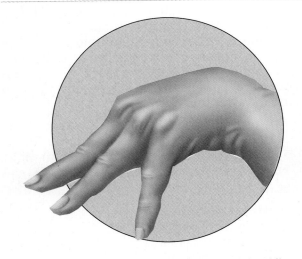

**Figure 12–13** ▸ Tetany of the hand in hypoparathyroidism.

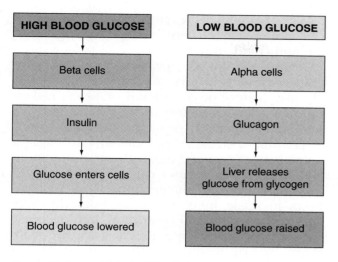

| HIGH BLOOD GLUCOSE | LOW BLOOD GLUCOSE |
|---|---|
| ↓ | ↓ |
| Beta cells | Alpha cells |
| ↓ | ↓ |
| Insulin | Glucagon |
| ↓ | ↓ |
| Glucose enters cells | Liver releases glucose from glycogen |
| ↓ | ↓ |
| Blood glucose lowered | Blood glucose raised |

**Figure 12–14** ► Control of blood glucose level.

## ► Hyposecretion of the Pancreas

## Diabetes Mellitus (Hyperglycemia)

Diabetes mellitus (DM) is an endocrine disease of impaired glucose regulation and hyperglycemia caused by complex interactions of genetics, environmental factors, and lifestyle choices. Depending on the underlying etiology of DM, factors contributing to hyperglycemia may include an absolute insulin deficiency, reduction in insulin secretion, decreased glucose utilization, and increased glucose production.

DM is classified on the basis of the underlying pathology that leads to hyperglycemia. The two broad categories of DM are designated as type 1 and type 2. **Type 1 diabetes** is characterized by an absolute insulin deficiency and often results from autoimmune destruction of the insulin-producing beta cells of the pancreas. **Type 2 diabetes** often develops later in life and is associated with variable degrees of insulin resistance, impaired insulin secretion, and increased glucose production, and is associated with obesity. Diabetes may develop during pregnancy, a condition called **gestational diabetes.** Resistance to the effects of insulin is related to the metabolic changes of pregnancy associated with increased requirements for insulin.

Approximately 6.3% of the U.S. population, or 18.2 million people, is estimated to have diabetes. Type 1 diabetes accounts for approximately 5% to 10% of cases; type 2 diabetes accounts for 90% to 95% of diabetic cases. Gestational diabetes occurs in approximately 4% of pregnancies annually in the United States. Most women revert to normal glucose tolerance following pregnancy but continue to have a considerable risk for developing diabetes later in life.

*Type 1 Diabetes* **Type 1 diabetes mellitus (T1DM)** is characterized by total or near total absence of insulin production. This type of diabetes has also been referred to as "juvenile-onset diabetes," as the peak incidence of this disease is between the ages of 10 to 14 years. Patients with T1DM require continuous insulin supplementation and glucose monitoring to sustain life.

T1DM occurs when an autoimmune process develops in individuals who are genetically susceptible and exposed to some unknown environmental trigger. In T1DM, the immune system attacks and destroys beta cells. This destruction typically occurs over several months, although it may be more rapid or last for years. Once 80% or more of beta cell function is destroyed, patients no longer have sufficient insulin capacity to control blood glucose, so they develop the hyperglycemia of diabetes. Eventually, patients lose the ability to produce insulin and depend on insulin injections to survive. Because type 1 diabetics cannot produce insulin, they are susceptible to severe metabolic derangements such as **diabetic ketoacidosis (DKA).**

Symptoms of T1DM include **polyuria**, or excessive urination, **polydipsia**, or excessive thirst; and **polyphagia**, or excessive hunger and weight loss. Because of water's movement by concentration gradients, water is lost through the kidneys as glucose concentrations rise. To compensate for fluid loss, patients develop extreme thirst. Although blood glucose levels are high, the body's tissues are unable to take up the glucose and use it effectively as an energy source due to the lack of insulin. Patients develop extreme hunger in the presence of hyperglycemia, leading to excessive eating with a paradoxical weight loss. Patients experience rapid weight loss despite increased food intake.

As T1DM progresses without treatment, alternative metabolic pathways are stimulated, causing depletion of protein and fat stores. Metabolism of fat produces molecules called **ketones**. During starvation, ketones serve as an alternative energy source; however, in T1DM these molecules accumulate to dangerous levels due to excessive fat metabolism. Diabetic ketoacidosis results when ketone buildup is associated with blood glucose levels greater than 250 mg/dL. Diabetic ketoacidosis can lead to coma and death if not treated immediately as a medical emergency. See the discussion of DKA in the section "Complications of Diabetes Mellitus."

***Type 2 Diabetes*** Unlike T1DM, type 2 diabetes (T2DM) is not associated with destruction of pancreatic beta cells. T2DM results from defects in insulin secretion by the pancreas and insulin utilization in target tissues. Insulin resistance occurs when the tissues' normal response to insulin is impaired. This insulin resistance leads to increased insulin secretion by the beta cells, with eventual insulin decline or insulin deficiency relative to blood glucose levels.

Insulin resistance can be induced by hormones such as cortisol, growth hormone, and epinephrine, or target tissue defects. Insulin receptor defects include disruption of glucose transport by free fatty acid accumulation common in obesity. Glucotoxicity, or high levels of blood glucose, results in structural and functional damage to the beta cells, reducing the ability of the beta cells to secrete sufficient insulin in response to glucose.

Type 2 diabetics retain some insulin-producing capacity. The primary defects leading to T2DM are insulin resistance in liver, muscle, and fat cells and reduced insulin secretion by the pancreas, and increased glucose production by the liver. Obesity contributes to insulin resistance, and weight reduction may help improve insulin resistance and lower blood glucose in obese patients. As T2DM progresses, insulin

levels eventually decrease due to the inability of the pancreas to continue producing large amounts of insulin.

Risk factors for the development of T2DM include a family history of diabetes, older age, obesity, history of gestational diabetes, sedentary lifestyle, and history of high blood pressure and high cholesterol, or hyperlipidemia.

Treatment of T2DM includes diet and weight management and oral medications, and insulin for patients who cannot control their diabetes with diet and oral medications. Oral medications increase insulin release from the beta cells, improve insulin utilization, and decrease insulin resistance. Patients often require more than one oral medication to control their diabetes, and some progress to lifelong insulin injections.

## Complications of Diabetes Mellitus

Acute complications of diabetes are related to excessive hyperglycemia and include DKA and hyperosmolar hyperglycemic state (HHS). DKA occurs in patients with T1DM, whereas HHS is a rare complication of T2DM.

DKA can be the initial presenting problem in a newly diagnosed patient with T1DM. More commonly, DKA is caused by acute illnesses such as the flu or common cold or physical and emotional stress. During stress, the production of stress hormones such as epinephrine and norepinephrine inhibits insulin action and stimulates glucose production. Without adequate amounts of insulin, the body continues to break down all forms of stored energy to glucose. Eventually the liver uses fatty acids to produce ketone bodies. As ketone bodies accumulate, the blood becomes acidic. Symptoms of DKA include nausea, vomiting, polyuria, polydipsia, dehydration, mental status changes, and rapid breathing. DKA treatment includes continuous intravenous infusions of fluids, electrolytes, and insulin until the ketosisis is reversed and the acidity is corrected.

Hyperosmolar hyperglycemic state typically occurs in older, debilitated type 2 diabetic patients. Similar to DKA, HHS is associated with acute stress from infections, medical illnesses, or surgery. Because T2DM patients have some insulin function, ketone body formation is prevented; however, patients often present with hyperglycemia in the range of 250 mg/dL to 400 mg/dL. Treatment of HHS is aimed at rehydration and correction of hyperglycemia and electrolyte disturbances. Aggressive intravenous fluid and electrolyte replacement is necessary as patients can lose up to 10 liters, or 2.5 gallons, of fluid within a short period of time. Administration of intravenous insulin is essential to improve glucose utilization and correct the hyperglycemia.

Chronic complications of diabetes are due to chronic pathological insults to the microvasculature, or small blood vessels, and to the macrovasculature, or large vessels. Microvascular disease occurs primarily in the eyes, kidneys, and nerves. Hyperglycemia damages the endothelial cell lining of blood vessels, resulting in progressive narrowing and occlusion of large and small vessels. Cells die when vessel occlusion cuts off blood supply. Macrovascular damage leads to cardiovascular disease, the leading cause of death in patients with diabetes.

Microvascular disease of diabetes includes retinopathy, nephropathy, and neuropathy. Diabetic retinopathy is the leading cause of blindness among adults aged 20 to 74 years. Diabetic nephropathy occurs in approximately 20% to 30% of patients with diabetes and is the leading cause of end-stage kidney disease. About 60% to 70% of patients with diabetes have nerve damage or neuropathy. Typical symptoms of neuropathy include numbness or tingling in the hands and feet and or severe, burning muscle aches. The loss of sensation in the feet and poor circulation can lead to severe infections requiring amputations. More than 60% of nontraumatic limb amputations in the United States occur annually in people with diabetes.

Macrovascular disease includes the development of coronary vascular disease, peripheral vascular disease, and stroke. Death rates due to heart disease are two to four times higher for adults with diabetes compared to persons without diabetes; stroke is two to four times more likely. Approximately 75% to 80% of patients with diabetes die due to the complications of cardiovascular disease. Treatment of the underlying factors that lead to cardiovascular disease is essential for the long-term health of patients with diabetes. The National Diabetes Education Program (NDEP) and the American Diabetes Association have developed an education and treatment program called the ABCs of Diabetes Management. Research has shown that reducing blood glucose as measured by blood levels of hemoglobin A1C (A), blood pressure (B), and cholesterol (C) levels reduces morbidity and mortality from cardiovascular disease in patients with diabetes.

See Table 12–2 ▶ for warning signs of type 1 and type 2 diabetes.

**Table 12–2  ▶  Warning Signs of Diabetes**

| Type 1 or Insulin-Dependent Diabetes Mellitus | Type 2 or Non-Insulin-Dependent Diabetes Mellitus |
| --- | --- |
| Frequent urination | Any of the Type 1 symptoms |
| Excessive thirst | Frequent infections |
| Extreme hunger | Recurring skin, gum, or bladder infections |
| Weight loss | Blurred vision |
| Fatigue | Cuts and bruises that heal slowly |
| Irritability | Numbness or tingling sensations in the hands or feet |

*Source:* American Diabetes Association website: www.diabetes.org/risk-test.jsp. Accessed August 25, 2008.

# Prevention PLUS!

## Obese Children and Type II Diabetes

The number of overweight children is increasing in the United States. Obese children are at increased risk of developing Type 2 diabetes mellitus as young adults. They also have an increased lifetime risk for heart disease and cancer. These chronic diseases are largely preventable through proper diet, weight control, and adequate exercise appropriate for age; see the MyPyramid for Kids diagram below.

*Source:* http://www.mypyramid.gov/kids/index.html

## Prevention ✚ PLUS!

### Diabetes Control

Can control of blood sugar prevent complications of diabetes? Nearly three-fourths of adults with diabetes lack basic information that can help control their disease. Studies have shown that better control of diabetes helps prevent serious complications that may develop over time.

## Tests for Diabetes Mellitus

A simple urine test can show the presence or absence of glucose or ketones in the urine. Urine tests are helpful for initial screening and for those who are prone to ketoacidosis. Fasting blood glucose levels, glucose tolerance testing, and glycosylated hemoglobin testing are used to monitor and diagnose diabetes. For the fasting blood glucose level test, a sample of blood is taken after the person has fasted for 8 hours. The glucose tolerance test challenges the body's ability to secrete and use insulin. The test is performed after a 10-hour fast. The patient drinks a standard glucose solution, and blood and urine sample are taken and analyzed for the next three hours. No glucose should appear in the urine, and the blood glucose levels should not exceed 170 mg/dL of blood if insulin is being produced and utilized. Glycosylated hemoglobin determination is a simple blood test that is used to monitor long-term control of diabetes. It generally indicates the average blood glucose levels over the past 90 days. Normal values should be below 6, and levels for diabetics should be less than 7.

## Education of the Diabetic Patient

The American Diabetes Association, physicians, nurses, and dieticians have made a great effort to assist the diabetic patient in leading a normal life. The diabetic who understands the disease knows the importance of weight control, diet, exercise, and either insulin or oral agents in leading a normal life. A safety precaution advised by the American Diabetes Association is that anyone who takes insulin carry an identification card explaining the emergency treatment required if an insulin reaction occurs.

## ▶ Abnormalities in Secretion of Sex Hormones

The gonads (ovaries and testes) are endocrine glands as well as the source of the ova and sperm. They secrete the hormones estrogen and testosterone directly into the blood.

### Hypergonadism (Hypersecretion)

Abnormally increased functional activity of the gonads before puberty produces precocious sexual development in both sexes. In a male child, excessive production of testosterone may be caused by a tumor in the testes. This causes rapid growth of musculature and bones but premature uniting of the epiphyses and shaft of long bones. Normal height, therefore, is not attained. Hypersecretion of ovarian hormones in the female is rare because negative-feedback stimulation of gonadotropic hormones stops ovarian hormone secretion.

### Hypogonadism in the Male

Several factors can cause hypogonadism, or decreased functional activity of the gonads. A person may be born without functional testes, the testes may fail to descend and thus may atrophy, or the testes may be lost through castration.

Testes fail to develop because of lack of gonadotropic hormone.

Loss of the male gonads before puberty causes the condition of eunuchism, in which sexual characteristics do not develop. Development of male traits depends on testosterone secreted by the testes. Castration after puberty causes some regression of secondary sexual characteristics, but masculinity is retained. Hormonal therapy, the administration of testosterone, can be effective.

## Hypogonadism in the Female

Hyposecretion of hormones by the ovaries may be caused by poorly formed or missing ovaries. When ovaries are absent or fail to develop, female eunichism results. Secondary sexual characteristics do not develop. A characteristic of this condition is excessive growth of long bones because the epiphyses do not seal with the shaft of the bone, as normally occurs at adolescence.

## ▶ Age-Related Diseases

Some changes in endocrine function occur normally with aging. Of these, none are significant causes of disease. However, some changes make the aging person more susceptible to disease.

Growth hormone level decreases with age. This is manifested in men after age 30 as a decrease in lean body mass and decreases in thickness and strength of bone matrix. As the body fat level increases, the growth hormone level decreases further. Increased body fat is correlated with greater risk of diabetes, heart disease, and cancer. Decreased bone density makes bones more susceptible to fracture.

A slight decrease in $T_3 : T_4$ ratio is seen with age, resulting in decreased metabolic rate. The incidence of autoimmune disease of the thyroid among females increases with age.

Although aldosterone levels remain relatively steady, an age-related decline in the kidneys' sensitivity to aldosterone occurs, accompanied by a diminishing capacity of the kidneys to secrete renin when needed. The body is less able to deal with the stress of changes in blood pressure, dehydration, and disease in general. There is an increased incidence of abnormalities in blood pressure, sodium and potassium levels, acid-base balances, and osmotic pressure.

The pancreas retains the ability to secrete insulin at normal levels with age, but tissue responsiveness to insulin decreases. Insulin resistance leads to a greater incidence of T2DM. It is estimated that T2DM occurs in 10% of those over age 56, 20% of those between 45 and 76, and 40% of people over age 85. Although T1DM is somewhat less common than T2DM and its occurrence is unrelated to aging, it remains among the 10 leading causes of death among people over age 65.

Androgen and estrogen levels drop with age, although this is considered a normal process of aging.

## RESOURCES

American Diabetes Association, Diabetes Facts and Figures: www.diabetes.org/diabetes-statistics.jsp

National Diabetes Information Clearinghouse (NDIC): www.diabetes.niddk.nih.gov

# DISEASE AT A GLANCE

## Endocrine System

| DISEASE | ETIOLOGY | SIGNS AND SYMPTOMS |
| --- | --- | --- |
| Pituitary dwarfism | GH hyposecretion beginning in childhood due to pituitary damage or ischemia | Normal mental development, slow growth, sexual development lacking |
| Adult growth hormone deficiency | Damage to the pituitary or hypothalamus | Increased body fat, reduced exercise capacity, impaired heart function, reduced muscle mass and abnormal lipid profile |
| Gigantism | GH hypersecretion beginning in childhood due to adenoma of anterior pituitary | Bone length increases rapidly, delayed sexual development |
| Acromegaly | GH hypersecretion beginning in adulthood due to adenoma of anterior pituitary | Enlargement of feet, hands, face as bones grow in diameter; soft tissue growth; nose, lips, lower jaw protrude; tongue and skin thicken |
| Diabetes insipidus | Central: hyposecretion of ADH by hypothalamic nuclei due to vascular lesion, neoplasm, trauma to base of skull, or inherited abnormality on chromosome 20 Nephrogenic: kidney insensitive to ADH due to X-linked gene or due to polycystic disease or pyelonephritis | Polyuria, polydipsia |
| Hyperprolactinemia | Pregnancy, stress, infections, liver disease | Hypogonadism, and reduced fertility |
| Hypothyroidism | Primary disease of the thyroid gland, autoimmune disease, radioactive iodine, dietary iodine deficiency, lithium | Hypotension, weakness, fatigue, weight gain, complaints of cold in hands and feet |
| Congenital hypothyroidism | Excessive maternal iodine intake during pregnanacy | Physical and mental sluggishness, poor muscle tone, umbilical hernia, protruding abdomen, bradycardia, and growth retardation |
| Thyrotoxicosis | Autoimmune, pituitary tumors, pregnancy | Nervousness, restlessness, heat intolerance, increased sweating, fatigue, weakness, muscle cramps, and weight loss |

| DIAGNOSIS | TREATMENT | PREVENTION | LIFESPAN |
|---|---|---|---|
| Serum assay for GH | Hormone replacement therapy | Unknown | Diagnosed in childhood and persists though ones life |
| X-ray, serum assay for GH | Hormone replacement therapy | Unknown | Occurs in adults |
| Serum assay for GH | None | Unknown | Diagnosed in childhood, persists for life |
| Serum assay for GH | None | Unknown | Occurs in adults |
| Urinalysis in water deprivation vasopressin test | Administer ADH | Unknown | Can occur at any age |
| Serum assay for prolactin | Treatment of the underlying cause | Unknown | More common in women of child bearing years |
| Serum assay for thyroxine, and TSH | Thyroid hormone replacement | Prevention of iodine deficiency by consumption of iodized table salt | Can occur at any age |
| Serum assay for thyroxine and TSH | Thyroid hormone replacement | Unknown | Diagnosed in infancy |
| Serum assay for thyroxine and TSH | Radioactive iodine, surgery to remove tumors, radiation | Unknown | Usually diagnosed in adulthood, though can occur at any age |

# DISEASES AT A GLANCE

## Endocrine System (*continued*)

| DISEASE | ETIOLOGY | SIGNS AND SYMPTOMS |
|---------|----------|--------------------|
| Thyroiditis | Autoimmune, or viral infection | Pain, swelling, thyroid tenderness, goiter |
| Addison's disease | Damage to the adrenal cortex, infections, opportunistic infections associated with AIDS, cancer, hemorrhage of the adrenal gland | Weight loss, fatigue, anorexia, abdominal discomfort, vomiting, diarrhea |
| Cushing's syndrome | Benign pituitary adenomas | Hyperglycemia, hyperlipidemia, fluid retention, weight gain, weakness, fatigue, hypertension |
| Pheochromocytoma | Tumor | Hypertension |
| Hyperparathyroidism | Neoplasm | Weak bones deform and fracture easily, kidney stones, pain in bones, depressed nervous system, weak muscles, slow heart rate, abdominal pain, vomiting, constipation |
| Hypoparathyroidism | Complication of thyroidectomy; also rare X-linked syndrome | Overexcited muscular and nervous system, characteristic tetany in hands, laryngeal spasm |
| Type 1 diabetes mellitus | Autoimmune destruction of the beta cells of the pancreas | Polyuria, polydipsia, polyphagia, weight loss |
| Type 2 diabetes mellitus | Obesity, hypertension, hyperlipidemia | Polyuria, polydipsia, |
| Hypergonadism | Hypersecretion of sex hormones caused by tumors | Precocious sexual development |
| Hypogonadism | Hyposecretion of sex hormones caused by undeveloped gonads | Lack of sexual development, eunuchism |

| DIAGNOSIS | TREATMENT | PREVENTION | LIFESPAN |
|---|---|---|---|
| Swelling and pain in neck region of thyroid gland | Anti-inflammatory medications, pain medications | Unknown | Can occur at any age |
| 24-hour urine assay for cortisol | Replacement of glucocorticoids and mineralocorticoids | Unknown | Can occur at any age, though more common in adults |
| Serum assay for diabetes, electrolyte disturbance, x-rays to diagnose tumor | Surgery, radiation, medications to treat hypertension, diabetes, and hyperlipidemia | Unknown | Occurs in adults |
| X-ray, CT scan, MRI | Antihypertensive medication | Unknown | Occurs mostly in adults |
| High serum calcium, patient history, kidney stones | Surgical removal of tumor, medication to lower calcium | Unknown | Can occur at any age, though mostly diagnosed in adults |
| Low serum calcium, patient history | Administer vitamin D and calcium | Unknown | Can occur at any age, though mostly diagnosed in adults |
| Serum assay for glucose, hemoglobin A1C | Insulin | Unknown | Can occur at any age, though mostly diagnosed prior to the age of 20 years |
| Serum assay for glucose, hemoglobin A1C | Weight loss, exercise, oral antidiabetic medication, insulin | Control of weight, healthy eating, exercise | Diagnosed in adulthood |
| Serum sex hormones | Administration of sex hormones | Unknown | Can occur at any age |
| Serum sex hormones | Administration of sex hormones | Unknown | Can occur at any age |

# Interactive Exercises

## Cases for Critical Thinking

1. A mother brings her 5-year-old son to the pediatrician with complaints that her son has been wetting the bed consistently. The child has a good appetite, drinks a lot of water, and has a high metabolism, according to the mother. On examination, the doctor notes that the child has lost 10 pounds since his last physical 6 months ago. What diseases should be ruled out?

2. A 59-year-old woman reports to the doctor's office with a chief complaint of terrible headaches, especially between her eyes. Her blood pressure, blood sugar, and cholesterol level are high. The doctor also notes a terrible bruise on her leg that was there since her last examination 2 months ago. What diseases should be ruled out?

3. A 45-year-old man reports to the emergency room with terrible dehydration. He has a yellowish appearance and can hardly stand without assistance. His blood level of potassium is extremely high and his legs feel tingly. His heartbeat is very rapid, and his breathing is shallow. What diseases might this man have?

## Multiple Choice

1. Acromegaly results from hyperactivity of the
   _____.
   a. thyroid
   b. parathyroid
   c. anterior pituitary
   d. posterior pituitary

2. Which hormone increases the blood calcium level?
   a. glucagon
   b. parathormone
   c. androgen
   d. insulin

3. Hypoglycemia is a sign in _____.
   a. Cushing's disease
   b. Addison's disease
   c. diabetes
   d. Graves' disease

4. The trunk is obese in _____.
   a. Graves' disease
   b. Cushing's disease
   c. Addison's disease
   d. Conn's disease

5. A deficiency of ADH is the cause of
   _____.
   a. IDDM
   b. NIDDM
   c. diabetes insipidus
   d. ketoacidosis

6. Which of these is associated with hypersecretion of thyroxine?
   a. Graves' disease
   b. gigantism
   c. cretinism
   d. myxedema

7. Which gland secretes epinephrine and norepinephrine?
   a. pancreas
   b. parathyroid
   c. testes
   d. adrenal

8. A deficiency in corticosteroids is associated with
   _____.
   a. Addison's disease
   b. Conn's disease
   c. diabetes insipidus
   d. pheochromocytoma

9. An absolute insulin deficiency is characteristic of
   _____.
   a. type 1 diabetes
   b. gestational diabetes
   c. type 2 diabetes
   d. all of the above

10. Iodine is required for the body to make
    _____.
    a. bone
    b. insulin
    c. thyroxine
    d. glucose

## True or False

_____ 1. Kidney stones are likely to form in hypoparathyroidism.

_____ 2. Hypercalcemia causes tetany.

_____ 3. Glucagon prevents hyperglycemia.

_____ 4. Steroids that suppress the inflammatory response, as in arthritis, are produced by the thyroid.

_____ 5. Hypertension accompanies Addison's disease.

_____ 6. Myxedema results from thyrotoxicosis.

_____ 7. A person with Graves' disease is very sensitive to cold.

_____ 8. Dehydration can develop in diabetes mellitus.

_____ 9. Cushing's syndrome results from an excess of glucocorticoids.

_____ 10. Glucagon elevates blood glucose level.

## Fill-Ins

1. Overproduction of growth hormone before puberty is called _____.

2. An overproduction of growth hormone after puberty is called _____.

3. The posterior pituitary secretes _____ and _____.

4. Microvascular disease is a chronic complication of _____.

5. A tumor of the adrenal medulla, or _____, causes overproduction of epinephrine and norepinephrine.

6. Insulin is secreted by cells of the pancreas called _____ _____.

7. Elevated blood levels of calcium are associated with excess _____ hormone.

8. Tropic hormones are secreted by the _____ _____.

9. Dwarfism is associated with hyposecretion of _____ _____.

10. Sexual characteristics do not develop in the rare condition called _____ _____.

## Labeling Exercise

Use the blank lines below to label the following image.

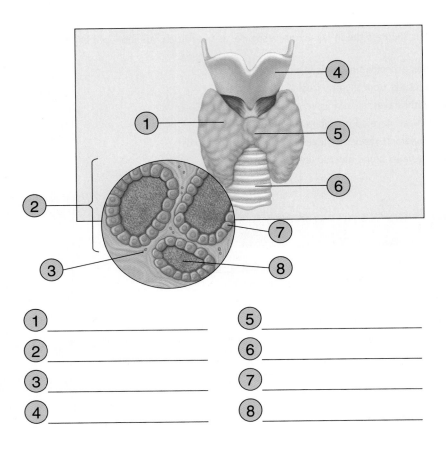

1 _____

2 _____

3 _____

4 _____

5 _____

6 _____

7 _____

8 _____

# Multimedia Preview

Additional interactive resources and activities for this chapter can be found on the Companion Website. For videos, audio glossary, and review, access the accompanying DVD-ROM in this book.

## ▶ DVD-ROM Highlights

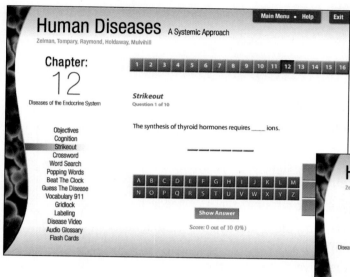

### Strikeout

Click on the alphabet tiles to fill in the empty squares in the word or phrase to complete the sentence. This game quizzes your vocabulary and spelling. But choose your letters carefully because three strikes means you're out!

### Labeling Exercise

A picture is worth a thousand words, but only if it's labeled correctly. Review anatomy by clicking and dragging the terms that correlate to a figure from this chapter. The correct labels will lock into place beside the picture.

## ▶ Website Highlights—www.pearsonhighered.com/zelman

### Audio Glossary

Take advantage of the free-access online study guide that accompanies your textbook. You'll find an audio glossary with definitions and audio pronunciations for every term in the book. By clicking on this URL you'll also access a variety of quizzes with instant feedback and links to current news articles.

CHAPTER

# 13

# Diseases of the Nervous System and the Special Senses

## Learning Objectives

After studying this chapter, you should be able to

- Recognize the basic structure and functions of the nervous system and major sensory elements

- Describe the etiology, signs and symptoms, diagnostic tests, and treatment of different types of headache

- Compare and contrast different types of headache

- Describe the etiology, signs and symptoms, diagnostic tests, and treatment of infectious diseases of the nervous system

- Describe degenerative diseases of the central nervous system, including multiple sclerosis, Parkinson's disease, and amyotrophic lateral sclerosis

- Discuss inherited and congenital diseases of the nervous system

- Describe the effects of trauma on the brain and sensory organs

- Discuss the etiology, signs and symptoms, diagnostic tests, and treatment of seizure disorders

- Discuss the etiology, signs and symptoms, diagnostic tests, and treatment of CVA (stroke) or related cerebrovascular disorders

- Describe the etiology, signs and symptoms, diagnostic tests, and treatment of selected eye and ear diseases

## Fact or Fiction?

Benign brain tumors are not very serious and therefore are not cause for concern.

*Fiction:* Benign tumors tend to grow and crowd out precious cranial space and, thus, apply pressure or restrict blood flow to particular brain regions. If these benign growths are inoperable or uncontrolled, they will kill the victim. Malignant brain tumors may be lethal, but they may also be surgically removed or reduced with medication or radiation. All brain tumors require attention and may be lethal if left untreated. Treatment with surgery, medication, or radiation is most successful for slowly growing, encapsulated tumors.

# Disease Chronicle

## Death to a Killer

**N**ot so long ago, your great-grandparent or grandparent may have suffered from this tragic disease or feared it within his or her community. Your parents' generation began to break free from the grip of this disease, and for today's generation this disease has been nearly eradicated. What is this devastating killer disease? Polio. Polio thrived in the United States and around the world until the 1950s, especially impacting the postwar "baby boom" generation. By 1955, Dr. Jonas Salk and Dr. Albert Sabin had formulated vaccines that put this disease on the shelf. How was that incredible feat accomplished?

Dr. Jonas Salk's vaccine consisted of inactivated poliovirus injected intramuscularly, which stimulated production of antibodies against poliovirus. With the institution of broad-scale immunization programs, cases of polio dropped immediately. Dr. Albert Sabin developed an oral vaccine more convenient to administer, particularly to large groups, and it is extremely effective. The Sabin vaccine is taken orally and stimulates the production of antibodies within the digestive system, where the viruses reside. Unlike the Salk vaccine, the Sabin vaccine basically destroys the viruses in the digestive system, thus preventing transmission and eliminating carriers. Many researchers believe, however, that the Salk vaccine is the better choice because it employs killed virus and ensures that the vaccine itself will not transmit polio, especially secondarily to compromised patients like those with HIV. In 2000, the Centers for Disease Control and Prevention changed course and recommended only the Salk vaccine in order to eliminate any exposure from live viruses.

The World Health Organization projects that in the near future polio will be eradicated worldwide. Between 1988 and 1998, polio declined 85% worldwide, and today, polio has been eliminated in the United States and from much of the world. The last case of polio in the United States occurred in 1979. In 2003, only 700 cases of polio were found in the world, and three-fourths of these cases were in Nigeria, India, and Pakistan, where undervaccination has enabled numerous outbreaks to occur. Clearly, it remains important to continue immunization, both locally and globally, to end this devastating disease.

# ▶ Structural Organization of the Nervous System

The nervous system monitors the external and internal environment of the body and, along with the endocrine system, controls many of the body's functions, like breathing rate and alertness.

The basic organization of the nervous system includes two major divisions: the central nervous system (CNS) and the peripheral nervous system (PNS). The CNS is composed of the brain and spinal cord. It integrates information and controls the peripheral nervous system. The PNS comprises all those nerves outside the CNS, beginning with the 12 pairs of cranial nerves and 31 pairs of spinal nerves. The nerves carry information to and from the CNS. Nerves consist of motor nerves, which carry information to muscles and glands, and sensory nerves, which carry sensory information from sense receptors to the CNS.

Certain organs are highly specialized for gathering sensory input; these are called organs of the special senses and include the eyes, ears, and nose. Diseases of the eye and ear will be discussed in this chapter; diseases of the nose were described in Chapter 8.

The basic unit of the nervous system is the **neuron**, or nerve cell. The neuron consists of a cell body with attached filamentous extensions called dendrites that carry information toward the cell body and a filamentous axon that carries information away from the cell body. A neuron is shown in Figure 13–1 ▶. Receptors attached to sensory neurons are capable of detecting environmental changes and transmitting messages to the brain or spinal cord (e.g., touch or pain). Motor neurons convey messages from the central nervous system out to muscles, causing contraction, or to glands, triggering secretion. The axons of sensory and motor neurons are insulated by a lipoprotein covering called **myelin** that forms a sheath, which insulates and protects the neuron. Deterioration of this sheath decreases the impulse velocity and impairs function. When the myelin degeneration becomes profuse it characteristically causes a misfiring or incomplete impulses as in multiple sclerosis.

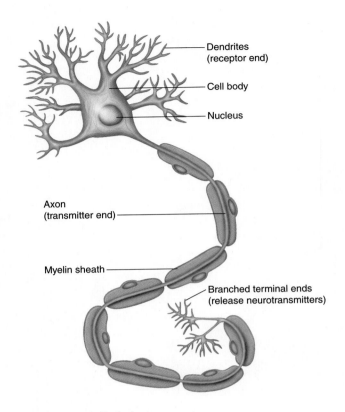

**Figure 13–1** ▶ Typical neuron.

## The Brain

Three membranous coverings, called the **meninges**, protect the delicate nerve tissue of both the brain and spinal cord. The innermost covering is the pia mater, the middle layer is the arachnoid, and the toughest, outermost covering is the dura mater. Meningitis is a potentially life-threatening disease caused by an inflammation of these coverings.

The brain has three major anatomical areas: the cerebrum, cerebellum, and brain stem. The largest portion of the brain is the cerebrum, comprised of two cerebral hemispheres. The cerebral surface is highly convoluted with many elevations (gyrus) and depressions (sulcus). The outer surface of the brain, the cortex, consists of gray matter, where nerve cell bodies are concentrated. The inner area consists mostly of white matter, the nerve fiber tracts. Deep within the interior of the white matter are clusters of nerve cell bodies known as **basal ganglia**, also called basal nuclei, which help control position and subconscious movements. It is the basal ganglia (also gray matter) that are defective in Parkinson's disease, because they fail to produce sufficient quantities of the neurotransmitter dopamine.

Within the brain are four cavities called ventricles, where **cerebrospinal fluid** (CSF) is formed. These ventricles all interconnect and are continuous with the central canal of the spinal cord. CSF is derived from plasma and flows out of the ventricles through small openings to circulate over the brain and spinal cord, forming a watery, protective cushion. CSF is reabsorbed into the venous sinuses of the dura mater, and new fluid is formed. Obstruction of cerebrospinal fluid circulation results in hydrocephalus, a condition commonly called "water on the brain" in the newborn.

The cerebellum controls voluntary movements, such as riding a bicycle. The brain stem is called the "vitals center" because it regulates heart and breathing rates. These three major brain areas will be examined as part of the CNS survey along with the spinal cord.

## The Spinal Cord

The spinal cord is housed within the vertebral column and is continuous with the brain stem (Figure 13–2▶). Numerous tracts of nerve fibers within the spinal cord ascend to and descend from the brain, carrying messages to and from muscles, organs, and glands.

## The Autonomic Nervous System

One division of the PNS is the autonomic nervous system (ANS). This system controls internal functioning of the body. The ANS houses the sympathetic and the parasympathetic nervous systems, which often work antagonistically to each other. The **hypothalamus**, located within the brain, controls certain activities of the ANS and is known as the center for homeostasis. Homeostasis is the foundation of all fundamental principles in the study of physiology. The ANS controls arterial blood pressure, heart rate, gas-trointestinal functions, sweating, temperature regulation, and many other involuntary actions. Whereas some peripheral nerves affect skeletal or voluntary muscle, the ANS acts on smooth or involuntary muscle and cardiac muscle. Diseases of the digestive system such as stress ulcers, regional enteritis, and ulcerative colitis (Chapter 9) are influenced by the ANS. As mentioned earlier, the overall function of the nervous system is to monitor and regulate the various body systems. This monitoring allows the body to adjust to the surrounding environment both internally and externally, and much of this is done by the ANS.

## The Sensory Nervous System

Sensations detected by receptors and carried by sensory neurons from specialized organs such as the eye and ear, as well as in skin, muscles, tendons, and internal organs, are transmitted to the central nervous system. The spinal cord receives simple sensations and directs simple reflex responses, as when one touches a hot stove and quickly withdraws the hand. Complex sensory information must travel to specialized parts of the brain. Impulses reaching the brain stem and cerebellum bring about many unconscious automatic actions, but sensory information involving thought processes must reach the highest area of the brain, the cerebral cortex.

The cerebral cortex has specialized areas to receive sensory information from all parts of the body, such as the feet, the hands, and the abdomen. Visual impulses are transmitted to the posterior part of the brain, whereas olfactory and auditory impulses are received in the lateral parts. Association areas of the brain interpret deeper meaning of the sensations, and many of the sensory messages are integrated and stored as memory. Creative thought becomes possible through use of sensory input.

## The Motor Nervous System

Just as the cerebral cortex has areas specialized for the reception of sensory information, it also has areas that govern motor activity. The primary motor cortex is the frontal lobe that controls discrete movements of skeletal muscles.

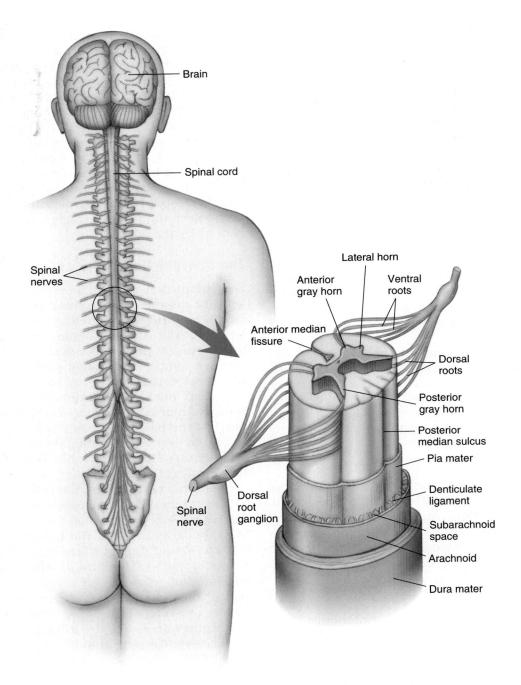

**Figure 13–2** ▶ The brain, spinal cord, and spinal nerves. An expanded view of the spinal cord is shown.

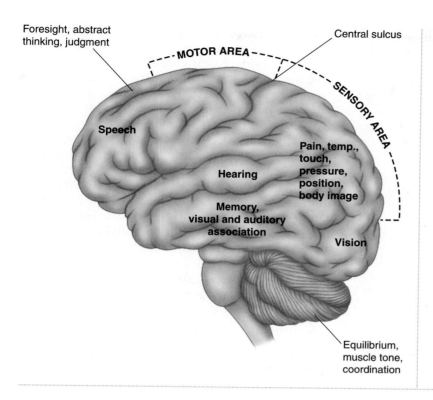

Foresight, abstract thinking, judgment

--- MOTOR AREA ---

Central sulcus

SENSORY AREA

Speech

Pain, temp., touch, pressure, position, body image

Hearing

Memory, visual and auditory association

Vision

Equilibrium, muscle tone, coordination

Figure 13–3 ▶ Specialized areas of the brain.

Because the nerve fibers cross over in the medulla or spinal cord, stimulation on one side of the cerebral cortex affects particular muscles on the opposite side of the body.

Anterior to the primary motor cortex is the premotor cortex, which controls coordinated movements of muscles. This process is accomplished by stimulating groups of muscles that work together. The speech area is located here and is usually on the left side, especially in right-handed people. Specialized areas of the brain are shown in Figure 13–3▶.

## ▶ Diagnostic Procedures for the Nervous System

Neurologic laboratory tests include CSF examination obtained by a lumbar (puncture) spinal tap, as previously described. Angiography allows visualization of the cerebral circulation through the injection of radiopaque material.

Computed tomographic (CT) scans are particularly valuable for diagnosing pathologic conditions such as tumors, hemorrhages, hematomas, and hydrocephalus. **Electromyelography (EMG)** is a radiographic process by which the spinal cord and spinal subarachnoid space are viewed and photographed after injection of contrast medium into the lumbar subarachnoid space. Myelography is used to identify spinal lesions caused by trauma or disease, such as amyotrophic lateral sclerosis (ALS). **Electroencephalography (EEG)** records the electrical activity of the brain (brain waves). It is used to diagnose lesions or tumors, and seizures, in impaired consciousness. Magnetic resonance imaging (MRI) uses magnetic fields in conjunction with a computer to view and record tissue characteristics at different planes. MRI is excellent for visualizing brain soft tissue, spinal cord, white matter diseases, tumors, and hemorrhages. Where a disease is idiopathic or without cure, the diagnosis is directed at relief of symptoms, as in Parkinson's disease.

For the eye, ophthalmoscopy is used for routine eye exams that may determine cataracts, when viewing through the slit-lighted feature of the scope. Tonometry procedures are for glaucoma determination. Audio exams with tuning fork and electronic audio signals help discover tone quality and hearing loss. Cochlear implants help to restore sounds and a better life for people of all ages.

## ▶ Diseases of the Nervous System

### Common Headache

Moderate to severe head pain characterizes the common headache. Tension or inflammation of muscles in the head, eyes, neck, and shoulders may cause the common headache. Other causes include dilation or constriction of cerebral blood vessels, allergies, chemical fumes, extreme temperatures, and constipation. Simple unintended actions like coughing and laughter may trigger a headache, as may an intracranial mass of tumors or lesions. Nausea, vomiting, and sensitivity to noise and light may accompany the common headache and more severe cases.

Common household treatments are rest and NSAIDs (nonsteroid anti-inflammatory drugs) such as aspirin, ibuprofen (Advil), and acetominophen (Tylenol). Resting in a dark, quiet room and applying a cold compress may be beneficial for many sufferers, especially if time and space are available. Two of the more intense and episodic forms of headache are the cluster headache and the migraine.

### Cluster Headache

Cluster headache affects 1 to 4 per 1000 individuals, and men, especially middle-aged men, are five times more likely to be affected than women. The cluster headache occurs suddenly, producing severe, sharp, and stabbing pain particularly near one eye or temporal area. The headaches are caused by blood vessel abnormalities and may occur two to three times per day for weeks, or may occur intermittently over a span of 1 to 3 months, subside, and recur months or years later. The pain may develop at any time but usu-

ally occurs at night and tends to last from 30 minutes to several hours. The pain is so severe that many individuals cannot lie down or be idle and may pace about. In contrast with migraine, however, light intensity, sounds, or strange odors do not elicit nausea or vomiting.

Often there is no family history of cluster headache, although this condition tends to run in families. As of this writing, genetic factors have not been determined. Alcohol and nicotine tend to trigger these painful headaches, along with stress, indigestion of specific foods, and glare. Treatment requires medications like subcutaneous or intranasal sumatriptan (Imitrex), and inhalation of 100% oxygen and dihydroergotamine works well, as well as biofeedback and reduction of stress. Ergotamine tartrate is used as a prophylactic agent given in various modes of delivery.

### Migraine Headache

Migraine headaches are more common in women than in men and usually begin in the teen years or early twenties. The symptoms are throbbing (moderate) pain on one or both sides of the head plus sensitivity to light and noise or certain odors. Because migraines tend to cause nausea and vomiting, they are referred to as a "sick headache." Sometimes an aura or premonition precedes the migraine onset. Additional symptoms include numbness, dizziness, and visual blurring. The headaches last from a few hours to a few days and may recur once a month or once every few years. A history of the symptoms helps diagnose migraine. Daily or weekly patient logs of activities, especially timing of migraine onset and subsequent events, helps reduce episodes and the need for medication.

Specific causes have not been identified, although there may be a natural abatement in some women when they discontinue birth control pills or attain menopause. The concentration of the neurotransmitter serotonin appears to have a role in the pathogenesis of migraines, and nitric oxide (NO), a vasodilator, may be implicated as well. When NO or serotonin are blocked, migraine pain subsides.

One of the most recently discovered causes related to migraine headache is a developmental or congenital defect in the heart that occurs as much as 25% of the time in those affected. The normal connection between the two atria in a fetal heart, the foramen ovale, happens to remain open (at least partially) instead of slapping shut at the time of birth. This fetal remnant is called a *patent foramen ovale* (PFO). Surgeons found that when this defect was closed in their adult patients, migraine episodes were resolved. Clinical trials are currently scheduled to evaluate this new development.

Heredity is now known as a primary factor in the case of migraine. It has been documented that a gene on chromosome 1 contributes to sensitivity of sound; on chromosome 5 a gene is recognized as one that allows pulsating headaches and sensitivity to light; and a gene on chromosome 8 is related to vomiting and nausea.

Bed rest and sleep in a dark, quiet room seems to benefit most migraine sufferers. Drug treatment is aimed at prevention and relief of symptoms. NSAIDs may not provide adequate relief, but prescription drugs like opioids, codeine, and mependine are often effective. Imitrex, mentioned previously, helps relieve pain and reduce nausea and sensitivities to light and sound. Cardiac medications like beta blockers (Atenolol) or calcium channel blockers (Diltiazem) help, but the exact mechanism is not fully understood, and tricyclic antidepressants have shown positive results as well.

## ▶ Infectious Diseases of the Nervous System

Certain pathogenic microorganisms are neurotropic in that the virus or bacterium has an affinity for nervous tissue. Pathogens obtain access to the nervous system by many routes, including wounds or trauma, and systemic infections entering from the thinner paranasal sinuses or mastoid regions.

## Meningitis

**Meningitis** is an acute inflammation of the first two meninges that cover the brain and spinal cord: the pia mater and the arachnoid mater. A contagious disease, it usually affects children and young adults and may have serious complications if not diagnosed and treated early.

There are many forms of meningitis, and some are more contagious than others. The most common bacterial causes are *Haemophilus influenzae; Neisseria meningitidis*, also called meningococcus; and *Streptococcus pneumoniae*. However, other bacteria, as well as viruses, cause meningitis. **Enteroviruses** account for most of the cases when the virus is identified; in aseptic meningitis no bacterium is found and thus it usually is considered a viral condition. The infecting organisms can reach the meninges from the middle ear, upper respiratory tract, or frontal sinuses; they can also be carried in the blood from the lungs or other infected sites. Healthy children may be carriers of the bacteria and spread the organisms by sneezing or coughing. Viral or aseptic meningitis is considered the cause in 30% of the cases involving nonimmunized individuals, primarily caused by contracted mumps, and it affects males two to five times more frequently than females. This form is normally a mild case of meningitis that may not require specific treatment. Other cases may be caused by the waning polio viruses and occasionally by herpes simplex, and noninfectious cases may result from lymphoma, brain cancer, or leukemia.

In the United States the bacterial cases of meningitis range from 0.6 to 4 per 100,000 individuals, or 1400 to 2800, while viral cases affect about 10 per 100,000 individuals. Causative agent, the geographical region, and accessibility to medical coverage influence prevalence; in addition, some agents become resistant to penicillin (*S. pneumoniae*) and others have been reduced because of the vaccine (Hib) for *Haemophilus influenzae* type B.

The symptoms of meningitis are high fever, chills, and a severe headache caused by increased intracranial pressure. A key symptom is a stiff neck that holds the head rigidly. Movement of neck muscles stretches the meninges and increases head pain. Nausea, vomiting, and a rash may also be symptomatic. The high fever often causes delirium and convulsions in children, and they may lapse into a coma.

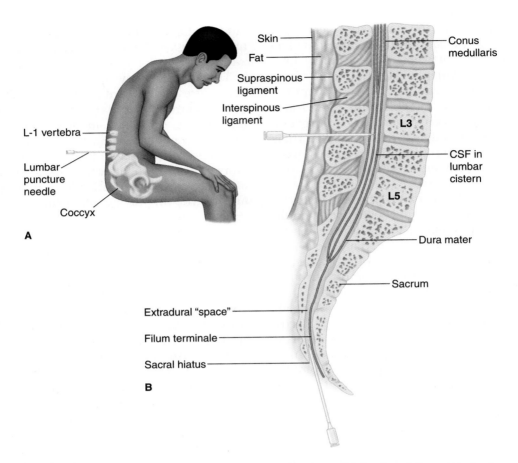

Figure 13–4 ▶ (A) Lumbar puncture, also known as spinal tap. (B) Section of the vertebral column showing the spinal cord and membranes. A lumbar puncture needle is shown at L3–4 and in the sacral hiatus.

Diagnosis of meningitis is made by performing a **lumbar puncture** (Figure 13–4▶) or spinal tap, in which a hollow needle is inserted into the spinal canal between vertebrae in the lumbar region. This procedure is possible because the spinal cord terminates at or near the first lumbar vertebra, although a sac containing cerebrospinal fluid extends down to the sacrum. In addition, a spinal tap may reveal the relative pressure of cerebrospinal fluid. The infected fluid contains an elevated protein level, numerous polymorphs/leukocytes, and infecting agents. When the level of glucose in the cerebrospinal fluid is below normal, bacteria may have used the sugar for their own growth and metabolism.

The prognosis depends on the cause of meningitis and a prompt diagnosis and treatment. Treatment with antibiotics like Rifampin, ciprofloxacin, or ceftriaxone is very effective if the meningitis is bacterial. If not treated, about 15% of those affected suffer permanent brain damage that manifests by sight or hearing loss, paralysis, mental retardation, or death. Another complication is blockage of the fourth ventricle by a pyogenic (bacteria) infection, which results in the accumulation of cerebrospinal fluid in the brain, a form of **hydrocephalus**. Preventive measures include viral vaccines like Hib or MPSV4 (meningococcal polysaccharide vaccine, recommended for ages above 2 years) and a conjugate vaccine (MCV4) for ages 11 to 55.

## Encephalitis

**Encephalitis**, an inflammation of the brain and meninges, is caused by several types of viruses. Some of these viruses may be harbored by wild birds and transmitted to humans by mosquitoes, commonly called arborviruses (carried by arthropods-insects). These cases are mostly seasonal and are represented by regional variations that occur within the United States, like Western, California, St. Louis, and Eastern. Along with West Nile, the California and St. Louis varieties of encephalitis seem to dominate in the United States. In 2003, West Nile caused an outbreak of 9800 cases and 250 deaths.

Symptoms of encephalitis range from mild to severe, such as headache, sudden fever, stiff neck, and drowsiness, to more severe cases that include cerebral dysfunction, disordered thought patterns, and seizures in 5% of the cases. Most cases resolve themselves within 1 to 2 weeks with no specific treatment required except for mild, flu-like symptoms. In serious cases involving extensive brain damage, convalescence is slow and requires prolonged physical rehabilitation. Some nerve damage may cause paralysis, as occurs in 10% of these cases. Personality changes or other emotional disturbances may occur that require therapy.

Diagnosis of encephalitis is made by lumbar puncture. Brain imaging CT or MRI may be used to check for brain swelling, and a blood test will determine the presence of West Nile. Treatment is essentially aimed at controlling high fever and intracranial pressure, maintaining fluid and electrolyte balance, and carefully monitoring respiratory and kidney function. In individuals generally in good health except for the virus, the prognosis is positive with supportive treatment.

There are many forms of the disease, and they may occur in epidemics. Lethargic encephalitis, or "sleeping sickness," is one type of encephalitis characterized by persistent drowsiness and delirium that sometimes results in coma. Secondary encephalitis may develop from

viral childhood diseases such as chicken pox, measles, and mumps, or herpes. In the case of herpes simplex encephalitis (HSE), type I is most common, but type II may cause infection in newborns or immunocompromised people like those with HIV or who have received an organ transplant. In the latter case, the patient may be treated with acyclovir or valacyclovir medications.

Prevention depends on control of mosquitoes and deterring contact through use of repellents, clothing, and timing of outdoor activities. Other sources may be unavoidable, but early treatment is crucial in order to reduce neurological severity and deficits or death.

## Poliomyelitis

**Poliomyelitis**, commonly called polio, is an infectious disease of the brain and spinal cord caused by an enterovirus. Motor neurons of the medulla oblongata and pons, which houses the respiratory center, and the spinal cord are primarily affected. As a result, muscle tissue is not stimulated; it weakens and finally atrophies. If the respiratory muscles are depressed, then an artificial means of respiration is required.

Symptoms of poliomyelitis are stiff neck, fever, headache, sore throat, and gastrointestinal disturbances. When diagnosed and treated early, severe damage to the nervous system and paralysis can be prevented. Those who survive paralytic polio may be left with a limp or need a walking aid such as crutches or a wheelchair. Excessive fatigue, muscular weakness, pain, and other difficulties such as muscle atrophy and scoliosis may occur 20 to 30 years after the onset of the disease. The recurrence of these symptoms is known as postpolio syndrome (PPS). Age seems to be an integral factor, although PPS's exact cause remains unknown. Additional rest seems to offer some necessary relief from PPS symptoms.

In the 1940s and early 1950s, polio was a highly prevalent disease around the world and the United States that crippled or killed thousands, primarily children. This devastating disease has nearly been eradicated worldwide through the development of the Salk and Sabin vaccines (see the Disease Chronicle at the start of this chapter).

## Rabies

**Rabies** is an infectious disease of the brain and spinal cord caused by a virus that is transmitted by secretions (saliva, urine) of an infected animal. Rabies is very rare in the United States due to animal and human vaccines in addition to animal control efforts. However, rabies can be lethal, and numerous pets are not vaccinated as required by local or state laws. Along with urban spread, outbreaks are common especially at seasonal times (summer). Rabies is primarily a disease of warm-blooded animals such as dogs, cats, raccoons, skunks, wolves, foxes, and bats, but it can be transmitted to humans through bites or scratches from a rabid animal that licks its fur or feet. (The virus may be airborne as a mist from urine in caves and in fecal matter, allowing for transfer to fur, feet, or saliva.)

The virus passes from the wound site along peripheral nerves to the spinal cord and brain, where it causes acute encephalomyelitis. The incubation period is long, one month to perhaps a year, depending on the distance of the wound from the brain or degree of breached surface. Bites on the face, neck, and hands are the most serious. The mode of tetanus and rabies transmission to the central nervous system is illustrated in Figure 13–5 ▶.

Symptoms of rabies include fever, pain, mental derangement, rage, convulsions, and paralysis. Rabies affects the areas of the brain that control the muscles in the throat required for swallowing and also muscles for breathing. As a result, spasms occur within the throat and voice box, causing a painful paralysis. Because of the inability to swallow or clear the throat ef-

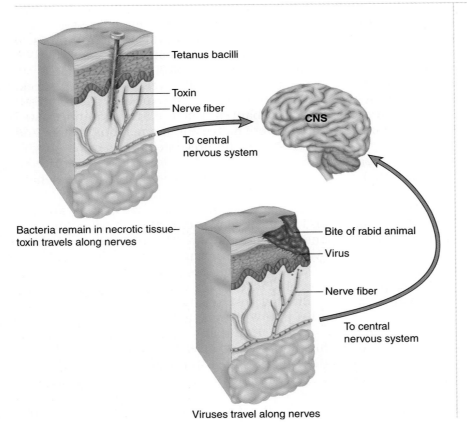

Bacteria remain in necrotic tissue–
toxin travels along nerves

Viruses travel along nerves

- Tetanus bacilli
- Toxin
- Nerve fiber
- To central nervous system
- CNS
- Bite of rabid animal
- Virus
- Nerve fiber
- To central nervous system

**Figure 13–5** ▶ Nerve involvement in tetanus and rabies.

fectively, the infected animal or human produces a profuse, sticky saliva, and thus tends to "foam" at the mouth. Hydrophobia is an aversion to water often linked to rabies. The disease is fatal in humans once it reaches the central nervous system and the symptoms described have developed. However, in 2004 a high school sophomore in Wisconsin, who postponed treatment for a month—it took that long for clinical rabies to develop after a bat bite—and then spent two months in intensive care, much of that time in a coma, has survived.

In the case of an animal bite, it is extremely important to know if the animal is rabid, and a detailed investigation of the animal must be made as soon as possible. If rabies is suspected, immunization and globulin injections are started on the infected person. The victim receives repeated injections of an altered virus to stimulate antibody production and an immune serum to provide a substantial passive immunity. The severity of rabies explains the critical need for the vaccination of dogs and cats against the disease.

Prevention of rabies is achieved by taking a series of three vaccinations over 28 days. The vaccine is required for field workers and medical associates who work with animals and tissues that may carry the rabies virus.

## Shingles (*Herpes zoster*)

**Shingles** is an acute inflammation of sensory neurons caused by the latency effect of the chicken pox virus, *Herpes zoster*. It may even be caused by shingles exposure itself without a reactivation of the chicken pox virus, but that scenario is less common. Shingles is manifested by pain and a rash characterized by small water blisters surrounded by a red area. The lesions follow a sensory nerve, forming a streak toward the midline of the torso, generally across the shoulder, chest, or trunk area. The rash is usually confined to one side of the body and does not cross the midline. Blisters fade and the lesions dry up and become encrusted. The encrusted areas cause severe itching and pain and may result in scaring; this after-effect is called **postherpetic neuralgia** and is caused by the release of substance P (pain agent). The optic nerve can be affected, causing severe conjunctivitis. If not properly treated, ulcerations can form on the cornea, especially from *Zoster keratitis*, and cause scarring or blindness.

Shingles can develop from exposure to a person with shingles in the infectious stage. It may also develop from exposure to chicken pox, which has an incubation period of about 2 weeks. It sometimes accompanies other diseases, such as pneumonia or tuberculosis. Shingles may also result from trauma or reaction to certain drug injections.

Treatment of shingles is directed toward relieving the pain and itchiness. Dry ice pads and lotions such as calamine may provide relief. Glucocorticoids may also be prescribed to suppress the inflammatory reaction, and antiviral agents like acyclovir (Zovirax) are used. About half a million cases of shingles are reported each year in the United States, according to the National Institutes of Allergy and Infectious Diseases, although the incidence is closer to 1 million and is projected to increase with the aging population. Two-thirds of the cases of shingles occur in those over the age of 50, and one half of the cases in those age 85 or more. Repeat occurrences are mostly found in immunocompromised patients.

Prevention includes immunization against chicken pox. For adults 60 and older, a vaccine called Zostavax prevents onset or reduces severity.

## Reye's Syndrome

**Reye's syndrome** is a potentially devastating neurological illness that sometimes develops in children after a viral infection. Viruses associated with Reye's syndrome include Epstein-Barr, influenza B, and varicella, the group which causes chicken pox. Use of aspirin during these infections is associated with Reye's syndrome. The actual cause of the disease is unknown.

Manifestations of Reye's syndrome include persistent vomiting, often a rash, and lethargy about 1 week after a viral infection. Neurologic dysfunction can progress from confusion to seizures to coma. The encephalopathy includes cerebral swelling with elevated intracranial pressure.

Management is geared toward lowering intracranial pressure and monitoring of vital signs, blood gases, and blood pH. The outcome is very satisfactory when diagnosed and treated early, with a recovery rate of 85% to 90%.

## Tetanus

Tetanus is an acute infectious disease, commonly called "lockjaw," characterized by rigid, contracted muscles that are unable to relax. Tetanus is caused by the tetanus toxin, which is produced by a rodlike tetanus bacillus that lives in the intestines of animals and human beings. The organisms are excreted in the fecal material and persist as spores indefinitely in the soil. The bacilli are prevalent in rural areas and in garden soil fertilizer containing manure, especially from horse farms or racetracks. About 45 cases of tetanus occur annually in the United States, but in developing countries neonatal tetanus kills about 250,000 per year and is called "the silent death" because the infants die before the birth is recorded.

A laceration, puncture, or animal bite introduces the bacterium deep into the tissues, where it flourishes in the absence of oxygen. Thus, deep wounds with ragged, lacerated tissue contaminated with fecal material (manure or contaminated soils) are the most dangerous type.

Tetanus has an incubation period ranging from 1 week to a few weeks. The toxin travels slowly, so the distance from the wound to the spinal cord is significant. The tetanus toxin (see Figure 13–5) anchors to motor nerve cells and stimulates them, which in turn stimulate muscles. Muscles become rigid, and painful spasms and convulsions develop. The jaw muscles are often the first to be affected (hence the name

lockjaw, also called **trismus** in the clinical setting). Because these muscles cannot relax, the mouth clamps tightly closed. The neck is stiff, and swallowing becomes difficult. If the muscles of respiration are affected, asphyxiation occurs. Death can result from even a minor wound if the condition is not treated.

Treatment includes a thorough cleansing of the wound and removal of dead tissue and any foreign substance. Immediate immunization to inactivate the toxin before it reaches the spinal cord is crucial. The type of immunization administered depends on the patient's history. If the patient has had no previous immunization, tetanus antitoxin is given. If 5 years have elapsed since the previous tetanus injection, the person receives a booster injection of **tetanus toxoid** to increase the antitoxin level.

Additional treatment includes the administration of antibiotics like metronidazole (Flagyl) or penicillin G and erythromycin to prevent secondary infections. Sedatives may be used to decrease the frequency of convulsions. Oxygen under high pressure is also used because the bacillus is anaerobic; that is, it thrives in the absence of oxygen.

Tetanus may be prevented by adequate immunization. Tetanus toxoid, which stimulates antibody formation, should be given to infants and small children at prescribed times. This inoculation may be done in combination with the diphtheria toxoid and pertussis vaccine (the latter prevents whooping cough).

## Abscesses of the Brain

Pyogenic organisms such as streptococci, staphylococci, ameobae, and *E. coli* can travel to the brain from other infected areas and cause a

## Prevention ✛PLUS!

### Reye's Syndrome

Reye's syndrome (RS) appeared in the 1950s and virtually disappeared by the 1980s. It has been suggested that the disappearance of RS is related to the recognition of metabolic inborn errors that parallel RS in various clinical manners. Reye's syndrome may be misdiagnosed because of mitochondrial dysfunction that allows various metabolites to increase (e.g., liver enzymes and ammonia) that cause RS-type symptoms and conditions. However, prescribing acetaminophen instead of aspirin will prevent this syndrome.

brain abscess. Infections of the middle ear, skull bones, or sinuses, including the mastoid, as well as pneumonia and endocarditis are potential sources for brain abscess. Figure 13–6► shows abscesses of the brain.

The symptoms of brain abscess may be misleading, because the symptoms may include fever and headache, which can suggest a tumor. Analysis of cerebrospinal fluid shows increased pressure and the presence of neutrophils and lymphocytes, indicating infection.

Once the diagnosis of a brain abscess has been made, the abscess must be opened surgically and drained, and the patient must be treated with penicillin-like antibiotics. Brain abscesses are not as common today in the developed world because most infections are held in check by antibiotics. Prevention may be unavoidable due to accidental trauma situations, but monitoring current infectious situations helps prevent the spread of any disease.

## ► Degenerative Neural Diseases

Some diseases of the nervous system involve the degeneration of nerves and brain tissue. Abnormalities in muscle and sensory function often result from degeneration of nervous tissue. For example, note that Alzheimer's disease is also discussed in Chapter 14, although it, too, can be considered a type of neurodegenerative disease. Therefore, the description of Alzheimer's in this section focuses on the degenerative aspects of nervous tissue.

## Alzheimer's Disease

The most common cause of **dementia** (a syndrome of brain abnormalities) in the elderly is Alzheimer's disease (AD), a progressive degenerative brain disease. The incidence of AD rises with age, and the prevalence doubles about every 5 years. Those aged 60 to 64 have a prevalence of at least 1%, while that number rises to 30% to 40% for those individuals older than age 85.

The root cause of Alzheimer's disease is genetic, although most cases seem to appear random or sporadic. Familial cases, or those linked within families, account for about 5% to 10% of the cases. Chromosomes 1, 10, 12, 14, 19, and 21 have shown genes which affect protein production for specific enzymes or structural components within nerve cells. In the neuron, a support scaffolding of microtubules helps the cell maintain its integrity and to be functionally

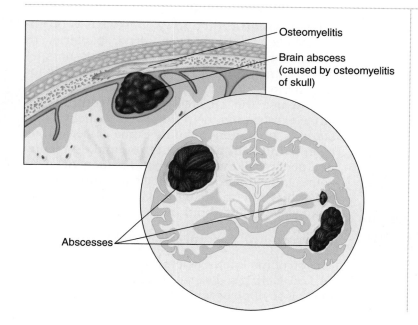

Osteomyelitis

Brain abscess (caused by osteomyelitis of skull)

Abscesses

Figure 13–6 ► Abscesses of the brain.

sound. The directional protein making these microtubules may be corrupted by a malformed compound known as the *tau* protein. This corruption causes a malformation of microtubules that normally form the linear feature of a neuron and results in a contracted mass known as neurofibrillary tangles. These tangles are not unique to Alzheimer's disease but do indicate a significant breakdown of functioning. These elements are apparent upon autopsy inspection, which is required to confirm a diagnosis of Alzheimer's disease.

Although autopsy is the confirming manner for this devastating disease, a combination of clinical assessment, modern imaging methods, and family history can accurately diagnose AD in 80% to 90% of the cases. Within 5 to 10 years of onset, the person tends to become disabled, immobile, and muted; the person usually dies of pneumonia.

## Multiple Sclerosis

Multiple sclerosis (MS) is a chronic, progressive, degenerative disorder of the central nervous system. It usually affects young adults between the ages of 20 and 40. MS frequency of occurrence is rare, at about 0.1%, currently afflicts about 400,000 in the United States and 1 million worldwide.

At first, the disease manifests itself by muscle impairment, beginning with a loss of balance and coordination. Tingling and numbness ensue and are accompanied by a shaking tremor and muscular weakness. Walking is reduced to a shuffle or use of a cane, and occasionally a wheelchair or a more permanent assistance is required. Speech becomes difficult, and urinary bladder dysfunction often develops.

Vision may suddenly become impaired, and double vision frequently occurs. Lesions on the optic nerve can lead to blindness. The individual acquires **nystagmus**, an involuntary, rapid movement of the eyeball. Emotional changes are common due to less independence and functional control. Signs and symptoms of MS waffle between periods of remission and exacerbation and proceed at different rates as the disease progresses.

The disease is difficult to diagnose in the early stages, as many disorders of the nervous system have similar symptoms. Diagnosis is based on the specific tissue changes that accompany MS.

The degeneration of nervous tissue in MS involves the breaking up or erosion of the neuronal (myelin) sheath due to chronic inflammation. The nerve tracts do not degenerate in a regular pattern or to the same degree. Therefore, patchy areas of demyelination appear and become sclerotic. A myelin sheath protects the neuron and acts as an insulator to insure the direction and velocity of the nerve impulse transmission. Any degradation of myelin impairs nerve conduction. MRI demonstrates plaques of demyelinated nerve fibers.

The disease basically takes one of four potential directions once established: relapsing-remitting involves about 85% of those affected, where flare-up episodes of worsening conditions are followed by partial or complete recovery periods; primary-progressive is exhibited by a slow, gradual deterioration at variable rates of speed with minor plateaus of improvement and involves about 10% of patients; secondary-progressive, or progressive-relapsing involves about 5% of patients and is characterized by steadily progressing deterioration and acute relapses with or without recovery.

The cause of MS is still uncertain, and although it is considered an autoimmune disease, it has been attributed to various viruses or immunologic reactions to a virus, bacteria, or trauma and heredity. To date, there is no specific treatment for MS that works effectively for long periods. Physical therapy enables the person to use the muscles that are controllable. Muscle relaxants help reduce spasticity, and steroids are often helpful. Some success has been found with beta interferon, and exercising in a pool of cold water seems to be beneficial for some individuals. Psychological counseling is advantageous in dealing with the emotional changes brought about by the disease.

## Amyotrophic Lateral Sclerosis

Amyotrophic lateral sclerosis (ALS), also known as Lou Gehrig's disease, is a chronic, terminal neurological disease noted by a progressive loss of motor neurons and supportive astocytes. ALS occurs late in life, most commonly in the fifties and sixties, and is slightly more common in men than in women. The prevalence of ALS is 2 to 3 per 100,000, with an incidence of 3 per 100,000 in the United States.

ALS is characterized by disturbances in motility and atrophy of muscles of the hands, forearms, and legs because of degeneration of neurons in the ventral horn of the spinal cord. Also affected are certain cranial nerves, particularly the trigeminal (V), facial nerves (VII), and hypoglossal (XI), which impair muscles of the mouth and throat. Swallowing and tongue movements are affected, and speech becomes difficult or impossible.

The cause of amyotrophic lateral sclerosis is not known. ALS is diagnosed by an electromyogram (EMG), which shows a reduction in the number of motor units active with muscle contraction. Motor units are motor neurons and their connection to a host of muscle fibers. Also observed are *fasciculations*, the spontaneous, uncontrolled discharges of motor neurons seen as irregular twitchings.

ALS requires early education of the patient and the patient's family so that a proper management system may be provided to anticipate and prevent certain hazards. Specifically, the prevention of upper airway obstruction and pathologic aspiration—drawing of vomitus or mucus into the respiratory tract—is the main focus. Aspiration can occur from weakened respiratory musculature and ineffective cough. Death usually occurs within 3 to 5 years after onset of symptoms and generally results from pulmonary failure. However, as the renowned British scientist Stephen Hawking attests, survivorship of ALS does vary.

Prevention of ALS is uncertain because 90% of the cases are undetermined as to origin, while 10% have an autosomal dominant gene on chromosome 21. Currently, about 20,000 to 30,000 individuals have ALS in the United States.

## Parkinson's Disease

Parkinson's disease (PD) is a degenerative disease that affects muscle control and coordination. PD normally strikes at midlife, about age 45. Approximately 1.5 million people are affected in the United States. More men than women are affected, and as the cause of Parkinson's disease is still unknown, environmental factors, particularly undetected viruses, are suspected. A very small percent of PD cases are hereditary as either autosomal dominant or recessive genes. The resultant cause is related to a loss of a neurotransmitter called dopamine produced in the substantia nigra of the basal nucleus within the core of the brain. Dopamine suppresses undesired movements that skeletal muscles may be instructed to do but are normally held in check or dormant. Therefore, when dopamine is not present, the unrestrained signals call for an uncoordinated, "shakey" tremor.

Symptoms are progressive and include tremor, rigid muscles, and loss of normal reflexes. The tremors are called "tremors at rest," meaning they occur while the patient is inactive and subside when the muscles are put into motion. A masklike facial expression is noticed along with faltering gait and mental depression in approximately 10% to 15% of patients.

In the earlier stages, physical therapy and exercise help maintain flexibility, motility, and mental well-being. Relaxation is particularly important for PD patients because stressful situations worsen the condition. Figure 13–7 ▸ summarizes possible effects of PD.

Treatment includes the administration of levadopamine (L-dopa), a form of dopamine similar to the natural form that passes the blood–brain barrier. The drug does not stop the degeneration, but it restores dopamine levels in the brain and reduces symptom severity. Other similar drugs like pergolide (Permex) and carbidopa-levodopa (Sinemet) may be used, as well as anticholinergic medications like diphenhydramine (Benadryl) for treatment.

In later stages, physical therapy, including heat and massage, helps reduce muscle cramps and relieve tension headaches caused by the rigidity of neck muscles. Psychological support is needed while learning to cope with the disability. In terminal stages, an increased risk for suicide has been noted.

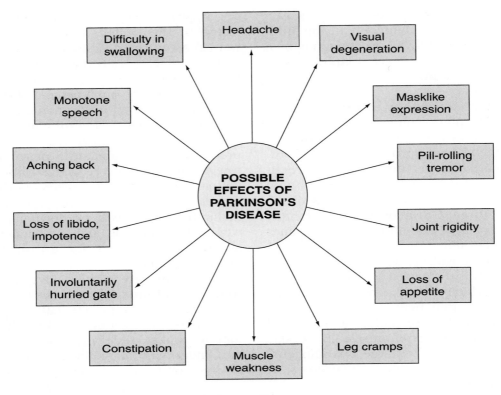

**Figure 13–7** ▶ Summary of Parkinson's disease effects.

Deep brain stimulation with electrodes implanted into the thalamus has become an additional tool for controlling tremors. The patient may turn on/off the implanted pulse generator by passing a magnet over it. The small, pacemaker-like device is implanted under the collarbone. Normally, a constant trickle of charge is sent to the thalamus in order to interrupt tremor-causing signals, similar to surgical techniques that destroy part of the thalamus to limit involuntary movements.

Another treatment suggested is a sort of "brain transplant," in which dopamine-producing neural tissue from a mouse or pig is implanted in the brain to replenish the missing dopamine. Most PD patients are unaware of the initial agent(s) that bring about this disorder, and prevention is not an option in hereditary cases. Pesticides are suspected causative agents.

## Essential Tremor

About 2 million people in the United States have essential tremor. This disorder is often confused with Parkinson's disease even though it usually becomes symptomatic in adolescence. Like PD, essential tremor progresses with the passage of time; at rest the problem abates. Moving or shaking of the head and hands and a halting or quivering voice are characteristic of this condition. There is a familial pattern, but the genetics are not clear. Drugs like beta blockers, known for heart regulation; tranquilizers like Valium; and botox injections help approximately 40% of the patients, and a noticeable improvement occurs in about 60% of the patients receiving brain implant devices. Still, some of those afflicted choose to leave the disease untreated until it interferes with the basic routines of living.

Prevention is basically uncertain and there may be familial links, but these associations are not clearly identified at this time.

## Huntington's Disease (Huntington's Chorea)

**Huntington's chorea** is a progressive degenerative disease of the brain that results in the loss of muscle control. *Chorea* refers to involuntary and ceaseless, rapid, jerky movements. The disease affects both the mind and body. Physical disabilities include speech loss and a difficulty in swallowing, coupled with involuntary jerking, twisting motions, and muscle spasms. Personality changes include carelessness, poor judgment, and impaired memory, ultimately deteriorating to total mental incompetence.

World prevalence is about 5 per 100,000 people. Huntington's disease is an inherited disease, but symptoms may not appear until middle age (ages 30 to 50). If either parent has the disease, the children have a 50% chance of inheriting it because it is an autosomal dominant trait (see Chapter 5 for a discussion of genetic transmission). The responsible gene has been identified on chromosome 4. The abnormality causes the neurotransmitter dopamine to be produced in excess, and insufficiencies of acetylcholine underlie the dementia and abnormal muscle activity. To reduce dopamine action, the receptors are blocked by drugs like phenothiazines and haloperidol; however, the choline-promoting-type agents have not been as effective. Given its genetic component, prevention is not an option. There is no cure for Huntington's chorea. When desired, carriers can be identified with gene testing. Following onset, death normally occurs 15 to 20 years afterward, with a progressive deterioration.

## ▶ Convulsions

A convulsion is a sudden, intense series of uncontrollabe muscular contractions and relaxations. Causes of convulsions include accumulation of waste products in the blood, such as occurs in uremia, toxemia of pregnancy, drug poisoning, or withdrawal from alcohol. Infectious diseases of the brain, such as meningitis and encephalitis, and high fevers, especially in young children, are frequently accompanied by convulsions. The basis for convulsions is abnormal electrical discharges in the brain, which abnormally stimulates muscles to contract.

## Epilepsy

Epilepsy is a group of uncontrolled cerebral discharges that recurs at random intervals. The seizures associated with **epilepsy** are a form of convulsion. Brain impulses are temporarily disturbed, with resultant involuntary convulsive movements. Epilepsy can be acquired as a result of injury to the brain, including birth trauma, a penetrating wound, or depressed skull fracture. A tumor can irritate the brain, causing abnormal electrical discharges to be released. Alcoholism can also lead to the development of epilepsy. Most cases of epilepsy are idiopathic, but a predisposition to epilepsy may be inherited.

Epilepsy is one of the more common, yet controllable, neurological disorders and affects 0.5% to 2% of the U.S. population at an incidence rate of about 181,000 per year. Childhood prevalence is rather high, at 4 to 9 per 1000, and involves proportionally more boys than girls.

Epilepsy may manifest itself mildly, particularly in children. Loss of consciousness may last only a few seconds, during which time the child appears in a state of shock or absent-mindedness (amnesia). Some muscular twitching may be noticed around the eyes and mouth, and the child's head may sway rhythmically, but the child may not fall to the floor. This form of epileptic seizure is known as absence (or petit mal) and usually disappears by the late teens or early twenties.

Major seizures, called tonic-clonic or grandmal, involve a sudden loss of consciousness during which the person falls to the floor. *Tonic* refers to the increased muscle tone or contraction phase, while *clonic* involves alternating contracting and relaxing muscle activities. Absence and tonic forms are considered generalized convulsions and range from mild to severe, with violent shaking and thrashing movements lasting about one minute. Hypersalivation causes a foaming at the mouth. The individual tends to lose control of the urinary bladder and sometimes bowels. Sometimes there are repeated seizures, without a recovery period, that may last 30 minutes. This condition is known as status epilepticus.

Individuals sometimes have a warning of an approaching seizure that gives them time to lie down or reach for support. This warning, known as an **aura**, may come as a ringing sound in the ears, a tingling sensation in the fingers, spots before the eyes, or various odors. The signs described are characteristic of the absence or clonic form of seizure. After a seizure, the person is fatigued, groggy, and unaware of what happened. Seizures last for varying lengths of time and appear with varying frequencies.

Epileptic seizures may take different forms. The International Classification of Epileptic Seizures, adopted by the World Health Organization, classifies seizures into four categories:

1. Partial seizures begin locally and may or may not involve a larger area of brain tissue.
2. Generalized seizures are bilaterally symmetrical and without local onset.
3. Unilateral seizures generally involve only one side of the brain.
4. Unclassified epileptic seizures are less defined in origin and degree.

Diagnosis of epilepsy can be made on the results of an electroencephalogram (EEG), a recording of brain waves. X-ray films are also used to identify any brain lesions. Family histories of epilepsy are very important in diagnosing the condition. The diagnosis of epilepsy and the seizure type has become more accurate with new techniques for imaging the brain. CT scans, using x-rays, and MRI, using magnetic fields, visualize brain anatomy.

Medication is very effective in controlling epilepsy, particularly anticonvulsant drugs, such as Dilantin or Tegretol and a more recent medication called Retigabine. Alcohol must be avoided with these types of medication. Molecular neurobiology research is providing new information on how nerve cells control electrical activity, thus making development of more effective anti-epileptic drugs possible. It is now known which drugs are best for treating the various kinds of seizures. Assistance or treatment during a seizure is directed toward preventing self-injury. Finally, epilepsy does not appear to interfere with mental prowess or creative talents for those afflicted. A consistent medication regimen usually prevents epileptic episodes.

## ▶ Developmental Errors or Malformations

### Spina Bifida

**Spina bifida,** a neural tube defect (NTD), is a developmental error in which one or more vertebrae fail to fuse, leaving an opening or weakness in the vertebral column. The consequences of spina bifida depend on the extent of the opening and the degree to which the vertebral column, usually in the lumbar area, is exposed and the involvement of the spinal cord. One form of spina bifida, spina bifida occulta (hidden), may not be apparent at birth. In this mildest case, a slight dimpling of the skin and tuft of hair over the vertebral defect indicates the site of the lesion.

Lesions of spina bifida occulta show internal weakness or backbone breaks that can be readily seen on x-ray films. Other malformations, such as hydrocephalus, cleft palate, cleft lip, club foot, and **strabismus** (crossed eyes), tend to accompany this developmental error and may occur simultaneously or separately. Any single malformation may point to spina bifida and trigger closer observations of the individual even without noticeable disability. Muscular abnormalities, such as incorrect posture, inability to walk, or lack of urinary bladder and bowel control, appear later.

A second form of spina bifida noticeable at birth is a **meningocele**. In this condition, meninges protrude through the opening in the vertebra as a sac filled with cerebrospinal fluid. The spinal cord is not directly involved in this case.

**Meningomyelocele** is a serious anomaly in which the nerve elements protrude into the sac and are trapped, thus preventing proper placement and development. The child with this defect may be paralyzed, fail to develop, lack sensation, and experience mental retardation. The consequences of the defect depend on the region and size of the spinal cord affected. Surgical corrections of the various forms of spina bifida have been very effective. Some procedures are intrauterine, to repair the defect of the fetus, and these new operations look promising. Physical rehabilitation may allow for a more normal lifestyle, depending on severity.

The most severe form of spina bifida is **myelocele**, in which the neural tube itself fails to close and the nerve tissue is totally exposed and disorganized. This condition is usually fatal. The various forms of spina bifida are shown in Figure 13–8 ▶.

Hereditary and environmental influences or idiopathic instances are possible causes of spina bifida. Before 1992 the occurrence rate of spina bifida in the United States was 3% to 4% annually, but since the introduction of folate into the neonatal care regimen, that number has been cut in half. Spina bifida and other NTD

cases may be detected by ultrasonagraphy and elevated blood levels of alpha fetoprotein.

## Hydrocephalus

**Hydrocephalus** is a consequence of excess CSF trapped within the brain. The formation, circulation, and absorption of CSF were described earlier in this chapter. In hydrocephalus, this fluid and pressure increases abnormally, causing the ventricles to enlarge and press the brain against the skull, which forces it to enlarge greatly, especially in the case of newborns.

An obstruction in the normal flow of CSF is the usual cause of hydrocephalus. A congenital defect causes stenosis (narrowing) of an exit opening from the ventricles, or an acquired lesion can block the CSF flow. Meningitis, a tumor, or birth trauma may result in acquired hydrocephalus. The error may also be a failure to absorb the fluid into the circulatory system.

There are two types of hydrocephalus: *communicating* and *noncommunicating*. In the communicating type, the excess CSF enters the subarachnoid space. In the noncommunicating

**SPINA BIFIDA OCCULTA**

Nerve fibers

Meninges

Tuft of hair

Dimpling of skin

Cleft in vertebra

**MENINGOMYELOCELE**

Skin

Spinal cord

Cerebrospinal fluid

Spinal nerves

Skin

Meninges

Spinal cord

Cerebrospinal fluid

**MENINGOCELE**

**MYELOCELE**

Spinal cord open-nerve tissue disorganized

Intervertebral disk

Cerebrospinal fluid

Figure 13–8 ▶ Forms of spina bifida.

hydrocephalus, the increased pressure of the CSF is confined within the ventricles and is not evident in a lumbar puncture (LP).

The head of a child born with hydrocephalus may appear normal at birth, but it will enlarge rapidly in the early months of life as the fluid accumulates. The brain is compressed, the cranial bones are thin, and the sutures of the skull tend to separate under the pressure. The appearance of a hydrocephalic infant exhibits a prominent forehead, bulging eyes, and a facial expression of fright or pain. The scalp is stretched, and the veins of the head are prominent. The weight of the excessive fluid in the head makes it impossible for the baby to lift its head. Infant growth is stunted, as is mental development.

There have been cases of self-arrested hydrocephalus in which expansion of the head stops. A balance is reached between production and absorption of the CSF fluid. The cranial sutures knit together and the skull bones thicken. The extent of brain damage before the arrest determines the degree of mental retardation.

The number of cases involved is difficult to attain due to causes, ages, and matters of degree, especially when tabulated in combination with other diseases. For example, an obvious case at birth is noted, but trauma or a tumor or encephalitis cases may not be accounted for and may simply be considered cerebral edema. The incidence of hydrocephalus is approximately 1.8 per 100,000. Success in relieving the excessive CSF has been achieved by placing a shunt between the blocked cerebral ventricles and the jugular vein (Figure 13–9 ▶), to the heart or placed into the peritoneal cavity. This connection facilitates the reduction in cranial pressure and allows the fluid to enter the general circulation. Prevention is difficult due to the uncertainty of events that gradually lead to this crucial disorder.

## ▶ Brain Injury

### Cerebral Palsy

Cerebral palsy (CP) is not a disease but a functional disorder of the brain manifested by motor impairment that may induce varying degrees of mental retardation and usually becomes apparent before age 3. The assault causing brain damage may be due to injury at or near the time of birth, a maternal infection such as rubella (German measles), or infection of the brain even after birth. Reduced levels of oxygen, primarily due to reduced blood flow or incompatible blood type or Rh, may cause brain injury. For example, a pinched umbilical cord against the birth canal may shut off blood and starve the fetus of necessary oxygen. With incompatibilities, an $Rh^-$ mother may produce antibodies against the blood of an $Rh^+$ fetus. The result is excessive destruction of fetal blood cells that causes hyperbilirubinemia; bilirubin is toxic to the brain and causes damage. Often, cerebral palsy is idiopathic. Cerebral palsy affects 2 to 4 per 1000 infants in the United States and is 10 times more often found in premature and low-weight babies.

There are four recognized forms of cerebral palsy: spastic, choreoathetoid, atactic, and mixed. However, it is not easy to diagnose a specific type before the infant is at least 18 months old because the signs may be subtle and attributed to immature development. The largest percentage of cerebral palsy type (70%) is the spas-

Figure 13–9  ▶  Hydrocephalus.

Enlarged ventricles

Blocked aqueduct

Catheter tip in ventricle

Valve

Shunt

## SIDE by SIDE ■ Hydrocephalus

▲ Normal ventricles.

▲ Enlarged ventricles in hydrocephalus.

tic version in which muscles are tense and re-flexes are exaggerated. In the athetoid form, constant, purposeless movements are uncontrollable. A continuous tremor or shaking of the hands and feet is common. Cerebral palsy sufferers with the atactic form have poor balance and are prone to fall. Poor muscular coordination and a staggering gait are characteristic of this form of CP.

Depending on the area of the brain affected, there may be seizures along with visual or auditory impairment. If the muscles controlling the tongue are affected, speech defects result. Intelligence may be normal, but often there is reduced mental capacity.

Treatment depends on the nature and the severity of the brain injury. Anticonvulsant drugs reduce seizures, and casts or braces may aid walking. In addition, muscle relaxants can relieve spasms along with traction or surgery, which is necessary in some cases. Muscle training is the most important therapy, and the earlier it is started, the more effective it is. Prevention may depend on circumstances such as sterile environment and strict monitoring of fetal status at the time of birth.

## ▶ Stroke or Cerebrovascular Accident (CVA)

The main cause of cerebral hemorrhage is hypertension. Prolonged hypertension tends to result from atherosclerosis, which leads to arteriosclerosis, explained in Chapter 6. The combination of high blood pressure and hard, brittle blood vessels is a predisposing condition for cerebral hemorrhage. **Aneurysms**, weakened areas in vascular walls, are also susceptible to rupture (Figure 13–10 ▶). Surrounding the pituitary gland is the circle of Willis, a major crossroads of cerebral vascularity, vulnerable to weakness, especially aneurysms. If the rupture or leakage occurs here, the collection of blood within the cranial cavity mounts, and the intracranial pressure increases proportionally to dangerous levels. When this pressure increase is controlled or alleviated early, brain damage and death is unlikely. The pressure relief may come in the form of medication or emergency surgical procedure. Any subsequent hemorrhage into the brain tissue damages the neurons, causing a sudden loss of consciousness.

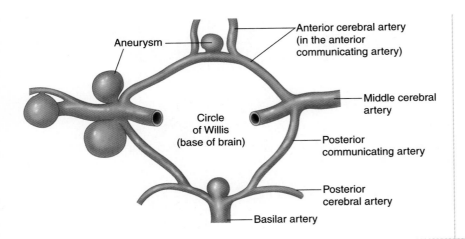

Figure 13–10 ▶ Aneurysms.

Anterior cerebral artery (in the anterior communicating artery)

Aneurysm

Middle cerebral artery

Circle of Willis (base of brain)

Posterior communicating artery

Posterior cerebral artery

Basilar artery

Death can follow, or, if the bleeding stops, varying degrees of brain damage can result. When detected, swift surgical repairs of aneurysms save lives.

**Cerebrovascular accident (CVA)** is the third leading cause of death in the United States. Prevention includes not smoking, maintaining proper diet and exercise, and monitoring blood pressure; some people take an 81-mg aspirin each day if they are not taking blood thinners like coumadin. Cerebrovascular accidents are basically of two varieties; those due to a hemorrhage or to a blood clot. Most CVAs result from the blood clot or occlusion and will be addressed in the next section.

## Thrombosis and Embolism

Blood clots that block the cerebral arteries cause infarction of brain tissue. **Thromboses** are blood clots that develop on walls of atherosclerotic vessels, particularly in the carotid arteries. These clots take time to form, and some warning may precede the occlusion of the vessel. The person may experience blindness in one eye, difficulty in speaking, or a generalized state of confusion. When the cerebral blood vessel is completely blocked, the individual may lose consciousness.

An **embolism** is a traveling clot that may suddenly occlude a blood vessel and cause ischemia. The embolism is most frequently a clot from the heart, aorta, or carotid artery, but it can travel from another part of the body, such as the deep veins of the leg. Consciousness may be lost suddenly. When this event occurs, tissue plasminogen activator (TPA), called a "clot buster," may be used to dissolve clots and restore blood flow in occluded vessels. However, if TPA is given in hemorrhagic cases of **cerebrovascular accidents (CVAs)**, intracranial bleeding and increasing pressure would continue, and the individual could die. Crucial decisions must be made in acute cases, and because most cerebrovascular accidents are of the ischemic form, TPA is a reliable and available agent for the physician.

The site and extent of the brain damage, regardless of its cause, determines the outcome for the patient. Gradually consciousness is regained, but immediately after the **stroke**, speech is often impaired. Loss of speech, or **aphasia**, is normally temporary but may require therapy to assist in a full recovery.

Damage to the motor nerves at the point passing down the spinal cord causes weakness **(paresis)** or paralysis on the side of the body opposite the brain lesion due to the crossover of nerve tracts in the brain stem. Paralysis on one side of the body is referred to as **hemiplegia**.

Various procedures make it possible to determine the site of blockage in a cerebral blood vessel. Angiography, a process in which radiopaque material is injected into cerebral arteries, allows x-rays to locate the lesion.

A blockage in a carotid artery can be treated surgically. **Endarterectomy**, the more common procedure, removes the thickened area of the inner vascular lining. Carotid bypass surgery removes the blocked vascular segment, and a graft is inserted to allow blood flow to the brain. Other vascular replacement may be done in other areas like the inferior aorta to reduce the risk of hemorrhage.

## Transient Ischemic Attack

Transient ischemic attacks (TIAs) are caused by brief but critical periods of reduced blood flow in a cerebral artery. TIAs may be thought of as "mini" strokes resulting from blood clots occluding vessels or vessel spasms that interrupt blood flow and thus impair neurological functioning. The individual may lose feeling in the face or extremity or have tingling sensations for a brief time. Factors influencing the constrictions are similar to CVA, and with prior TIAs there is a ten-fold chance of a stroke. Reduced flow may be due to an atherosclerotic narrowing of the blood vessel or to small emboli that temporarily lodge in the vessel. The attacks may last less than a minute or two or up to several hours, with the average attack lasting 15 minutes. Manifestations are often abrupt and can include visual disturbances, transient hemiparesis (muscular weakness on one side), or sensory loss on one side. Lips and tongue may become numb, causing slurred speech. Multiple TIAs often precede a complete stroke and may serve as warning of a cerebral vascular disturbance. Further diagnostic testing, such as a cerebral angiogram or CT scan, may be indicated. Prevention of a TIA is uncertain, but their occurrence may alert the person to see a doctor and prevent further damage caused by a full-scale stroke by taking "blood thinning" medications.

## ▶ Traumatic Disorders

## Concussion of the Brain

A **concussion** is a transient disorder of the nervous system resulting from a violent blow to the head or a fall. The person typically loses consciousness and cannot remember the events of the occurrence. Although the brain may not actually be damaged, the whole body is affected; the pulse rate is weak, and when consciousness is regained, the person may experience nausea and dizziness. A severe headache may follow, and the person should be watched closely, since a coma may ensue, and that could be life threatening.

Every year about 1.5 million trauma brain injuries (TBIs) occur, and concussions, occurring at over 300,000 per year, are a major contributing form. About 50,000 TBI victims die per year, and TBI is a leading cause of death for those under age 45. However, concussions account for only about 1.5 deaths per year in the United States. There are many causes of concussion, from falling, vehicle accidents, and sports injuries to firearms accidents.

A person suffering from a concussion should be kept quiet, and drugs that stimulate or depress the nervous system, such as painkillers, are contraindicated. The condition usually corrects itself with time and rest. Prevention is difficult because of the unpredictability of some situations, but vehicular accident-related concussions are down due to use of seatbelts and child car seats and helmet laws for bicycle riding.

## Contusion

In a **contusion**, there is an injury, a bruise, to brain tissue even though the skin at the site of the trauma may not be broken, as it is in a skull fracture. The brain injury may be on the side of the impact or on the opposite side, where the brain is forced against the skull. Blood from broken blood vessels may accumulate in the brain, causing swelling and pain. The blood clots and necrotic tissue form and could block the flow of CFS, causing a form of hydrocephalus.

Efforts must be made to reduce intracranial pressure, and surgery may be necessary to alleviate pressure and to remove clotted blood areas. Simple pain reduction measures, such as ice packs, may help until professional help arrives. Along with observation, rest will be necessary for full recovery, although some pain medications may be prescribed if needed.

## Skull Fractures

The most serious complication of a skull fracture is damage to the brain. A fracture at the base of the skull is likely to affect vital centers in the brain stem. The pressure that increases due to accumulation of CSF or blood must be reduced by medications like mannitol. Another danger of skull fractures is that bacteria may be able to directly access the brain.

## Hemorrhages

Hemorrhages can occur in the meninges, causing blood to accumulate between the brain and the skull. A severe injury to the temple can cause an artery just inside the skull to rupture. The blood then flows between the dura mater and the skull; this is known as an **extradural** or **epidural** hemorrhage (Figure 13–11▶). The increased pressure of the blood causes the patient to lose consciousness. Surgery is required immediately to seal off the bleeding vessel and remove the blood. No blood would be found in a lumbar puncture because the blood accumulation is outside the dura mater.

A hemorrhage under the dura mater, a **subdural** hemorrhage or hematoma (Figure 13–12▶), is a rupture of a cranial vein, or the large venous sinuses of the brain, rather than an artery. This breach may occur from a severe blow to the front or back of the head. The blood clots and CSF accumulates in a cystlike formation. Intracranial pressure increases, but the cerebral symptoms may not develop for a time. Subdural hemorrhages are sometimes chronic occurrences in cases of alcoholic abuse (due to

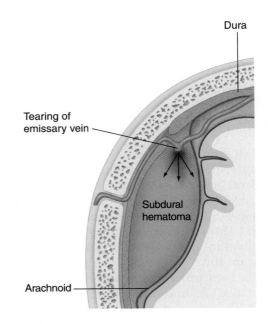

Figure 13–12 ▶ Subdural hematoma.

falling accidents) and in battered or violently abused individuals.

The surface membrane of the brain may be torn by a skull fracture, causing a **subarachnoid** hemorrhage. Blood flows into the subarachnoid space, where CSF circulates. Blood is found in the CSF with a lumbar puncture. Rupture of an aneurysm can also cause a subarachnoid hemorrhage.

Many hemorrhages are accidental and unpredictable. Therefore, prevention is not easy to project, but prior symptoms may be used as indicators to reduce occurrences.

## ▶ Brain Tumors

Tumors of the brain may be malignant or benign. Because benign tumors may grow and compress vital nerve centers, they are considered serious growths. Benign tumors are usually encapsulated, and they can be completely removed surgically. Malignant tumors have extensive roots and are extremely difficult or impossible to remove in their entirety. Most malignant tumors of the brain are metastatic from other organs, especially the lung and breast.

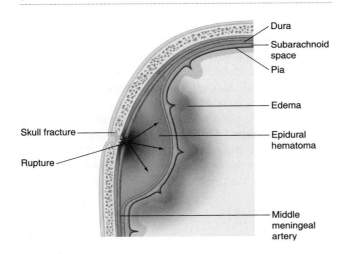

Figure 13–11 ▶ Extradural hematoma.

Primary malignant tumors of the brain are called **gliomas**, tumors of the glial cells that support nerve tissue rather than growths of the neurons themselves.

Brain tumors manifest themselves in different ways depending on the site and growth rate of the tumor. **Astrocytomas** are basically benign, slow-growing tumors. **Glioblastomas** multiforma are highly malignant, rapidly growing tumors. Brain function is affected by the increased intracranial pressure. Mannitol, corticosteroids, and cranial shunts help relieve those pressure symptoms. Blood supply to an area of the brain may be reduced by an infiltrating tumor or by edema, and that causes dysfunctional activity as well as causing the tissue to become necrotic.

Symptoms of brain tumors typically include a severe headache because of the increased pressure of the tumor. Personality changes, loss of memory, or development of poor judgment may give further evidence of a brain tumor. Visual disturbances, double vision, or partial blindness often occur, and the ability to speak may be impaired. An upright person may be unsteady while standing or become drowsy. Seizures often develop and may progress into a coma.

Diagnostic measures include MRI and CT scans plus a full array of skull x-rays. Treatment depends on growth type and location. When possible, surgery (see Chapter 4) is followed by radiation and/or chemotherapy. Radiosurgery uses a gamma knife, and the radiation is beamed through designated holes in a helmet that directs the radiation specifically to the target. A limitation of gamma knife surgery is that a special nuclear facility is required for this procedure.

## ▶ Cranial Nerve Disease

## Trigeminal Neuralgia

Any one of the twelve pairs of cranial nerves may be subject to impairment. Individual cranial nerves may be affected by degeneration or unknown causes and thus involved with various ailments. The fifth (V) cranial nerve, or trigeminal nerve, may become inflamed, causing severe intermittent pain, usually on one side of

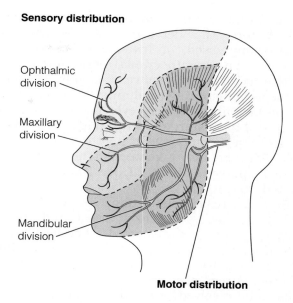

**Sensory distribution**

Ophthalmic division

Maxillary division

Mandibular division

**Motor distribution**

**Figure 13–13** ▶ Sensory and motor distribution of the trigeminal nerve. There are three sensory divisions: opthalmic, maxillary, and mandibular.

the face. This condition, known as trigeminal neuralgia or *tic doulourex,* affects 1 individual per 25,000 (Figure 13–13▶). The cause of *tic doulourex* is often idiopathic but may be caused by stress, tumors compressing the nerve, or, in young individuals, may be an indication of multiple sclerosis barring other neurological signs. Those affected are usually age 40 or older and complain of severe pain, especially around the oral cavity (the tongue, lips, and gums). This recurring pain may or may not respond readily to pain medication. Anticonvulsive agents like phenytoin or valproate, and baclofen for muscle spasm, are generally prescribed. In very severe and resistant cases, drugs or agents like alcohol or phenol may be injected directly into the nerve as it exits the skull to reduce the pain, or surgery may be required to cut sensory root elements and give relief in a procedure called **rhizotomy**.

## Bell's Palsy

Bell's palsy involves the inflammation of the seventh (VII) cranial nerve, or facial nerve. The etiology is usually unknown, but viruses, autoimmunity, and vascular ischemia are probable factors. This nerve may also be traumatized, compressed, or invaded by pathogens. Because the seventh cranial nerve innervates facial muscles and salivary glands, attacks cause sagging of the facial muscles on one side of the face and a watery eye. The person may drool and have slurred speech (Figure 13–14 ▶). In these cases, massage or heat treatment may help. Recovery may take weeks. The occurrence of Bell's palsy is about 23 per 100,000 in the United States.

Some corticoid medications like prednisone or antiviral agents (acyclovir) are given if herpes simplex I (HSVI) is suspected. Therefore, relief of symptoms may not always be quick or simple. Bell's palsy is rare in children. Usually it strikes between ages 25 and 50. If the situation fails to be resolved, a facial contracture develops. The prognosis is generally good, although complete healing may take many months to a year.

**Figure 13–14** ▶ Bell's palsy, showing typical drooping of one side of the face. (NIH/Phototake NYC)

## ▶ Pain

Pain and pain perception are integral parts of nervous system function. In this section, we will discuss the following:

- Definition of pain
- The function or purpose of pain
- Types and characteristics of pain
- The physiology of pain
- Pain assessment
- Pain management
- Other methods of pain control

Pain means different things to different individuals. Pain includes a major degree of perception and therefore is subjective. This symptom requires a level of threshold and therefore acts as a gauge of tolerance, plus learned behaviors, that rely on past experience and culture. Threshold accounts for the initial level of pain that an individual acknowledges, while tolerance suggests the point at which the same individual requires treatment in dealing with the pain. Thus, pain may be thought of as an individualistic occurrence.

In neurophysiology, pain is described as a result of some form of tissue damage. However, this simple definition does not account for emotional pain or pain resulting from some functional disorders. When physical breakdowns or lesions are apparent, it is easier to ascertain an accompanying pain criterion. Functional disparities are not always found or determined through superficial observation (e.g., a microscope), but many forms of psychogenic pain are well recognized and treated.

Regardless of definition, perception, or understanding, pain is a sensation of hurt or a strong discomfort, typically from some form of noxious stimulus. Therefore, pain is caused by injury or disease and transmitted throughout the body to associated cortical areas in the brain for interpretation and prospective recourse.

Pain does have a purpose and function. Its primary purpose is to warn the person of an abnormal state, like inflammation, infection, body trauma, or injury. Second, it is a signal not to pursue any activity that causes additional pain and thus may cause any more damage. This pause will assist the healing process by allowing the body to rest and conserve resources for recovery and homeostasis. Pain is considered the most common cause that forces individuals to the doctor's office or health treatment center.

There is a rare alternative to pain sensation, known as "congenital insensitivity to pain," found in individuals who are born without a sense of pain. In these cases, the nervous system is not equipped to instruct the person about injurious conditions or accidents and may allow continual walking on broken limbs or permit advanced infections to go untreated. There is a natural reluctance to pain, but without it life may be less safe.

## Categories and Characteristics of Pain

Various categories of pain usually refer to origination or duration. The pain origin includes areas such as cutaneous (skin), somatic (body), visceral (organ), neuropathic, or referred (redirected site). Somatic pain involves blood vessels, nerves, muscles, and joints (e.g., sprained ankle), while cutaneous pain may emanate from a pinprick or sunburn. Visceral pain may be diffuse or poorly localized. In the case of appendicitis, pain is referred to the surface of the right lower quadrant of the abdomen, even though the problem is internal. (See Table 13–1 ▶.)

Neuropathic pain may not be caused by a commonly held noxious agent but tends to be delayed and induce a generalized burning sensation and occasionally stabbing pain, as found in the legs of some diabetics.

Pain duration is acute (immediate) or chronic. Acute pain has a relatively short time of activity (e.g., within 6 months), whereas chronic pain exceeds the 6-month time frame and may last for years. Severity and specific descriptions, like pounding, throbbing, and sharp or dull, help to qualify the situation as well.

Pain importance may be ascribed to the fact that pain receptors (**nociceptors**) are the most abundant sensory receptor in the skin; there are as many as 1300 per square inch. Compared to touch or thermal receptors, pain reception is

| Table 13–1 ▶ | Body Regional Pain |
|---|---|
| **Body Region** | **Pain Manifestations** |
| Cranial | Headache—common, migraine<br>Oral—toothache, canker sore<br>Facial—Bell's palsy |
| Cervical—neck | Whiplash—may become chronic pain |
| Torso | Chest—heart pain, lung<br>Abdominal—gastric (e.g., ulcer)<br>Appendix, gallbladder—stones<br>Lumbar—Lower back, pinched nerve<br>Pelvic—ovary, urinary bladder |
| Extremities—limbs | Muscle and joint pain (e.g., arthritis) |

scattered around to insure basic protection and homeostatic balance. Nociceptors consists of free nerve ending elements (not encapsulated) attached to a sensory neuron. Pain receptors are found in the viscera, or internal organs, as well, as noted by gas pains or gastric burning sensations, and in the muscles and joints.

## Physiology of Pain

Pain, like other sensations and actions, is interpreted and delegated to the brain cortex. Different areas known as cerebral lobes interpret and inform the individual as to various sensations (e.g., sound is interpreted by the temporal lobe). In addition to body location, type and degree of a particular pain stimulus; it is primarily registered in the parietal lobe. In addition, the thalamus, which is known as a major sensory relay center, helps discriminate rudimentary sensations and their location and subsequently relays its input to the respective cerebral lobe. The hypothalamus responds to coping mechanisms, as does the medulla oblongata. The well-recognized "fight or flight" response induces the adrenal cortex to release corticosteroids for endurance.

At the same time, the adrenal medulla releases epinephrine to heighten cardiovascular and respiratory responses in preparation for escape or elevated alertness. These acts of awareness are most valuable when facing fear or major injury and are also coordinated with the brain stem (medulla oblongata and pons), known as the vitals center.

## Pain Theory Concept

The most commonly supported theory by which pain is exhibited is called the gate control theory. It begins with a primary afferent nociceptor complex that has three levels of design and thus influences their role in when, where, and how pain might be dispensed, if at all. The primary differences are in the size or diameter of the neuronal fibers and if they are insulated with myelin or unmyelinated and thus cause a variance in the conduction velocity of their impulse. The largest-diameter fiber type is the A-beta form, which responds to light touch in the skin primarily and therefore normally does not cause a pain response. The small-diameter myelined A-delta and unmyelinated C fibers are found in nerves of the skin and deeper somatic (body) and visceral structures. These fibers are missing in individuals with congenital insensitivity to pain. Some designated areas, like the cornea, have only A-delta and C fiber neurons because they respond maximally only to intense and painful stimuli. For the most part, primary afferent nociceptors respond to heat and intense mechanical stimuli (e.g., pinching and noxious or irritating chemicals). When these fibers are blocked from responding, then no pain sensation is expressed.

The gate control theory holds that pain impulses are transmitted from specialized nociceptors within the skin, muscle, or joints to the spinal cord. These impulses are carried by large A and small C fibers to a specialized area within the superior horn of the spinal cord known as the substantia gelatinosa. This area acts as a gate that regulates transmission for impulses to the CNS. Stimulation of the larger fibers (A) causes cells within substantia gelatinosa to "close the gate" and therefore diminish pain per-

ception. The smaller fiber elements (C) do the reverse and thus enhance pain perception. Depending on the degree of opening and closing, the CNS regulates pain output. Similarly, the thalamus, functioning as a relay station, tends to delegate or transmit some pain activity and alternately inhibit other pain transmission. The quick-acting myelinated large nerve fibers (A) tend to carry impulses for well-localized, sharp pain, while the unmyelinated C fibers carry sensations more slowly, as in a diffuse burning or aching feeling. (See Figure 13–15▶.) Note that amplified or continual outside impulses would interfere with pain input, as when we bang our head against a wall or pound our fist; the force of the activity delays or diverts the pain sensation.

Another concept, known as the nociceptor pain process, extends the gate control theory. It consists of four primary features: *transduction, transmission, reception of pain,* and *modulation;* these will be discussed here. These features parallel physiological nerve conduction operations.

In transduction, the nociceptors distinguish among the various stimuli as to noxious or harmful versus innocuous inputs. Transduction also converts the noxious stimuli into sensory nerve ending impulses to the spinal cord and basically describes how pain is perceived by the body. Transmission is the movement of the transduced stimuli into impulses that ascend up the spinal cord to the brain stem and thalamus. From here the dispatched impulse proceeds to the proper cortical lobe or area (e.g., parietal lobe) for pain interpretation. Some impulses may be challenged or blocked from relay as well. Perception of pain means the sensation has become a conscious feeling. The overall perception and response process is not well understood, especially among different individuals. Again the reminder here is that pain is an individual-type sensation. Modulation is the manipulation that the brain imposes on signals to modify or inhibit pain impulses. In this case, the brain naturally releases compounds that produce relief (analgesia) called **endorphins** and **enkephalins**. These compounds are often referred to in the case of marathon runners who feel a sense of euphoria miles into a race. Both of the prevailing concepts of pain attempt to in-

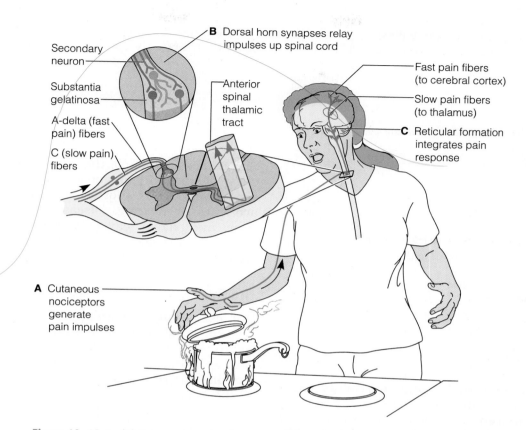

**Secondary neuron**

**Substantia gelatinosa**

**A-delta (fast pain) fibers**

**C (slow pain) fibers**

**B** Dorsal horn synapses relay impulses up spinal cord

Anterior spinal thalamic tract

Fast pain fibers (to cerebral cortex)

Slow pain fibers (to thalamus)

**C** Reticular formation integrates pain response

**A** Cutaneous nociceptors generate pain impulses

**Figure 13–15** ▶ (A) Cutaneous nociceptors generate pain impulses that travel via A-delta and C fibers to the spinal cord's dorsal horn. (B) Secondary neurons in dorsal horn pass impulses across spinal cord to anterior spinothalamic tract. C, Slow pain impulses ascend to the thalamus, while fast pain impulses ascend to the cerebral cortex. The reticular formation in the brainstem integrates the emotional, cognitive, and autonomic responses to pain.

corporate basic neurological processes or principles with a means to envision a mechanism for interpretation and control.

## Pain Assessment and Management

The most reliable indicator of the presence and degree of pain is reported by the person experiencing it. Pain must also be assessed. During the assessment process, there are a variety of considerations: language barriers, children and developmental stage, and those with hearing limitations or who are intubated. A variety of tools are used to assess pain. These tools include simple pictorial or numeric scales or mnemonics that can help convey vital information from the patient to the healthcare assistant or clinician (Figure 13–16▶). Culture, age, and past experience with pain can also influence assessment findings.

Chronic pain causes fatigue and interferes with the routines of working, eating, sleeping, and concentrating. In the case of cancer, chronic pain may become the central concern. The cancer may become secondary to pain for some stricken individuals, because it may be exacerbated by treatment and fear. Cancer-related pain can be acute or chronic, but accurate assessment of pain is essential as it influences treatment. Counseling and group therapy may

**Figure 13–16** ► Examples of commonly used pain scales.

help relieve some anxiety and uncertainty, especially in cases of little or no family support.

Pain management depends on a number of variables, but the focus is to control pain without serious side effects. Over-the-counter (OTC) drugs and prescription forms such as opiates are often needed to treat acute or chronic pain. See Table 13–2► for a summary of alternative treatments.

The body has its own endogenous opioid agents, called **endorphins** or **enkephalins**, to counteract pain-causing symptoms such as induced by substance P, an agent that is thought to be released from a pain source. However, it is the OTC and prescription medications that tend to act on a specific target. Aspirin is a widely used drug; others include NSAIDs, like acetaminophen (Tylenol), ibuprofen (Advil), or naproxsyn (Aleve), all of which work to reduce or stop pain primarily in the PNS. Opiates or narcotic-type drugs work best in the CNS by blocking or interfering with pain receptors or pathways (e.g., OxyContin or Roxicet). Chronic pain requires stronger remedies like morphine for surgical wounds and Demerol for birth labor or persistent headache. The drug Fentanyl is currently considered the best agent to fight

chronic pain, but because it depresses the respiratory system, its use is closely monitored.

## ► Diseases of Special Senses: Eye and Ear

Special senses include the nose for olfaction or sense of smell; the tongue for gustatory or taste sensations; the eyes for vision; and the ears for acoustics or hearing. Diseases related to the nose and nasal cavity were discussed in Chapter 8; diseases of the eye and ear are covered in the sections that follow.

### The Eye

Our discussion starts with protective coverings of the eye, called eyelids and associate glands, and continues to the eye surface or conjunctiva; the clear area known as the cornea; the photoreceptors and the retina; and the optic nerve (Figure 13–17►). The ear disorders will also be covered from the external to internal components.

*Eyelids and Associate Glands*   One of the most noticeable lesions found on the eyelid is the common **stye** or **hordeolum**. This reddish tender lump is caused by a local staphylococcus abscess on the upper or lower lid. Smaller styes tend to be external to the lid surface and on the margin, while internal styes tend to jut toward the eye surface. Sometimes they resolve themselves, but when the lesion is large enough to cause irritation or a reduced field of vision, treatment is required. A warm compress or application of bacitracin ointment usually resolves the situation. Because of oversight or lack of attention, these common bumps tend to recur, especially in youngsters.

Similar to the stye is a hardened internal lesion called a **chalazion**. This inflammation impacts a deeper oil gland (**meibomian**) and feels tender and irritated. The oil secreted by the meibomian gland is necessary to prevent the watery tear fluid from evaporating. When the oil is absent, a dry eye develops, which causes pain and potential for a coarse scleral and corneal sur-

| Table 13–2  ▶  **Alternative Pain Therapies** | |
| --- | --- |
| **Therapy** | **Methodology** |
| Acupuncture | Ancient Eastern method may stimulate release of endorphins |
| Aromatherapy | Oils and scents along with bath or massage |
| Biofeedback therapy | Electrothermal devices plus training for pain (e.g., migraine) |
| Heat and cold packs | Traumas such as sprains and burns |
| Humor | Acts as a distraction and comfort, at least temporarily |
| Hypnosis | Extends pain relief or blocks pain perception |
| Imagery | Induces relaxation; may induce endorphins and reduce stress |
| Massage | Promotes muscle relaxation and blood flow for comfort |
| Music and art | Provide soothing atmosphere in clinics and help to calm patient fears |
| Relaxation techniques | Reduce muscle tension and increase pain threshold; reflexology is an example |
| Transcutaneous electrical nerve stimulation (TENS) | Electrical stimulation through skin patches to interfere with pain release and timing activities |
| Transcendental meditation (TM) | Solitary introspection for calming relaxation |
| Yoga | Body manipulation, mind relaxation, and mind control technique |

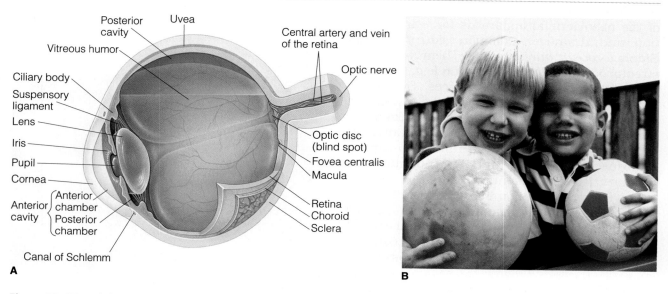

**Figure 13–17** ▶ (A) Human eye anatomy and (B) normal vision image. (National Eye Institute)

face or superficial cracks. As in cases of exoph-thalmia, found in Graves' disease (Chapter 12), eye drops like Restasis (cyclosporine in a castor oil base) help relieve the dryness. When given extended, albeit untreated, time, the condition may resolve itself, but hot compresses normally help, with a gentle message, repeated twice daily for best results. If the condition does not improve, vision may be impaired and a corticos-teroid injection may be needed or the cyst may need to be lanced to let it drain. Once resolved, the problem seems to subside, and with in-creased awareness the occurrence is reduced.

**Blepharitis** is a common chronic inflammation, with or without ulcers, often involving both eyelid margins and perhaps becoming bilateral (occur-ring in both eyes). This bacterially initiated prob-lem resembles seborrhea of the scalp and eye-brows or perhaps acne rosacea (see Chapter 16). Itching and burning sensations are due to oozing pus, and a thick crust develops, especially after sleep. The potential for ulceration of the cornea is serious, and treatment is warranted. Antibiotic ointment like bacitracin plus polymixin B or sul-facetamide may be used for known microbe types, and if other skin conditions are factors, they should be addressed as well. Preventive measures include good hygiene, with consis-tency, and proper training to keep hands away from nose, mouth, and especially eyes.

**Dacryocystitis** is an infection and obstruction of the nasolacrimal apparatus for tear produc-tion and drainage. Common skin flora like *Staphylococcus aureus* or the beta version of streptococcus and yeast infection (e.g., *Candida albicans*) are all potential sources. Symptoms include swelling, tenderness, and pain. If chronic, tearing and pus discharge are cause for surgical relief, and antibiotics may continue, al-though they may have been unable to dry up the ducting network initially. Spontaneous healing can occur in some patients.

Prevention of common infectious conditions is achieved through hygiene and retraining of old habits, like unnecessary finger and hand contact with the eye. If known allergies are recognized, they must be avoided or eliminated if possible.

*Conjunctivitis* Conjunctivitis is an inflammation of the conjunctiva, the superficial covering of the visible sclera (white of the eye) and the inner lin-ings of the eyelids. Red, swollen eyes with dis-charge and some discomfort are the usual symp-toms. About 30% of all eye complaints are for conjunctivitis, commonly called "pink eye," yet many cases go unreported, and children are the primary source group.

Various fumes, such as from peeled onions or bathroom cleansers, may initiate an inflamma-tory or basically allergic response. However, viruses and various bacteria, including the nor-mal bacterial flora such as *Staphylococcus au-reus,* or fungi commonly cause conjunctivitis. Unfortunately, these viral and bacterial infec-tions are quite contagious, and therefore pa-tients, usually children, are instructed to stay home from school or social activities. Reinfec-tions may occur due to lack of hygiene and to rubbing or touching the eye unnecessarily. Often the inflammation subsides on its own ac-cord, but it may progress into *inclusion conjunc-tivitis,* which is caused by particular bacteria (e.g., *Chlamydia trachomatis*) and is longer last-ing. For diagnosis and determination of infective agents, ocular swabs or scrapings are taken to culture and suggest favorable antidotes. Topical antibiotics or eye drops, such as sulfonamides (even in viral cases, to prevent secondary infec-tion) or antihistamines and cold compresses help control the "pink eye." See Figure 13–18►.

Chronic conjunctivitis, or **trachoma**, results when the infecting agent invades the **conjunc-**

Figure 13–18 ► Conjunctivitis. (©Dorling Kindersley)

**tiva.** These cases tend to be highly contagious and when severe may disrupt the corneal surface and impair vision. The infective agent in this case is *Chlamydia trachomatis,* mentioned previously, the same organism responsible for the STD chlamydia (chapter 11). Infected mothers pass on this infection to the newborn. An erythromycin ointment or tetracycline is usually administered to resolve trachoma.

Prevention of conjunctivitis is best achieved by reducing hand to eye contact, disposing of contaminated materials such as contact lenses and beauty products (e.g., mascara), and avoiding known allergic agents or persons with conjunctivitis.

*Glaucoma*  Glaucoma is an insidious, painless disease that typically results from pressure building up in the anterior chamber of the eye or the space in front of the lens. This condition is known as chronic glaucoma and will be discussed here; however, there is acute glaucoma, which is accompanied by intense pain and blurriness. In acute cases intraocular pressure must be relieved immediately to reduce pain and to save vision.

The aqueous humor made by the ciliary body apparatus is produced at a fairly constant rate and normally drains away. But in glaucoma, fluid accumulates and increases pressure within the eye. Pressure exceeding twice the normal intraocular pressure (8–21 mm Hg) causes the retina to start losing its ability to distinguish images clearly. This progression of events continues until a partial to total blindness develops. Peripheral vision is severely reduced if the condition is untreated; then it is lost, and "tunnel vision" ensues as the photoreceptors on the retina are destroyed and continue to deteriorate visual quality (eyesight) (Figure 13–19▶).

A glaucoma gene, GLCA1 on chromosome 1, may account for 10% of the 80,000 to 100,000 new cases per year in the United States. Worldwide, glaucoma affects about 66.8 million individuals. Most congenital glaucoma is hereditary, while secondary glaucoma is caused by systemic diseases, such as infections, or drugs like corticosteroids. The incidence of glaucoma among black Americans is four times that of white Americans. This disease affects nearly 2% of the population over age 35, or about 3 million

**Figure 13–19** ▶ Glaucoma visual image reveals tunnel vision. (National Eye Institute)

persons in the United States. In Southeast Asia glaucoma is quite common, considering a host of tropical infections and lack of treatment. Individuals with a family history or with diabetes should have frequent eye checkups.

The ophthalmoscope is the primary portable tool used by the optical agent to view the interior of the eyeball for general inspection. However, to diagnose glaucoma, a noncontact ("airpuff") **tonometer** helps to screen for the disease by bouncing a puff of air off the cornea that flattens it slightly and allows a quick register of intraocular pressure. After first using numbing droplets on the eye, a more accurate measurement is done with **applanation tonometry**, which allows the instrument to touch the cornea lightly. The pressure required to indent the corneal surface is measured, and using a slit lamp (magnifying) device allows the ophthalmologist to explore the whole interior of the eye with bright light and get a three-dimensional view. In this case, the lighted interior tends to show a cupping of the optic disc, where the optic nerve enters the back of the eye.

Drugs like timolol reduce fluid production, and pilocarpine promotes aqueous humor flow. Surgery involves piercing the anterior chamber with a laser, which promotes draining and reduction in pressure and improves vision. Prevention is basically genetically determined but includes a healthy diet with adequate intake of vitamin A, and good vision care (e.g., reducing infections via limited hand–eye contact, and wearing eye protection such as sunglasses).

*Uveitis* The uvea is the second layer of the eye known as the vascular or pigmented layer and includes the ciliary body and the colored part of the eye known as the iris. Inflammation of the uvea may be caused by infectious agents, especially in reduced immune conditions, but uveitis itself has an immunological or neoplastic basis. Symptoms include pain, redness, photophobia, and blurred vision. Depending on if the inflammatory attack is in front of the lens (anterior) or behind it (posterior), different approaches are taken to insure the best outcome. Anterior inflammation accounts for about 90% of the cases and usually lends itself to topical corticosteroids. Posterior uveitis requires systemic (internal) medications or intravitreal (in uvea) corticosteroid therapy, and if bacterial agents are present, then the appropriate antibiotics would be used. This primarily immune disorder is related to or accompanies many other conditions or diseases, from psoriasis to Crohn's disease. Prevalence is estimated at 8 per 100,000, with approximately 38,000 new cases per year in the United States.

### Light and Refractory Distortions

**Astigmatism** Light enters the clear curved cornea. If the cornea is pitted from prior ulceration or is unsymmetrical or has thick and thin sections, it would transmit light to the lens and retina in irregular wavelengths. Similarly, if the lens is warped or irregular, the transmitted light is uneven. Both scenarios give a blurry or unclear image when the light (image) strikes the retinal surface. This refractory condition is called **astigmatism**. It may be associated with any other eye condition, like myopia, and may affect one eye or both. The objects viewed might be basically recognizable, but there is always some degree of distortion to the overall image. Corrective lenses, including contact lenses, help but may

not fully repair the condition, especially if the irregularities are with the internal lens. Cornea adjustments may be made surgically, or the lens could be replaced. Most individuals tend to ignore the minor deficiency and adjust to it.

***Myopia and Hyperopia (Nearsightedness and Farsightedness)*** The more common types of eye problems involve distance. An acuity test done by the famous Snellen chart (E letters) allows determination of a 20/20 (normal) or a range from 20/200 to 20/10 reading for different distance levels. Nearsightedness, or **myopia**, and farsightedness, or **hyperopia**, as well as astigmatism, described earlier, are outlined in Figure 13–20▶.

Compared to normal vision, myopia or nearsightedness is noticed when close objects are clear and sharp while more distance objects are blurred. The eyeball is longer than normal, so the image falls short (thus the term *short/near sightedness*) and does not reach the retina sufficiently, leaving a blurry image. It may be that the lens is too thick and thus the image would fall in front of the retina. To correct myopia, a concave lens is required to stretch incoming light rays to reach the retina and give a clear picture. Approximately 70 million adult Americans have myopia.

In the case of hyperopia, objects at a distance are clear, but those images close up are blurry. About 1 in 4 Americans share this disorder, or almost 61 million people. The eyeball appears too short, or a lens may be too thin. A convex lens is required to bend the light waves more quickly or shorter to strike the retina in a clearly focused fashion. Contact lenses work well, and laser treatments may shave layers off the cornea or lens to improve sight. LASIK surgery, a type of cornea surgery, holds great promise for long-term relief. LASIK surgery eliminates or reduces use of eyeglasses or contact lenses for most normal activities requiring near- or far-sighted vision. For some tasks, reading glasses may still be required. With either case, astigmatism may be an additional part of the visual correction, and that would require a special lens or glasses to offer a sharper image at the retinal surface. The astigmatism may be in one or both eyes and be of varying degree.

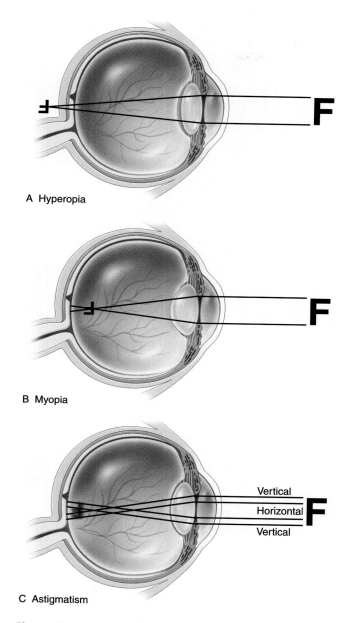

A Hyperopia

B Myopia

Vertical
Horizontal
Vertical

C Astigmatism

**Figure 13–20** ► In hyperopia light rays focus behind the retina, making it difficult to focus on objects at close range. In myopia light rays focus in front of the retina, making it difficult to focus on objects that are far away. In astigmatism light rays do not uniformly focus on the eye due to abnormal curvature of cornea or lens.

***Presbyopia*** Presbyopia is an age-related and refractive disorder. About 1 per 11 or 9% of Americans have this condition. At about age 45, the crystalline lens of the eye loses its flexibility and causes a reduction in the ability to focus images on the retina. This may happen rather suddenly, but the lens has been growing from birth and continues to grow throughout life, so by the time of death the lens has increased in weight by about four times. This change is a normal modification to the eye due to aging, and individuals notice the problem when they hold pictures and written material at arm's length to get a better view. Optometrists can fit corrective lens like bi- or trifocals or contact lenses for better vision. Because things continue to change, so must the corrective lenses.

***Cataracts*** **Cataracts** are the result of a clouding of the lens. There are three types of cataracts that correspond to the three layers of the lens. The outer layer is a clear membrane or capsule, the middle zone is composed of soft clear material called the cortex, and the core is the least flexible site called the nucleus. The cause of cataracts is not known, but they have been attributed to a congenital defect, eye trauma, the effects of toxins, and aging. The main symptom is fading and distortion of vision. Additional lighting is useful early on, especially for printed material, and this helps clue the person as to an impending visual impairment.

By age 65, almost half of all Americans have some degree of cataracts and thus impaired vision, and after age 75 the figure is close to 70%. Usually by the eighth decade, cataracts have become more evident or ripe. A routine (general) eye exam, using ophthalmoscopy, normally detects early stages of cataracts. This detection allows planning for treatment if needed or preventative measures to reduce the progression of cataract development, such as avoiding bright light and wearing sunglasses. A new measuring device called an **aberrometer** allows a better record of the status of the eye and assists the preparation of LASIK surgery to match or exceed what glasses or contact lenses do for sight. The patient looks at a pattern of faint red lights, and the machine makes detailed optical measurements as it inspects the interior of the eyeball. This procedure is simple, painless, and is done in the doctor's office. In the past, treatment was usually nonspecific or withheld, and with time the lens was surgically replaced. Outpatient surgery for lens replacement including lenses for 20/20 vision or bifocals, has become a routine procedure, and vision is restored to normal in patients 95% of the time. Prevention is almost impossible for an age-related condition or in the face of a concurrent disease (e.g., diabetes or syphilis). However, avoiding harmful drugs or chemicals and direct sunlight can postpone this common disorder. (See Figure 13–21 ▶.)

### Retinal Image Defects

**Macular Degeneration**   Macular degeneration is the reduction or loss of acute vision. Macular degeneration develops in 10% of the elderly and affects both eyes, affecting only central vision and leaving peripheral vision intact. There are two forms of macular degeneration: the atrophic (dry) version, comprising 70+% of the cases, and the exudative (wet, hemorrhagic) type, a more destructive version. (See Figure 13–22 ▶.)

Causes for this degeneration are not well understood, but it is known that obstructed blood flow, followed by revascularization (as occurs in atherosclerosis), compromises the area of the

Figure 13–22 ▶ Age-related macular degeneration demonstrating loss of central vision. (National Eye Institute)

retina responsible for acute vision. Other contributing factors are injury, inflammation, infection, and heredity.

Diagnosis is by direct eye exam with ophthalmascope and fluorescein angiography, which reveal leaking vessels in the subretinal area. There is no cure for the atrophic case, but 5% to 10% reduction in the exudative condition can be accomplished by using an argon laser to cause photocoagulation.

**Diabetic Retinopathy**   About 40% of the diabetes type 1 patients will be diagnosed with diabetic retinopathy (DR) within 3 years of diabetes diagnosis. Depending on the intensity of the diabetes and patient's age, it may be a mild abnormality or a major factor causing loss of eye sight. It is the leading cause of new blindness in adults aged 20 to 65; as diabetes diagnoses continue to rise in the United States, related diseases will increase as well. In type 2 diabetes, about 20% of the cases have DR at the time of diagnosis. Screening involves dilated pupils and ophthalmoscopy, which may become routine annual

Figure 13–21 ▶ Cataracts show the whole image as blurry. (National Eye Institute)

events with eye checkups. Special attention must be given to those pregnant or attempting to become pregnant. This monitoring is done primarily through diabetes control measures, like blood glucose levels, and kidney functioning plus blood pressure measurements. In exudative cases, leakage can be abated by using an argon laser to cause photocoagulation. Prevention is unlikely considering the universal effect over the body that diabetes mellitus presents.

***Retinitis Pigmentosa*** Retinititis pigmentosa is a genetic disease either as a recessive or dominant trait on the X chromosome. Other forms may exist, but it is a rare, progressive retina degeneration that eventually causes blindness. The symptoms of weakened sight start in childhood and slowly encroach peripherally and cause tunnel vision, somewhat like glaucoma. A special electroretinogram that measures the retina and its response to light determines the disease and its status. No particular treatment is known, although some success has been noted with fetal retinal tissue transplant. Retinal detachment is possible here as well, and that causes more complications for treatment.

The optic nerve may be a part of the visual disturbance pattern, and that may be caused by physical strain, such as trauma or pressure (stretching) in the event of exophthalmos, as found in hyperthyroidism. With various toxins (especially heavy metals), low oxygen levels, and drugs (including Viagra), the optic nerve is sensitive to many factors injurious to eye sight. Blindness normally develops when light is blocked to the retina as in cataracts and when there is increased intraocular pressure as in glaucoma, optic nerve damage, or image failure recognition by the occipital cortex. Regardless of cause, the best way to prevent visual impairment is to practice good hygiene (e.g., avoid unnecessary hand-eye contact), observe safety precautions, and seek medical help with any noticeable eye problem.

## The Ear

Hearing loss is a major problem for those with normal acoustic function, and there are three categories of hearing loss: conductive, mainly a blockage or physical problem; sensory loss due to inner ear elements being lost or compromised; and neural hearing loss from damage to the auditory nerve (VIII). Age can be a major factor in hearing disabilities along with the environmental workplace and modern instrumentation, like cell phones and personal audio devices, that put a significant stress on hearing abilities. More than 28 million Americans are deaf or have hearing loss, and each year sudden deafness occurs among 1 per 5000, particularly the elderly.

Conductive hearing loss is commonly caused by excess ear wax buildup (cerumen impaction), a tumor, or pus buildup in the auditory canal or middle ear from infection (external otitis, otitis media). The middle ear bony ossicles may stiffen as in arthritis, called **otosclerosis,** and a perforated ear drum is a frequent occurrence. All of these situations reduce hearing abilities and require different modes or procedures to correct them. External and middle ear infection are common events, especially in children, and these dysfunctional disorders are now addressed.

***External Ear*** The visible part of the external ear is known as the **auricle** or **pinna** and it enhances hearing perception by a small percent (2% to 4%). It assists hearing by collecting sound waves and funneling them down the auditory canal and is subject to skin cancer, primarily from sun exposure, and trauma from accidents or athletic activities. Skin cancer is treated mainly by surgery. Trauma cases may require surgery as well and to prevent disfigurement (such as a "cauliflower" appearance). Cosmetically, auricle design or size may be an issue, especially for children when the auricles are extra large or protrude and appear unsymmetrical. Infections can occur when pierced earring sites are not properly cleaned, and some metals cause allergic reactions. Protecting the ear from severe environmental extremes and using ear plugs for noise reduction are effective preventive measures for reducing hearing loss. (See Figure 13–23 ▸.)

***Cerumen Impaction*** Wax is necessary for the soft texture and flexibility of the ear drum. However, cerumen impaction or excess wax buildup may recur, especially in youngsters or the elderly.

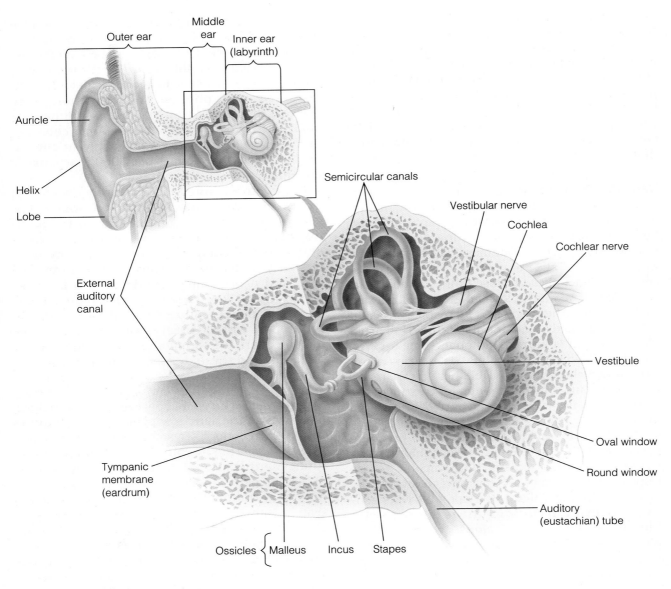

**Figure 13–23** ► Human ear anatomy.

Upon first appearance of wax building, better hygiene is required. The buildup is usually alleviated by heated water, oil treatment, hydrogen peroxide (3%), or alcohol drops as simple remedies. However, on occasion a suction action or mechanical removal is necessary. It is imperative to have an intact ear drum when performing any treatment, and be sure to dry the ear area completely following treatment. Prevention is possible through routinely checking the ear canal for signs of wax accumulation.

***External Otitis*** External otitis, or "swimmer's ear," is an infection caused by bacteria and fungi. Symptoms and signs include pain, pruritis, fever, and (temporarily) hearing loss.

The pathogens responsible for external otitis are found in contaminated swimming pools or beaches. Drying the external ear opening after bathing or swimming and cleaning earphones, earplugs, and earmuffs can prevent it. Treatment with antibiotics is effective for bacterial infections, but some fungus infections may be more stubborn to control.

***Otitis Media*** Acute otitis media is a middle ear infection that affects primarily infants and children because of weak immune systems and perhaps the lack of breast feeding. Symptoms include pain and edema, with pus, and left unchecked the condition may cause perforation of the tympanic membrane (ear drum). Otitis media often follows pneumonia or an upper respiratory infection (URI), such as sinusitis. Most often, bacteria are the cause. Children are more susceptible than adults to middle ear infections because their nearly horizontal auditory tubes prevent adequate drainage. Diagnosis is primarily done by observation of pus in the ear canal and complaint of earache. Pain can be controlled with analgesics, and swelling is reduced by use of decongestants. To relieve pressure and allow pus to drain, small ear tubes like tiny cylinders are placed through the ear drum (tympanic membrane) to allow air into the middle ear. They are called tympanostomy tubes or myringotomy tubes, or simply ventilation tubes. In recurrent cases, scarring of the ear drum, auditory ossicles, and inner ear components can occur. There is potential for invasion of the nearby mastoid area, a honeycombed sinus area, and this penetration results in **mastoiditis**. With mastoiditis comes a fever and the possibility of brain infection or abscess formation because of the relatively thin membrane between the sinus area and the brain vault. In undeveloped countries with inadequate access to health care and antibiotics, chronic otitis media and its complications are very common among both adults and children. Penicillin-type antibiotics help, but in some resistant cases like *Pseudomonas aeruginosa*, stronger agents are required.

For chronic otitis media there may be relief. A clinical test study funded by NIH and published in 2005, using a device called the EarPopper, had an efficacy (effectiveness) rate of about 85% for those tested. This tool sends a gentle stream of air into the nasal cavity, and as the individual swallows, it forces open the Eustachian tube (or auditory tube) and equalizes the pressure within the middle ear. If fluid is present, it may take two treatments per day for a few weeks, but the benefit is that ear surgery is not required. This device is safe, basically pain free, and can used by anyone, including children.

***Inner Ear*** The inner ear consists of the semicircular canals (which, along with the cerebellum, maintain equilibrium) and the snail-like device called the cochlea. The semicircular canals work like a carpenter's level, with a bubble floating in a sea of fluid, to give the sense of balance and being upright. In addition, at the base where the three semicircular canals meet and form a connection with the cochlea, stiff ciliated (brushlike) elements attached to neurons line a common chamber. In this same chamber of fluid are grains of "sand," called **otoliths,** that tumble or float down like an hourglass and thereby stimulate the sensory elements to signal the brain as to body positioning or orientation (e.g., turned head). Along with the cerebellum and visual cues, the body maintains a normal standing or sitting posture or comprehends body location.

Some infections may interfere with the functioning of semicircular canals. In the case of fever or various drug interactions and electrolyte imbalances, the viscosity of the internal fluid may be altered. Vertigo or dizziness may cause nausea or headache and may cause accidential stumbling or falling. Acute cases of imbalance that may become episodic or longer-term vertigo would need to be addressed.

The cochlea houses coiled tubes filled with fluid that rushes over miniature "harps" called an *organ of Corti* and triggers signals to the auditory nerve. When these organs of Corti are damaged or lost, the hearing loss is permanent. Loud noises or sounds from heavy equipment, airplanes, and loud music; or ototoxic drugs like some chemotherapy drugs; and various infective agents leave a scar on the hearing apparatus.

As with sight and age, hearing too has its limitations, called **presbycusis**. This conditition is the most common cause of sensorineural hearing loss in adults. The actual cause is not known, but the condition tends to run in families and progresses with age. Constant exposure to loud noises gives ample reason to wear devices (earplugs) to protect the natural hearing mechanism. About 25% of those age 65 to 75 have measurable hearing loss, in part due to age, and about half those over age 75 have presbycusis. Hearing aids help restore some sound, but clarity is somewhat sacrificed.

Neural loss involving the eighth cranial nerve (vestibulocochlear) or auditory nerve has many possibilities. If the nerve is damaged by trauma, high fever, toxins, or other agents, the loss may be permanent. Experiments have used nerves located in the back and other areas, but without the auditory nerve connection to the temporal lobe of the brain, it is basically impossible to have the sounds clearly interpreted.

Deafness has its genetic component, as when a baby is born deaf, and cochlear implants are often used to overcome deafness. Inheritance of deafness may be either dominant or recessive, and over 100 genes have been identified as instrumental in this deficiency. The *connexin*-26 mutation has been suggested as a prevalent form of recessive hearing loss. Mitochondrial (cell organelle) disorders and hearing loss also play a significant role in the complex mechanism of auditory challenge. Whatever the circumstance, it is critical to save and protect all areas of the auditory pathway for the melodies of sound; cochlear implants are a viable alternative when hearing is lost.

***Ménière's Disease*** The occurrence of **Ménière's disease** is at 0.5 to 7.5 per 1000 and usually occurs in the mid- to late forties. Primarily considered idiopathic, some cases may be initiated by trauma, tumor, or autoimmune diseases that impact the cochlear apparatus whereby fluid and delicate sensory hairs are altered or degenerated. Ménière's disease is characterized by intermittent hearing loss, tinnitus (see below), and episodes of vertigo or dizziness. Therapy is focused on vertigo. Diuretics and restricted salt intake control fluid levels, and short-term glucocorticoids reduce inflammatory activity. Surgery may be a later option, but some loss of hearing may occur. Many individuals live with this disease if dizzy spells are reasonably under control.

***Tinnitus*** **Tinnitus** is defined as the perception of ringing, buzzing, or roaring sounds from an environment void of sound. The cause or pathophysiology of tinnitus is not well known, perhaps because there are many causes and tinnitus may be just one indication among many of other disease attributes. At least 12 million Americans have tinnitus, and 1 million have it severely enough that it interferes with daily life. This development may involve either conductive or sensorineural hearing loss. A full examination is required of the ear, nose, and throat to discern problems like infection, trauma, or growths, plus family history and and any drug regimen. Diagnosis is similar to other ear investigation and begins with the **Weber and Rinne tuning fork** test. Not only are the frequencies or pitch of the sound noted, but more so, whether the limitation is conductive or sensorineural. The stem of the vibrating fork is placed on the skull near the mastoid process (just behind and under the ear), or maybe the teeth, to tell if a sound is louder or softer compared to the sound in air. If the sound is louder in air versus the contacted bone, then it appears to be a sensorineural insufficiency, and if louder by bone contact, it appears to be a conduction defect.

Tinnitus is known to be affected by, or is part of, a hearing loss problem because of excesive loud noise exposure, poor reaction to some medications, or various other health concerns. Treatment by the **otolaryngologist** includes hearing aids to overpower the background sounds, sound-masking devices to cancel or reduce the ringing noises, amplifier devices on phones, or eletronic equipment to pick up better-quality sound, plus medications and relaxing techniques. People with tinnitus should avoid loud sounds and be patient; some may find that lipoflavanoid supplementation is helpful. Lipoflavanoid is a dietary supplement used since the 1960s to specifially improve the microcirculation within the inner ear. Therefore, the flexibility of the sensory hair cells responsible for sound transmission to the brain is maintained and the fluid within the cochlear canals flows easier. Lipoflavanoid improves inner ear health and reduces the intensity of ear ringing found in tinnitus as well as symptoms found in Ménière's syndrome.

All senses make for a more enjoyable life. Any reduced stress promotes better homeostasis, and that means a healthier and better existence. The olfactory sensation, mentioned in Chapter 8, may add pleasure or displeasure to the environment and thus necessary for detecting methane gas or rotten odors from spoiled food sources; thus a the sense of smell could help prevent illness or save a life, both of which could be fatal. Similarly, the sense of taste (gustatory) is necessary to detect rotten, toxic, or pleasurable attributes of our living arena. Taste and smell often diminish with age, disease, and drugs like chemotherapy treatments. Zinc supplements seem to offer some relief in the case of reduced gustatory abilities and allow for a more pleasant taste of life.

## ▶ Age-Related Diseases

Neurological disease affects individuals at all stages of life. Glaucoma and cataracts are age-related visual problems, as is presbyopia, a lens condition that occurs usually in the mid-40s. In presbyopia, the lens becomes less resilient and remains relatively flat, leaving distance vision intact but impairing near vision. Corrective lenses are very common after age 43 to 45. Macular degeneration typically comes along with age, as do cataracts and difficulty hearing (called presbycusis). Tinnitus, an ear ringing sensation, normally develops in later years due to environmental or unknown factors. Cranial nerve dysfunction usually occurs in young and middle-aged adults. Alzheimer's disease (see Chapter 14) is a prominent concern for seniors. The incidence of dementia and of Parkinson's disease increases with age. In trisomy 21 (Down syndrome), patients who live past age 45 tend to have AD.

Finally, with age, the 3-pound brain reduces in weight and size, with concurrent loss of neurons and synapses. Thus, it is understandable that functional losses in hearing, sight, and coordination will be experienced in the elderly. Reaction times are reduced, and so is agility, which increases risks for injury.

## RESOURCE

National Institutes of Allergy and Infectious Diseases: www.nei.nih.gov

# DISEASES AT A GLANCE

## Nervous System and Special Senses

| DISEASE | ETIOLOGY | SIGNS AND SYMPTOMS |
|---|---|---|
| Glioma, glioblastoma | Idiopathic | Severe headache, personality changes, loss of speech, unsteady movement, seizures, coma |
| Meningitis | Bacterial, viral | High fever, chills, severe headache, stiff neck, nausea, vomiting, rash, delirium, convulsions, coma |
| Encephalitis | Viral | Mild to severe headache, fever, cerebral dysfunction, disordered thought, seizures, persistent drowsiness, delirium, coma |
| Poliomyelitis | Viral | Stiff neck, fever, headache, sore throat, GI disturbances, paralysis may develop |
| Tetanus | Clostridium tetani | Rigidity of muscles, painful spasms and convulsions, stiff neck, difficulty swallowing, clenched jaws |
| Rabies | Viral | Fever, pain, mental derangement, rage, convulsions, paralysis, profuse sticky saliva, throat muscle spasm produces hydrophobia |
| Shingles | Varicella, herpes zoster | Painful rash of small water blisters with red rim, lesions follow a sensory nerve, confined to one side of body, severe itching, scarring |
| Reye's syndrome | Idiopathic or viral; Epstein-Barr, influenza B, varicella | Persistent vomiting, rash, lethargy about 1 week after a viral infection, may progress to coma; linked with use of aspirin |
| Abscess | Pyogenic bacteria | Fever, headache |
| Multiple sclerosis (MS) | Idiopathic, suspect viral or autoimmune | Muscle impairment, double vision, nystagmus, loss of balance, poor coordination, tingling and numbing sensation, shaking tremor, muscular weakness, emotional changes, remission and exacerbation |
| Amyotrophic lateral sclerosis (ALS), or Lou Gehrig's disease | Idiopathic | Disturbed motility; fasciculations; atrophy of muscles in hands, forearms, and legs; impaired speech and swallowing; death from pulmonary failure in 3 to 4 years |

| DIAGNOSIS | TREATMENT | PREVENTION | LIFESPAN |
|-----------|-----------|------------|----------|
| CT scan, MRI | Surgery, chemotherapy, radiation | Uncertain | Any age, usually adult |
| Lumbar puncture (spinal tap) | Antibiotics if bacterial infection | Be aware, avoid contact | Can occur at any age |
| Lumbar puncture (spinal tap) | Control fever, control fluid and electrolyte balance, monitor respiratory and kidney function | Depends on circumstance | Can occur at any age |
| Physical exam | Supportive; preventive vaccination | Vaccine | Usually younger to early adult |
| Physical exam, patient history | Antitoxin, symptom relief, preventive vaccination | Vaccine | Can occur at any age |
| Physical exam, history of animal bite | Vaccination before disease develops; fatal once CNS involved | Vaccine, be alert | Can occur at any age |
| Physical exam | Alleviation of symptoms and pain relief, steroids | Avoid contact, vaccine | Usually 50+ |
| Patient history, liver enlargement, hypoglycemia, ammonia in blood | Supportive; close monitoring necessary | Avoid aspirin, Seek care | Infants, young children |
| Lumbar puncture (spinal tap) | Surgical draining of abscess, antibiotics | Quick treatment | Can occur at any age |
| Physical exam, patient history, MRI | None effective; physical therapy and muscle relaxants, steroids, counseling | Basically autoimmune and polygenetic | Midlife |
| Electromyelography (EMG) | Supportive | Uncertain | Midlife |

# DISEASES AT A GLANCE

## Nervous System and Special Senses (*continued*)

| DISEASE | ETIOLOGY | SIGNS AND SYMPTOMS |
|---------|----------|--------------------|
| Huntington's disease (Huntington's chorea) | Genetic | Involuntary, rapid, jerky movements; speech loss; difficulty swallowing; personality changes; carelessness; poor judgment; impaired memory; mental incompetence |
| Convulsion: epilepsy | Trauma, chemical, idiopathic | Involuntary contractions or series of contractions; a seizure is a sign of illness, not a disease. Petit mal: brief loss of consciousness, "absence seizure" Grand mal: often preceded by aura (various sensations), total loss of consciousness, generalized convulsions, hypersalivation; incontinence may occur |
| Spina bifida | Congential, lack folate | Opening in vertebral canal; spina bifida occulta: hidden; meningocele: meninges protrude; meningomyelocele: nerve elements protrude; myelocele: nerve tissue disorganized |
| Hydrocephalus | Congenital, idiopathic | Enlarged head develops |
| Cerebral palsy | Birth trauma, rubella infection | Seizures, visual or auditory impairment, speech defects. Spastic: muscles tense, reflexes exaggerated. Athetoid: uncontrollable, persistent movements, tremor. Atactic: poor balance, poor muscular coordination, staggering gait |
| Transient ischemic attacks (TIA), "mini strokes" | Ischemia, aneurysm, hypertension | Visual disturbances, transient muscle weakness on one side, sensory loss on one side, slurred speech; attacks last minutes to hours, average 15 minutes |
| Cerebrovascular accident (CVA) stroke, brain attack | Trauma | Severe, sudden headache; muscular weakness or paralysis; disturbance of speech; loss of consciousness |
| Alzheimers's disease | Idiopathic, but genetically connected | Memory loss, moody, indigent |

| DIAGNOSIS | TREATMENT | PREVENTION | LIFESPAN |
|---|---|---|---|
| Patient history (inherited disease) and physical exam | No cure; genetic counseling for family | Totally genetic | Age 35+ |
| Observation of seizure, electroencephalogram (EEG), x-ray, family history, CT scan, MRI | Removal of cause once detected; anticonvulsive drugs | Avoid cranial trauma; use helmet or headgear | Can occur at any age |
| Physical exam, CT scan, MRI, EEG | Surgical, physical therapy | Variable, folate supplements | Middle-aged mother |
| Physical exam, CT scan, MRI, spinal tap | Implant shunt to drain CSF | Variable to pathogen exposure | Can occur at any age, but more prevalent among newborns |
| Physical exam | Muscle relaxants, anticonvulsive drugs, casts, braces, traction, surgery, physical therapy | Variable, birth caution | Can occur at any age |
| Cerebral angiogram, CT scan | Depends on cause; surgical treatment of blocked vessels | Blood pressure monitoring, uncertain | Usually middle age |
| Angiography, CT scan, MRI | Clot-dissolving drugs, surgery, endarterectomy | Uncertain, family history, keep low blood pressure levels | Usually mid life+ |
| Behavioral, clinical screening | Care facilities, medications to stay calm | None with long survival | Onset-mid age, progressive with time |

# DISEASES AT A GLANCE

## Nervous System and Special Senses (*continued*)

| DISEASE | ETIOLOGY | SIGNS AND SYMPTOMS |
|---|---|---|
| **Special Senses: Eye** | | |
| Conjunctivitis | Viral, bacterial | Inflamed eye surface, oozing |
| Glaucoma | Poor aqueous fluid drainage | Elevate intraocular pressure, dim vison |
| Uveitis | Infectious agents | Eye discharge, pain, low vision |
| Astigmatism | Irregular cornea or lens | Blurry vision |
| Cataracts | Cloudy lens | Blurred, dim vision |
| Macular degeneration | Idiopathic | Central vision lost |
| Diabetic retinopathy | Diabetes | Blurred, cloudy vision to blinded |
| Retinitis pigmentosa | X chromosome | Weakened sight gradual blindness |
| **Special Senses: Ear** | | |
| External otitis | Infection | Discharge, pus |
| Otitis media | Infection | Internal fluid pressure,fever |
| Presbycusis | Increased age | Hard of hearing |
| Ménière's disease | Idiopathic, trauma, autoimmune? | Vertigo, disoriented, tinnitus |
| Tinnitus | Idiopathic, may be blood pressure related, loud sounds | Ringing, roaring internal sounds without real sounds externally |

| DIAGNOSIS | TREATMENT | PREVENTION | LIFESPAN |
|---|---|---|---|
| Eye inspection, environment, eye fluids | None or ointment or eye drops | Contagious, avoid contact | Usually young child, but not determined by age |
| Ophthalmoscope and slit-scope | Eye drops | None, 10% genetic | Mid age+ |
| Eye exam | Corticoids | Basically autoimmune | Variable |
| Chart exam, eye inspection | Corrective lenses | None | NDA |
| Ophthalmoscope | Some laser, lens replacement | None, avoid sunlight, STDs | Usually elderly |
| Ophthalmoscope | Nonspecific | None | Older persons |
| Ophthalmoscope and fluorescein angiography | Some laser, control diabetes and blood pressure | Perhaps control diabetes | More likely with aging |
| Electroretinogram | Nonspecific | None | From birth |
| Ear inspection | Antibiotic, cleanse area | Depends, use good hygiene, keep ear canal dry | Can occur at any age |
| Ear inspection | Drain tube, antibiotics | Depends, use good hygiene | Children + |
| Audio testing | Hearing aids | None | Worse with age |
| Hearing test and exam | Glucocoricoid, low salt diet | Uncertain | Age 40+ |
| Hearing test | Sound aids, low sound makers for interference | Depends | Usually middle aged, but expected in younger people following loud music performances |

# Interactive Exercises

## Cases for Critical Thinking

1. J. A. has had a severe headache for the last 12 hours, a fever of 102, plus a stiff neck. Following a lumbar puncture, *Streptococcus pneumoniae* was found in culture along with low sugar levels and higher protein values. What disease best explains these findings? What is the prognosis and treatment?

2. At age 78, K. B. started rubbing her eyes and constantly cleaning her (old) glasses for a better view. The right eye particularly was not very good, and she hoped the problem, which she first noticed months ago, would finally go away.

   The vision in the right eye was foggy, dim, and not focused. There was essentially no pain. What do the symptoms suggest? What are the prognosis and treatments for this woman?

3. T. C. complained of an earache, and after a recent bout with a bad cold, he was rather irritable. The ear was "beet red" and felt warm. He could hardly hear on that side, but he knew there was nothing intentionally or accidentally poked into the ear. What disease best explains these symptoms? Give some recommendations for treatment.

## Multiple Choice

1. What is the infective agent for rabies?
   a. bacterium      b. virus
   c. fungus         d. tick

2. Which of the following may cause epilepsy?
   a. a birth trauma
   b. injury to the brain
   c. a penetrating wound
   d. all of these

3. What functions are controlled by the brain stem?
   a. sensory function    b. muscle action
   c. memory              d. heart rate and breathing

4. What is called an acute inflammation of the first two meninges of the brain and spinal cord, the pia mater and the arachnoid?
   a. thrombophlebitis    b. meningitis
   c. prostatitis         d. encephalitis

5. Which of the following is true of polio?
   a. is caused by a virus
   b. affects sensory neurons
   c. is found in most people by age 80
   d. was wiped out in 1976

6. Which of the following applies to MS?
   a. occurs only in males
   b. occurs primarily in east European cultures
   c. results from a damaged myelin sheath
   d. strikes adults age 20 or beyond

7. Within 3 to 4 hours, what clot-buster may be used to treat the most common form of CVA?
   a. aspirin    b. TPA
   c. ATP        d. hemolase

8. What disease has a seizure symptom known as petit mal?
   a. polio      b. MS
   c. epilepsy   d. encephalitis

9. What is the lesion in Parkinson's disease?
   a. no dopamine     b. no myelin
   c. autoimmunity    d. cerebral blood clot

10. Pauly, a first-grader, woke one morning to discover a blood-shot right eye and a yellowish mass near the medial corner of his eye. What is the correct diagnosis?
    a. common cold     b. trachoma
    c. conjunctivitis  d. osteitis

## True or False

_____ 1. Rabies is a viral infection.

_____ 2. The Sabin vaccine works in the digestive tract.

_____ 3. Oxygen under high pressure is effective in treating rabies.

_____ 4. Blood is not normally found in cerebrospinal fluid.

_____ 5. Dopamine deficiency causes epilepsy.

_____ 6. Transient ischemic attacks are characterized by loss of consciousness.

_____ 7. An aura is a flashback of previous contusion events.

_____ 8. Viral meningitis requires quarantine isolation procedures.

_____ 9. Excess Dilantin may cause Parkinson's disease.

_____ 10. Conjunctivitis is usually a viral attack in adults.

## Fill-Ins

1. _____, commonly called lockjaw, is an infection of nerve tissue caused by the tetanus bacillus that lives in the intestines of animals and human beings.

2. Amyotrophic lateral sclerosis is diagnosed by _____.

3. _____ _____ is a chronic, progressive disease of the central nervous system with myelin destruction.

4. _____ _____, also known as shaking palsy, is a disease of brain degeneration that appears gradually and progresses slowly.

5. The common drug given to victims of Parkinson's disease is _____.

6. _____ headaches are severe, are unilateral, involve the periorbital and orbital area, and typically occur in men.

7. Tic douloureau, or _____ _____, causes severe pain elicited from cranial nerve V.

8. _____ _____ is a unilateral dysfunction of muscles in the face that leaves the person with slurred speech and a watery eye.

9. _____ is called Lou Gerhig's disease.

10. _____ is the worst form of spina bifida.

## Labeling Exercise

Use the blank lines below to label the following image.

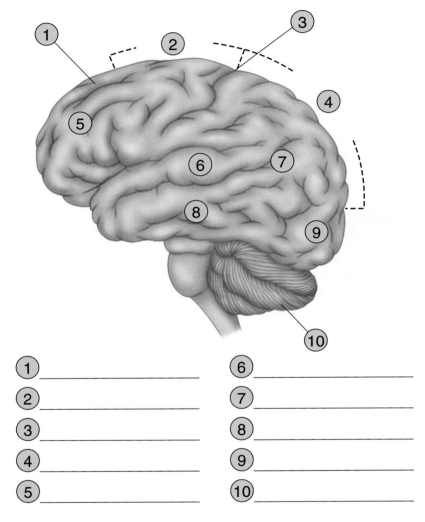

1 _____

2 _____

3 _____

4 _____

5 _____

6 _____

7 _____

8 _____

9 _____

10 _____

# Multimedia Preview

Additional interactive resources and activities for this chapter can be found on the Companion Website. For videos, audio glossary, and review, access the accompanying DVD-ROM in this book.

## ▶ DVD-ROM Highlights

### Beat the Clock

Do you know your diseases? Test your smarts against the clock in this game of knowledge, spelling, and speed. Can you correctly answer 20 questions before the final tick?

### Vocabulary 911

Someone call 911, it's a human disease emergency! Test your knowledge by helping the injured word into the correct ambulance.

## ▶ Website Highlights—www.pearsonhighered.com/zelman

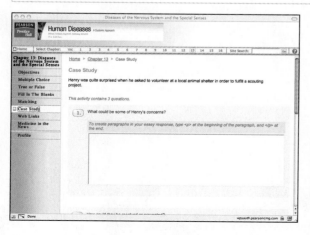

### Case Study

Take advantage of the free-access online study guide that accompanies your textbook. Put your understanding of human diseases to the test with this real-world scenario. You'll be presented with a clinical case followed by a series of questions that challenge your grasp of the situation. By clicking on this URL you'll also access links to current news articles and an audio glossary.

CHAPTER

14

# Mental Illness and Cognitive Disorders

## Learning Objectives

After studying this chapter, you should be able to

- Describe the warning signs of mental illness
- Identify signs, symptoms, etiology, and treatment of the following:
  - Developmental disorders
  - Disruptive behavior disorders
  - Mood disorders
  - Substance use disorders
  - Schizophrenia
  - Anxiety disorders
  - Eating disorders
  - Personality disorders
- Recognize environmental, genetic, and biological factors associated with mental illness
- Describe diagnostic approaches for mental illness
- Identify the warning signs of suicide

## Fact or Fiction?

Mental illness is a weakness of character.

*Fiction: Mental illness has physical and/or biological causes, just as do the diseases of the other systems discussed in this text. For every 100 people, one ends up with schizophrenia, one develops bipolar disorder, and 20 experience some form of depression. Heredity may account for as much as 80% of the risk for these illnesses.*

# Disease Chronicle

## Post-Traumatic Stress Disorder and Modern Psychiatry

The human brain has evolved to cope with intermittent ordinary stressors, such as hunger, pain, and isolation, but the brain is not well adapted to handle stressors that are outside the realm of normal human experience. Certainly such extreme stressors occurred occasionally in the human evolutionary past; however, the modern world presents humans with abundant opportunities to experience extreme stress, the sort of stress associated with post-traumatic stress disorder. These experiences include war; rape or sexual abuse; being hit or harmed by someone in your family; violent crime; airplane or car crashes; hurricane, tornado, or fire; any event in which you thought you might be killed; or witnessing any of these events. Today we know that post-traumatic stress disorder is a real disorder with severe consequences; to appreciate the significance of this, remember that until recently this disorder and many mental illnesses were misunderstood. Prior to the twentieth century, mental illnesses were primarily attributed to human fault and hostility, magic, or divine forces. The mentally ill were treated by confinement in prisons and asylums. Reforms in the treatment of the mentally ill started after the French Revolution with Franz Mesmer, an Austrian physician, who established rapport with patients. Emil Kraepelin began the modern classification of psychiatry in the nineteenth century. Modern psychiatry, founded in the twentieth century by Sigmund Freud, is credited with a comprehensive approach to understanding development, emotion, behavior, and psychiatric illness. Psychological theory, treatment options, and scientific advancements continue to evolve, contributing to further understanding of the biological, chemical, environmental, social, and behavioral mechanisms of mental illness.

## ▶ Mental Illness

Mental illness refers to a group of **psychiatric** disorders characterized by severe disturbances in thought, mood, and behavior. **Psychiatry** is the medical specialty that diagnoses and prescribes medical treatment for mental illness, whereas **psychology** is the discipline that studies normal and abnormal behavior and applies counseling methods to treat mental illness.

Mental illness affects one of every four Americans and is associated with social stigma, disability, and death. Many people suffering from mental illness may not look as though they are ill, while others may appear detached and withdrawn from society. Warning signs of mental illness are listed in Box 14–1 ▶.

Over 200 psychiatric diagnoses for adults and children are categorized in the *Diagnostic and Statistical Manual of Mental Disorders*, or DSM. The DSM-IV is the most recent edition and is used internationally to classify, assess, and guide treatment for mental illness. Because it is difficult to provide a single definition that accounts for all mental illness, disorders are categorized in the DSM-IV according to groups of symptoms or diagnostic criteria. Psychiatric disorders are assigned a diagnosis in one of five

---

### Box 14–2 ▶ The Five-Axis System of Psychiatric Diagnoses

Axis I:   Primary diagnosis (clinical disorders and other conditions that may be a focus of clinical attention)

Axis II:   Primary diagnosis (personality disorders, mental retardation, learning disabilities)

Axis III:   General medical conditions

Axis IV:   Psychosocial and environmental problems

Axis V:   Global assessment of functioning

Primary Psychiatric Diagnosis is indicated on Axis I or II.

*Source: Diagnostic and Statistical Manual Text Revision IV. American Psychiatric Association, 2000.*

---

axes, and each axis is a grouping of developmental, medical, psychosocial, and overall adaptive disorders (Box 14–2 ▶). All DSM-IV diagnoses require evidence that the symptoms impair academic achievement, occupational performance, and social relationships.

## ▶ Causes of Mental Illness

### Biological Basis for Mental Illness

Current biological theories of mental illness implicate anatomical differences, genes, and chemical messengers or **neurotransmitters** in mental illness. Anatomical differences such as brain size and altered neural connections develop from physical insults to the brain, degenerative processes, and genes. Genes within the brain's DNA are inherited from both parents and contain all the necessary information to build the structures that mediate the specialized function of neurotransmitters.

Neurotransmitters are produced, stored, and released from **neurons**, or nerves cells, within the central and peripheral nervous system. Voluntary and involuntary physical and psychological processes, such as heart rate and blood pressure, behavior, emotions, mood, sleep, and sex drive, are regulated by intricate neurotransmitter activity. Inadequate regulation of neurotransmitters and excess neurotransmitter activ-

---

### Box 14–1 ▶ Warning Signs of Mental Illness

- Aggression
- Changes in eating or sleeping habits
- Confusion
- Decline in school or work performance
- Depression
- Euphoria alternating with depression
- Excessive fear
- Frequent complaints of physical illnesses
- Hearing voices
- Substance abuse
- Thoughts of suicide
- Withdrawal from family and friends

*Source: Diagnostic and Statistical Manual Text Revision IV. American Psychiatric Association, 2000.*

ity in distinct areas of the brain are associated with mental illness. The regulatory action of neurotransmitters and their associated mental illnesses are listed in Table 14–1 ▶.

## Environment and Mental Illness

Environmental causes of mental illness have informed the diagnosis and treatment of mental illness for many years. Family interactions, age, gender, race, culture, and socioeconomic status alter biological and psychological vulnerability for mental illness and define learned behaviors, attitudes, and perception of health and illness.

Age and gender are determining factors for some mental health problems and illnesses. Mood disorders such as depression, anxiety disorders, and eating disorders occur more frequently in women, whereas disorders with outwardly directed behaviors such as antisocial personality disorder and associated substance abuse are more common in males. Attention deficit hyperactivity disorder (ADHD) is a development behavioral disorder that appears more commonly in males prior to the age of 7 years. Degenerative disorders involving memory and dementia, such

as Alzheimer's disease and Huntington's chorea, occur most commonly among older adults.

Mental illness affects all cultures, races, and socioeconomic classes. Access to medical care and acceptance of psychiatric illness is also influenced by race, cultural beliefs, and socioeconomic status. The highest rates of mental illness are found among the lowest socioeconomic classes, which are associated with adverse living conditions, increased social stress, and limited access to medical and psychiatric care.

## Mental Illness in Children and Adolescents

Mental illness in childhood can have far-reaching academic, social, developmental, and physical consequences. Common complications of childhood-onset mental illness include learning delays and poor performance in school, low self-esteem, impaired relationships with family and friends, and social rejection and withdrawal.

Although many psychiatric disorders begin in childhood, they may not be diagnosed until adulthood. In the United States, about 20% of children and adolescents have a mental disorder.

**Table 14–1** ▶ **Neurotransmitters, Regulatory Actions, and Associated Psychiatric Disorders**

| Neurotransmitter | Regulatory Action | Mental Illness |
| --- | --- | --- |
| Dopamine | Mood, behavior, thought process, muscle movement, physical activity, heart rate, blood pressure, feeding, appetite, satiety | Schizophrenia, depression, ADHD, bipolar disorder, eating disorder, autism, Tourette syndrome |
| Norepinephrine | Mood, anxiety, vigilance, arousal, heart rate, blood pressure | Depression, anxiety disorders, ADHD, bipolar disorder |
| Serotonin | Perception of pain, feeding, sleep–wake cycle, motor activity, sexual behavior, temperature regulation | Depression, aggression, suicidality, bipolar disorder, eating disorders |
| Acetylcholine | Learning, memory, muscle tone | Alzheimer's disease, Parkinson's disease, Huntington's chorea, Tourette syndrome |
| Gamma aminobutyric acid (GABA) | Interacts with a wide range of neurotransmitters to enhance inhibition | Anxiety disorders, alcoholism, Tourette syndrome, sleep disorders |

*Source:* Kaplan, G. B. and Hammer R. P. *Brain Circuitry and Signaling in Psychiatry: Basic Science and Clinical Applications.* American Psychiatric Association, 2002.

Some disorders have slightly adapted criteria for children. Unlike adults, children often do not verbalize their feelings and may present with behavioral problems such as boredom, irritability, and conduct problems. The outcome of childhood mental illness depends on the ability of the family to cope and seek treatment, the severity of the illness, and the ability of the child to compensate for and adapt to mental health deficits.

## ▶ Diagnostic Tests for Mental Illness

Comprehensive evaluations, including a medical history and physical exam, psychosocial history, mental health exam, and family history, are essential for diagnosis of mental illness. A thorough medical history and physical exam should identify physical illnesses and metabolic and hormonal stresses that mimic symptoms of mental illness. A patient history obtained from family and friends with major timelines of life events can help form a diagnosis. Observation of the patient alone or within a family environment is used to assess emotional responses, physical appearance and reactions, speech and language abilities, clinical estimate of intelligence, and level of judgment and insight. A number of standardized questionnaires and rating scales supplement the clinical evaluation by providing a systematic review and standard score to describe behaviors and emotions.

## ▶ Disorders of Infancy, Childhood, or Adolescence

### Disruptive Behavior Disorders

Disruptive behavior disorders, including **conduct disorder** and **oppositional defiant disorder**, are characterized by willful disobedience. Conduct disorders affect males more often than females and commonly overlap with other psychiatric disorders. A single cause cannot be identified; however, many of these children come from unstable or dysfunctional families and are exposed to domestic violence, poverty, and shifting parental figures. The risk for disruptive behavior disorders increases with inconsistent parenting and puni-

tive disciplinary techniques, parental alcohol and drug abuse, and parental antisocial personality disorder. Harsh parental discipline with physical punishment appears to lead to aggressive behavior; however, genetic heritability of antisocial and aggressive behaviors has been identified.

Signs include defiance of authority, fighting, school failure, and destruction of property. During adolescence, fire setting, theft, sexual promiscuity, and criminal behaviors may develop. Treatment involves individual and family counseling as well as medication if appropriate.

### Attention Deficit Hyperactivity Disorder

**Attention deficit hyperactivity disorder (ADHD)** is characterized by prominent symptoms of inattention and/or hyperactivity and impulsivity. ADHD affects males more often than females and persists into adolescence and adulthood. The cause is unknown, but family and twin studies provide evidence of genetic susceptibility, and molecular DNA studies implicate the role of genes in ADHD. Imaging techniques show anatomic and metabolic differences in the brains of ADHD subjects compared to non-ADHD subjects.

The DSM-IV defines three subtypes of ADHD: predominantly inattentive, predominantly hyperactive-impulsive, and combined inattentive, hyperactive, and impulsive. Children with the inattentive subtype tend to be described as "spacey" and socially withdrawn, and they have fewer conduct and behavioral problems than the hyperactive-impulsive subtype. The term *ADD* (attention deficit disorder) was once used to describe children with these symptoms, but ADD is no longer a DSM diagnosis. Even so, at times ADD is still used informally today to describe children with the predominantly inattentive subtype of ADHD. Hyperactive ADHD children tend to run around excessively, fidget, and have difficulty playing or engaging in quiet activities. Impulsivity in ADHD is characterized by the inability to wait turns, blurting out answers, and interrupting others.

Contrary to common belief, ADHD is not limited to childhood. ADHD has a chronic lifelong course and, if untreated, results in school and work failure, substance use disorders, legal difficulties, car accidents and fatalities, and sexual indiscretions. ADHD commonly occurs with de-

| Table 14–2 ► Clinical Specialists in Treatment and Diagnosis of ADHD | | | |
|---|---|---|---|
| **Clinical Specialty** | **Can Diagnose** | **Can Prescribe Medication If Needed** | **Provides Counseling or Training** |
| Psychiatrists | Yes | Yes | Yes |
| Psychologists | Yes | No | Yes |
| Pediatricians or Family Physicians | Yes | Yes | No |
| Neurologists | Yes | Yes | No |
| Clinical Social Workers | Yes | No | Yes |

*Source:* National Institutes of Mental Health: www.nimh.org

pressive disorders, anxiety disorders, conduct disorder, oppositional defiant disorder, and learning disorders. Like many psychiatric disorders, ADHD often requires multimodal treatment that may include medication, cognitive-behavioral therapy, counseling, and collaboration among a variety of clinical professionals (Table 14–2►). The majority of children with ADHD are effectively treated with stimulant medications. Stimulant medications are the oldest and most established pharmacological agents in children with ADHD (Table 14–3►). Behavior therapy can

| Table 14–3 ► Medications Used in Treatment of ADHD | | |
|---|---|---|
| **Trade Name** | **Generic Name** | **Approved Age** |
| Adderall | amphetamine | 3 and older |
| Concerta (long acting) | methylphenidate | 6 and older |
| Cylert* | pemoline | 6 and older |
| Dexedrine | dextroamphetamine | 3 and older |
| Dextrostat | dextroamphetamine | 3 and older |
| Focalin | dexmethylphenidate | 6 and older |
| Metadate ER (extended release) | methylphenidate | 6 and older |
| Metadate CD (extended release) | methylphenidate | 6 and older |
| Ritalin | methylphenidate | 6 and older |
| Ritalin SR (extended release) | methylphenidate | 6 and older |
| Ritalin LA (long acting) | methylphenidate | 6 and older |

*Because of its potential for serious side effects affecting the liver, Cylert should not ordinarily be considered as first-line drug therapy for ADHD. The Food and Drug Administration recently approved a medication for ADHD that is not a stimulant. The medication Strattera®, or atomoxetine, works on the neurotransmitter norepinephrine; whereas the stimulants primarily work on dopamine. Both of these neurotransmitters are believed to play a role in ADHD. More studies will need to be done to contrast Strattera with the medications already available but the evidence to date indicates that over 70% of children with ADHD given Strattera manifest significant improvement in their symptoms.

*Sources:* National Institutes of Mental Health: www.nimh.org; Food and Drug Administration: www.fda.gov

improve academic achievement and reduce targeted conduct problems, especially in children with a co-occurring conduct disorder.

## ▶ Developmental Disorders

### Mental Retardation

Mental retardation is defined by the presence of low intelligence accompanied by deficits in social and language skills and adaptive functioning. The most common biological cause of mental retardation is fragile X syndrome, an inherited defect of the X chromosome that affects 1 in 4000 males and 1 in 6000 females in the United States. However, in some cases the exact cause cannot be identified. Treatment focuses on occupational therapy to maximize the development of cognitive and behavioral skills.

### Autistic Disorder

**Autistic disorders** (autism) include deficits in reciprocal language and social interactions and are characterized by repetitive stereotyped behaviors. Autism affects approximately 3.4 in 1000 children in the United States. Autism often goes unrecognized during infancy and first becomes apparent after 3 years of age. The cause of autism is unknown. Central nervous system changes have been postulated, but no definitive links have been made to autism and no genes are yet strongly associated with the disorder.

The concordance rate for autism in twins is about 90%, and the rate of autism is higher in families with a history of language-related disorders.

The most notable deficits in autism are severe deficits in reciprocal social interactions. These include minimal eye contact with caregivers, delayed language development, and disinterest in social interactions with peers, usually first observed during the toddler years. When speech does develop, it usually is illogical and echolike, as words that are heard are repeated. Repetitive and stereotypic behaviors include odd posturing, hand flapping, self-injurious behavior, abnormal patterns of eating and drinking, and unpredictable mood changes.

Widely accepted as effective when begun early, applied behavior analysis (ABA) has been shown to improve behavior and communication skills. ABA utilizes intensive and frequent one-on-one interaction with a therapist. No medications are approved for treatment of children with autism. Medications for behavior and mood have been used and these include antidepressants, anxiolytics, and antipsychotics. As with other childhood illnesses, parental guidance and assurance is critical for obtaining appropriate medical and psychosocial support. Informed parents contribute to the child's learning of self-care and adaptive skills and to positive long-term outcomes.

### Tic Disorders

A **tic** is a sudden, rapid, involuntary stereotyped movement or vocalization that may be temporarily suppressed by conscious efforts. Tics are exacerbated by stress, anxiety, boredom, or fatigue, and typically decrease in severity when the child is concentrating on an enjoyable task. Tics occur more commonly in boys than girls and are presumed to result from a neurotransmitter imbalance. Tourette syndrome is a common tic disorder characterized by patterns of motor and vocal tics and affecting 1 to 10 of every 1000 children and adolescents in the United States.

Complications of tic disorders include embarrassment and impaired self-esteem that results from being teased and rejected by peers and adults. Severe symptoms may interfere with forming intimate friendships. The unemployment rate in adults with tics has been reported as high as 50%.

Transient tics usually do not require treatment. Complicated tic disorders require carefully titrated medication therapy. No medication eliminates tics, but some can modulate tic severity. The dopamine blockers risperidone and haloperidol can reduce the severity of tics.

### Dementia

Dementia is a degenerative syndrome characterized by deficits in memory, language, and mood. The most common form of dementia is

**Alzheimer's disease**, which develops gradually and occurs most commonly after the age of 60 years. **Vascular dementia** has a more abrupt onset and is caused by physical insults from high blood pressure, diabetes, and strokes. Poor nutrition, head injuries, with chronic alcohol intake may result in alcohol-related dementia. Parkinson's disease is a degenerative neurological movement disorder characterized by dementia in late stages of the disease (see Chapter 13).

## Alzheimer's Disease

In 1906 Dr. Alois Alzheimer first recorded certain abnormalities in the brain of a woman who died from dementia. Alzheimer's disease is a degenerative and progressive form of dementia that seriously disrupts daily living activities, behavior, and mood.

The two most significant risk factors for Alzheimer's disease are advanced age and family history. Up to 4.5 million people annually are affected by Alzheimer's disease in the United States. The prevalence of Alzheimer's disease increases with age, with the risk increasing over age 60, but Alzheimer's disease is not a normal part of aging. Alzheimer's affects about 5% of men and women age 65 to 74 and about 50% of those over age 80. Causes remain unknown, but certain mutations in chromosomes and inheritance of two high-risk genes are associated with a greater risk for developing Alzheimer's disease.

Alzheimer's disease can only be diagnosed definitively by autopsy. However, it is important to recognize the disease early, and so a tentative diagnosis is made using a number of different sources of information. The patient, caretakers, and family members should be interviewed to determine the patient's history, information about the person's general health, past medical problems, and ability to carry out daily activities. Standard psychological tests are given to assess memory, problem solving, attention, counting, and language. Finally, brain scans (positron emission tomography, or PET scans) can evaluate brain function.

The earliest manifestation of Alzheimer's disease is loss of short-term memory. Psychosis, aggression, and profound personality changes are associated with advanced disease. With severe disease, judgment is lost, personal care is neglected, and physical illnesses ultimately may lead to death.

Physical findings in Alzheimer's disease include degeneration of neurons and plaque formation on and around neurons. Plaques or deposits of proteins build up around neurons and interrupt communication between neurons by neurotransmitters. Abnormal collections of proteins form **neurofibrillatory tangles** that are detected by brain scans. **Acetylcholine** is the neurotransmitter that is most affected by Alzheimer's disease. Decreases in acetylcholine are correlated with memory loss. Alterations in norepinephrine, GABA, and serotonin have been documented and may play a role in mood, behavior, and aggression.

Medications can slow the progression of early and middle stages of Alzheimer's disease, but they do not cure the disease or stop its progression. These medications include Aricept, Exelon, Razadyne, and Namenda. Associated symptoms of depression, aggression, and anxiety may be treated with antidepressants and anxiolytics. Social support is needed to improve the quality of life and maximize personal care. Vitamin E may prevent the progression of Alzheimer's disease by decreasing oxygen-free radicals that accelerate cell death. In spite of treatment, the disease remains progressive, often ending in death 8 to 10 years after onset of symptoms.

## ▶ Substance Abuse Disorders

**Substance abuse disorders** include drug and alcohol abuse and addiction. Drug and alcohol abuse and addiction have many adverse medical, emotional, and economic outcomes. Commonly abused substances include alcohol, cocaine, amphetamines, LSD, PCP, prescription drugs like benzodiazepines and painkillers, barbiturates, opiates like codeine and morphine, and marijuana (Table 14–4 ▶). Substance abuse and addiction occur at all ages, affect all socioeconomic groups, and worldwide are among the most common causes of disability and death.

| Table 14–4 ▸ **Commonly Abused Drugs** | |
|---|---|
| **Stimulants** | **Street Names** |
| Cocaine | Coke, snow, crack, crank |
| **Amphetamines** | |
| Amphetamine sulfate | Bennies, grennies, cartwheels |
| Methamphetamine | Speed, meth, crystal |
| Dextramphetamine sulfate | Hearts, oranges, dexies |
| **Hallucinogens** | |
| LSD (lysergaic acid diethylamide) | PCP, angel dust, rocket fuel, elephant tranquilizer, peace pill |
| **Depressants** | |
| Alcohol | Beer, wine, distilled drinks like whiskey, gin, vodka |
| Benzodiazepines | Dolls, yellow jackets |
| Barbituates | Barbs, downers, reds |
| Opiates | Heroin: junk, horse, H, smack; Morphine: M, morph |
| **Cannabinoids** | |
| Marijuana | Pot, grass, weed, reefer, joint, THC |

Symptoms of drug and alcohol dependence include compulsive use, physical and psychological cravings and dependence, tolerance, and withdrawal. The addict cannot function without the use of drugs and/or alcohol, and daily activities center on obtaining the substance. The key sign of substance abuse is persistent use that is physically damaging and continues in spite of adverse medical, social, economic, and legal consequences.

Some signs and symptoms are specific to the type of substance abused and include behavioral and physical changes. Long-term alcohol abuse and addiction are characterized by denial and attempts to hide the addiction and temporarily lead a functional life. A patient history reveals a pattern of alcohol use to maintain normal functioning and the inability to refrain from drinking or becoming intoxicated. The physical effects of long-term alcohol abuse include mal-nutrition, cirrhosis, neuropathy, brain damage, and cardiomyopathy. See Chapter 9 for more on the physical effects of alcohol addiction.

Behavioral and physical changes accompanying addiction and abuse involving other substances also depend on the type of substance abused, and this lies beyond the scope of this text.

Causes and risk factors that lead to substance abuse include stressful events, untreated mental illness, genetic predisposition, and, in children and adolescents, peer pressure, poor self-esteem, depression, and even boredom. Legitimate medicinal use of drugs rarely leads to abuse or addiction. Underlying addiction and abuse are seeming alterations in the dopamine reward centers of the brain where alcohol or drugs simulate pleasure and reward in susceptible individuals. Family and twin studies have implicated genes in addiction.

## Treatment of Alcohol and Substance Abuse

Treatment of alcohol abuse and addiction must include total abstinence from drinking. Supportive individual and group therapy and counseling, including Alcoholics Anonymous (AA), is effective for some alcoholics. Medical treatments such as acamprosate (Campral) reduce craving for alcohol and are effective at reducing relapses when used in combination with supportive therapy. Treatment of other types of substance abuse and addiction depends on the type of substance but must also include a treatment plan that leads to complete abstinence.

## ▶ Schizophrenia

Schizophrenia is a complex mental illness that affects over 1% of the U.S. population. The onset of **schizophrenia** is often first noted in late teenage years or early adulthood. Signs and symptoms of schizophrenia include hallucinations, delusions, disordered thinking, movement disorders, flat affect, social withdrawal, and cognitive deficits. These symptoms fall into three categories: positive, negative, and cognitive, and include fairly complex and pervasive disturbances in behavior and thinking (Box 14–3▶). The suicide rate among schizophrenics is 10%, and the average life expectancy is lower than that of the general population.

Schizophrenia diagnosis is based on a detailed history and family interviews. Medical causes such as tumors or endocrine disorders may be ruled out. The pattern of characteristic signs and symptoms are key to diagnosis. The characteristic signs of schizophrenia are a gradual withdrawal from people, activities, and social contacts, with increasing concern for abstract and sometimes eccentric ideas. Some patients experience only a single episode and remain symptom free for most of their lives. The course of the illness can fluctuate over many years and can get worse if episodes reoccur. Depression, anxiety, suspiciousness, difficulty in concentrating, and restlessness are among the early symptoms of schizophrenia, and they intensify or diminish as the illness progresses.

Disturbances in perception, or **hallucinations**, and false beliefs, or **delusions**, are reflected in behavior and thoughts that are vague and detached from reality. Schizophrenics may experience auditory or visual hallucinations in which they may hear or see things that are not present. Delusions are commonly **persecutory** (belief that they are being watched, followed, or plotted against), **grandiose** (belief that they have special powers, influence, or wealth), or **somatic** (physical belief that something is rotting inside their bodies).

**Affect**, or "feeling tone," refers to the outward expression of emotion. The schizophrenic affect may be extremely unstable, with rapid shifts from sadness to happiness for no obvious reason, or it may be flattened, with no signs of emotion in tone of voice or facial expression. Patients may state that they no longer respond to life with normal intensity or that they are "losing their feelings."

Motor disturbances in schizophrenia may be **catatonic** or rigid, or disorganized or agitated. Catatonic features may range from a total reduction in movement, or "zombie-like state," to a wild, aggressive, and agitated state. Disorganized conduct is usually **blunted** or dull, bearing no relationship to social signals. The causes of schizophrenia are complex and include genetics and environment. While schizophrenia occurs in 1% of the population, it occurs in 10% of those who have a first-degree relative with schizophrenia and occurs at a high rate among identical twins. In spite of these observations of genetic risk for developing schizophrenia, no genes have been definitively linked to schizophrenia. Environmental risks include exposure to viruses or malnutrition in the womb, problems during birth, and psychosocial factors, like stressful environmental conditions. Levels of the neurotransmitters dopamine and glutamate and changes in brain metabolism and structure point to the biological basis for schizophrenia.

Treatment includes antipsychotic medications such as risperidone and olanzapine.

---

**Box 14–3** ► **Signs and Symptoms of Schizophrenia**

**Positive Symptoms**

Positive symptoms are easy-to-spot behaviors not seen in healthy people and usually involve a loss of contact with reality. They include hallucinations, delusions, thought disorder, and disorders of movement. Positive symptoms can come and go. Sometimes they are severe and at other times hardly noticeable, depending on whether the individual is receiving treatment.

- Hallucinations
- Delusions
- Thought disorders
- Disorders of movement

**Negative Symptoms**

The term *negative symptoms* refers to reductions in normal emotional and behavioral states.

- Flat affect (immobile facial expression, monotonous voice)
- Lack of pleasure in everyday life
- Diminished ability to initiate and sustain planned activity
- Speaking infrequently, even when forced to interact.
- Neglect basic hygiene
- Need help with everyday activities

**Cognitive Symptoms**

Cognitive symptoms are subtle and are often detected only when neuropsychological tests are performed.

- Poor "executive functioning" (the ability to absorb and interpret information and make decisions based on that information)
- Inability to sustain attention
- Problems with "working memory" (the ability to keep recently learned information in mind and use it right away)

Source: *Diagnostic and Statistical Manual Text Revision IV.* American Psychiatric Association, 2000 and the National Institute of Mental Health, www.nimh.gov

---

Treatment must include illness management therapy, psychosocial therapy, and cognitive behavioral therapy and must often include family therapy.

## ► Mood Disorders

Mood disorders are characterized by marked periods of sadness and euphoria. While it is normal for people to experience ups and downs, those who have **major depression** or **bipolar disorder** experience debilitating symptoms that result in vocational failure, social withdrawal, and dysfunctional relationships.

## Major Depression

Complaints of sadness and hopelessness are commonly expressed by depressed individuals. Major depression occurs at any age and, if untreated, may result in suicide. At least one depressive episode affects up to 80% of the U.S. population annually. Women are diagnosed with major depression about twice as often as men. Depression in the elderly is often masked by concurrent physical illness and is attributed to normal aging processes. Poor performance in school, irritability, loss of appetite, social withdrawal, and pretending to be sick are signs of depression in children.

A major depressive disorder consists of at least one episode of serious mood depression accompanied by a number of changes in behavior. Complaints frequently include a loss of interest and pleasure, and withdrawal from activities. Feelings of guilt, worthlessness, anxiety, and shame are reported because individuals with major depression view their illness as a moral deficiency. Physical symptoms that suggest emotional distress include unexplained weight loss or weight gain, disturbed sleep, decreased energy, poor eye contact, monosyllabic speech, and indifference to pleasure or joy.

Subcategories of depression include **seasonal affective disorder**, **postpartum depression**, **dysthymia**, and **premenstrual dysphoric disorder**. Seasonal affective disorder is believed to be due to decreased sunlight exposure during the winter months. Postpartum depression usually occurs 2 weeks to 6 months following the birth of a child. Persistent care of the newborn, sleep deprivation, social stresses, and hormonal changes all play a role in the development of postpartum depression. Chronic depression or dysthymia is diagnosed when symptoms persist for more than 2 years. Cyclic depressive symptoms prior to menstruation may occur regularly for some women.

Heredity is currently the most important predisposing factor for major depression. The risk for major depression is higher in families with a history of mood disorders. Depression in a parent contributes to depression in genetically vulnerable children. While stressful life events trigger sadness, despair, and grief, stressful factors alone do not cause major depression (Box 14–4 ▶).

The most prominent theory for depression focuses on regulatory disturbances in neurotransmitters. The neurotransmitters serotonin, norepinephrine, and dopamine are widely distributed in the central nervous system and are implicated in regulation of mood, arousal, movement, and sleep. Medications that increase serotonin, norepinephrine, and dopamine effectively reduce symptoms of depression.

Major depression may occur with a number of physical and psychological disorders. Physical disorders such as thyroid disease or Cushing's disease induce depression by altering hormone levels. Chronic heart disease or cancer produce depressive symptoms from associated disability, fatigue, and physical pain. Direct physical causes of depression include HIV infections and seizure disorders that damage the brain and central nervous system. Psychological disorders such as anxiety disorders, eating disorders, and developmental disorders are often referred to as **co-morbid disorders** because they commonly occur with major depression.

Various prescription medications and substance abuse induce depression by altering brain function and regulation of hormones and neurotransmitters. Heart medications, for example, alter neuronal responses to norepinephrine, leading to fatigue and depressive symptoms. Corticosteroid medications induce behavioral changes, psychosis, and major depression especially in susceptible individuals.

---

**Box 14–4 ▶ Symptoms of Major Depression**

- Prolonged sadness or unexplained crying spells
- Significant changes in appetite and sleep patterns
- Irritability, anger, worry, agitation, anxiety
- Pessimism, indifference
- Loss of energy, persistent lethargy
- Unexplained aches and pains
- Feelings of guilt, worthlessness, and/or hopelessness
- Inability to concentrate
- Indecisiveness
- Inability to take pleasure in former interests
- Social withdrawal
- Excessive consumption of alcohol or use of chemical substances
- Recurring thoughts of death or suicide

Source: *Diagnostic and Statistical Manual Text Revision IV.* American Psychiatric Association, 2000.

Alcoholic beverages as well as many commonly abused substances depress the central nervous system.

A trial of antidepressant medication that restores regulation of norepinephrine, dopamine, and/or serotonin is indicated for most cases of major depression. These drugs elevate the levels of these neurotransmitters; the drugs are commonly called selective serotonin reuptake inhibitors (SSRIs), noreprinephrine reuptake inhibitors (NRIs), serotonin and norepinephrine reuptake inhibitors (SNRIs), and dopamine agonists. Optimal reduction of symptoms is usually noticed 14 to 21 days after starting medication. Psychosocial treatment is often required to improve social functioning and to change depressive thought processes. Depression that is resistant to drug treatment may respond to electroconvulsive therapy, in which electrodes apply current to the brain. Severe depression may be accompanied by psychosis, which requires the use of antipsychotic medications.

## Bipolar Disorder

Bipolar disorder, or manic-depressive illness, is a mood disorder that causes unusual shifts from depression to **mania**, or an overly elevated, energetic, irritable mood. Periods of highs and lows are called *episodes* of mania and depression. Bipolar disorder affects more than 2 million American adults annually. Bipolar disorder typically develops in late adolescence or early adulthood. However, some people have their first symptoms during childhood, and some develop them late in life. Bipolar disorder is often not recognized as an illness, and people may suffer for years without a diagnosis or proper treatment (Box 14–5▸).

Mania can vary from extreme elation, hyperactivity, and irritability to extreme aggression, with little need for sleep, and risky behaviors that are later regretted. An overly enthusiastic mood at times may attract others; however, mood shifts with delusions may lead to alienation of friends and family and to irresponsible behaviors such as spending one's life savings or engaging in sexual indiscretions.

A distinct period of an abnormally elevated mood that is not induced by the physiologic ef-

---

**Box 14–5 ► Symptoms of Mania**

- Increased physical and mental activity and energy
- Heightened mood, exaggerated optimism and self-confidence
- Excessive irritability, aggressive behavior
- Decreased need for sleep without experiencing fatigue
- Grandiose delusions, inflated sense of self-importance
- Racing speech, racing thoughts, flight of ideas
- Impulsiveness, poor judgment, distractibility
- Reckless behavior such as spending sprees, rash business decisions, erratic driving, and sexual indiscretions
- In the most severe cases, delusions and hallucinations

*Source: Diagnostic and Statistical Manual Text Revision IV.* American Psychiatric Association, 2000.

---

fects of a drug substance followed by a distinct period of depression is central to diagnosis of a bipolar disorder. Different categories of bipolar disorder are determined by patterns of symptoms or severity of highs and lows. Bipolar I disorder is associated with periods of intense mania and depression that last for several weeks. Bipolar II disorder is associated with less severe episodes of mania, but depression may continue for several weeks. A chronic fluctuating mood, with mild symptoms of both depression and mania, or cyclothymic disorder, often is undiagnosed and may eventually result in a more severe form of bipolar disorder.

The causes of bipolar disorder are unclear, though genetic, biochemical, and environmental causes have been identified. Like other mental illnesses, several genes acting together may ultimately identify patients who will develop bipolar disorder. Bipolar disorder runs in families, and stressful experiences may trigger some symptoms. Changes in neurotransmitter regulation that lead to bipolar disorder may be affected by the presence of another illness, stress, substance abuse, changes in diet and exercise, and hormonal changes.

Medical treatment of bipolar disorder is complex. Patients often require prolonged treatment with medications called mood stabilizers, such as lithium or certain antiepileptic medications, antidepressants, sedative medications or "sleep aids," and major tranquilizers or antipsychotic medications. Family and individual patient counseling improves social functioning by providing psychological support and treatment that stabilizes extreme characteristics of mania or depression.

▶ **Anxiety Disorders**

**Anxiety disorders** include a number of disorders in which the primary feature is abnormal or inappropriate anxiety that interferes with daily school, work, recreational, and family activities. Anxiety is a normal phenomenon in which our mind and body reacts to flee from danger, also known as "fight or flight." Heart rate, respiratory rate, blood pressure, and muscle tension increases at the onset of a stressful event. Symptoms of anxiety become a problem when they occur without any recognizable cause or when the cause does not require an intense response.

Anxiety disorders affect adults and children and may persist for many years without proper treatment. As with many other mental illnesses, family and friends often label those that suffer anxiety disorders as weak and unable to "snap out of their condition." Some people's lives become so restricted that they avoid normal, everyday activities such as grocery shopping or driving. In some cases, they become housebound.

The genetic basis for anxiety disorders originates from family studies. Anxiety disorders are common among relatives of affected individuals. The risk for phobias is greater in relatives of individuals with both depression and panic disorder. In cases of PTSD, genetic factors may explain why only certain individuals exposed to trauma develop PTSD.

Head injuries, an overactive thyroid gland, cardiovascular disease, respiratory disease, altered regulation of neurotransmitters, and certain medications may cause anxiety disorders. Individuals with anxiety disorders are more sensitive to medications that increase heart rate, blood pressure, and fear behaviors. Abnormal neurotransmission of the neurotransmitter serotonin as a cause of obsessive-compulsive disorder (OCD) is recognized by a reduction of symptoms with medications that increase serotonin.

## Types of Anxiety Disorders

Physical symptoms and behaviors vary slightly with each subtype of anxiety disorder. Panic disorder, generalized anxiety disorder, phobic disorders, social phobia, obsessive compulsive disorder, and post-traumatic stress disorder share the common theme of excessive, irrational fear.

*Panic Disorder*   A panic attack involves a sudden onset of fear and terror accompanied by physical symptoms in vital organs such as the heart and lungs. Shortness of breath, chest pains, and palpitations peak within 10 minutes and usually resolve within 30 to 60 minutes. Because of the unpredictability of a panic attack, people who have them develop anticipatory anxiety, or a persistent pattern of worry regarding when and where the attack will take place. Physical complaints often lead patients to seek emergency medical care.

*Generalized Anxiety Disorder*   Severe persistent worries that are out of proportion to the circumstance describe a typical day for sufferers of generalized anxiety disorders. Common worries related to work, money, health, and safety are difficult to control. Additional complaints of restlessness, fatigue, muscle tension, impaired concentration, and disturbed sleep may often be misdiagnosed as depression.

*Phobic Disorders*   An irrational fear of something, or a specific phobia, that poses little or no danger is the most common type of anxiety disorder. Some phobias, such as a fear of the dark, of strangers, or of large animals, begin in childhood and disappear with age. Hyperventilation, or rapid breathing, may accompany a fear of heights, flying, closed spaces, insects, and rodents. Although adults with phobias realize that these fears are irrational, they often find that facing the feared object or situation brings on a panic or severe anxiety attack.

*Social Phobia*   Social phobia involves excessive worry and self-consciousness in everyday social situations. Intense fears of being humiliated in social situations interfere with ordinary activities. Physical symptoms that accompany social anxiety include blushing, profuse sweating, nausea, and difficulty talking.

*Obsessive-Compulsive Disorder* Anxious, irrational thoughts and images, also known as obsessions, lead to the need to perform rituals to prevent or get rid of the obsessive stimulus. Rituals are patterns of irrational behaviors, or compulsions, that provide temporary relief from the anxiety. Obsessions centered on cleanliness and fear of germs, for example, may lead to compulsive hand washing. Other rituals may include the need to repeat certain words and phrases to ward off danger, or repetitive counting of objects. Patients with obsessive-compulsive disorder (OCD) are aware that their compulsion and corresponding ritual is irrational but cannot stop it. OCD affects both men and women, and symptoms may ease over time with appropriate treatment.

*Post-traumatic Stress Disorder* Exposure to an overwhelming traumatic incident such as the events of September 11, 2001, or encounters of trauma such as rape, violence, child abuse, or war, may lead to symptoms and diagnosis of post-traumatic stress disorder (PTSD). Victims of trauma develop persistent frightening thoughts and memories months or years after the event. The traumatic event is repeatedly experienced as nightmares and flashbacks or numbing recollections of the event throughout the day. The individual avoids reminders of the event, startles or feels frightened easily, and may feel detached and numb. PTSD sufferers may lose interest in things they used to enjoy, avoid affection, and become irritable or aggressive. Individuals with PTSD often feel guilty about surviving the event or about behaving destructively, as in case of veterans of war.

Imaging techniques have focused on the role of brain structures that mediate communication and process information to memory. The **amygdala** is an almond-shaped structure located deep within the brain, and it may play a role in fear and phobias. The **hippocampus** is a structure of the brain that processes and stores information to memory. The size of the hippocampus appears smaller in post-traumatic stress disorder, which may explain the memory deficits and flashbacks in individuals with PTSD.

## Treatment of Anxiety Disorders

Anxiety, as a learned response to a stimulus and corresponding biochemical changes in brain chemistry, responds to treatment with medications and psychotherapy. Medications that increase serotonin are effective in the treatment of OCD, though psychotherapy is often required to gain understanding of underlying emotional conflict. Antianxiety medications that increase the effect of the neurotransmitter gamma aminobutyric acid (GABA) have a calming effect and work quickly. The use of antianxiety medications is limited, however, by their potential for addiction.

## ▶ Eating Disorders

Eating disorders involve serious disturbances in eating behavior. Fashion trends, ad campaigns, social attitudes, and athletics promote leaner body weight and a preoccupation with body shape and weight. Extreme attitudes surrounding weight and food, combined with psychological and medical complications, define the disabilities that meet the criteria for eating disorders.

## Symptoms of Eating Disorders

**Anorexia nervosa** and **bulimia nervosa** occur primarily in young women who develop a paralyzing fear of becoming fat. In anorexia nervosa, fear of obesity causes excessive restriction of food, resulting in emaciation. Bulimia involves massive binge eating followed by purging or excessive dieting and exercise to prevent weight gain.

*Anorexia Nervosa* *Anorexia* means "lack of appetite." Ironically, individuals with anorexia nervosa are hungry and yet are preoccupied with dieting and limiting food intake to the point of starvation. There is an intense fear of gaining weight or becoming fat even though anorectics become dangerously thin. The process of eating becomes an obsession, with rituals centered on meal plans, calorie counts, compulsive exercise, and self-induced vomiting despite little food intake.

The typical anorectic is an adolescent female who has lost 15% of her body weight, fears obesity, stops menstruating, and otherwise looks healthy. Other notable signs include low blood pressure, decreased heart rate, and **edema**, or swelling of tissues. Metabolic changes, including dehydration and depletion of electrolytes (sodium, potassium, and chloride), can result in abnormal heart rhythm, heart failure, sudden cardiac arrest, and death.

Usually described as the honor-roll student or state champion, the individual denies that anything is wrong and typically does not seek medical care until prompted into treatment by friends and family. Depression is common as anorectics withdraw from social affairs involving food and festivities.

*Bulimia Nervosa* Similar to anorexia nervosa, bulimics are excessively concerned with body weight and physical shape. Unlike anorectics, bulimics **binge** by eating an excessive amount of food within a restricted period of time, followed by compensatory **purging** behavior such as self-induced vomiting or misuse of laxatives or diuretics. Rigorous dieting and exercise may also follow binges to prevent weight gain. There is a feeling of loss of control during the binging episode, followed by intense distress and guilt. Body weight may be normal, which makes it easy for bulimics to hide their illness.

The medical consequences of bulimia nervosa can be devastating. Stomach acid and digestive enzymes from vomiting erode tooth enamel and cause injury and inflammation to the esophagus and salivary glands. Severe dental caries and gum disease eventually require removal of teeth. Vomiting and laxative and diuretic abuse lower blood potassium levels, causing muscle cramping and abnormal heart rhythms. In cases of severe potassium loss, death may result from cardiac arrest. Prolonged and excessive laxative abuse may severely damage the bowel. If the bowel ceases its function, surgery is required to form a **colostomy**, an opening from the bowel to the abdominal wall to allow removal of the feces into a bag attached to the outer abdominal wall.

Bulimics are aware of their behavior and feel intense guilt and shame. Bulimics are generally outgoing, impulsive, and prone to depression and alcohol or drug abuse. Unlike anorectics, bulimics are more likely to talk about their illness and desperately seek help from physicians and friends.

Patterns of psychological and interpersonal issues most consistently provide insight into the causes of eating disorders. Low self-esteem and persistent feelings of inadequacy shape attitudes of perfectionism for the anorectic and severe self-criticism for the bulimic. Troubled family relationships, difficulty expressing feelings and emotions, and a history of physical or sexual abuse are reported more often in bulimics than anorectics. Social attitudes that value thinness and limit beauty to specific body weight and shape influence body image and contribute to extreme dieting and exercise for both anorectics and bulimics.

The biological basis for eating behavior involves a complex network of brain structures and neurotransmitters. The hypothalamus regulates hunger, monitors fullness of the stomach, and determines how much food is eaten. The limbic system influences emotions and selection of foods to appease the appetite. The prefrontal region of the brain controls decisions about when, where, and how to eat. Future studies on the biology of appetite control and behavior may lead to development of new medications to treat eating disorders.

Successful treatment of and recovery from eating disorders requires the realization that starvation, binging, and purging is destructive. Medical treatment to restore nutrition and replace fluids and electrolytes is crucial to prevent death from organ failure. Medication to relieve depression and anxiety may improve mood and thought processes. Group, family, individual, and nutritional counseling provide support to break down delusions that shape eating behavior and distortions in body image.

## ▶ Personality Disorders

Persistent, inflexible patterns of behavior that affect interpersonal relationships describe **personality disorders**. Personality disorders appear in adolescence or early adulthood and remain stable throughout an individual's lifetime. The DSM-IV describes three major categories of personality disorders based on "clusters" of symptoms.

Personality disorders occur along with medical and psychiatric illnesses. Relations with family, friends, and caregivers are often strained by inflexible and maladaptive personality characteristics. People with severe personality disorders are more vulnerable to psychiatric breakdowns and are at risk for alcoholism, substance abuse, reckless sexual behavior, eating disorders, and violence.

## Symptoms of Personality Disorders

### Cluster A: Paranoid and Schizoid

**Paranoid Personality** The paranoid personality type is indifferent, suspicious, and hostile. His or her relationships are shallow because of a tendency to respond to positive acts or kindness with distrust. The paranoid personality type interprets positive statement such as "You look like a million bucks" to mean "My friend is after my money."

**Schizoid Personality** People with schizoid personality appear cold and isolated. Often called introverted, schizoid personality types appear self-absorbed and withdrawn. They often deal with their fears through superstitions, magical thinking, and unusual beliefs.

### Cluster B: Antisocial, Borderline, Histrionic, and Narcissistic

**Antisocial Personality** Callous disregard for others and manipulation of people for personal gratification characterize antisocial personality types. Antisocial personality may start as a conduct problem in childhood, manifested as disrespect for authority and for personal and public property. Adolescents and adults with antisocial personalities are at risk for alcoholism, drug abuse, sexual improprieties, and violence.

**Borderline Personality** Borderline personality disorders often occur in women who were deprived of adequate care during childhood. Their moods are unstable and characterized by crisis and anger alternating with depression. Threats of real or imagined abandonment elicit impulsive behaviors such as promiscuity and substance abuse. The individual with a borderline personality disorder is vulnerable to brief psychotic episodes, substance abuse, and eating disorders.

**Histrionic Personality** The histrionic personality is characterized by theatrical and exaggerated emotional behavior. Friendships are initially formed because others are attracted to the histrionic personality's energetic and entertaining behavior. Hysteria and flamboyant behaviors often result in negative responses and feelings of rejection.

**Narcissistic Personality** The narcissistic personality type has an exaggerated self-image and a tendency to think little of others. Narcissists expect others to admire their grandiosity and feel they are entitled to have their needs attended to. When rejected by others through criticism or defeat, the narcissist becomes enraged or severely depressed.

### Cluster C: Avoidant, Dependent, and Obsessive-Compulsive

**Avoidant Personality** Avoidant personality types appear shy and timid, as if they have a social phobia. They fear relationships, although they have a strong desire to feel accepted. They are hypersensitive to criticism and rejection and are susceptible to depression, anxiety, and anger for failing to develop social relationships.

**Dependent Personality** Dependent personality types have an extremely poor self-image. They appoint others to make significant decisions out of fear of expressing themselves or offending others. Extended illness may bring out a dependent personality in adults.

**Obsessive-Compulsive Personality** The obsessive-compulsive personality types are dependable, meticulous, orderly, and intolerant of mistakes. They are often high achievers, attending to details while failing to complete the task at hand. Individuals with an obsessive-compulsive personality avoid new situations and relationships because these new elements cannot be methodically controlled.

## Treatment of Personality Disorders

Most people with personality disorders do not see a need for treatment. Often, secondary medical and psychiatric illnesses force persons with personality disorders to seek treatment. Rigid thoughts and behavior often complicate compliance with treatment and are frustrating for healthcare providers. Individual, family, and group therapy is required to point out consequences of behavior. Antianxiety, antidepressant, and antipsychotic medications may be required to treat accompanying symptoms of anxiety, depression, and psychosis.

## ▶ Suicide

Suicide is almost always associated with mental illness. People consider suicide when they feel hopeless and are unable to see alternative solutions to confusion, mental and physical anguish, and chaos in their life. Risks for suicide include substance abuse, previous suicide attempts, a family history of suicide, a history of sexual abuse, and impulsive or aggressive character. More than four times as many men as women die by suicide; however, women attempt suicide more often. Suicidal behavior occurs most often when people experience major losses and stressful events such as divorce, loss of a job, incarceration, and chronic illness.

Unlike physical illnesses, mental illness has no visible wounds and so is associated with social stigma, isolation, and personal faults. Those with mental illness contemplating suicide may talk about their distress at the risk of being judged, ignored, and isolated. Warning signs of suicide include withdrawal, talk of death, giving away cherished possessions, and a sudden shift in mood. A severely depressed person may unexpectedly appear better, or a schizophrenic may progressively develop delusions about death prior to a suicide attempt. A suicide attempt or completed suicide is devastating to families, friends, and caregivers, who commonly experience remorse and guilt for failing to avert the suicide attempt or death.

## ▶ Age-Related Disorders

Mental illness can occur at any age. Some disorders occur first in childhood and adolescence, such as ADHD, conduct disorder, and oppositional defiant disorder. Others are developmental disorders usually first recognized in childhood but continue throughout life; these disorders include mental retardation, autistic disorders, and tic disorders. Some are strongly associated with adolescence, including bulimia nervosa and anorexia nervosa. Other disorders clearly associated with advanced aging include dementia and Alzheimer's disease. Many other disorders can first occur at any time during adulthood from young adult through advanced age. These include depression, anxiety, schizophrenia, and substance abuse disorders.

### RESOURCES

Food and Drug Administration: www.fda.gov

National Alliance for the Mentally Ill: www.nami.org

National Institutes of Mental Health: www.nimh.org

World Health Organization: www.who.org

## Prevention ✚ PLUS!

### Suicide Warning Signs

Mentally ill people may have self-destructive thoughts and may exhibit suicidal behaviors. Patients with depressive symptoms in particular are more likely to have suicidal thoughts. Thus it is important for healthcare workers and families of the patient to watch for suicide warning signs. The following are signs of suicidal behavior and require immediate attention:

- Withdrawal and isolation
- Saying good-bye to close friends and family
- Indirectly expressed suicide messages or wishes

- Depression
- Giving away or discarding personal possessions
- Explicit suicide messages

If you or someone you know exhibits these behaviors, call your doctor, or call 911, or go to a hospital emergency room to get immediate help, or ask a friend or family member to help you do these things. Call the toll-free, 24-hour hotline of the National Suicide Prevention Lifeline at 1-800-273-TALK (1-800-273-8255); TTY: 1-800-799-4TTY (4889) to talk to a trained counselor.

*Source:* National Institutes of Mental Health: www.nimh.org

# DISEASES AT A GLANCE
## Mental Illness and Cognitive Disorders*

| DISORDER | ETIOLOGY | SIGNS AND SYMPTOMS |
| --- | --- | --- |
| Disruptive behavior disorders | Genetics, biology, environment | Willful disobedience, defiance of authority, aggression |
| Attention deficit hyperactivity disorder | Genetics, biology, environment | Hyperactivity, impulsivity, inattention |
| Mental retardation | Genetics, biology, environment | Social language deficits, below-average intelligence |
| Autistic disorder | Genetics, biology, environment, toxins | Reciprocal language deficits, repetitive stereotypical behaviors |
| Tic disorder | Genetics, biology, environment | Rapid involuntary repetitive movement or vocalization |
| Dementia | Genetics, biology, environment, toxins | Language, memory, and mood deficits |
| Substance abuse disorders | Genetics, environment | Compulsive use, physical and psychological cravings, tolerance, and withdrawal |

*Prevention of a disorder and its complications depends on screening and intervention, especially in at-risk persons.

| DIAGNOSIS | TREATMENT | LIFESPAN |
|---|---|---|
| Psychosocial and medical evaluation, psychometric testing; diagnosed in childhood | Cognitive, behavioral psychotherapy, pharmacotherapy: stimulants, atypical antipsychotic medications, mood stabilizers | Onset in early childhood |
| Psychosocial and medical evaluation, psychometric testing; diagnosed prior to the age of 7, with approximately 50% persistence into adulthood | Cognitive, behavioral psychotherapy, pharmacotherapy: stimulants, atypical antipsychotic medications, certain antidepressants | Onset in early childhood; more prevalent in boys |
| Psychosocial and medical evaluation, psychometric testing; diagnosed usually before 3 years of age | Behavioral therapy, occupational therapy, social support services | Usually first recognized in childhood |
| Psychosocial and medical evaluation, psychometric testing; diagnosed usually around 3 years of age | Behavioral therapy, occupational therapy, social support services; pharmacotherapy or other supportive care to manage aggression or self-injurious behavior | Usually first recognized by age 3 |
| Psychosocial and medical evaluation, psychometric testing; diagnosed usually before adulthood | Behavioral therapy; pharmacotherapy: certain antidepressants or atypical antipsychotic medications | Can develop at any age; usually first recognized in childhood and adolescence |
| Psychosocial and medical evaluation; diagnosed most commonly after age 60 | Behavioral, cognitive, family psychotherapy; social supportive care services; pharmacotherapy: memory enhancers, atypical antipsychotic medications, antidepressants, and/or mood stabilizers | Onset in older adults |
| Diagnosis may follow social, medical, or legal consequences imposing psychosocial evaluation | Behavioral therapy, 12-step programs supporting abstinence (such as Alcoholics Anonymous or Narcotics Anonymous). Pharmacotherapy: antidepressants, atypical antipsychotic medications, or mood stabilizers | |

# DISEASES AT A GLANCE

## Mental Illness and Cognitive Disorders (*continued*)

| DISEASE | ETIOLOGY | SIGNS AND SYMPTOMS |
| --- | --- | --- |
| Schizophrenia | Genetics, biology, environment | Loss of contact with reality, severe disturbance in social functioning, bizarre thoughts, withdrawal from social interactions, hallucinations, delusions |
| Major depression | Genetics, biology, environment | Prolonged sadness, significant changes in sleep and appetite, irritability, feelings of guilt and anxiety |
| Bipolar disorder | Genetics, biology, environment | Mania (episodic elation, inflated sense of self) alternating with depression |
| Anxiety disorder | Genetics, biology, environment | Inappropriate fear response with avoidance of daily work, family, life, school, and recreational activities |
| Eating disorders | Genetics social trends, attitudes, and stresses | Anorexia: persistent dieting, starvation, excessive exercise, body weight less than 15% of ideal body weight<br>Bulimia: binge followed by purging behavior, overuse of laxatives, excessive dieting, body weight normal or thin |
| Personality disorders | Environment | Inflexible patterns of behavior with strained relationships; may occur with substance use disorders, reckless sexual behavior, eating disorders and violence |

| DIAGNOSIS | TREATMENT | LIFESPAN |
|---|---|---|
| Psychosocial and medical evaluation, psychometric testing, unpredictable behavior | Pharmacotherapy: antipsychotic medications primarily, antidepressants occasionally; behavioral therapy, occupational therapy, social support services | Usually first recognized in late adolescence and early adulthood |
| Psychosocial and medical evaluation, psychometric testing | Cognitive behavioral therapy, psychotherapy, social supportive care; pharmacotherapy: antidepressants, tranquilizers, sleep aids or sedative medications | Usually first recognized in late adolescence and early adulthood |
| Psychosocial and medical evaluation, psychometric testing | Cognitive behavioral therapy, psychotherapy, social supportive care; pharmacotherapy: mood stabilizers, atypical antipsychotic medications, sleep aids or sedative medications | First seen in young adults |
| Psychosocial and medical evaluation, psychometric testing | Cognitive behavioral therapy; pharmacotherapy: antianxiety medications and certain antidepressants | Usually first recognized in late adolescence and early adulthood |
| Psychosocial and medical evaluation, psychometric testing | Psychosocial therapy, pharmacotherapy | Most prevalent in late childhood and adolescence, young adulthood; mostly in girls and women |
| Psychosocial and medical evaluation, psychometric testing | Cognitive behavioral therapy, social support, social services; pharmacotherapy for coexisting depression, anxiety, agitation, aggression, delusions, or psychosis | Onset in early adulthood; more prevalent in females |

# Interactive Exercises

## Cases for Critical Thinking

1. J. R. is a 17-year-old male with above average intelligence. As an infant, he was colicky and difficult to put to sleep. He learned to walk around 12 months of age. At home, J. R. seemed to run on a motor: He scurried around the house, frequently bumping into furniture. J. R. had a hearing test at school at 5 years of age because teachers felt that he may have been hard of hearing, but the test was normal. His grades were average during the primary, intermediate, and junior high-school years. By his senior year in high school, J. R.'s grades dropped dramatically. He frequently appeared spacey, irritable, and angry. He preferred to eat lunch alone and spent much time in his room. His parents feared that he was abusing drugs because he had a history of a "poor choice for friends." His high school counselor recommended a psychiatric evaluation for J. R. His parents were offended at this recommendation.

   a. What are the advantages and disadvantages of a full mental health evaluation?
   b. What potential disorders do you suspect J. R. is experiencing?
   c. What are the potential causes of his disorders?

2. A. M. is a 10-year-old female with a history of bad school grades and fighting in class. She has a brother with ADHD. Her parents divorced when she was 5 years old, and she has been raised with a nanny because her mother travels frequently with her job. A. M. is very athletic—she is a member of the traveling soccer team and a competitive ballet dancer. She has voiced frustration over her grades, as she feels that although she works hard, she cannot "make the grades." She fears disappointing her mother by quitting dance and soccer, and she feels like a failure. Although A. M. is a very talented dancer, she trembles and feels her heart pound prior to competition. Her appetite has been poor, and she has been observed picking at her food. A. M.'s mother is concerned and has made an appointment with a doctor.

   a. Does A. M. have warning signs of a potential mental illness? What symptoms and behaviors point to a potential problem?
   b. Would you recommend an evaluation for A. M.?
   c. What type of treatments are available for A. M.?

3. D. T. is a 46-year-old male who recently moved his family across the state. His mother recently died of complications from Alzheimer's disease, and he is executor of her estate. D. T. moved his family because of a great job opportunity. Although he loves his job, he regrets moving his family from the town they lived in for 20 years. He has been spending much of his free time alone in his office and has been ignoring his wife and children. D. T.'s father was an alcoholic, and his wife fears that his recent stress may drive him to drink. He has lost interest in sex and recently declined an invitation to a golf outing that he had enjoyed in the past. D. T. has been talking to himself a lot and claims that at times he has seen his mother in his sleep. He awoke abruptly one night from sleep and has been complaining of having nightmares. D. T. sometimes appears frozen and indifferent to conversations and behaves as though something is bothering him. His wife feels that D. T. is mourning the loss of his mother, since his mother was never the person he always longed for. His mother had been abusive to D. T., who was conceived out of wedlock. His mother made sure that he had "proper" upbringing with strict discipline and often punished D. T. rather harshly if he failed to follow directions.

   a. What signs of mental illness does D. T. have?
   b. What condition do you think D.T. has?
   c. What recommendations would you give to D.T.'s wife?

## Multiple Choice

1. Reforms in the treatment of the mentally ill started after the French Revolution with an Austrian physician named _____.
   a. Sigmund Freud          b. Franz Mesmer
   c. Emil Kraepelin         d. Sybil Dorsett

2. Psychiatric diagnoses are categorized in a book named the _____.
   a. PDR                    b. AMA
   c. DSM                    d. Axis

3. Which of the following neurotransmitters is implicated in schizophrenia, depression, and ADHD?
   a. epinephrine
   b. serotonin
   c. gamma aminobutyric acid (GABA)
   d. dopamine

4. Which of the following regarding ADHD is false?
   a. ADHD is limited to children.
   b. ADHD is a neurobiological disorder.
   c. ADHD is more common in males than in females.
   d. There are three subtypes of ADHD.

5. Medications that replace _____ are effective in improving memory in persons with Alzheimer's disease.
   a. dopamine               b. serotonin
   c. acetylcholine          d. GABA

6. A false belief that one is being watched or punished is also known as a _____ delusion.
   a. persecutory            b. somatic
   c. grandiose              d. affective

7. Binge eating followed by purging behavior such as self-induced vomiting most commonly occurs in _____.
   a. anorexia nervosa
   b. bulimia nervosa
   c. binge eating disorder
   d. all of the above

8. Periods of intense mania and depression that last for several weeks is also known as _____.
   a. cyclothymic disorder
   b. bipolar I
   c. bipolar II
   d. all of the above

9. Adults with bipolar illness may be treated with all of the following types of medications except _____.
   a. sedatives
   b. antidepressant medications
   c. stimulant medications
   d. antipsychotic medications

10. Anxious, irrational thoughts and images are also called _____.
    a. compulsions            b. delusions
    c. hallucinations         d. obsessions

## True or False

_____ 1. Bipolar disorder is a behavioral disorder with extreme highs and lows.

_____ 2. ADHD is an emotional disorder associated with depression, anxiety, and hyperactivity.

_____ 3. Persons of different age groups are at risk for different types of mental illness.

_____ 4. Childhood conduct disorder is also known as childhood antisocial personality.

_____ 5. People with high blood pressure and diabetes have a higher risk for dementia.

_____ 6. Substance abuse is a conscious choice to use drugs or alcohol.

_____ 7. Hallucinations and delusions are symptoms of posttraumatic stress disorder.

_____ 8. Children are at risk for major depression.

_____ 9. Individuals with a schizoid personality disorder are distant, introverted, and tend to hallucinate.

_____ 10. Primary psychiatric diagnoses are indicated in all the five axis of diagnosis according to the *DSM*.

## Fill-Ins

1. _____ is the medical specialty that diagnoses and prescribes medical treatment for mental illness.

2. Chemical messengers, or _____, are implicated in mental illness.

3. Mood, thought processes, appetite, movement, heart rate, and blood pressure are regulated by the neurotransmitter _____.

4. Below average intelligence accompanied by deficits in language and adaptive functioning is diagnostic for _____.

5. Rapid stereotyped movements that may be suppressed by conscious effort are known as _____.

6. Alzheimer's disease is mostly due to impaired regulation of _____ neurotransmitters.

7. Core symptoms of drug and alcohol abuse include _____, _____, _____, and _____.

8. An individual's emotional state in mental illness is referred to as _____.

9. _____ is due to decreased sunlight exposure during the winter months.

10. Decreased need for sleep, with excessive irritability and grandiosity, is symptomatic for _____.

# Multimedia Preview

Additional interactive resources and activities for this chapter can be found on the Companion Website. For videos, audio glossary, and review, access the accompanying DVD-ROM in this book.

## ▶ DVD-ROM Highlights

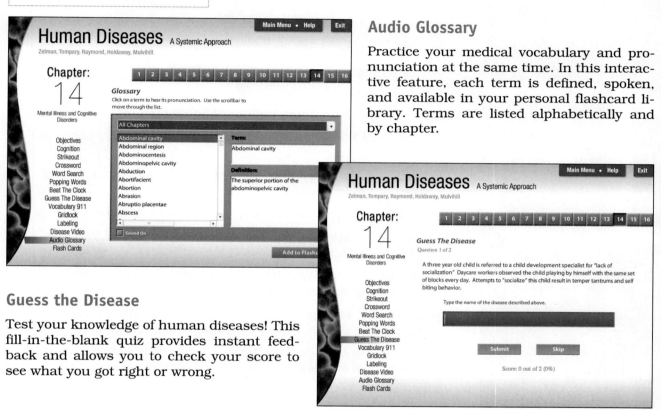

### Audio Glossary

Practice your medical vocabulary and pronunciation at the same time. In this interactive feature, each term is defined, spoken, and available in your personal flashcard library. Terms are listed alphabetically and by chapter.

### Guess the Disease

Test your knowledge of human diseases! This fill-in-the-blank quiz provides instant feedback and allows you to check your score to see what you got right or wrong.

## ▶ Website Highlights—www.pearsonhighered.com/zelman

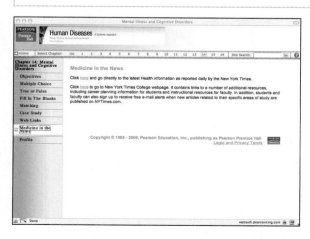

### Medicine in the News

Take advantage of the free-access online study guide that accompanies your textbook. You'll be able to stay current with a link to medical news articles updated daily by *The New York Times*. By clicking on this URL you'll also access a variety of quizzes with instant feedback and an audio glossary.

CHAPTER

# 15

# Diseases of the Musculoskeletal System

## Learning Objectives

After studying this chapter, you should be able to

- Understand the normal structure and function of bones, joints, and muscle

- Describe the etiology, signs and symptoms, diagnostic tests, and treatment of infectious diseases of bone

- Explain how vitamin and mineral deficiencies lead to bone disease

- Describe the etiology, signs and symptoms, diagnostic tests, and treatment of bone cancer

- Describe the etiology, signs and symptoms, diagnostic tests, and treatment of the common types of arthritis, gout, and bursitis

- Identify the etiology, signs and symptoms, diagnostic tests, and treatment of dislocations, sprains, strains, and carpal tunnel syndrome

- Describe the etiology, signs and symptoms, diagnostic tests, and treatment of muscular dystrophy and myasthenia gravis

- Understand age-related changes and diseases of the musculoskeletal system

## Fact or Fiction?

Rest is best for rheumatoid arthritis.

*Fiction: Unless pain is too severe, daily low-impact exercise maintains mobility and range of motion.*

# Arthritis

**A**rthritis in its various forms has long plagued humans. Lack of understanding of medical science, coupled with a desperate search for relief, produced unusual prescriptions in American traditional and folk medicine. One folk healer suggested that relief from gout could be obtained by cutting a hole in a tree, holding the affected body part to it, and sealing the hole with sand, trapping the disease. Another nineteenth-century prescription required the sufferer to carry a potato in the hip pocket. Treating "like with like" was the basis for treating gout with an earthworm, whose curled shapes resemble gnarled gout-afflicted appendages. How the earthworm was administered is not clear. A home remedy from Texas called for ingestion of wintergreen oil. These ineffective treatments were benign compared to some prescriptions. Citing bad blood as the culprit, some people were subjected to regular bleedings. Cashing in on the public's misunderstanding of uranium's powers in the 1950s, predatory entrepreneurs recommended baths in uranium pools or ingestion of uranium-laced water. Our understanding and treatment of arthritis has progressed significantly. Still, unscrupulous individuals and companies espouse ineffective and expensive treatments that prey upon vulnerable people.

## ▶ Interaction of Bones, Joints, and Muscles

Bones, joints, and muscles work together. The bones of the skeleton provide the body with a sturdy framework. Bones are held together by a variety of joints, some of which permit movement at portions of the skeletal framework. Because skeletal muscle is attached via tendons to bones, when muscle contracts, or shortens, it moves the skeleton. Thus, the muscles that span a joint bring about action at that joint. Groups of muscles may have opposite or antagonistic actions on a joint. For example, one group of muscles extends (straightens) the knee, while another group flexes (bends) the knee. Still other muscles stabilize joints, preventing undesired movements. In this chapter, the principal diseases and disorders of bone, joints, and muscles—the musculoskeletal system—are explained.

## ▶ Structure and Function of Bone, Joints, and Muscle

Bone may appear inert, but changes constantly occur within it. Bone development, growth, and homeostasis rely on interplay among its constituent minerals, proteins, and living cells. **Calcium** and **phosphate**, bone's primary minerals, are embedded in **collagen**, bone's main protein. The minerals confer hardness and rigidity to bone, while the collagen imparts flexibility. Mature bone cells, **osteocytes**, along with bone-forming cells, **osteoblasts**, and bone-resorbing cells, **osteoclasts**, reside within this bony matrix. The cells receive nutrients by an organized system of blood vessels that course throughout the bone.

Bones are long, flat, or irregularly shaped, but most are covered with a layer of a type of bone tissue called **compact bone**. The cells, minerals, proteins, and blood vessels of compact bone are arranged in a regular, organized fashion. Another type of bone tissue, **spongy bone**, contains many bone-marrow-filled spaces. This

red-colored marrow is found at the ends of long bones and is the site of blood cell formation.

The long bones found in the arms and legs contain a hollow cavity, the **medullary cavity**, filled with yellow bone marrow primarily consisting of fat. The growth of long bones occurs at the growth plate, an area of cartilage near each expanded end of the bone (Figure 15–1 ▶). At this site, new bone is formed, pushing the ends apart from each other until full growth is achieved, at which time the cartilage turns into bone, a process called **ossification**. Damage to the growth plate before maturity tends to prevent the bone from reaching its mature length.

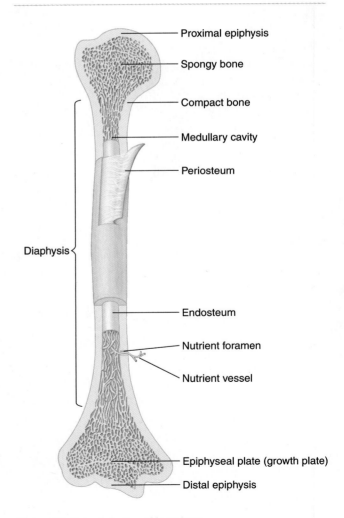

Figure 15–1 ▶ Cut view of long bone.

The **periosteum** is a highly vascular layer of fibrous connective tissue that covers the surface of bones. It contains cells that are capable of forming new bone tissue and serves as a site of attachment for tendons or muscles.

Joints are the articulating sites between bones. Various degrees of movement, called *range of motion,* are possible in different kinds of joints. The amount and type of movement at a joint is defined by the shapes of bones and the type of connective tissue holding the bones together at the joint. The shoulder (joint between humerus and scapula) is the most freely movable joint, but it is also the one most easily dislocated.

Articulating bones are held together by **ligaments**. Dense strands of collagen impart great strength to ligaments. A joint capsule consisting of ligaments and connective tissue surrounds the bone ends. The inner surface of the capsule is lined with a **synovial membrane** that secretes **synovial fluid**, which lubricates the joints. Sacs of this fluid, the **bursae**, are situated near some joints, such as the shoulder and knee, where they reduce friction during movement. The articulating surfaces of the bone ends are covered with a layer of cartilage, which also reduces friction. A typical joint is illustrated in Figure 15–2 ▶.

**Skeletal** or **voluntary muscle** tissue is found in muscles that are firmly attached to bones by **tendons**. Some voluntary muscles (the muscles of facial expression, for example) are attached to soft tissue. Muscles consist of bundles of muscle fibers held together by connective tissue. When stimulated by nerves at the myoneural junction, muscle fibers contract, and because muscles are attached to bones, the shortening of the muscles moves the bones.

The diseases of muscle described in this chapter are diseases of voluntary muscle. Because muscle action requires nerve stimulation, some nervous system diseases are manifested in muscles. Those diseases are discussed with the nervous system in Chapter 13. This chapter discusses a few muscle diseases that are not directly caused by nervous system disease. Smooth muscle, or involuntary muscle, is a different type of muscle found in the walls of the internal organs and the walls of blood vessels. Cardiac muscle is an involuntary striated muscle and is present only in the heart (Chapter 6). This chapter does not address cardiac or smooth muscle disease.

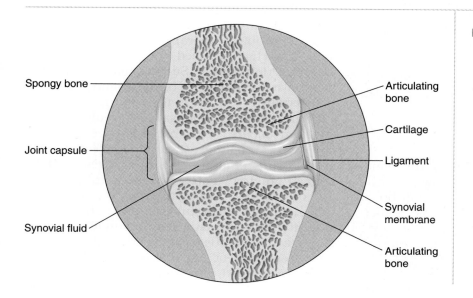

Figure 15–2 ▶ Typical joint.

Spongy bone

Joint capsule

Synovial fluid

Articulating bone

Cartilage

Ligament

Synovial membrane

Articulating bone

## ▶ Diagnostic Tests for Musculoskeletal Diseases

X-rays can reveal fractures, joint dislocations, bone deformities, and calcification; measure bone density; and detect signs of other bone damage. MRI (magnetic resonance imaging) uses strong magnetic fields to visualize details of joint anatomy and can show trauma and arthritis damage. CT (computed tomography) scans show details of soft tissues like tendons and ligaments as well as muscle. Arthroscopy is used to visualize the inside of a joint cavity such as the knee. Joint fluid can be aspirated for microscopic and chemical analysis. Myelography detects abnormalities of the spinal cord by visualizing the distribution of a radio opaque dye injected into the subarachnoid space. Myelography can detect tumors and herniated discs. Electromyography measure electrical activity of muscles and reveals some abnormalities of muscle function. Biopsy can show muscle tissue abnormalities.

## ▶ Diseases of Bone

Bone can be affected by disease in various ways. Infectious agents can enter bone through a compound fracture, transmission in the blood, or extension from an adjacent infection. Mineral and vitamin deficiencies prevent proper formation or maintenance of bone structure. Bones **atrophy** with disuse and fracture, or spontaneously in certain diseases. Tumors can also develop in bone.

### Infectious Diseases of Bone

**Osteomyelitis** is an inflammation of the bone, particularly of the bone marrow in the medullary cavity and the spaces of spongy bone. Osteomyelitis affects 2 in 10,000 people, principally children and adolescents, mostly boys, whose bones are still growing. In children, the long bones—the femur, the tibia, and the humerus—are most frequently affected near their ends at the growth plate. In adults, osteomyelitis usually affects the pelvis and vertebrae following trauma and surgery. The main risk factor for developing osteomyelitis is a recent bacterial infection that may have escaped treatment, permitting the bacteria to become blood-borne.

Osteomyelitis is caused by bacteria, usually *Staphylococcus aureus* and occasionally *Streptococcus pyogenes, Pneumococcus,* or *Escherichia coli.* The bacteria are carried by blood to the bone from some other site in the body, such as infection adjacent to the bone. Hence, the chief risk factor for osteomyelitis includes infections, including open wounds of a compound fracture.

In osteomyelitis, the infection develops into an abscess in the bone, which compresses small blood vessels, reduces circulation, and causes bone necrosis. Infections may spread under the periosteum, lifting sections of it from bone surface, further reducing circulation to bone. In an attempt to heal, bone may be deposited around this area of necrosis.

Local symptoms of bone infection include pain, redness, and heat. Systemic symptoms of chills, fever, and leukocytosis, tachycardia, nausea, and anorexia also occur. Diagnosis begins with history and physical exam and can be confirmed with white blood cell count, an elevated erythrocyte sedimentation rate, blood culture of causative microorganism, and magnetic resonance imaging or bone scans. An x-ray will not reveal early infections.

Early antibiotic therapy is an effective treatment and has reduced the incidence of advanced serious cases. Surgery may be required to remove necrotic bone tissue (Figure 15–3 ▶).

**Tuberculosis** of bone is rare and is associated with untreated pulmonary tuberculosis. This infection occurs when bacteria spread to the bones from the lungs. Commonly affected areas are the ends of long bones and knees. Usually seen in children, Pott's disease is tuberculosis of the vertebrae, leading to deformity and paralysis. As in the lungs, tuberculosis of bone leads to cavitation and tissue destruction (Chapter 8). The infection can be treated with antibiotics, although strains of *Mycobacterium tuberculosis* have developed multiple-drug resistance. Surgery may be able to correct bone deformities.

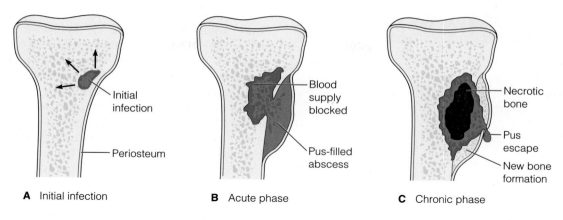

| **A** Initial infection | **B** Acute phase | **C** Chronic phase |

**Figure 15–3** ▶ Three phases of bone infection.

## Bone Disease and Vitamin and Mineral Deficiencies

Vitamins and minerals are key to bone health. Calcium and phosphorus are required in appropriate quantities for proper bone formation and maintenance. However, dietary calcium cannot be absorbed from the digestive tract without vitamin D. Thus, mineral or vitamin D deficiencies may result in soft, malformed, or fragile bones.

**Rickets** is a disease of infancy or early childhood in which the bones do not properly ossify, or harden. Rickets is rare in the United States but occurs occasionally in infants fed unfortified formula. A child with rickets develops bones that are soft and tend to bend. Over time the weight-bearing bones of the body become deformed: The legs become bent ("bow-legged" or "knock-kneed") and the vertebral column becomes misaligned. The sternum projects forward, and bony nodules form on the ends of ribs and at wrists, ankles, and knees. The skull is large and square. The pelvic opening in a girl may narrow, leading to problems with childbirth later. Other signs and symptoms of rickets include flaccid muscles, delayed teething, and a characteristic potbelly. Each of these symptoms can be explained by calcium deficiency.

Rickets can be prevented with vitamin D–fortified milk and exposure to sunlight. Sunlight converts a substance (dehydrocholesterol) in the skin to vitamin D in the body. This need for

sunlight explains the higher incidence of rickets in large, smoky cities where buildings are close together and shut out the sun. Children with rickets respond well to sunlight exposure and treatment with vitamin D concentrate.

**Osteomalacia** is the softening or decalcification of bones in adults. Osteomalacia is rare in the United States. It is most prevalent in Asia among women who have had multiple births, eat a cereal-based diet, and have little exposure to sunlight. Symptoms include muscle weakness, weight loss, and bone pain. Bones of the vertebral column, legs, and pelvis become susceptible to bending and fracturing with mild stress.

Osteomalacia is caused by inadequate dietary vitamin D and dietary deficiency of calcium or phosphorus; it is treated with vitamin D supplements and adding adequate calcium and phosphorous to the diet.

Both rickets and osteomalacia may be secondary to malabsorption syndrome because vitamin D is not absorbed from the intestine.

**Osteoporosis** is a disease characterized by porous bone that is abnormally fragile and susceptible to fracture. Eighty percent of those affected by osteoporosis are women. While some bone loss is expected with aging, the cause of the accelerated bone loss observed in osteoporosis is unknown. However, risk factors for osteoporosis have been identified, and these include being female, advanced age, and having a small frame (Box 15–1 ▶).

### Box 15–1 ► Risk Factors for Osteoporosis

Low bone mass
Low calcium intake
Female
Vitamin D deficiency
Small frame
Sedentary lifestyle
Family history
Cigarette smoking
Postmenopausal
Excessive alcohol use
Hysterectomy
Caucasian or Asian
Amenorrhea

Unfortunately, osteoporosis can quietly become advanced because no symptoms accompany bone loss until bones weaken enough to fracture. Weight-bearing bones of the vertebrae and pelvis are especially susceptible, and accumulated compression fractures in these bones cause a decrease in height and bending of the spine (Figure 15–4 ►). Compressed vertebrae press on spinal nerves, causing great pain. Fractures are common in the hip and wrists.

Osteoporosis is diagnosed using patient history and bone density tests. No cure exists, so prevention is strongly recommended. A lifelong diet rich in calcium and vitamin D along with weight-bearing exercise stimulates the development of dense and strong bone and slows progression of the disease. Smoking should be avoided, and alcohol and caffeine consumption

Height
5'6"
5'3"
5'
4'9"
4'6"
4'3"

Age      40          60          70

**Figure 15–4** ► Spinal changes caused by osteoporosis.

## SIDE by SIDE ■ Osteoporosis

▲ X-ray of pelvis in 18-year-old female showing normal bone density. (© B. Bates/Custom Medical Stock Photo)

▲ X-ray of female pelvis with osteoporosis. Note greatly decreased bone density especially visible in hip bones. (© Custom Medical Stock Photo)

should be minimized. Treatment requires medication. Various medications facilitate calcium uptake in bone and include estrogens, calcitonin, parathyroid hormone, as well as estrogen-receptor modulators and bisphosphonates.

## Other Bone Deformities

**Paget's disease**, or **osteitis deformans**, results in overproduction of bone, particularly in the skull, vertebrae, and pelvis. Paget's disease is rare worldwide, but in the United States it affects approximately 2.5 million people, mostly men over 40. The cause of Paget's disease is unknown, but approximately 20% to 30% of cases are genetically based.

The disease begins with bone softening, which is followed by bone overgrowth. The new bone tissue is abnormal and tends to fracture easily. The excessive bony growth causes the skull to enlarge, which often affects cranial nerves; thus, vision and hearing are affected. Abnormal bone development causes curvatures in the spinal column and deformities in legs.

Another complication of this disease is **osteogenic sarcoma**; see discussion following.

Paget's disease is diagnosed by examination, x-rays, bone scan, and bone biopsy. Treatment requires calcitonin and etidronate, which reduce bone resorption, and mithramycin, which decreases calcium.

**Scoliosis** is an abnormal lateral curvature of the spine that occurs to varying degrees of severity and is usually first identified during childhood. Scoliosis may be caused by abnormal development that results in fusion of the vertebrae. Scoliosis may also have a neuromuscular origin. Weak or asymmetric muscle development can pull the spine laterally. This can result from diseases such as polio, muscular dystrophy, spina bifida, or cerebral palsy. Finally, scoliosis may be idiopathic. Symptoms may include lower back pain and fatigue. Diagnosis is based on history, physical exam, and x-rays. Mild curvatures of less than 20 degrees are common in adolescents and may require no treatment. More severe curvatures of 30 degrees in growing adolescents must be treated with braces to prevent further curving of the vertebrae. Curves of 40 degrees require surgery to correct the misalignment. The outcomes are promising following treatment. However, neuromuscular scoliosis may be more difficult to treat because it is usually accompanied and caused by another disease, such as polio, muscular dystrophy, spina bifida, or cerebral palsy.

**Kyphosis**, an exaggerated posterior curve of the thoracic spine, sometimes called hunchback, occurs most commonly in adults and becomes more noticeable in the elderly (Figure 15–5►). It is most often caused by collapse of vertebrae affected by osteoporosis and by degenerative changes associated with arthritis of the vertebrae. Symptoms include mild back pain, back fatigue, perhaps tenderness, and, in severe cases, difficulty breathing because of compression of the thoracic cage. It can be diagnosed with physical exam and x-rays. Treatment options are few and provide no cures.

Treatment of the underlying osteoporosis can slow progression of kyphosis. Treatment of underlying arthritis can relieve pain and immobility but only to a limited degree.

**Lordosis**, "swayback," is an inward curvature of the lumbar vertebrae. Some degree of curvature is normal and most cases of lordosis are benign. Any unusual pain or curvature should be evaluated.

## Bone Cancer

*Malignant Bone Tumors* Bone cancer is rare, comprising 1% of malignancies. Most bone cancer is secondary and results from metastasis from a tumor located elsewhere in the body. Primary malignancy of bone occurs most often in males, especially children and adolescents. One type of bone cancer, **osteogenic sarcoma**, arises in the bony tissue itself and frequently affects the ends of long bones, frequently at the knee, where enlargement of the bone is observed. The cause

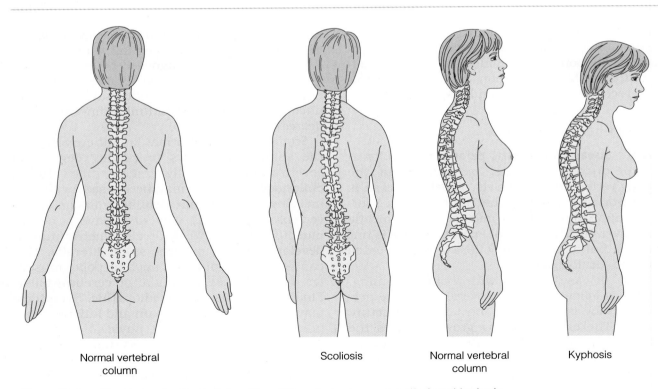

Normal vertebral column          Scoliosis          Normal vertebral column          Kyphosis

Figure 15–5 ► The two most common deformities of the spinal column are scoliosis and kyphosis.

of osteogenic sarcoma is unknown. Signs and symptoms include dull localized bone pain that intensifies at night. Masses may be noted and fractures accompany sarcomas. Bone cancer is diagnosed with biopsy. X-rays and CT scans are used to locate and measure tumors. Treatment may involve chemotherapy to reduce tumor size followed by surgical removal. See Chapter 4 for a discussion of cancer.

## Bone Trauma: Fractures

Several diseases and disorders discussed in this chapter may result in bone loss or other damage that can result in fracture. Trauma, however, is also a common cause of bone fractures. Excessive force, twisting, or compression can lead to

bone fractures. The chief signs and symptoms of a fracture include

- Visibly out-of-place or misshapen limb or joint
- Swelling, bruising, or bleeding
- Intense pain
- Numbness and tingling
- Broken skin with bone protruding
- Limited mobility or inability to move a limb

These signs and symptoms require diagnosis and medical attention in order to promote healing and to prevent infections. A variety of fractures can occur (Figure 15–6▶). Most fractures require immobilization with a splint or cast, while others, like compound fractures, require surgery, pins, and plates to promote healing.

| FRACTURE TYPE | DESCRIPTION | COMMENTS |
| --- | --- | --- |
| Closed | Bone breaks cleanly but does not penetrate skin. | Also called a simple fracture. |
| Open | Broken ends of bone protrude through soft tissues and skin. | Serious; may result in osteomyelitis. Also called a compound fracture. |
| Comminuted | Bone fragments into many pieces. | Common in those with conditions causing brittle bones, such as osteogenesis imperfecta |
| Compression | Bone is crushed. | Common in clients with osteoporosis. |
| Impacted | Broken ends of bone are forced into each other. | Commonly results from falls; also common in hip fracture. |

| FRACTURE TYPE | DESCRIPTION | COMMENTS |
| --- | --- | --- |
| Depressed | Broken bone is pressed inward. | Common in skull fractures. |
| Spiral | Jagged break due to twisting force applied to bone. | Common fracture due to sports injuries. |
| Greenstick | Bone breaks incompletely, much in the way a green twig breaks. | Common in children, whose bones have proportionally more organic matrix and are more flexible than those of adults. |

**Figure 15–6** ▶ Fractures. Adapted from Marieb, E.N. (1998). *Human anatomy and physiology* (4th ed., (p. 180). Menlo Park, CA: Benjamin Cummings.)

## ▶ Diseases of the Joints

Joints permit movement of the skeleton; thus diseases of the joints cause pain and limit mobility. Joints that bear weight—the lower vertebrae, hips, and knees—receive a great deal of stress and are especially susceptible to the diseases and disorders discussed in this chapter. Even the muscles, nerves, and bones may be affected by joint disease.

### Arthritis

**Arthritis** means "inflammation of a joint." Symptoms of arthritis include persistent joint pain and stiffness. Joints may be swollen and may lose mobility and become deformed to the point of losing function. Commonly affected joints include the lower vertebrae, hips, fingers, and knees.

***Rheumatoid Arthritis*** A chronic and debilitating autoimmune disease, rheumatoid arthritis is a systemic inflammatory disease that affects several joints and the surrounding muscles, tendons, and ligaments. Rheumatoid arthritis affects 1.3 million Americans and affects nearly three times more females than males, usually beginning between ages 30 and 60. No risk factors have been linked to rheumatoid arthritis and the cause of rheumatoid arthritis remains unknown, but it appears to be an autoimmune disease. **Rheumatoid factors**, such as antiglobulin antibodies, combine with immunoglobulin in the synovial fluid to form antibody complexes. Neutrophils are attracted to the joint space and cause destruction. The condition is aggravated by stress, and there is a genetic predisposition toward development of the disease.

Symptoms include joint pain and stiffness, particularly on waking. The joints are swollen, red, and warm. The same joints are often affected on both sides of the body. As the disease is systemic, the patient experiences fatigue, weakness, and weight loss. Rheumatoid arthritis begins with an inflammation of the synovial membrane that lines the joints, particularly the small joints of the hands and feet. The membrane thickens and extends into the joint cavity, sometimes filling the space with a thickened granulation tissue, called a pannus, which eventually erodes and scars the articular cartilage of the bone ends. When this scar tissue turns to bone, the ends of the bones fuse, a condition called **ankylosis**. The fusion immobilizes and deforms the joint. Figures 15–7▶ and 15–8▶ illustrate the crippling swan neck deformity and ulnar deviation characteristic of advanced rheumatoid arthritis in the hands. Rheumatoid nodules may form under the skin, usually near the joints, but they sometimes develop on the white of the eye, too.

Diagnosis is based on physical exam, x-rays showing joint changes, a rheumatoid factor test, and synovial fluid analysis. Early diagnosis and a comprehensive treatment program that includes medicine and exercise can reduce pain and the amount of damage done to the joints. Anti-inflammatory medications are effective when prescribed by a physician, with aspirin (salicylates) and similar drugs being the most commonly used. Other nonsteroidal anti-inflammatory medications commonly used include indomethacin, fenoprofen, and ibuprofen. Immunosuppressants such as corticosteroids and methotrexate are now administered in early stages of the disease. COX-2 inhibitors like Celebrex have also been used. A balance between exercise and rest should be achieved.

Figure 15–7 ▶ Contractures of rheumatoid arthritis.

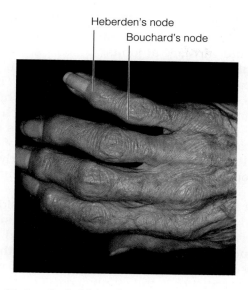

Heberden's node

Bouchard's node

**Figure 15–8** ► Typical joint changes associated with osteoarthritis. (Courtesy of the American College of Rheumatology)

In an acute phase, the joint should be rested to prevent further inflammation. Physical therapists can teach patients how to perform range-of-motion exercises that help preserve joint mobility. Exercises for good posture are directed toward removing stress on weight-bearing joints.

*Osteoarthritis*  Osteoarthritis is the most common form of arthritis. Osteoarthritis affects 27 million Americans, including 14% of those over age 25 and 34% of those over age 65. Men and women are affected equally, usually after age 40. Osteoarthritis may be described as primary or secondary. They are the same disease, but with slightly different origins. Primary osteoarthritis occurs with normal aging. Secondary osteoarthritis is associated with joint injury, trauma, or obesity. Other than injury, risk factors and causes are not well understood.

Unlike rheumatoid arthritis, osteoarthritis may affect only one joint. Signs and symptoms include pain and stiffness in the joint. Muscle tension and fatigue contribute to the aches and pain of osteoarthritis. Arthritis in the lower

back may pinch a spinal nerve, such as the sciatic nerve, in which case pain radiates down the back and leg. Affected joints lose their range of motion, and associated muscles become weak.

Degeneration occurs at the articular cartilage of the joint. This cartilage caps the bone surface where bone meets another bone in a joint. This cartilage erodes, exposing the underlying bone, which degenerates and leads to new bone deposits in and around the joint. The bone ends thicken and develop sharp irregular bony surface structures called spicules and **spurs**. Small joints such as the knuckles enlarge and become knobby (Figure 15–9 ►).

Diagnosis of osteoarthritis is made principally by x-rays that show the joint damage and a history of the symptoms. There is no cure for osteoarthritis, but treatment can greatly relieve the pain. A combination of rest and mild exercise to maintain range of motions, medication, and heat applications is generally prescribed. Nonsteroidal anti-inflammatory medications commonly used include aspirin, indomethacin, fenoprofen, and ibuprofen. Steroids such as cortisone are sometimes injected into the joint capsule to relieve pain. Surgical replacement of

© ACR

**Figure 15–9** ► Acute gouty arthritis of the finger joints. (Courtesy of the American College of Rheumatology)

a damaged joint like the hip and knee has become very effective, although factors such as age are important considerations.

*Gout* Also called gouty arthritis, **gout** affects the joints of the feet, particularly those of the big toe, and sometimes of the hand, fingers, wrist, or knee. Gout affects an estimated 3 million Americans, is most prevalent among men over age 40, but also affects postmenopausal women. The cause of gout is unknown. It sometimes follows a minor injury or excessive eating or drinking, and there may be no explanation for its occurrence, but heredity seems to play a role. The pathogenesis of gout is better understood than its cause. Gout attacks are related to excess uric acid in blood, which results either from a defect in metabolism of purines (a component of nucleic acids), or from abnormal retention of uric acid, or both. The high uric acid level leads to deposits of uric acid crystals in the joints. Uric acid crystals also deposit in the kidneys, stimulating kidney stone formation and irritating the kidney.

The onset of an acute attack of gout is generally sudden. The affected joints exhibit typical signs of inflammation: pain, heat, swelling, and redness (see Figure 15–9). Signs and symptoms may last from days to many weeks. Resolution of an acute attack may be followed by symptom-free periods of 6 months to more than 2 years before recurrence. A chronic form of gout also occurs in which a person experiences persistent arthritis.

Gout can be diagnosed by microscopic examination of aspirated joint fluid, which reveals needle-like urate crystals. High serum level of uric acid is consistent with gout. X-rays of af-fected joints may initially appear normal until repeated attacks of chronic gout damage the bone and cartilage at joints.

Acute gout attacks can be treated with rest, application of hot or cold compresses, analgesics, colchicine, and corticosteroids. Chronic gout may be treated with colchicine, which prevents acute attacks, and uricosuric agents such as probenecid that promote excretion of uric acid. If diagnosed early and treated properly, the development of chronic gout can be prevented.

*Septic Arthritis* Septic arthritis is considered a medical emergency. It develops as a result of bacterial infection of a joint. Cartilage and bone destruction may lead to ankylosis and life-threatening septicemia (blood-borne bacterial infection). Streptococci and staphylococci cause septic arthritis by invading a joint following trauma or surgery. *Neisseria gonorrhea*, the cause of gonorrhea, may spread to joints via blood from a primary infection site. Antibiotics are required to control the joint infection and to prevent septicemia.

## Bursitis

Bursae are small, fluid-filled sacs located near the joints that cushion and reduce friction on movement. **Bursitis** is an inflammation of these bursae, and it is a very painful condition. The bursae of the shoulder joint are the most frequently affected, although bursitis can develop at any joint. Repeated irritation or injury of a bursa can cause bursitis. Limitation of movement results from the pain of the inflammation. Treatment includes rest, anti-inflammatories,

## Prevention ■■PLUS!

### Bones, Joints, and Muscles Benefit from Exercise

In a healthy aging body, muscles lose strength and coordination, bones become thin and brittle, and joints stiffen and lose flexibility. The consequences include greater risk of falls and fractures. These can result in immobility, disability, diminished quality of life, and susceptibility to depression and disease. A vigorous exercise program benefits the bones, joints, and muscles as well as the cardiovascular and respiratory system. However, such a program should not be undertaken without physician guidance. A systematic vigorous program of exercise may not be feasible due to health or may not be appealing to the individuals. Nonetheless, significant physical and psychological benefits can be reaped from daily activities that engage the musculoskeletal system: walking, gardening, doing laundry, and climbing stairs.

and moist heat applications. Steroids are sometimes injected into the joint to reduce the inflammatory response.

## Dislocations, Sprains, and Strains

A **dislocation** is a displacement of bones from their normal position in a joint. Dislocations are most common in the shoulder and finger joints, but they can occur anywhere. The dislocation causes pain and reduced mobility at the involved joint. The bone must be reset and immobilized to allow healing of torn ligaments and tendons. Congenital dislocations of the hip result from an improperly formed joint, and they are treated in infancy with a cast or surgery.

**Sprains** result from the wrenching or twisting of a joint such as an ankle that injures the ligaments. Blood vessels and surrounding tissues, muscles, tendons, and nerves may also be damaged. Swelling and discoloration due to hemorrhaging from the ruptured blood vessels occur. A sprain is very painful, and the joint should not be used while it is severely inflamed. Immobilization with a splint or cast might be necessary for more severe sprains. Cold compresses reduce the swelling immediately after the injury, whereas later, heat applications relieve discomfort and speed healing. A "whiplash" is a sprain in which the cervical (neck) ligaments and tissues are injured. Whiplash injuries are often the result of rear-end motor vehicle accidents.

**Strains**, also called pulled muscles, result from a tearing of a muscle and/or its tendon from excessive use or stretching. Conditioning and warm-up before exercise prevent strains. Strains should be treated with rest, initially with ice to reduce inflammation, and later with warm compresses to encourage blood flow and healing. Severe strains may require many months to heal before safely resuming activity.

## Carpal Tunnel Syndrome

A painful condition of the hand known as carpal tunnel syndrome (CTS) affects up to 10% of the working population in the United States, causing disability and lost work time. It is actually one of a larger class of problems known as repetitive strain injuries (RSIs). Women are three times more likely to develop CTS than in men. Many women report the symptoms during pregnancy, which is attributed to accumulation of fluid within the tissues. Risk factors for CTS include the performance of repetitive manual tasks such as knitting, driving, typing, computing, and piano playing (Figure 15–10 ►). It usually begins as numbness or tingling in the hand but progresses to pain that can radiate up the arm to the shoulder; the pain is most severe at night. Simple tasks requiring finger movements become difficult.

A physician may diagnose carpal tunnel syndrome by requiring certain hand maneuvers. The diagnosis is confirmed by an **electromyogram**. The test measures the velocity of sensory and motor nerve conduction. If electrical impulses are slowed as they travel through the carpal tunnel, compression of the nerve is indicated.

Conservative treatments begin with avoiding the repetitive action where possible, at least temporarily. Immobilizing the hand and wrist with a lightweight, molded plastic splint is often

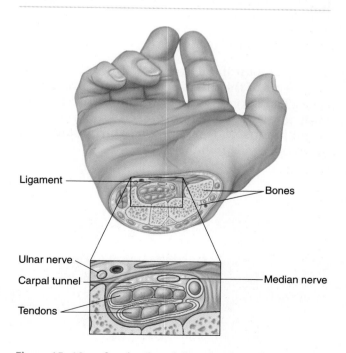

**Figure 15–10** ► Crosssection of the wrist showing tendons and nerves involved in carpal tunnel syndrome.

adequate for the inflammation to subside. Injection of a steroidal anti-inflammatory drug into the carpal tunnel is sometimes effective. For some individuals, nonsteroidal anti-inflammatory drugs such as aspirin and ibuprofen can reduce symptoms. Surgery may be required to divide the transverse ligament, which is compressing the median nerve. The procedure generally provides permanent relief without affecting hand movement or strength.

## ▶ Diseases of the Muscles

Skeletal muscle moves the body and provides much of the body's heat. Skeletal muscle function is intimately associated with nervous system function. Muscles cannot function unless they are stimulated by nerves. In Chapter 13, diseases in which the nerves fail to innervate muscles were discussed. Muscles themselves can also be diseased and lose their ability to contract. Another cause of muscle failure is the improper transmission of the impulse for contraction at the myoneural junction, the site at which a nerve ending sends its signal to a muscle cell.

### Muscular Dystrophy (MD)

The term **muscular dystrophy (MD)** includes several forms of the disease, all of which are hereditary. The various forms are transmitted differently and affect different muscles, but all forms result in muscle degeneration, which totally disables the individual.

The most common and serious type is Duchenne, which is caused by a sex-linked gene and affects approximately 2 per 10,000 people. Muscular dystrophy can appear at any age, but generally signs appear in the third to fifth year. In Duchenne's muscular dystrophy, a cytoskeletal protein called **dystrophin** is missing. As a result of this defect, muscle fibers die and are replaced by fat and connective tissue. Because neither of these tissues has the ability to contract, skeletal muscles weaken. A severe form can progress rapidly and affect the muscle of the heart, causing death; other forms progress slowly. In the most severe form of muscular dystrophy, the calf muscles enlarge as a result of fat deposition. The shoulder muscles are weak, which causes the arms to hang limply. A child with this form of muscular dystrophy is very weak and thin and does not usually live to adulthood.

The diagnosis is based on electromyography, which shows weak muscle contractions. Biospy of muscle shows abnormal muscle fibers: variation in sizes, fat deposits, and absence of dystrophin. Immunologic and molecular biology techniques can diagnose the disease prenatally as well as at birth.

No cure exists. Treatment includes physical and occupational therapy, exercise, and use of orthopedic appliances.

### Myasthenia Gravis (MG)

**Myasthenia gravis (MG)** is a disorder of the myoneural junction in which the nerves fail to transmit an impulse for contraction to the muscles. Lack of stimulation and use leads to mus-

## Prevention ✚PLUS!

### Carpal Tunnel Syndrome: An Occupational Hazard

Carpal tunnel syndrome, caused by damage to the median nerve, is a common problem of data processors, computer users, typists, beauticians, and dentists, who often maintain a flexed wrist position. Frequent rest and splinting may help prevent the complications of carpal tunnel syndrome. If surgery is required to relieve pressure on the nerve, a new technique is greatly reducing recovery time and lost work. A tiny video camera enables the surgeon to make two tiny incisions in the wrist and palm, each requiring only one stitch. Recovery is therefore much faster than with the traditional longer incision.

cle atrophy and muscle weakness. The cause is unknown, but myasthenia gravis may be classified as an autoimmune disease. Antibodies attach near the myoneural junction and destroy acetylcholine or its receptors. Myasthenia gravis is rare, affecting about 3 per 10,000 and occurring more frequently among women than men. No risk factors are known. An autoimmune disease, myasthenia gravis is probably genetic in origin.

The principal symptoms of this disease are fatigue and the inability to use the muscles. The voluntary muscles of the body are affected, including the muscles of facial expression, rendering the person's face expressionless. Eyelid control is lost, and simple actions such as chewing and talking become difficult. The greatest danger in this disease is respiratory failure because the muscles required for respiratory ventilation are unable to contract.

Treatment includes drugs that increase acetylcholine levels at the myoneural junction. The thymus gland, which is involved in the immune response, is often enlarged in myasthenia gravis patients. Removal of this gland sometimes brings about a remission but not a cure.

## Tumors of Muscle

Muscle tumors are rare, but when they occur, they are usually highly malignant. A malignant tumor of skeletal muscle is a **rhabdomyosarcoma**. The tumor requires surgical removal, and the prognosis is poor. The rhabdomyosarcoma metastasizes early and is usually an advanced malignancy when it is diagnosed. Muscle malignancy is rare because muscle cells do not continually divide like blood or skin cells.

## ▶ Age-Related Diseases

## Bones

Osteoblast activity declines with age. Because these cells build bone tissue in response to stress, for remodeling or repair, this results in age-related thinning of bones. In addition, aging bone has more minerals and less protein, making the tissue more brittle. Overall, the total amount of bone declines steadily with age. At menopause, bone loss accelerates, making women more susceptible to osteoporosis and its effects. More than 80% of those with osteoporosis are women, and a majority of women over age 60 have osteoporosis.

## Joints

Joint mobility decreases with age because cartilage in movable joints becomes stiffer, ligaments lose flexibility and elasticity, and synovial membranes become fibrous and stiff and produce less synovial fluid. These changes begin at age 20 and become significant by age 30, especially if the joints and muscles are not regularly exercised and stretched. The incidence of arthritis increases with age: While fewer than 20% of young adults have arthritis, 60% of adults over age 60 have some form of arthritis. Most of these cases are osteoarthritis.

## Muscles

Muscles become less sensitive to stimulation with age, meaning that they take longer to contract when stimulated. Recovery following contraction becomes slow, diminishing the ability to sustain repeated contractions and reducing endurance. With age, the number of muscle fibers decreases, and they become shorter and thinner, reducing muscle strength and range of motion. Exercise reduces the rate of these changes and helps maintain muscle mass, strength, and flexibility.

## RESOURCES

American Academy of Orthopedic Surgeons: www.aaos.org

American College of Sports Medicine: www.acsm.org

American Physical Therapy Association: www.apta.org

# DISEASES AT A GLANCE

## Musculoskeletal System

| DISEASE | ETIOLOGY | SIGNS AND SYMPTOMS |
|---|---|---|
| Osteomyelitis | Infection by staphylococci | Pain, redness, heat, chills, fever, tachycardia, nausea, weight loss |
| Rickets | Vitamin D deficiency in childhood | Deformation of bones, knock-knee, bow-leg, curved spine, nodular swellings at rib ends and joints, enlarged and square head, flaccid muscles |
| Osteomalacia | Vitamin D deficiency in adults | Muscular weakness, weight loss, pain in bones, deformation of bones, easily fractured bones |
| Osteoporosis | Calcium deficiency, decreased bone density | Decreased height from vertebral compression fractures, curvature of spine, easily fractured bones |
| Paget's disease | Idiopathic, genetic | Enlarged skull, nerve compression curvatures in spine, and deformed legs |
| Bone tumors | Idiopathic; commonly metastatic | Painless lump in bone tissue, fracture without trauma |
| Rheumatoid arthritis | Autoimmunity | Pain and stiffness in joints, swollen, red, warm joints, bilateral involvement, exacerbation and remission, rheumatoid nodules, crippling deformities |
| Osteoarthritis | Idiopathic; may follow joint injury or chronic irritation | Aches, pain, stiffness in joints, limited range of motion, muscle weakness around affected joint, enlarged joints, bone spurs; may involve only one joint |

| DIAGNOSIS | TREATMENT | PREVENTION | LIFESPAN |
|---|---|---|---|
| Bone scan, CT scan, MRI, WBC count | Antibiotics, surgery | Antibiotics for compound fractures or other infected wounds | Any age |
| Physical exam, x-ray | Vitamin D–fortified milk, sunlight, cod liver oil | Vitamin D–fortified milk, sunlight, cod liver oil | Children |
| Physical exam, x-ray | Vitamin D–fortified milk, sunshine, cod liver oil, calcium and phosphorous supplements | Vitamin D–fortified milk, sunshine, cod liver oil, calcium and phosphorous supplements | Adults |
| X-ray and bone scan | Pain relief, fracture treatment, some medical treatment (estrogens, calcitonin, bisphosphonates) | Calcium supplements, weight-bearing exercises | Postmenopausal women |
| Physical exam | Surgical, limited | None | Older men |
| X-ray, biopsy | Surgery | None | Children and adolescents |
| Physical exam, presence of rheumatoid factor in blood | Mild exercise, anti-inflammatories, steroids | None | Adults |
| X-ray, history | Pain relief, mild exercise and rest, heat applications, steroids, surgery | None | Adults |

# DISEASES AT A GLANCE

## Musculoskeletal System (*continued*)

| DISEASE | ETIOLOGY | SIGNS AND SYMPTOMS |
|---|---|---|
| Gout | Inherited defect in uric acid metabolism leads to high levels of urate and uric acid deposition in joints | Severe pain, heat, swelling, redness in affected joint; acute onset |
| Septic arthritis | Bacterial infection of joint | Pain, redness, swelling, bone and joint destruction |
| Bursitis | Overuse of joint | Pain at joint, especially during use |
| Carpal tunnel syndrome | Repetitive use of wrist | Numbness and tingling of hand, pain radiating to shoulder, limited finger movement, severe at night |
| Muscular dystrophy | Defect in X-linked gene for muscle protein dystrophin | Weakened muscles, muscles may enlarge as fat is deposited; muscles degenerate |
| Myasthenia gravis | Autoimmunity interferes with nerve transmission to muscles | Fatigue, muscle paralysis |

| DIAGNOSIS | TREATMENT | PREVENTION | LIFESPAN |
|---|---|---|---|
| Uric acid level in blood, x-ray | Analgesics, hot and cold compresses, colchicine, probenecid | Avoid triggers, which may be dietary | Men over age 40 |
| History, blood and synovial cultures | Antibiotics | Treat infected wounds or other infections with antibiotics to prevent sepsis | Any age |
| Physical exam and history | Moist heat, analgesics, steroids, rest | Reduce or avoid triggering activities | Adults |
| Physical exam, electromyography | Splinting hand and wrist, surgery | Reduce or avoid triggering activities | Adults and adolescents |
| Physical exam, serum enzymes, muscle biopsy | Physical therapy, orthopedic procedures | None; screening helps detect early onset | Onset in young adults |
| Antibody level, response to anticholinesterase drugs, electromyography | Thymectomy, anticholinesterase drugs, steroids, immune suppression | None | Onset in young adult women |

# Interactive Exercises

## Cases for Critical Thinking

1. A 68-year-old woman visits her physician and reports that her back hurts. Physical exam finds kyphosis and that she has lost height since her last visit a few years ago. What is a likely diagnosis for this case? Name two treatment possibilities that the physician might suggest. Name something that might have helped prevent this condition, especially if it had been initiated and applied at an earlier age.

2. A 55-year-old carpenter reports persistent swelling and pain in the knuckles of his right hand. What information do you need to determine the type of joint disease he has?

3. A 20-year-old woman has worsening pain in her leg below the knee. She says she feels "a little weak and out of sorts" and has stopped her jogging routine. How can you determine whether she has a type of arthritis, a bone infection, a fracture, or a joint sprain?

## Multiple Choice

1. Bones are soft in rickets due to a _____ deficiency.
   a. vitamin A
   b. vitamin C
   c. vitamin D
   d. vitamin K

2. Osteomalacia affects which of the following?
   a. the joints of young children
   b. the joints of adults
   c. the bones of children
   d. the bones of adults

3. Carpal tunnel syndrome is caused by damage to the _____.
   a. wrist
   b. fingers
   c. median nerve
   d. forearm muscles

4. Biopsy in addition to electromyography is a diagnostic test for _____.
   a. gout
   b. sprain
   c. carpal tunnel syndrome
   d. Duchenne's MD

5. _____ is the most common form of arthritis.
   a. Rheumatoid arthritis
   b. Osteoarthritis
   c. Septic arthritis
   d. Gout

6. Ankylosis and immobility results in severe _____.
   a. rheumatoid arthritis
   b. osteoarthritis
   c. septic arthritis
   d. gout

7. Colchicine and corticosteroids are used to treat acute cases of _____.
   a. rheumatoid arthritis
   b. osteoarthritis
   c. septic arthritis
   d. gout

8. Which of these is NOT due to calcium deficiency?
   a. osteoporosis
   b. osteomalacia
   c. osteogenic sarcoma
   d. rickets

9. Which of these is a type of autoimmune disorder?
   a. rhabdomyosarcoma
   b. Duchenne's MD
   c. myasthenia gravis
   d. osteitis fibrosa cystica

10. Streptococci and staphylococci are associated with _____.
    a. Pott's disease
    b. tuberculosis
    c. osteomyelitis
    d. osteoporosis

## True or False

_____ 1. Osteomyelitis affects principally children and adolescents.

_____ 2. Women with large bone mass are most prone to osteoporosis.

_____ 3. An osteoma is a malignant bone tumor.

_____ 4. Rheumatoid arthritis is the most crippling form of arthritis.

_____ 5. Osteomyelitis is a local and systemic infection.

_____ 6. Osteoarthritis is the most common form of arthritis.

_____ 7. Muscular dystrophy is a hereditary disease.

_____ 8. Myasthenia gravis is an infectious disease of the muscles.

_____ 9. Rhabdomyosarcoma is a malignant bone tumor.

_____ 10. There is no cure for osteoarthritis.

## Fill-Ins

1. A special form of tuberculosis that affects the vertebral column of children is called _____.

2. A disease of infancy and early childhood in which the bones do not properly ossify, or harden, is called _____.

3. The word _____ means increased porosity of the bone, which makes the bone abnormally fragile.

4. A very painful condition caused by deposits of uric acid crystals in the joints is called _____.

5. The principle minerals in bone are _____ and _____.

6. Bone is deposited by cells called _____.

7. The _____ membrane becomes inflamed in rheumatoid arthritis.

8. Antibodies against acetylcholine receptors are the cause of _____ _____.

9. Colchicine is an effective treatment for _____.

10. Vitamin D is required for dietary absorption of _____.

## Labeling Exercise

Use the lines below to label the following images.

1 _____    4 _____

2 _____    5 _____

3 _____    6 _____

# Multimedia Preview

Additional interactive resources and activities for this chapter can be found on the Companion Website. For videos, audio glossary, and review, access the accompanying DVD-ROM in this book.

## ▶ DVD-ROM Highlights

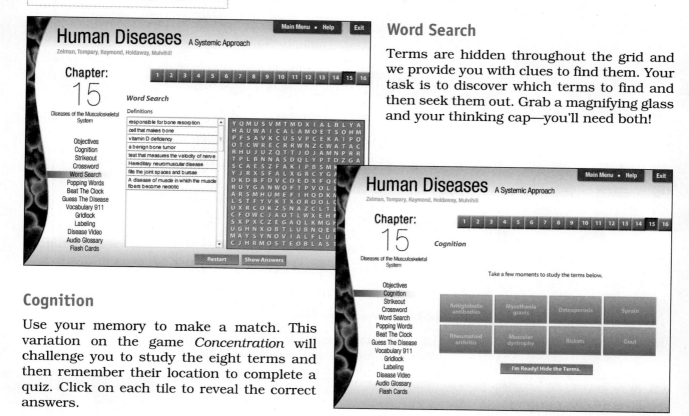

### Word Search

Terms are hidden throughout the grid and we provide you with clues to find them. Your task is to discover which terms to find and then seek them out. Grab a magnifying glass and your thinking cap—you'll need both!

### Cognition

Use your memory to make a match. This variation on the game *Concentration* will challenge you to study the eight terms and then remember their location to complete a quiz. Click on each tile to reveal the correct answers.

## ▶ Website Highlights—www.pearsonhighered.com/zelman

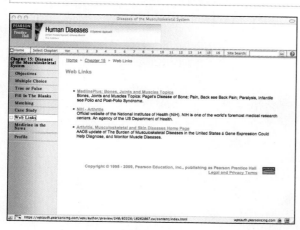

### Web Links

Take advantage of the free-access online study guide that accompanies your textbook. This online activity challenges you to visit selected web links where you can explore important issues to reinforce your understanding. By clicking on this URL you'll also access links to current news articles and an audio glossary.

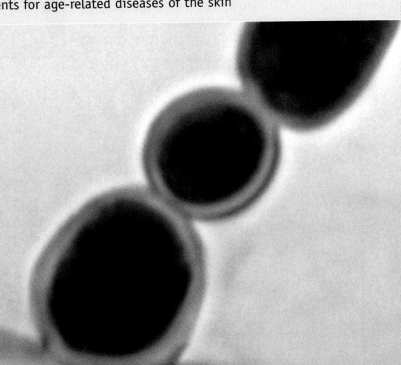

Macroconidia of the dermato-phytic fungus, *Epidermophyton floccosum*. (Courtesy of the CDC/Dr. Libero Ajello, 1972)

CHAPTER

# 16

## Diseases of the Integumentary System

### Learning Objectives

After studying this chapter, you should be able to

- Describe the normal structure and function of skin
- List the etiology, signs and symptoms, diagnostic tests, and treatments for infectious diseases of the skin
- Explain hypersensitivity, or immune disorders of the skin
- Identify benign tumors of the skin
- Compare and contrast the different types of nonmelanoma skin cancer
- Describe sebaceous gland disorders
- Compare and contrast pigment disorders
- Define trauma to the skin
- List the etiology, signs and symptoms, diagnostic tests, and treatments for age-related diseases of the skin

## Fact or Fiction?

Everyone can get a suntan.

*Fiction: People with the most sensitive skin type always burn and never tan. However, everyone can develop skin cancer. Limit your exposure and protect yourself from UV radiation.*

# Disease Chronicle

## Trench Foot

**S**oldiers in World War I suffered from trench foot, a fungal infection that thrived in the skin and tissues of feet damaged by chronic exposure to cold, wet, unsanitary conditions. Although healthy skin can resist fungal infections, soldiers stood for hours in waterlogged trenches without removing wet socks or boots, which caused their feet to go numb. Reduced circulation caused the skin to turn blue or red and, more importantly, made it difficult to fight infections. Left untreated, gangrene developed and amputation was necessary. British soldiers were ordered to have three pairs of socks with them and to dry their feet and change their socks at least twice per day. Soldiers were also told to cover their dry feet with grease made from whale oil. It is estimated that a battalion at the front used 10 gallons of whale oil every day.

## ▶ Functions of the Skin

Skin is the largest organ in the human body, with a surface area of approximately 2 square meters. The integumentary system, includes the skin, hair, nails, and sweat and **sebaceous** glands. The skin is much more than an external body covering. The skin protects deeper tissue from mechanical, chemical, thermal, ultraviolet, and bacterial damage. It insulates and cushions the deeper body organs. Skin regulates temperature, senses pain, protects against dehydration, aids in the excretion of urea and uric acid, and synthesizes vitamin D.

The skin indicates malfunction within the body through color changes. **Cyanosis**, a blue coloration of the skin, signals a lack of oxygen and indicates a cardiovascular or pulmonary problem. Jaundice indicates liver disease, bile obstruction, or hemolysis of red blood cells, in which case an accumulation of the bilirubin in the blood produces a yellowish coloration. An abnormal redness accompanies polycythemia (Chapter 7), carbon monoxide poisoning, and fever. **Pallor,** or whitening of the skin, may indicate anemia.

Skin color, texture, and folds identify people as individuals. Anything that disrupts skin function or appearance can have important consequences for physical and mental health.

## ▶ Structure of the Skin

Each layer of the skin performs specific tasks. The outermost layer of the skin is the **epidermis** and consists of stratified or layered squamous epithelium. The top portion of the epidermis, the stratum corneum, contains **keratin**. Keratin is a tough, fibrous protein produced by cells called **keratinocytes**. Keratin protects the skin from harmful substances and prevents water loss. At the bottom of the epidermis are the **melanocytes**, or the cells that produce **melanin**. Melanin is the dark pigment of the skin that protects the body from the harmful rays of the sun.

The **dermis** lies below the epidermis. The dermis is composed of connective tissue that sup-

ports blood and lymph vessels, elastic fibers, nerves, hair follicles, sweat glands, and sebaceous or oil glands. The subcutaneous tissue lies under the dermis and connects the skin to underlying structures. Adipose tissue or fat cells in the subcutaneous tissue help insulate the body from heat and cold. Figure 16–1 ▶ shows the structure of the skin.

## ▶ Diagnostic Procedures for Skin Diseases

Skin diseases are usually identified by visual examination. Blood and urine tests may be used to rule out underlying diseases. Diagnosis may include microscopic examination of skin scrapings. Cultures, DNA testing, or blood tests for antibodies may be used to identify the causative organism in skin diseases.

In hypersensitivity skin disorders, a complete medical history, including prior outbreaks and locations of outbreaks, may help identify the allergen. Sensitivity testing or blood tests for antibodies may be used to identify the allergen.

Biopsies are used to diagnose benign tumors and nonmelanoma skin cancer. Types of biopsies performed include punch, incisional, or total excisional.

## ▶ Skin Lesions

Skin diseases are identified and classified according to characteristic lesions. **Pruritus** (itching), edema (swelling), **erythema** (redness), and inflammation usually accompany lesions and are helpful in making a diagnosis. A **macule**, or freckle, is a discolored spot of the skin. A **wheal**, or hive, is a localized elevation in the skin that is often accompanied by pruritus. A **papule**, or pimple, is a solid, elevated area on the skin. A **nodule** is a larger papule. A **vesicle**, or blister, is a small, fluid-filled sac. A **bulla** is a larger vesicle. A **pustule** is a small, elevated lesion filled with pus. An **ulcer**, or erosion, is an eating away of the tissue. Figure 16–2 ▶ shows various skin lesions.

**Figure 16–1** ▶ Structure of the skin.

Keratinized layer

Hair

Receptor

Sebaceous gland

Hair follicle

Touch nerve fibers

Hair root

Artery

Vein

Deep connective tissue

Epidermis

Free nerve endings

Dermis

Capillary network

Smooth muscle

Subcutaneous fatty tissue

Sweat gland

Adipose tissue

Muscle fibers

## ▶ Epidermoid and Pilar Cysts

A cyst is a sac that is filled with a fluid or semifluid material. Two of the most common types of cyst that occur under the skin surface are epidermoid and pilar cysts. These cysts were previously called sebaceous cysts, but this term is no longer correct as they do not originate from the sebaceous glands in the skin. Both epidermoid and pilar cysts are smooth, round lumps just beneath the skin surface. In both cases, the semifluid contents of the cyst include keratin.

An epidermoid cyst sac forms from cells in the epidermis. Epidermoid cysts occur in an estimated 1% to 5% of the population. Epidermoid cysts can affect anyone, but risk factors include age (thirties or forties), gender (men are twice as likely to have epidermoid cysts), a history of acne, and traumatic or crushing injury to the skin. They can appear anywhere on the skin, but they develop most commonly on the face, neck, chest, and upper back. A pilar cyst sac forms from cells in the bottom of hair folli-

cles. Pilar cysts occur in an estimated 5% to 10% of population and usually occur in clusters on the scalp. Pilar cysts can affect anyone but are most common among middle-aged women.

Both epidermoid and pilar cysts usually cause no signs or symptoms. Occasionally they may become infected, leak, or form in an uncomfortable place such as in the genital skin folds or beside a nail. Epidermoid and pilar cysts form when there is abnormal cell proliferation. This may occur following an injury to the skin or damage to a hair follicle or sebaceous gland. The cells that multiply form into a sac and produce the keratin that they would normally make on the top layer of the skin. The keratin becomes trapped in the sac. A tendency to form pilar cysts runs in some families. Epidermoid cysts in themselves are not hereditary, and most form for no apparent reason in healthy people.

Epidermoid and pilar cysts are diagnosed by visual examination. If required, the cyst can usually be removed easily by excision. There is no way to prevent epidermoid or pilar cysts from forming.

**Figure 16–2** ► Skin lesions.

A macule is a discolored spot on the skin; freckle

A pustule is a small, elevated, circumscribed lesion of the skin that is filled with pus; varicella (chickenpox)

A wheal is a localized, evanescent elevation of the skin that is often accompanied by itching; urticaria

An erosion or ulcer is an eating or gnawing away of tissue; decubitus ulcer

A papule is a solid, circumscribed, elevated area on the skin; pimple

A crust is a dry, serous or seropurulent, brown, yellow, red, or green exudation that is seen in secondary lesions; eczema

A nodule is a larger papule; acne vulgaris

A scale is a thin, dry flake of cornified epithelial cells; psoriasis

A vesicle is a small fluid filled sac; blister. A bulla is a large vesicle.

A fissure is a crack-like sore or slit that extends through the epidermis into the dermis; athlete's foot

# ▶ Drug Eruptions

Adverse drug reactions manifest more often on the skin than in any other organ system. About 2% to 5% of patients suffer from cutaneous drug eruptions. Although any medication can cause eruptions, the most common types of medications that cause a drug eruption include antibiotics (penicillin or sulfa drugs), anti-inflammatory medicines (ibuprofen, naproxen, or indomethacin), painkillers (codeine or morphine), anticonvulsants (phenytoin or carbamazepine), chemotherapy drugs, psychotropic medications, diuretics, and iodine (especially that found in radiographic contrast dye). Drug eruptions can appear as various types of skin rashes, including pink-to-red papules, wheals, red patches, and pustules, or as sensitivity to sunlight. Drug rashes may involve the entire skin surface, or they may be limited to one or a few body parts. Pruritus is common in many drug eruptions. Skin reactions may be serious enough to cause anaphylaxis, shock, or death. A thorough medical history, including current medications, can help diagnose the adverse drug reaction and help determine the medication that must be changed.

# ▶ Infectious Skin Diseases

Bacteria, viruses, fungi, and parasites may cause infections of the skin. Normal microbes that reside on the skin cause the most common skin infections. Infections from less common microbes may develop in high-risk individuals (immunocompromised or diabetic individuals) and those who reside in nursing homes and hospitals. Most skin infections are not serious unless systemic involvement occurs.

## Bacterial Skin Infections

*Impetigo* **Impetigo** is an acute, contagious skin infection usually caused by *Staphylococcus aureus* or *Streptococcus pyogenes*. Impetigo affects mainly infants and children. Impetigo affects approximately 1% of children and accounts for approximately one-tenth of all cutaneous problems in pediatric clinics. Two clinical types of impetigo exist: nonbullous and bullous impetigo. The nonbullous type is more common and typically occurs on the face and extremities, initially with vesicles or pustules on reddened skin that eventually rupture to leave the characteristic honey-colored crust. Bullous impetigo, almost exclusively caused by *S. aureus*, exhibits vesicles with clear, yellow fluid that rupture and leave a golden-yellow crust. Fever and enlarged lymph nodes may accompany impetigo. Risk factors for contracting impetigo include direct contact with a person with impetigo, contact with a contaminated fomite (an inanimate object that can transmit infectious agents), warm and humid weather, and participation in sports that involve skin to skin contact. Diagnosis is made by visual examination and bacterial culture. The lesions should be washed with soap and water, kept dry, and exposed to air. Impetigo is treated with antibiotics. Prevention includes daily bathing, frequent handwashing, and prompt attention to minor wounds.

*Erysipelas and Cellulitis* **Erysipelas** is a superficial infection of the skin. **Cellulitis** is a deeper infection that extends to the subcutaneous tissue. *S. aureus* and *S. pyogenes* are the most common pathogens responsible for erysipelas and cellulitis. The bacteria enter through a break in the skin. Risk factors for erysipelas and cellulitis include circulatory problems, diabetes, and trauma to the skin. Mild erysipelas is common, but because it is often self-limited, patients rarely present to the doctor. Cellulitis is a common infection with an incidence of approximately 2 to 3 cases per 100 people per year.

Erysipelas and cellulitis infections usually appear on the face or the legs. The involved area is generally swollen, bright red, hot, and tender (Figure 16–3 ▶). Small vesicles may be present. Fever, chills, and swelling of lymph nodes may occur. Diagnosis may include visual examination and bacterial culture. When the infection is severe, treatment with antibiotics is required. Prevention of erysipelas and cellulitis includes prompt attention to wounds, moisturization of the skin, and careful trimming of nails.

*Folliculitis, Furuncles, and Carbuncles* **Folliculitis** is a superficial infection of the hair follicles characterized by erythema and follicular-based

**Figure 16-3** ▶ Cellulitis indicated by redness and swelling around the eye. (Courtesy of the CDC/Dr. Thomas F. Sellers/Emory University, 1963)

papules and pustules. **Furuncles**, or boils, are a deeper infection of the hair follicle. **Carbuncles** are clusters of furuncles. Folliculitis, furuncles, and carbuncles are caused by infection with staphylococci.

Folliculitis is common, but because it is often self-limited, patients rarely present to the doctor. This condition commonly occurs in young men and affects thighs, buttocks, head, and scalp (Figure 16-4▶). Risk factors for folliculitis include obesity, trauma to the skin, impaired immunity, long-term antibiotic therapy for acne, living in a warm and humid climate, and topical corticosteroid therapy. Diagnosis is based on visual examination and bacterial culture. Folliculitis is effectively treated with daily cleansing with an antiseptic soap. Severe cases require treatment with oral antibiotics. Keeping skin clean, dry, and free from abrasions or irritation can help prevent folliculitis.

Furuncles appear in hair follicles located on the face, neck, breasts, or buttocks. The core of the furuncle becomes necrotic and liquefies,

**Figure 16-4** ▶ The lesions of folliculitis are pustules surrounded by areas of erythema.

forming pus (Figure 16-5▶). Carbuncles develop and heal more slowly than furuncles. They appear mostly in men and are commonly located on the back of the neck. Risk factors for furuncles and carbuncles include minor trauma to the skin, preexisting skin disease, poor hygiene, and impaired immunity. Diagnosis is based on visual examination and bacterial culture. Furuncles and carbuncles may be treated with application of moist heat, antiseptic skin cleansing, antibiotics, and incision and drainage. Keeping skin

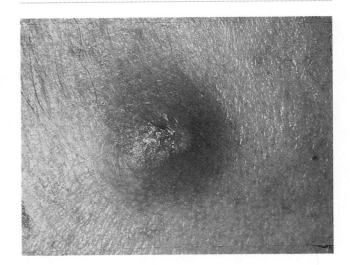

**Figure 16-5** ▶ A furuncle or boil.

clean, dry, and free from abrasions or irritation may help prevent furuncles and carbuncles.

## Viral Skin Infections

*Herpes*　Herpes is a large family of viruses that cause clusters of fluid-filled vesicles on the skin. Herpes simplex type I (HSV-1) causes cold sores or fever blisters (Figure 16–6▶). Eighty-five percent of the population has antibody evidence of HSV-1 infection. The vesicles generally form near the mouth or lips, as in Figure 16–6. Some patients have a burning or tingling sensation that precedes the appearance of vesicles by a few hours or a day or two. The virus goes latent, but a cold, flu, fever, sun exposure, stress, trauma to the skin, and changes in the immune system can stimulate a recurrence. HSV-1 is spread from person to person by kissing, close contact with herpetic lesions, or even contact with apparently normal skin that is shedding the virus. Diagnosis may include visual observation of the herpetic vesicles, viral culture, and testing for HSV-1 DNA. The outbreaks are usually self-limiting, but antiviral drugs can be used for treatment. Cold sores can be prevented by avoiding contact with HSV-1 and recurrence triggers (e.g., sunlight, stress, fatigue, weakened immune system) and frequent handwashing.

Herpes simplex type II causes genital herpes (see Chapter 11 for more information). Herpes varicella-zoster causes chicken pox (see Chapter 3 for more information). If an adult develops limited immunity to herpes varicella-zoster, the virus may lie dormant for years after recovery from chicken pox. The virus may flare up during periods of stress, diseases, trauma, or immunosuppression, causing painful vesicles called shingles (see Chapter 13).

*Warts*　Warts, or **verucca vulgaris**, are caused by the human papillomavirus (HPV). HPV infection of keratinocytes causes them to proliferate, forming a benign neoplasm with a rough, keratinized surface. Warts are spread by direct contact with HPV. There are few reliable, population-based data on the incidence and prevalence of nongenital warts. Prevalence probably varies widely among different age groups, populations, and periods of time. Two large population-based studies found prevalence rates of 0.84% in the United States. Prevalence is highest among children and young adults. Warts are most common at sites of trauma, such as the hands and feet, and probably result from inoculation of virus into minimally damaged areas of epithelium. There are several types of warts, including common, plantar, flat, filiform, and periungual.

Common warts grow most often on the hands, but they may occur anywhere on the body. Common warts are rough, shaped like a dome, and gray-brown in color (Figure 16–7▶). Plantar warts grow inward on the soles of the

**Figure 16–6** ▶ Cold sores or fever blisters. (Courtesy of the CDC/Dr. Herrman, 1964)

**Figure 16–7** ▶ Common warts.

feet. One observational study of 146 adolescents found that the prevalence of warts on the feet was 27% in those who used a communal shower room and 1.3% in those who used only locker rooms without showers. Plantar warts look like hard, thick patches of skin with dark specks. Pressure on the soles of the feet makes them very painful, and they are often difficult to remove permanently. Flat warts usually grow on the face, arms, or legs. They are small (usually smaller than the eraser on the end of a pencil), have flat tops, and can be pink, light brown, or light yellow. Filiform warts usually grow around the mouth, nose, or beard area. They are the same color as the skin and have growths that look like threads sticking out of them. Periungual warts grow under and around the toenails and fingernails and can affect nail growth. They look like rough bumps with an uneven surface and border.

Warts are diagnosed by visual examination. One study of 1000 children found that two-thirds of warts resolved without treatment within a 2-year period. Warts can be removed by medications, electrocautery, cryosurgery, and laser surgery. To prevent HPV infections, avoid touching warts, walking barefoot on warm moist surfaces, and incurring trauma to the skin.

## Fungal Skin Infections

Fungi, or **dermatophytes**, that infect the skin tend to live on the dead, top layer of the skin. Superficial fungal infections are among the most common skin diseases, affecting millions of people throughout the world. The estimated lifetime risk of acquiring a dermatophyte infection is between 10% and 20%. Fungal transmission occurs through direct contact with infected persons, animals, soil, or fomites. Fungi usually reside on moist areas of the body where skin surfaces touch. The skin folds of the breast, groin, and toes are the most common areas affected. Obese people, with excessive skin folds, are more susceptible to fungal infections.

*Tinea* **Tinea**, or ringworm, is classified by its location on the body (Table 16–1 ▶). Tinea corporis, or body ringworm, affects smooth areas of skin on the arms, legs, and body. It is characterized by a pink to reddish rash that sometimes forms round patches with clear areas in the center (Figure 16–8 ▶).

Scales and fissures on the soles of the feet and between the toes characterize tinea pedis, or athlete's foot (Figure 16–9 ▶). Tinea pedis is the most common type of tinea worldwide. A foul odor usually accompanies the lesions.

| Table 16–1 ▶ | Ringworm or Tinea Classification and Symptoms |
|---|---|
| **Tinea** | **Symptoms** |
| Tinea corporis | Body ringworm; pink to reddish rash sometimes forms round patches with clear areas in the center |
| Tinea pedia | Athlete's foot; scales and fissures occur on the soles of the feet and between toes; a foul odor usually accompanies lesions |
| Tinea cruris | Jock itch; red, ringlike areas with blisters |
| Tinea capitis | Scalp ringworm; mild, scaly rash or patch of hair loss without a rash |
| Tinea unguium | Nail fungus; white patches on nails, eventually turn the nail brown; nail thickens and cracks and may be destroyed |
| Tinea barbae | Barber's itch; deep, inflammatory pustules and crusting around hairs |

Figure 16–8 ► Tinea corporis, or body ringworm. (Courtesy of the CDC/Lucille K. Georg, 1964)

Tinea pedis is highly contagious and is spread by direct contact with contaminated surfaces.

Tinea cruris, or jock itch, generally affects the groin and upper and inner thighs. The fungi cause red, ringlike areas with vesicles (Figure 16–10 ►). Tinea cruris develops more frequently

Figure 16–9 ► Tinea pedia, or athlete's foot. (Courtesy of the CDC/Dr. Lucille K. Georg, 1964)

Figure 16–10 ► Tinea cruris, or jock itch. (© Custom Medical Stock Photo)

during warm weather. Tinea capitis (Figure 16–11 ►), or scalp ringworm, is highly contagious and most commonly occurs in children. This fungus may produce a mild, scaly rash or a patch of hair loss without a rash.

Tinea unguium, or nail fungus, typically affects toenails and rarely affects fingernails. This fungus is difficult to treat because it resides under the nail. The infection begins at the nail

Figure 16–11 ► Tinea capitis, or scalp ringworm. (Courtesy of the CDC, 1959)

tips, causing white patches and eventually turning the nail brown. The nail thickens and cracks. If left untreated, the fungus may destroy the entire nail and tends to spread to other nails (Figure 16–12▶).

Tinea barbae causes barber's itch. The fungus affects bearded areas of the face and neck. This fungus may produce deep, inflammatory pustules and crusting around hairs (Figure 16–13▶).

Diagnosis of tinea may include visual examination, scraping the affected area of skin, and examining the cells under a microscope. Treatment includes keeping the affected area clean and dry and using antifungal medications.

Prevention of tinea includes keeping the skin clean, cool, and dry and wearing sandals or shoes at gyms, locker rooms, and pools.

### Seborrheic Dermatitis

Seborrheic dermatitis, or chronic dandruff, is a chronic inflammatory skin disorder generally affecting areas of the head and trunk where sebaceous glands are prominent. The prevalence rate of seborrheic dermatitis is 3% to 5% worldwide. For infants, seborrheic dermatitis of the scalp is known as cradle cap. Common signs and symptoms of seborrheic dermatitis include dry or greasy scaling of the scalp with variable pruritus. Severe disease may include yellow or red scaling papules. Infants develop thick, yellow-crusted scalp lesions.

The exact cause of seborrheic dermatitis isn't known, although many factors have been impli-

**Figure 16–13** ▶ Tinea barbae, or barber's itch. (Courtesy of the CDC, 1975)

cated. *Pityrosporum ovale* yeast has been implicated in the development of seborrheic dermatitis. *P. ovale* is part of the normal flora; why some people develop seborrheic dermatitis and others do not is unclear. It has been suggested that seborrheic dermatitis is an inflammatory response to this organism, but this remains to be proved. The fact that seborrheic dermatitis responds to antifungal medications suggests that yeast probably plays a role in seborrheic dermatitis. People with neurological conditions frequently develop seborrheic dermatitis. It has been postulated that seborrheic dermatitis in these patients is a result of increased pooling of sebum caused by immobility. This increased sebum pool permits growth of *P. ovale*, which induces seborrheic dermatitis.

Diagnosis of seborrheic dermatitis may include visual examination and biopsy to confirm the diagnosis and rule out other types of dermatitis. There is no cure for seborrheic dermatitis, but treatments can control its signs and symptoms. Proper hygiene plays a key role in controlling seborrheic dermatitis. Frequent cleansing with soap removes oils from affected areas. Treatment may include medicated shampoo, antifungal medication, and corticosteroids. There is no way to prevent seborrheic dermatitis.

### Candidiasis

Candidiasis is a fungal infection that is caused by the fungus *Candida*. *Candida albicans* is commonly responsible for candidiasis.

**Figure 16–12** ▶ Tinea unguium, or nail fungus. (Courtesy of the CDC/Dr. Edwin P. Ewing, Jr., 1997)

*Candida* species are ubiquitous fungi found throughout the world as normal body flora. *Candida* species colonize over 50% of healthy individuals. Candidiasis is the most common mycotic infection and causes a variety of diseases. Usually, *Candida* is kept under control by the normal flora and by the body's immune defenses. If the mix of normal flora is changed by antibiotics, the body moisture that surrounds normal flora can also have subtle changes in its acidity or chemistry. This can cause yeast to grow and to stick to surfaces, so that the yeast causes signs and symptoms. *Candida* infections can cause occasional symptoms in healthy people. If a person's immune system is weakened by illness (especially AIDS or diabetes), malnutrition, or certain medications (e.g., corticosteroids or anticancer drugs), *Candida* fungi can cause signs and symptoms more frequently. Candidiasis can go systemic; up to 14% of patients with immunocompromising disease develop systemic candidiasis.

Vaginal *Candida* infections are common in pregnant women, diabetics, or those who are immunocompromised. During a lifetime, 75% of all women are likely to have at least one vaginal *Candida* infection, and up to 45% have two or more. Women may be more susceptible to vaginal yeast infections after antibiotic therapy or from the use of birth control pills. Signs and symptoms include a white "cottage cheese"–like discharge from the vagina, accompanied by burning, pruritus, and erythema (Figure 16–14►). Diagnosis is usually made by visual examination but may also include microscopic examination and culture. Vaginal candidiasis is effectively treated with vaginal antifungal creams or oral antifungal agents.

Creamy white patches on the tongue or side of the mouth often characterize a *Candida* infection of the mouth, or thrush. The patches are often painful and can easily be scraped off. Thrush is common in young healthy children, immunosuppressed adults, and diabetics. Diagnosis is usually made by visual examination but may also include microscopic examination and culture. Long-term treatment of oral thrush with topical liquids or oral antifungals is generally required.

*Candida* can cause skin infections in areas of skin that receive little ventilation and are un-

**Figure 16–14** ► Vaginal candidiasis.

usually moist. Common sites include the diaper area; the hands of people who routinely wear rubber gloves; the rim of skin at the base of the fingernail, especially for hands that are exposed to moisture; areas around the groin and in the crease of the buttocks; and the skin folds under large breasts. Cutaneous candidiasis causes patches of red, moist, weepy skin, sometimes with small pustules nearby. Diagnosis is usually made by visual examination but may also include microscopic examination and culture. Cutaneous candida can be effectively treated with a variety of antifungal powders and creams. The affected area must be kept clean and dry and protected from chafing.

Prevention of *Candida* infections includes keeping skin clean and dry, using antibiotics exactly as prescribed, and following a healthy dies. Diabetics should keep their blood sugar under control.

## Parasitic Infestations

***Pediculosis*** A **pediculosis**, or louse, infestation is extremely common; more than 12 million Americans are infested each year. Hundreds of millions of cases of louse infestation are reported annually worldwide, with an apparent increase over the past few decades. Lice are ectoparasites that live on the body. The three types of lice that parasitize humans are *Pediculus humanus capitis* (head louse), *Pediculus humanus corporis* (body louse), and *Pthirus pubis* (pubic louse). Lice have claws on their legs that are adapted for feeding and clinging to hair or clothing; they spread from person to person by close physical contact, and overcrowding encourages the spread of lice. Lice are also spread through fomites (e.g., combs, clothes, hats, linens). Lice are blood-sucking insects and feed on humans approximately five times per day for about 35 to 45 minutes each time. Pruritus, the most common symptom of the infestation, results from the saliva of lice as they penetrate the skin and engorge on human blood. The scratching that follows can open the skin to other invading organisms. Multiple erythematous papules (bites) are usually present.

*Pediculus humanus capitis,* or head lice, are common among schoolchildren, and, although annoying, these parasites are not dangerous and do not carry epidemic disease. Adult head lice are difficult to see, but their nits (eggs) can be located on the hair shaft. The average life span of head lice is 30 days. The female head louse lays as many as 10 eggs per 24 hours, usually at night. The female louse cannot survive for more than 3 days off the human head.

*Pthirus pubis,* or pubic lice, infest pubic hair of both men and women and are generally spread by sexual contact. The lice do not spread other sexually transmitted infections. The pubic louse gets the nickname of "crab" from its shorter, broader body and large front claws, which give it a crablike appearance. Their large claws enable pubic lice to grasp the coarser pubic hairs in the groin, anal, and armpit areas. The average life cycle of pubic lice is 35 days. The average female pubic louse lays only one to two eggs per day. Pubic lice cannot survive off the human host for more than 1 day.

*Pediculus humanus corporis,* or body lice, are most common among underprivileged, transient people. This type of infestation can be prevented with proper grooming and hygiene. Body lice can spread serious disease; the body louse is the vector of typhus, trench fever, and relapsing fever. Unlike the head louse and the pubic louse, the body louse does not live on the human body, it prefers cooler temperatures. Body lice live in human clothing, crawling onto the body only to feed, predominantly at night. Body lice lay 10 to 15 eggs per day some distance from the human body on the fibers of clothing, mainly close to the seams. The adult female body louse, unlike the head louse, can survive as long as 10 days away from the human body without a blood meal.

A diagnosis of any type of pediculosis requires the finding of live specimens of lice and/or a viable nit. Treatment includes use of pediculicidal medication. Washing fomites in temperatures exceeding 131°F (55°C) for more than 5 minutes and machine drying kills nits and lice. Items that cannot be washed in hot water should be dry cleaned or sealed in a plastic bag for 5 days. Prevention includes proper hygiene and safe sex practices.

*Scabies*  **Scabies**, commonly called "the itch," is a contagious skin disease usually associated with poor living conditions. Worldwide, an estimated 300 million cases occur annually. Scabies occurs frequently in homeless populations, and epidemics occur in healthcare facilities and other institutions. No recent published data are available on its incidence in the United States. Scabies is caused by the parasitic mite *Sarcoptes scabiei*. Mites are unable to fly or jump; therefore, transmission is predominantly through direct skin-to-skin contact. Indirect contact through fomites such as infested bedding or clothing is possible, although not usual. Scabies mites can survive up to 4 days off the human body. The female mite burrows into skin folds in the groin, under the breasts, and between fingers and toes. As she burrows, she lays eggs in the tunnels, the eggs hatch, and the cycle starts again. Intense pruritus is caused by hypersensitivity to the mite. Vesicles and pustules develop, and the tunnels in the skin appear as grayish lines. Scratching opens the lesions to secondary bacterial infection.

The combination of a history of pruritus (especially at night) and a classic rash is adequate for the diagnosis of scabies. Mites seen on microscopic examination of skin scrapings confirm the diagnosis. Treatment includes use of scabicidal medication. Pruritus may persist while treatment is being administered. Washing fomites in temperatures exceeding 131°F (55°C) for more than 5 minutes and machine drying kills scabies and their eggs. Items that cannot be washed in hot water should be dry cleaned or sealed in a plastic bag for 5 days. Prevention includes proper hygiene.

## ▶ Hypersensitivity, or Immune Disorders of the Skin

The skin frequently manifests allergic or hypersensitivity reactions. This fact serves as a basis for the patch tests given to determine specific allergies. Some diseases of the skin develop in atopic people, persons with a genetic predisposition to allergies. Others occur in anyone who has been sensitized to an allergen, such as poison ivy. Emotional stress frequently triggers or exacerbates an allergy-caused skin disease.

### Insect Bites

Insect bites and stings can produce local inflammatory reactions that may vary in appearance. Acute reactions may appear as hives, whereas more chronic reactions may appear as papules or bullous. See Chapter 2 for more information on allergy to insect bites.

### Urticaria (Hives)

**Urticaria**, or hives, results from a vascular reaction of the skin to an allergen. Urticaria is a common skin condition that affects 15% to 25% of the population at some point in their lives. The word *urticaria* is derived from a Latin word that means "plants covered with stinging nettles." The lesions are wheals, rounded elevations with red edges and pale centers. Urticaria is a rash of smooth, raised, pink or reddish wheals that comes on suddenly. Wheals usually appear first on the covered areas of the skin such as the trunk and upper parts of the arms and legs and appear in batches. Each wheal may last from a few minutes up to 6 hours. The allergic response causes damage to mast cells, which then release histamine. Histamine causes

blood vessels to dilate and become more permeable. Blood proteins and fluid ooze out of the capillaries into the tissues and result in edema. This irritation to the tissues causes intense pruritus.

At least half of the time, the specific cause of urticaria cannot be determined. Some of the most common triggers are allergies to food, medications, cosmetics, soap, and detergent; viral infections; insect stings and bites; transfusion of blood or blood products; emotional and physical stress; and physical agents such as sunlight, heat, cold, water, and pressure. Risk factors include a previous case of urticaria, a previous allergic reaction, and family members who have urticaria. Urticaria is diagnosed by visual examination and is generally treated with corticosteroids, antihistamines, and calamine lotion applied topically to reduce pruritus. If the cause of the allergic reaction can be determined, the allergen should be avoided. Reducing emotional and physical stress may also help.

### Dermatitis

Dermatitis is a broad term covering many different disorders that all result in a rash accompanied by pruritus and erythema.

**Allergic contact dermatitis** is a localized inflammation of the skin caused by contact with an allergen. There are an estimated 13.6 cases of allergic contact dermatitis per 1000 people. Allergic contact dermatitis is a type I hypersensitivity triggered by allergen binding to IgE on mast cells, which produces local severe inflammation (see Chapter 2). Unlike most allergic reactions, the trigger is external rather than internal. Initial exposure does not cause a rash; however, it sensitizes the skin so that it will react to the next exposure. Common plant allergens that cause allergic contact dermatitis include poison ivy, poison oak, and poison sumac. Many other substances can cause allergic contact dermatitis, including hair products; the metal nickel, which is found in jewelry and belt buckles; tanning agents in leather; latex rubber; and citrus fruit, especially the peel. Fragrances in soaps, shampoos, lotions, perfumes, and cosmetics can also cause a reaction (Figure 16–15 ▶). Even certain medications applied to

Figure 16–15 ► Allergic contact dermatitis, a type I hypersensitivity. (Bart's Medical Library/Phototake NYC)

the skin can cause allergic contact dermatitis. Allergic contact dermatitis is usually confined to the area where the trigger actually touched the skin. A rash accompanied by erythema is the usual reaction, but sometimes the rash does not appear for 1 to 2 days after the exposure. Pruritus and burning may accompany the rash.

Allergic contact dermatitis is diagnosed by visual examination. Treatment may include corticosteroids and antihistamines. Allergic contact dermatitis can be prevented by avoiding contact with the allergen. If contact does occur, the material should be washed off immediately with soap and water. If circumstances risk ongoing exposure, gloves and protective clothing may be helpful. Barrier creams are also available that can block certain substances, such as poison ivy, from contacting the skin.

**Atopic dermatitis**, also known as eczema, is one of the most common skin diseases, affecting 10% to 15% of children. In half of these children, atopic dermatitis will be gone by the teenage years. Doctors do not know what causes atopic dermatitis, but people who have it usually have many allergic disorders, particularly asthma, hay fever, and food allergies. The relationship between atopic dermatitis and these disorders is not clear because atopic dermatitis is not an allergy to a particular substance. Many conditions can make atopic dermatitis worse, including emotional stress, changes in temperature or humidity, bacterial skin infections, and contact with irritating clothing. In some infants, food allergies may provoke atopic dermatitis.

In babies, atopic dermatitis primarily affects the face, neck, ears, and torso. It also appears on the tops of feet or the outside of the elbows. Atopic dermatitis in older children, teenagers, and adults usually involves the skin inside the creases of the inward bend of the elbow, as well as the knee, ankle or wrist joints, the hands, and upper eyelids. Atopic dermatitis appears as irritated, red, dry, crusted patches on the skin (Figure 16–16►). If the skin becomes infected, it may develop a weeping look. Scratching causes more irritation and increases the risk of infection.

Atopic dermatitis may be diagnosed by visual examination. Atopic dermatitis is treated with

Figure 16–16 ► Atopic dermatitis. (ISM/Phototake NYC)

corticosteroids. There is no way to prevent atopic dermatitis.

## Rosacea

**Rosacea** is an inflammatory skin disease that causes facial erythema. Rosacea affects an estimated 14 million people in the United States and over 45 million people worldwide. Although rosacea can affect all segments of the population, individuals with fair skin who tend to flush or blush easily are believed to be at greatest risk. The disease is more frequently diagnosed in women; studies have shown that women are affected about two to three times more frequently than men. However, men have more severe signs and symptoms.

The primary signs of rosacea include flushing, persistent erythema, papules and pustules, and telangiectasias (tiny blood vessels dilate and become more visible through the skin). (See Figure 16–17▶.) Left untreated, rosacea tends to be progressive; however, in most people rosacea is cyclic. In severe cases the nose may grow swollen and bumpy from excess tissue. This condition, called rhinophyma, gave the late comedian W. C. Fields his trademark bulbous nose. Rhinophyma occurs mainly in men. Ocular problems, including burning and grittiness, occur in at least 50% of patients with rosacea. If untreated, a serious complication that can damage the cornea, rosacea keratitis, may impair vision.

Although the exact cause of rosacea is unknown, a number of factors can aggravate it or make it worse by increasing blood flow to the surface of the skin. Some of these include hot foods or beverages, spicy foods, alcohol, temperature extremes, sunlight, stress, anger or embarrassment, strenuous exercise, wind, hot baths or saunas, skin care products, and drugs that dilate blood vessels.

Diagnosis of rosacea is based on visual examination; there is no cure. The first step in treatment and for prevention is avoidance of rosacea triggers. Treatment may include antibiotics and topical vitamin A derivatives (retinoid). Telangiectasias can be treated with laser surgery.

## Psoriasis

**Psoriasis** is a chronic skin disease characterized by scaling and inflammation. Psoriasis affects an estimated 2% to 3% of the population worldwide. Psoriasis occurs in all age groups and equally in men and women. Psoriasis is characterized by skin cells that multiply up to 10 times faster than normal. As underlying cells reach the skin's surface and die, their sheer volume causes raised, red patches covered with white scales. Psoriasis typically occurs on the knees, elbows, and scalp and can also affect the torso, palms, and soles of the feet. There are many forms of psoriasis, including plaque, guttate, pustular, inverse, and erythrodermic psoriasis.

The most common type of psoriasis is plaque psoriasis. Approximately 9 out of 10 people with psoriasis have plaque psoriasis. Approximately 1% to 2% of people in the United States, or about 5.5 million, are affected. In plaque psoriasis, lesions have a reddened base covered by silvery scales (Figure 16–18▶). Plaque psoriasis may be caused by an abnormal immune system that produces too many T cells in the skin. These T cells trigger the inflammation and excessive skin cell reproduction, leading to inflammation and flaking of skin. Plaque psoriasis may worsen and then improve. Conditions that may cause flare-ups include changes in climate, infections, stress, and dry skin.

**Figure 16–17** ▶ Rosacea.

**Figure 16–18** ► Plaque psoriasis (Courtesy of the CDC/Dr. N.J. Fiumara, 1976)

Diagnosis of psoriasis is based on visual examination. Biopsy may be used to confirm the diagnosis and rule out other skin conditions. There is no cure for psoriasis, nor is it preventable. Three basic categories of treatment are used: Topical or external treatments include steroids, coal tar, and anthralin. Phototherapy, which employs lasers and UV light, is generally used for patients with moderate to severe psoriasis who are not responding to topical treatments or who have disease too extensive for topical treatment. Systemic drugs, including the organ-transplant-rejection drug cyclosporine, the cancer drug methotrexate, and oral retinoids, are usually reserved for patients with moderate to severe psoriasis.

## ► Benign Tumors

### Nevus (Mole)

A **nevus** is a small, dark skin growth that develops from pigment-producing cells or melanocytes. Most people have between 10 and 40 nevi. Although the typical nevus is a plain, brown spot, nevi come in a wide variety of colors, shapes, and sizes. It is unknown why nevi develop or what purpose they serve, if any.

The nevi themselves are usually harmless, but they can become malignant. Nevi should be examined by a physician if they are painful,

# Prevention ✚PLUS!

### Examining Your Skin

It's important to check your own skin, preferably once a month. A self-exam is best done in a well-lit room in front of a full-length mirror. You can use a hand-held mirror for areas that are hard to see. A spouse, close friend, or family member may be able to help you with these exams, especially for those hard-to-see areas like the lower back or the back of your thighs. The first time you inspect your skin, spend a fair amount of time carefully going over the entire surface of your skin. Learn the pattern of moles, blemishes, freckles, and other marks on your skin so that you'll notice any changes next time. Any trouble spots should be seen by a doctor.

Follow these step-by-step instructions to examine your skin:

### FACE THE MIRROR

Check your face, ears, neck, chest, and belly. Women will need to lift breasts to check the skin underneath. Check the underarm areas, both sides of your arms, the tops and bottoms of your hands, in between your fingers, and fingernail beds.

### SIT DOWN

Check the front of your thighs, shins, tops of your feet, in between your toes, and toenail beds. You will need a hand mirror for your thighs, back, and scalp. Now look at the bottoms of your feet, your calves, and the backs of your thighs, first checking one leg and then the other. Use the hand mirror to check the buttocks, genital area, lower back, upper back, and the back of the neck. Or it may be easier to look at your back in the wall mirror using a hand mirror. Use a comb or hair dryer to part your hair so that you can check your scalp.

*Source:* The American Cancer Society

itching or burning, oozing or bleeding, inflamed, scaly or crusty, or suddenly different in size, shape, color, or elevation.

Diagnosis of nevi may include visual examination and biopsy. Nevi can be removed by excision or cryosurgery. There is no way to prevent nevi, but the best way to catch potential problems at an early stage is to become familiar with the location and pattern of the nevi. Skin should be examined carefully on a regular basis.

## Hemangioma

**Hemangioma** is a benign tumor made of small blood vessels that form a red or purple birthmark. Hemangiomas are present in 62 of every 1000 newborns. At the age of 1 year, the prevalence is 120 per 1000 children. The cause of hemangiomas is unknown, and there is no way to prevent hemangiomas. Hemangiomas are diagnosed by visual examination and biopsy.

Port-wine stain (Figure 16–19 ▶) is a dark red to purple birthmark that occurs in 3 of every 1000 infants. Port-wine stain can appear anywhere on the body, and most are readily visible at birth. Port-wine stain can be flat or slightly raised and is usually permanent. Laser treatment can reduce color and improve skin texture.

Strawberry hemangioma (Figure 16–20 ▶) is a strawberry red, rough, protruding lesion on the face, neck, or trunk and is seen in approximately 0.5% of infants. The tumor may be present at birth or a few weeks after birth. Strawberry hemangioma will grow, start to fade, and turn gray in color, usually disappearing between the ages of 5 and 10. Surgery to remove the hemangioma might be necessary depending on size and location of the tumor. Other treatments may include compression and massage, steroids, x-ray therapy, laser therapy, cryotherapy, or injection of hardening agents.

Cherry hemangioma (Figure 16–21 ▶) is a small, red, dome-shaped tumor that appears most frequently after age 40. More than 70% of

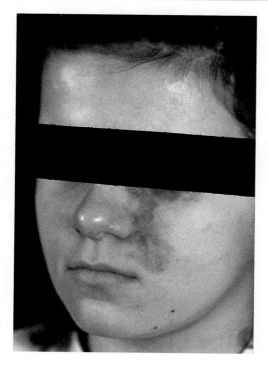

**Figure 16–19** ▶ Port-wine hemangioma. (© Custom Medical Stock Photo)

**Figure 16–20** ▶ Strawberry hemangioma. (© NMSB/Custom Medical Stock Photo)

Figure 16–21 ▶ Cherry hemangioma. (© Logical Images/Custom Medical Stock Photo)

people age 70 or older have cherry hemangiomas. Cherry hemangiomas can occur almost anywhere on the skin, but most commonly on the torso. When they first occur, cherry hemangiomas are about the size of a pinhead and do not protrude above the surface of the skin. However, some grow to one-quarter inch across or more and become spongy and dome shaped. Cherry hemangiomas can be removed by electrosurgery, cryosurgery, or laser or simply left alone.

## ▶ Nonmelanoma Skin Cancer

The American Cancer Society (ACS) estimates that more than 1 million people get nonmelanoma skin cancer each year in the United States. Men are about twice as likely to develop these cancers as women. The number of these cancers has been increasing. Perhaps this is due to a combination of increased detection, more sun exposure, and aging of the population. (Melanoma is covered in Chapter 4.)

## Basal Cell Carcinoma

The most common skin cancer is **basal cell carcinoma**, a slowly growing and generally nonmetastasizing tumor. Basal cell carcinoma begins in the lowest layer of the epidermis, called the basal cell layer. The ACS estimates that approximately 70% to 80% of all skin cancers in men and 80% to 90% in women are basal cell carcinomas. The ACS estimates that there are 800,000 to 900,000 cases per year in the United States. Within 5 years of being diagnosed with one basal cell cancer, 35% to 50% of people develop a new skin cancer. Basal cell carcinoma usually develops on sun-exposed areas, especially the head and neck. The lesion begins as a pearly nodule with rolled edges that may bleed and form a crust (Figure 16–22 ▶). Ulceration occurs and size increases if basal cell carcinoma is not treated.

Figure 16–22 ▶ Basal cell carcinoma. (© Caliendo/Custom Medical Stock Photo)

Risk factors for basal cell carcinoma include ultraviolet (UV) light exposure, fair skin, male gender (men are two times more likely than women to get basal cell carcinoma), exposure to certain chemicals (e.g., arsenic, industrial tar, coal, paraffin, certain types of oil), radiation exposure, and previous skin cancer. UV radiation damaging DNA is the cause of basal cell carcinoma. Diagnosis of basal cell carcinoma includes visual examination and biopsy. Basal cell carcinoma may be treated by surgery, chemotherapy, or radiation therapy. The best way to prevent basal cell carcinoma is to limit exposure to UV radiation. Examining the skin on a regular basis can help find cancer early.

## Squamous Cell Carcinoma

**Squamous cell carcinoma** is more serious than basal cell carcinoma because it grows more rapidly, infiltrates underlying tissues, and metastasizes through the lymphatic system. This cancer develops in any squamous epithelium of the body, including the skin or mucous membranes lining a natural body opening. The ACS estimates that there are 200,000 to 300,000 cases per year in the United States. Squamous cell carcinoma is a malignancy of the keratinocytes in the epidermis of people who have been excessively exposed to the sun. It commonly appears on sun-exposed areas of the body such as the face, ears, neck, lips, and back of the hands. The lesion is a crusted nodule that ulcerates and bleeds (Figure 16–23►).

Risk factors for squamous cell carcinoma include UV light exposure, fair skin, male gender (men are three times more likely than women to get squamous cell carcinoma), exposure to certain chemicals (e.g., arsenic, industrial tar, coal,

**Figure 16–23** ► Squamous cell carcinoma (Bart's Medical Library/Phototake NYC)

paraffin, and certain types of oil), radiation exposure, and previous skin cancer. UV radiation damaging DNA is the cause of squamous cell carcinoma. Diagnosis of squamous cell carcinoma includes visual examination and skin biopsy. Squamous cell carcinoma may be treated by surgery, chemotherapy, or radiation therapy. The best way to prevent squamous cell carcinoma is to limit exposure to UV radiation. Examining the skin on a regular basis can help find cancer early.

## ► Sebaceous Gland Disorders

## Acne (Vulgaris)

**Acne** affects more than 90% of adolescents and 25% of adults in the United States. There are two types of acne, noninflammatory acne and inflammatory acne. Several factors contribute

## Prevention ✚ PLUS!

### Limiting UV Exposure

The most important way to lower the risk of basal and squamous cell carcinoma is to limit your exposure to UV radiation. Practice sun safety when you are outdoors. Wear protective clothing and a hat with at least a 2- to 3-inch brim. Use sunscreen and lip balm with an SPF of 15 or higher. Wear sunglasses to protect your eyes and the skin around your eyes.

to acne development, including abnormal exfoliation of skin, bacteria, hormones, and possibly genetics.

Acne begins in the sebaceous hair follicles. Each hair follicle is connected to a sebaceous gland that secretes sebum. Sebum is an oily substance that lubricates hair and skin. Old skin cells are exfoliated to prepare for new skin. If old skin cells are not shed or are shed unevenly, they may clump and form a plug (or comedo) that traps sebum and bacteria inside the hair follicle. Noninflammatory acne includes closed comedones (whiteheads) and open comedones (blackheads).

If there is a break in the follicle wall (forming a papule), inflammation is triggered and inflammatory acne develops. Pustules form as white blood cells make their way to the surface of the skin. If the hair follicle totally collapses, a nodule is formed. Severe chronic acne, as seen in Figure 16–24 ▶, can lead to disfiguring and scarring. Acne is diagnosed by visual examination.

Treatment for acne may include topical antibiotics and antibacterials (benzoyl peroxide), retinoids (Retin-A), oral antibiotics, and oral contraceptives. Often, a combination of such products is required to achieve optimal results. Isotretinoin (Accutane) may be used to treat severe acne or acne that does not respond to other treatments. Isotretinoin is associated with severe birth defects if pregnancy occurs during the course of treatment or within several weeks of

concluding treatment. Isotretinoin may increase the levels of triglycerides and cholesterol in the blood and may increase liver enzyme levels.

Prevention of acne includes not overcleansing the skin, not using harsh scrubs, avoiding products with high concentrations of alcohol, and keeping the hands away from the face.

## ▶ Pigment Disorders

The main skin pigment, melanin, is interspersed among other cells in the epidermis. Skin color varies from light to dark depending on the number of melanocytes present. Melanin production normally increases with exposure to sunlight, causing tanning. Hypopigmentation is caused by an abnormally low amount or absence of melanin. The skin may be pale white to various shades of pink caused by blood flowing through it. Hyperpigmentation is caused by an abnormally high amount of melanin.

### Albinism

**Albinism** is a group of genetic conditions that cause a lack of pigment. Albinism affects people from all races. About 1 in 17,000 people has some type of albinism, although up to 1 in 70 is a carrier of albinism genes. People with albinism have visual issues, including rapid eye movements, eyes that do not track properly, photophobia, decreased visual acuity, or even functional blindness.

Ocular albinism affects only the eyes. People with ocular albinism usually have normal or only slightly lighter than normal skin. However, examination of the eye will show that there is no pigment in the retina. Ocular albinism is X-linked recessive.

Oculocutaneous albinism affects both the skin and the eyes. Common signs of oculocutaneous albinism include absence of pigment from the hair, skin, or iris of eyes. Oculocutaneous albinism is autosomal recessive.

Albinism may be diagnosed based on the appearance of the skin, hair, and eyes and genetic testing. Treatment includes improving vision, protecting eyes from bright light, and protecting the skin and eyes from the sun.

**Figure 16–24** ▶ Severe acne. (© Custom Medical Stock Photo)

Figure 16–25 ▶ Vitiligo. (© Custom Medical Stock Photo)

## Vitiligo

**Vitiligo** is a loss of melanin resulting in white patches of skin. An estimated 1 to 2 million Americans have vitiligo. Although any part of the body may be affected by vitiligo, depigmentation usually develops first on sun-exposed areas of the skin (Figure 16–25▶). Vitiligo affects both sexes and all races but is often more noticeable and more disfiguring in people with darker skin. Vitiligo usually starts as small areas of pigment loss that spread and become larger with time. The white patches are usually well demarcated and may cover large parts of the body. The cause of vitiligo is unknown, and there is no cure. Possible risk factors include immune system disorders, heredity, sunburn, and emotional distress.

Diagnosis is based on visual examination. Small areas of skin may be covered with tinted make-up, and sunscreen should always be applied to the skin to prevent sunburn. Treatment options include corticosteroids, Psoralen (contains chemicals that react with UV light to cause darkening of the skin), UV light therapy, depigmentation therapy, and surgical therapies. There is no way to prevent vitiligo.

## Ephelides and Lentigines

**Ephelides,** also known as macule or freckles, refer to flat spots that are red or light brown and typically appear during the sunny months and fade in the winter. They occur most often in people with light complexions. Ephelides are genetic and are related to the presence of the melanocortin-1 receptor gene variant, which is dominant. Ephelides can also be triggered by long exposure to sunlight. Ephelides are predominately found on the face, although they may appear on any skin exposed to the sun. The regular use of sunscreen helps suppress the appearance of ephelides.

**Lentigines** are a type of freckle that develop in older adults and are often called liver spots or age spots. Lentigines are small, brown lesions occurring on the face, neck, and back of the hands (Figure 16–26▶). Lentigines are not due to aging but are due to excessive sun exposure. Ephelides and lentigines pose no medical risks. Diagnosis is based on visual examination. Treatment may include bleaching creams, retinoids, cryosurgery, and laser treatment. Protecting the skin from sunlight is the best way to prevent ephelides and lentigines.

## Melasma

**Melasma,** also known as chloasma or pregnancy mask, is characterized by patches of darker skin on the face, especially over the cheeks. Melasma occurs in an estimated 5 to 6 million women in the United States. The cause of melasma remains unknown but is believed to be due to an increase in the production of melanin. What causes the increased production of

Figure 16–26 ▶ Lentigo. (© Zuber/Custom Medical Stock Photo)

melanin is not known. Possible triggers include hormones, prolonged sun exposure, use of birth control pills, and certain medications like tetracycline and antimalarial drugs. Melasma is diagnosed by visual examination. Treatment may include bleaching creams, chemical peels, or laser treatment. Protecting skin from the sun is key to preventing melasma.

## ▶ Skin Trauma

**Lacerations** are cuts in the skin caused by a sharp object. **Abrasions**, or scrapes, result from wearing away the upper layer of skin by friction; they are red, raw, and painful, and bleeding is minimal. **Punctures** are injuries caused by a pointed object piercing or penetrating the skin, with minimal bleeding. A possible complication of puncture is tetanus; the puncture creates the anaerobic environment preferred by the bacteria. Sutures or glue may be needed to close skin that has been split open or is gaping.

**Contusions**, or bruises, are caused when blood vessels are damaged or broken as a result of a blow to the skin. Blood leaks out of the damaged vessels into the surrounding tissues. A purplish, flat bruise that occurs when blood leaks out into the top layers of skin is known as an **ecchymosis**. In an **avulsion,** a portion of the skin has been torn away or is barely attached. Crushing injuries result when a body part is subjected to a high degree of force or pressure, usually after being squeezed between two heavy objects. Hemorrhage, contusions, lacerations, and fractures are possible complications of a crushing injury.

## Pressure Sores or Decubitus Ulcers

Pressure sores, or decubitus ulcers, usually occur in skin overlying bony projections such as the hips, heels, elbows, and ankles. Constant pressure against the skin reduces the blood supply to that area, and the affected tissue dies. At-risk patients can develop a pressure sore within 2 to 6 hours of the onset of pressure. An estimated 1.8 million people in the United States get a pressure sore each year, and 70% of pressure sores occur in patients older than 70 years,

probably due to a decrease in adipose tissue. The prevalence rate in residents of long-term care facilities is estimated to be 23%. Patients hospitalized with acute illness have an incidence rate of pressure sores between 9% and 13%. Disturbingly, even with current medical and surgical therapies, patients who achieve a healed wound have recurrence rates of as high as 90%. Treatment of pressure sores in the United States costs more than $1.3 billion annually.

The hip and buttock regions account for 67% of all pressure sores. The lower extremities account for an additional 25% of all pressure sores. The remaining 10% or so of pressure sores may occur in any location that experiences long periods of uninterrupted pressure. No surface of the body can be considered immune to the effects of pressure.

Risk factors for pressure sores include impaired mobility, skin atrophy, chronic conditions such as diabetes or vascular disease that prevent areas of the body from receiving proper blood flow, sensory loss, malnourishment, mental disability, older age, and urinary or bowel incontinence.

Pressure sores are categorized by severity. There are four stages, ranging from intact red or discolored skin to full-thickness loss of skin and subcutaneous tissue that extends into muscle or bone. Figure 16–27▶ shows a patient with several pressure sores.

**Figure 16–27** ▶ Pressure sores. (© Caliendo/Custom Medical Stock Photo)

Diagnosis is based on visual examination and may include bacterial culture if the sore is infected. The first step in treatment is eliminating the pressure. Specialized support surfaces and pressure reduction devices have been shown to reduce pressure. Regardless of support surface or device, turning and repositioning the patient remain the cornerstones of prevention and treatment. This should be performed every 2 hours, even in the presence of a specialty surface or bed.

## Corns and Calluses

**Corns** and **calluses** are areas of the skin that have grown thick in response to repeated pressure and friction and form to protect the skin. A callus (tyloma) involves a thickening of skin without distinct borders. Calluses usually form on feet and hands over bony spots. Calluses vary in color from white to gray-yellow, brown, or red. Calluses may be painless or tender and may throb or burn.

When a callus develops a mass of dead cells in its center (glassy core), it becomes a corn (heloma). Corns have distinct borders and usually form on the feet. Corns may be hard or soft and are usually painful. Causes of calluses and corns include ill-fitting shoes or socks, not wearing shoes or socks, manual labor, bony prominences on the feet, and biomechanical or gait abnormalities.

Diagnosis may include visual examination, biopsy, and x-rays. Treatment may include shaving or cutting off the hardened area on the skin, removing the corn or callus by medication or surgery, or surgically removing areas of protruding bone where corns and calluses form. Prevention includes wearing gloves to protect hands, making sure shoes and socks fit properly and do not rub, surgically correcting bony abnormalities, and keeping hands and feet moisturized.

## Burns

A burn is damage to the body's tissues caused by heat, chemicals, electricity, sunlight, or radiation. Thermal burns are the most common. When tissues are burned, fluid leaks into the tissue from the blood vessels, causing edema and pain. In addition, damaged skin and other body surfaces are easily infected because they can no longer act as a barrier against invading organisms. More than 2 million people in the United States require treatment for burns each year, and between 3000 and 4000 die annually as a result of burns.

The extent of damage depends on surface temperature and contact duration. Burns are classified according to the depth of skin involved. First-degree or superficial burns affect the epidermis The epidermis is red, swollen, and painful (Figure 16–28 ▶). First-degree burns heal in approximately 1 week and do not scar.

Second-degree, or partial thickness, burns affect the epidermis and the dermis. The epidermis is extremely red and blistered, and the area is very painful (Figure 16–29 ▶). Second-degree burns heal in a few weeks; some scarring and depigmentation may occur. Treatment includes antibiotic cream and pain relievers.

Third-degree, or full thickness, burns affect the epidermis, dermis, and subcutaneous tissue (Figure 16–30 ▶). The skin may appear white or black with a leathery appearance. The nerve endings are destroyed, so the burned area will not be painful. The patient may go into shock due to loss of fluids. Treatment may include antibiotics, IV fluids, pain relievers, surgical

Figure 16–28 ▶ First-degree burn.

Figure 16–29 ▶ Second-degree burn.

debridement, and grafting. Severe third-degree burns cause extensive scarring.

To determine the severity of a burn, doctors estimate what percentage of the body's surface has been burned. For adults, doctors use the rule of nines. This method divides almost all of the body into sections of 9% or 18% (Figure 16–31 ▶). Burns that involve more than 90% of the body surface, or more than 60% in an older person, usually are fatal. For children, doctors use charts that adjust these percentages according to the child's age (Lund-Browder charts; Figure 16–31). Adjustment is needed

because different areas of the body grow at different rates.

## Hypothermia and Frostbite

**Hypothermia** is an abnormally low body temperature resulting from prolonged exposure to cold air or water. Hypothermia occurs when more heat escapes from the body than the body can produce. Approximately 700 people in the United States die each year of hypothermia. Signs and symptoms of hypothermia include shivering (the body is attempting to generate heat), cold and pale skin, lack of coordination, disorientation, and decreased heart rate, respiration rate, and blood pressure that can lead to loss of consciousness or can lead to death. Diagnosis is based on body temperature. Risk factors for hypothermia include age (young or old), living in a cold climate, and alcohol use. Rewarming is the main treatment. Prevention includes dressing appropriately for the weather by wearing dry, loose-fitting, layered clothing that wicks moisture away from skin. It is important to wear a hat; 30% to 50% of body heat is lost through the head. Alcohol should be avoided because it causes the blood vessels in the skin to dilate, reducing circulation.

Frostbite is damage to the skin caused by freezing due to prolonged exposure to cold conditions. Freezing causes formation of ice crystals within cells, rupturing and destroying the cells. Signs and symptoms of frostbite may include pain, tingling, numbness, eventual loss of sensation, blistering, and tissue death.

Risk factors for frostbite include age (young or old), living in a cold climate, alcohol use, smoking, and circulatory problems. Diagnosis of frostbite is based on visual examination. Treatment may include rewarming, pain medication, antibiotics, and anti-inflammatory medication. Tissue affected by severe frostbite may require surgery or amputation.

Prevention includes dressing adequately for the weather by wearing loose-fitting, layered clothing; keeping clothes dry; refraining from smoking; and avoiding alcohol.

Figure 16–30 ▶ Third-degree burn.

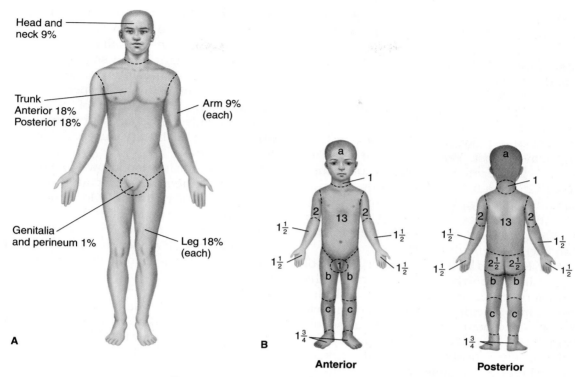

Relative percentage of body surface area (% BSA) affected by growth

| Body Part | 0 yr | 1 yr | 5 yr | 10 yr | 15 yr |
|---|---|---|---|---|---|
| a = $\frac{1}{2}$ of head | $9\frac{1}{2}$ | $8\frac{1}{2}$ | $6\frac{1}{2}$ | $5\frac{1}{2}$ | $4\frac{1}{2}$ |
| b = $\frac{1}{2}$ of 1 thigh | $2\frac{3}{4}$ | $3\frac{1}{4}$ | 4 | $4\frac{1}{4}$ | $4\frac{1}{2}$ |
| c = $\frac{1}{2}$ of 1 lower leg | $2\frac{1}{2}$ | $2\frac{1}{2}$ | $2\frac{3}{4}$ | 3 | $3\frac{1}{4}$ |

**Figure 16–31** ► Determining the extent of a burn: (A) rule of nines (adult); (B) Lund-Browder chart (children).

## ► Age-Related Diseases

The structure and function of skin changes with age. Skin loses some of its elasticity with age due to a decrease in elastic fibers, and the skin appears wrinkled and saggy. Touch sensation of the skin decreases with aging, making burns and frostbite more likely. Stem cell production declines with aging, causing slower epidermal cell reproduction and thinner, more translucent skin that is more prone to injury and infection and re-

tains less water. Migration of cells to the top of the epidermis slows. As a result, skin heals more slowly; healing time may be more than twice as long in the elderly as in younger people. This longer healing time increases the risk of secondary infections. A decrease in the blood supply to the dermis and a decrease in sweat production lead to impaired thermoregulation. The elderly have an increased risk for hypothermia. The number of macrophages and other cells of the immune system decrease and these cells are less efficient, increasing the risk of infection.

Melanocyte number and activity declines with aging, causing the skin to become paler and the hair to turn gray or white. This also causes an increased susceptibility to sunburn and skin cancer. In addition, selected melanocytes increase their production in areas exposed to the sun, resulting in lentigines. Sebaceous gland activity decreases, as does sebum production. The skin becomes dry and flaky. Hair becomes brittle, thin, and may be lost. Vascularity and circulation decrease in the subcutaneous tissue, causing drugs that are administered in this manner to be absorbed slowly. Vascular supply to the nails and hair decreases, resulting in slowed growth. Nails become dull, brittle, hard, and thick and become difficult to trim.

**Seborrheic keratosis** is a benign overgrowth of epithelial cells. Seborrheic keratoses are the most common benign tumor in older individuals. Most people develop at least one seborrheic keratosis at some point in their lives. A seborrheic keratosis has a characteristic "pasted on" look and typically appears on the head, neck, or trunk of the body. Seborrheic keratoses range in color from light tan to black, are round to oval shaped, are flat or slightly elevated with a scaly surface, and range in size from very small to more than 1 inch across (Figure 16–32▶). Seb-

orrheic keratosis may cause pruritus. The exact cause of seborrheic keratoses is unknown. They tend to run in some families, so genetics may play a role. UV light may also play a role in their development. Diagnosis is made by visual examination; a biopsy may be performed to rule out skin cancer. Treatment of seborrheic keratoses usually isn't necessary; however, they can be removed by cryosurgery, curettage, or electrocautery.

**Actinic keratosis**, also known as solar keratosis, is a precancerous skin condition caused by exposure to UV radiation. More than 5 million people in the United States have at least one actinic keratosis lesion. The prevalence of actinic keratosis increases dramatically with age. Multiple wartlike lesions develop on areas of the body exposed to the sun such as the face, arms, and legs (Figure 16–33▶). Actinic keratoses are small (usually less than one-fourth inch) rough spots that may be pink-red or flesh colored. If actinic keratosis is not treated, 10% to 15% may develop into squamous cell carcinoma. Even though most actinic keratoses do

**Figure 16–32** ▶ Seborrheic keratosis. (Courtesy of the CDC/Dr. Steve Kraus, 1981.)

**Figure 16–33** ▶ Actinic keratosis. (Medical On-Line, Ltd.)

not become cancers, they are a warning that the skin has suffered sun damage and should be checked regularly. Diagnosis of actinic keratosis is made by visual examination and may include biopsy. Treatment of actinic keratosis may include surgery, acid chemical peels, and topical chemotherapy. The best way to prevent actinic keratosis is to limit exposure to UV radiation.

## RESOURCES

The American Academy of Dermatology: www.aad.org

American Cancer Society: www.cancer.org

Centers for Disease Control and Prevention: www.cdc.gov

The National Organization for Albinism and Hypopigmentation: www.albinism.org

The National Psoriasis Foundation: www.psoriasis.org

The National Rosacea Society: www.rosacea.org

Vascular Birthmarks Foundation: www.birthmark.org

# DISEASES AT A GLANCE

## Integumentary System

| DISEASE | ETIOLOGY | SIGNS AND SYMPTOMS |
|---|---|---|
| Epidermoid and pilar cysts | Abnormal cell proliferation | Smooth, round lump just beneath the skin surface |
| Impetigo | *S. pyogenes, S. aureus* | Vesicles and pustules that rupture forming a crust, fever, swollen lymph nodes |
| Erysipelas, cellulitus | *S. pyogenes, S. aureus* | Swollen, bright red, hot, and tender area of the skin, small vesicles, fever, chills, swelling of lymph nodes |
| Folliculitis | Staphylococci | Erythema, follicular-based papules and pustules |
| Furuncles, carbuncles | Staphylococci | Furuncles—large, tender, swollen, pus-filled lesion<br>Carbuncles—cluster of furuncles |
| Herpes | Herpes virus family | Small, fluid-filled, painful vesicles |
| Warts | Human papillomavirus | Benign neoplasms with rough, keratinized surface |
| Tinea | Fungi | Mild scales, rash, fissures |
| Seborrheic dermatitis | Unknown | Adults: Dry or greasy scaling with variable pruritus<br>Infants: Thick, yellow-crusted scalp lesions |
| Candidiasis | *Candida albicans, Candida tropicalis, Candida parapsilosis, Candida guilliermondi, Torulopsis glabrata* | Vaginal: white cottage-cheese discharge, burning, pruritus, erythema<br>Oral: Creamy white, painful patches<br>Cutaneous: patches of red, moist, weepy skin |
| Pediculosis | *Pediculus humanus capitis, Pediculus humanus corporis, Pthirus pubis* | Pruritus, multiple erythematous papules |
| Scabies | *Sarcoptes scabiei* | Pruritus, vesicles, pustules, grayish lines (tunnels) |
| Urticaria (hives) | Hypersensitivity | Wheals with rounded elevations and pale centers, pruritus |

| DIAGNOSIS | TREATMENT | PREVENTION/LIFESPAN |
|---|---|---|
| Visual examination | Removal by excision if required | None |
| Visual examination, bacterial culture | Antibiotics | Proper Hygiene |
| Visual examination, bacterial culture | Self-limiting, antibiotics | Prompt attention to wounds, moisturizing the skin, careful trimming of nails |
| Visual examination, bacterial culture | Self-limiting, daily cleansing with antiseptic soap, antibiotics | Keep skin clean, dry, and free from abrasions or irritation |
| Visual examination, bacterial culture | Moist heat, antiseptic skin cleansing, antibiotics, incision and drainage | Keep skin clean, dry, and free from abrasions or irritation |
| Visual examination, viral culture, DNA testing | Self-limiting, antiviral drugs | Avoid contact with HSV-1, frequent handwashing, avoid recurrence triggers |
| Visual examination | Removal by medication, electrocautery, cryosurgery, laser surgery | Avoid touching warts, walking barefoot on warm moist surfaces, trauma to the skin |
| Visual examination, microscopic examination of skin scrapings | Keeping area clean and dry, antifungal medication | Keep skin clean, cool, and dry; wear sandals or shoes at gyms, locker rooms, and pools |
| Visual examination biopsy | Medicated shampoo, antifungal medication, corticosteroids | None |
| Visual examination, culture | Antifungal medication | Keeping skin clean and dry, proper use of antibiotics, healthy lifestyle, controlling blood sugar |
| Finding lice or nits | Pediculosidal medication | Proper hygiene, safe sex practices |
| Pruritus, rash, microscopic examination of skin scrapings | Scabicidal medication | Proper hygiene |
| Visual examination | Corticosteroids, antihistamines, calamine lotion | Avoid allergen, reduce emotional and physical stress |

# DISEASES AT A GLANCE

## Integumentary System (*continued*)

| DISEASE | ETIOLOGY | SIGNS AND SYMPTOMS |
| --- | --- | --- |
| Allergic contact dermatitis | Type I hypersensitivity | Rash with erythema, pruritus, burning |
| Atopic dermatitis | Unknown | Red, dry, crusted patches on the skin |
| Rosacea | Unknown | Flushing, persistent erythema, papules pustules, telangiectasias |
| Psoriasis | Hereditary; too many T cells trigger inflammation | Red lesions with silvery scales |
| Nevus (mole) | Benign tumor | Small, dark skin growth |
| Hemangioma | Benign tumor | Red or purple birth marks |
| Basal cell carcinoma | UV radiation damaging DNA | Pearly nodule with rolled edges may bleed, form crust |
| Squamous cell carcinoma | UV radiation damaging DNA | Crusted nodule, ulcerates and bleeds |
| Acne (vulgaris) | Abnormal skin exfoliation, bacteria, hormones, genetic factors | Comedones, papules, pustules, nodules |
| Albinism | Hereditary | Absence of melanin |
| Vitiligo | Unknown | White, well-demarcated areas of skin without melanin |
| Ephelides, lentigines | Hereditary, sun exposure | Red or brown macule |

## True or False

_____ 1. Impetigo is caused by a virus.

_____ 2. Basal cell carcinoma metastasizes rapidly.

_____ 3. Cold sores are caused by a bacterial infection.

_____ 4. Seborrheic dermatitis is a malignant skin tumor.

_____ 5. Warts are caused by bacteria.

_____ 6. A mole is a nevus.

_____ 7. Ringworm is a viral infection.

_____ 8. Erythema is whitening of the skin.

_____ 9. The cause of seborrheic dermatitis is unknown.

_____ 10. Rosacea is caused by fungus.

## Fill-Ins

1. _____ is the dark pigment of the skin that protects the body from the harmful rays of the sun.

2. _____ is a tough, fibrous protein that protects the skin from harmful substances.

3. The _____ is composed of connective tissue that supports blood and lymph vessels and elastic fibers.

4. _____ is a large family of viruses that cause clusters of fluid-filled vesicles on the skin.

5. _____ is a contagious skin disease usually associated with poor living conditions.

6. _____ is a chronic skin disease characterized by scaling and inflammation.

7. _____ are caused when blood vessels are damaged or broken as a result of a blow to the skin.

8. _____ is a benign tumor made of small blood vessels that form a red or purple birthmark.

9. _____ is loss of melanin resulting in white patches of skin.

10. _____ _____ causes scales and fissures on the soles of the feet and between toes.

## Labeling Exercise

Use the lines below to label each photo.

1 _____

2 _____

3 _____

4 _____

5 _____

# Multimedia Preview

Additional interactive resources and activities for this chapter can be found on the Companion Website. For videos, audio glossary, and review, access the accompanying DVD-ROM in this book.

## ▶ DVD-ROM Highlights

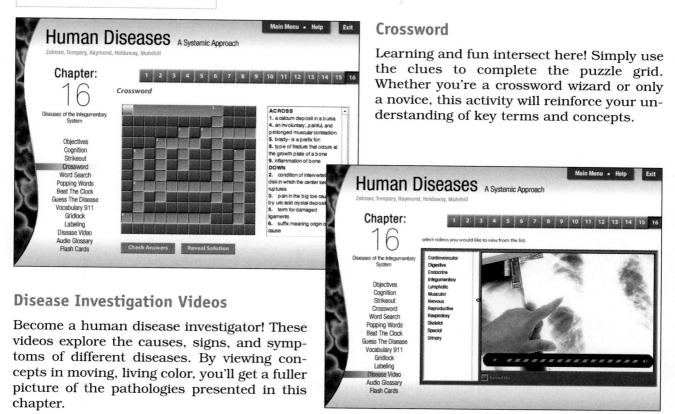

### Crossword

Learning and fun intersect here! Simply use the clues to complete the puzzle grid. Whether you're a crossword wizard or only a novice, this activity will reinforce your understanding of key terms and concepts.

### Disease Investigation Videos

Become a human disease investigator! These videos explore the causes, signs, and symptoms of different diseases. By viewing concepts in moving, living color, you'll get a fuller picture of the pathologies presented in this chapter.

## ▶ Website Highlights—www.pearsonhighered.com/zelman

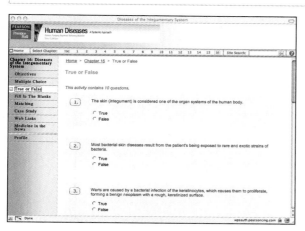

### True or False Quiz

Take advantage of the free-access online study guide that accompanies your textbook. You'll find a true or false quiz that provides instant feedback and allows you to check your score to see what you got right or wrong. By clicking on this URL you'll also access links to current news articles and an audio glossary.

# Appendix A
# Glossary

**Abruptio placentae.**  Premature separation of the placenta from the uterus prior to or during birth.

**Acetylcholine.**  Neurotransmitter of the parasympathetic nervous system.

**Achlorhydria.**  A condition in which hydrochloric acid is absent in the stomach.

**Achondroplasia.**  An autosomal dominant disorder of defective cartilage formation in the fetus.

**Achondroplastic dwarfism.**  A condition caused by defective cartilage formation that results in improper bone development.

**Acidosis.**  The condition in which the production of acids lowers the body's pH.

**Acne.**  Blackheads, pimples, and pustules that result from hormonal changes occurring most often during puberty.

**Acne rosacea.**  Tiny pimples and broken blood vessels on the cheeks, chin, and nose of some fair-skinned people.

**Acquired immunodeficiency syndrome (AIDS).**  The deadly disease caused by HIV that destroys an individual's immune system, making the victim remarkably susceptible to infection.

**Acrodermatitis enteropathica.**  A rare autosomal recessive disorder that results in defective malabsorption of zinc.

**Acromegaly.**  The condition that results from excessive production of growth hormone after puberty.

**Actinic keratosis.**  Wartlike lesions found on areas of the body that receive excessive sun exposure.

**Activated lymphocytes.**  White blood cells that have been stimulated by antigens that include B and T cells.

**Active immunity.**  A type of artificial immunity; the person is given a vaccine or toxoid as the antigen, and he or she forms antibodies to counteract it.

**Acute.**  A disease is that has a sudden onset and a short duration.

**Adenocarcinoma.**  A cancerous glandular tumor.

**Adenohypophysis.**  The anterior and larger portion of the hypophysis; it is glandular and maintains direct communication with the hypothalamus of the brain.

**Adenoma.**  A benign tumor of glandular tissue that often develops in the breast, thyroid gland, or mucous glands of the intestinal tract.

**Adhesion.**  Condition caused by connective tissue fibers that anchor adjacent structures together; a kinking of the intestine.

**Adipose.**  Fat tissue.

**Adrenalin.**  A hormone of the sympathetic nervous system; the most vital therapy in treatment of allergies and can be self-injected in an emergency.

**Adrenal virilism.**  Expression of secondary male sexual characteristics in females caused by a testosterone-secreting adrenal gland neoplasm.

**Adrenocorticotropic hormone (ACTH).**  The tropic horomone  that affects the adrenal cortex.

**Adult or (acute) respiratory distress syndrome (ARDS).**  Condition characterized by the development of sudden breathlessness within hours to days of an inciting event such as trauma, sepsis (microorganisms growing in a person's blood), or drug overdose.

**Affect.**  Emotional state or feeling tone used to describe one's emotional expression.

**Agglutinate.**  Clumping or aggregation, as occurs in some antibody-antigen reactions.

**Albinism.**  An autosomal recessive disorder in which no melanin is formed, causing a person to have white hair, pale skin, and pink eyes.

**Albuminuria.**  The presence of the plasma protein albumin in urine.

**Aldosterone.** The principle hormone from the adrenal cortex that causes sodium retention and potassium secretion by the kidneys.

**Alleles.** Alternative forms of a gene.

**Allergens.** Agents that initiate an allergic response.

**Allergy.** Abnormal immunologic response to allergens such as pollens, dust, animal dander, and certain foods.

**Alpha cells.** Glucagon-secreting cells of the endocrine pancreas.

**Alpha-feto-protein.** Fetal protein found in maternal blood, and sometimes detected in adults with various cancers.

**Alveoli.** Small air sacs in the lungs where gas exchange occurs.

**Alzheimer's disease.** A common form of dementia that generally affects people after age 65.

**Amenorrhea.** The absence of menstruation.

**Amniocentesis.** A diagnostic test for hereditary diseases performed on fetal cells withdrawn from amniotic fluid.

**Amoeboid.** A type of protozoa that moves with pseudopodia.

**Amygdala.** Almond-shaped structure located deep within the brain.

**Amylase.** A digestive enzyme that breaks down carbohydrates.

**Amyotrophic lateral sclerosis (ALS).** Also known as Lou Gehrig's disease; a chronic, terminal, degenerative disease of the motor nervous system.

**Analgesics.** Medications that reduce pain.

**Anaphylactic shock.** A severe inflammation brought on by a severe antigen-antibody reaction such as occurs in an incompatible blood transfusion.

**Anaphylaxis.** The condition of anaphylactic shock, a life-threatening state in which blood pressure drops and airways become constricted.

**Anatomy.** Study of the normal structure of the body.

**Androgenital syndrome.** A form of hyperadrenalism caused when the male hormone is secreted in excess.

**Androgen.** The sex hormone in males.

**Anemia.** A condition caused by a reduction of oxygen-carrying hemoglobin.

**Aneurysm.** A localized dilation caused by a weakening in the wall of a blood vessel.

**Angina pectoris.** The temporary chest pain or sensation of chest pressure caused by transient oxygen insufficiency.

**Angiocardiography.** An x-ray of the heart and great vessels in which a contrast indicator (dye) is injected into the cardiovascular system.

**Angioma.** A type of benign tumor composed of blood vessels, such as red birthmark or "port-wine" stain.

**Angioplasty.** A procedure by which a balloon-tip catheter is inserted into the coronary arteries and expanded to break and crush plaque buildup.

**Ankylosis.** Scar tissue formation at bone ends that can turn to bone, causing the ends to fuse.

**Anorexia.** A loss of appetite.

**Anorexia nervosa.** A disease of psychoneurotic origin in which an aversion to food leads to emaciation and malnutrition; found to be most common in teenage girls.

**Antibiotic resistance.** Resistance arising when bacteria adapt to antibiotics and the adaptation becomes common in the bacterial population, rendering the antibiotics ineffective.

**Antibiotics.** Drugs used to treat bacterial infections.

**Antibodies.** Proteins secreted by plasma cells that aid in defense against infectious agents.

**Anticoagulant.** Medication used to prevent intravascular clotting.

**Antidiuretic hormone.** One of two hormones secreted by the posterior pituitary.

**Antigen.** A substance, usually foreign to the body, which triggers the immune response.

**Antihistamine.** A drug to counteract the unpleasant effects caused by the release of histamines in the body due to allergies; has a drying effect on the mucous membranes of the mouth and throat.

**Antitussive.** A substance administered to suppress a cough.

**Anuria.** The total stoppage of urine production.

**Anxiety disorder.** General term for disorders in which the primary feature is abnormal or inappropriate anxiety that interferes with daily work, school, recreational, and family activities. Subtypes include panic disorder, generalized anxiety disorder, phobic disorders, social phobia, obsessive-compulsive disorder, and post-traumatic stress disorder.

**Aorta.** The largest artery in the body; carries blood away from the heart to the arteries.

**Aortic stenosis.** The narrowing of the valve leading into the aorta.

**Aphasia.** Loss of speech.

**Aphonia.** Inability to produce sounds from the larynx.

**Aplasia.** Developmental failure leading to the absence of a structure or tissue.

**Apnea.** Temporary cessation of breathing.

**Apoptosis.** Cell death or cell deletion by fragmentation into membrane particles, which are phagocytosed by other cells.

**Arrhythmia.** A deviation from the normal rhythm of the heartbeat.

**Arterial blood gas (ABGs).** A blood test that is performed to determine the concentration of oxygen, carbon dioxide, and bicarbonate, as well as the pH of the blood.

**Arteriosclerosis.** Progressive hardening of blood vessels, especially arteries.

**Arthritis.** The inflammation of a joint.

**Ascites.** Fluid that develops as a result of liver failure and accumulates in the peritoneal cavity.

**Aspermia.** Caused when there is no formation or emission of sperm due to the absence of the gonadotropic hormones in a male before puberty.

**Asthma.** A disease caused by increased responsiveness of the tracheobronchial tree to various stimuli, which tends to cause dyspnea and wheezing.

**Astigmatism.** Caused by the front surface of the eye, the cornea, having an irregular curvature or the lens having irregularities.

**Astrocytoma.** Basically benign, slow-growing tumors of the brain.

**Atelectasis.** A state in which the lung, in whole or in part, is collapsed or without air.

**Atherosclerosis.** The accumulation of fatty material under the inner lining of the arterial wall.

**Atresia.** The absence or closure of a normal body opening or tubular structure.

**Atrophic.** A degenerating, wasting condition.

**Atrophy.** The decrease in size or function of an organ.

**Attention deficit hyperactivity disorder (ADHD).** Neurobiological disorder characterized by prominent symptoms of inattention, hyperactivity, and impulsivity.

**Aura.** A warning signal such as the symptoms that precede an epileptic seizure.

**Auscultation.** Listening with a stethoscope for sounds within the body, such as heart valve sounds or the lungs, during an exam.

**Autistic disorder.** Developmental disorder of reciprocal language and social interactions, with stereotypical behavior.

**Autoantibodies.** Antibodies produced against self-antigens.

**Autoimmune diseases.** Failure of immune tolerance; activated T cells and antibodies attack the body's own tissue.

**Autosomes.** Name for 44 of the 46 chromosomes; does not include the sex horomones.

**B lymphocytes.** Lymphocytes that produce antibodies in cell-mediated immunity.

**Bacilli.** Rod-shaped bacterial cells.

**Bacteria.** A single-celled organism with simple structure and lacking a nucleus.

**Bartholin's glands.** Mucus-secreting glands situated at the vaginal entrance.

**Basal cell carcinoma.** Most common form of skin cancer.

**Basal ganglia (basal nuclei).** Nerve cell bodies deep within the white matter of the brain, which help control position and unconscious movements.

**Basophils.** A type of white blood cell that promotes inflammation and participates in allergic responses.

**Benign.** A noncancerous neoplasm or tumor.

**Benign prostatic hyperplasia.** Enlargement of the prostate gland in older men.

**Beriberi.** A thiamine deficiency; includes dry or wet syndromes, cerebral beriberi, and Wernicke-Korsakoff syndrome.

**Beta cells.** Insulin-secreting cells of the endocrine pancreas.

**Beta human chorionic gonadotropin.** Hormone secreted during pregnancy.

**Bile.** Substance secreted by the liver and necessary for fat digestion; consists of water, bile salts, cholesterol, and bilirubin.

**Biliary calculi.** Gallstones; consist mainly of cholesterol, bilirubin, and calcium.

**Biliary cirrhosis.** A form of cirrhosis resulting from cholecystitis.

**Bilirubin.** A colored pigment produced when hemoglobin breaks down.

**Binary fission.** Process in which bacteria reproduce by splitting in half.

**Binge.** Eating excessive amounts of food within a restricted period of time.

**Biopsy.** Procedure in which a small sample of a tissue is surgically removed and examined microscopically for abnormalities.

**Bipolar disorder.** Mood disorder associated with shifts from depression to mania. Includes three subcategories: bipolar I, bipolar II, and cyclothymic disorder.

**Blunted conduct.** Dull behavior bearing no relationship to social signals; may occur in persons with schizophrenia.

**Bowman's capsule.** A sac containing the glomerular capillaries; also called glomerular capsule.

**Bradycardia.** Heart rate of 60 beats per minute or less.

**Bradykinesia.** Slowness of movement.

**Bradykinin.** Substance released by damaged tissue that promotes inflammation.

**Bronchi.** Passageway that leads from the trachea to the lung.

**Bronchioles.** Small soft tissue tubules with smooth muscle wrappings that connect small bronchi to alveolar structures.

**Bronchitis.** Inflammation of the bronchi; may be acute or chronic.

**Bronchogenic carcinoma.** Most common type of lung cancer that arises from the bronchial tree.

**Bronchopneumonia.** Type of pneumonia that may develop as a result of small bronchi becoming obstructed because of infection or aspirated gastric contents.

**Bulbourethral glands.** A pair of glands that secrete into the urethra as it enters the penis.

**Bulimia nervosa.** Eating disorder characterized by episodes of excessive eating (binging), followed by purging, either through intentional vomitting or use of laxatives.

**Bundle of His.** The specialized tissue in heart muscle capable of sending the impulse for contraction to the ventricles.

**Bursa.** Sac of fluid situated near the joint to reduce friction on movement.

**Bursitis.** Inflammation of the bursa.

**Cachexia.** Condition caused when a patient becomes weak and emaciated in appearance due to the rapid growth of a malignant tumor; also accompanies many chronic diseases like cancer, HIV/AIDS, and tuberculosis.

**Calcium.** Mineral essential for bone and tooth structure and for cell physiology.

**Capsid.** Protein coat of viruses.

**Carbuncles.** Clusters of boils.

**Carcinogens.** Various chemicals that promote cancer development.

**Carcinoma.** Type of cancer affecting epithelial tissues, skin, and mucous membranes lining body cavities, or glandular tissue such as the breast, liver, or pancreas.

**Carcinoma in situ.** Premalignant lesion, the earliest stage of cancer in which the underlying tissue has not yet been invaded.

**Cardiac catheterization.** Procedure in which a catheter is passed into the heart through appropriate blood vessels to sample the blood in each chamber for oxygen content and pressure.

**Cardiac cycle.** The alternate contraction and relaxation of atria and ventricles.

**Cardiac sphincter.** Muscular gateway between the esophagus and stomach.

**Cardiogenic shock.** The result of extensive myocardial infarction; often fatal, but drugs to combat it are sometimes effective.

**Cardiopulmonary resuscitation (CPR).** Pertains to both heart and lung assistance by trained personnel to rhythmically compress the chest and breathe into victim's airway until medical services can be provided.

**Carotene.** A plant pigment from which vitamin A is derived.

**Caseous.** The term used to describe soft and cheese-like lung tissue in tuberculosis.

**Casts.** Molds of kidney tubules consisting of coagulated protein and blood.

**Cataracts.** Clouding of the eye lens to the point of opacity.

**Catatonia.** Motor disturbance that may occur in persons with schizophrenia.

**Cell walls.** A rigid layer of organic material surrounding delicate cell membranes of bacteria.

**Cell-mediated immunity.** Protection from infection provided by T cells.

**Cellulitis.** Spreading skin infection caused by streptococci.

**Cerebrospinal.** A term pertaining to the brain and spinal cord; cerebrospinal fluid bathes these organs.

**Cerebrovascular accident (CVA).** A stroke.

**Chancre.** An ulceration on the genitals in the primary stage of syphilis.

**Chemotaxis.** The attraction of white blood cells to the site of inflammation.

**Chemotherapy.** Systemic administration of medications to kill malignant cells.

**Chlamydial infection.** Sexually transmitted disease caused by *Chlamydia trachomatis*.

**Cholecystectomy.** The surgical removal of the gallbladder.

**Cholelithiasis.** The formation or presence of gallstones.

**Cholesterol.** A fatty substance found in animal cell membranes.

**Choriocarcinoma.** Malignant tumor of the placenta.

**Chorionic gonadotropin hormone.** The hormone that indicates a positive pregnancy test.

**Chorionic villus sampling.** Genetic test involving the removal of cells from the villi through the cervix.

**Chromosome.** A molecule of DNA found in the human cell. Each human cell contains 46 chromosomes divided into 23 pairs.

**Chronic.** A disease that may begin insidiously and be long-lived.

**Chronic fatigue syndrome.** A disease that produces flu-like symptoms, including severe and persistent fatigue, muscle and joint pain, and fever.

**Chronic obstructive pulmonary disease (COPD).** The term used to describe a number of conditions, including chronic bronchitis and emphysema, in which the exchange of respiratory gases is ineffective.

**Chronic ulcerative colitis.** A serious inflammation of the colon, the origin of which is unknown.

**Chymotrypsin.** A digestive enzyme that digests protein.

**Cilia.** The hairlike projections found in the mucous membrane that lines the respiratory tract.

**Ciliates.** A type of protozoa that moves using hairlike cilia.

**Cirrhosis.** A chronic destruction of liver cells and tissues with a nodular, bumpy regeneration.

**Coarctation.** A narrowing, or stricture, of the aorta that provides blood to the entire body.

**Cocci.** Spherical bacterial cells.

**Collagen.** A fibrous protein found in connective tissues, causing wounds to heal poorly.

**Colostomy.** An artificial opening in the abdominal wall with a segment of the large intestine attached.

**Communicable.** An infectious disease transmitted from human to human.

**Co-morbid.** The occurance of two or more concurrent illnesses or conditions.

**Compact bone.** Dense bone issue surrounding most bones.

**Complications.** Conditions that develop in a patient already suffering from a disease.

**Compression sclerotherapy.** A treatment for varicose veins in which a strong saline solution is injected into specific sites within the vessel tract.

**Computerized tomography (CT scan).** A diagnostic imaging technique used to make diagnosis and determine the location of lesions or growths inside the body.

**Concussion.** A transient disorder of the nervous system resulting from a violent blow on the head or from a fall.

**Conduct disorder.** Disruptive behavior disorder diagnosed in children.

**Cone biopsy.** Procedure in which a cone-shaped wedge of abnormal tissue is removed from the cervix and examined under a microscope

**Congenital diseases.** Diseases that appear at birth or shortly after but are not caused by genetic or chromosomal abnormalities.

**Conjunctiva.** The membrane that lines the eyelids and covers the eyeball.

**Conn's syndrome.** A form of hyperadrenalism in which aldosterone is excreted in excess.

**Contagious.** An infectious disease transmitted from human to human.

**Continuous positive airway pressure (C-PAP).** Nasal C-PAP delivers air into the airway through a specially designed nasal mask or pillow; the flow of air creates enough pressure when inhaled to keep the airway open.

**Contusion.** An injury to tissue without a breaking of the skin at the site of the trauma; also called a bruise.

**Cor pulmonale.** A serious heart condition in which the right side of the heart fails as a result of long-standing chronic lung disease.

**Coronary arteriography.** The selective injection of contrast material into coronary arteries for a film recording of blood vessel action.

**Corpus luteum.** The structure that develops from the ovarian follicle after ovulation.

**Cortisol.** The principal hormone in the group of steroid hormones, also known as hydrocortisone; stress increases production of cortisol.

**Cortisone.** A hormone of the adrenal gland that has anti-inflammatory properties.

**Creatinine.** Nitrogen-containing waste products of protein metabolism.

**Cri du chat syndrome.** A hereditary disease resulting from the deletion of part of the short arm of chromosome 5; the name comes from the characteristic cat-like cry.

**Cretinism.** A congenital thyroid deficiency in which thyroxine is not synthesized.

**Crohn's disease.** An inflammatory disease of the intestine in which the intestinal walls become thick and rigid.

**Croup.** Characterized by a loud cough that resembles the barking of a seal, difficulty breathing, and a grunting noise or wheezing during breathing.

**Cryosurgery.** A technique that uses extreme cold to freeze and destroy skin conditions and tumors.

**Cryptorchidism.** The failure of the testes to descend from the abdominal cavity, where they develop during fetal life, to the scrotum.

**CT scan.** Computed tomography scan; 3-D computer aided x-ray.

**Cushing's syndrome.** A condition resulting from excessive levels of glucocorticoid hormones.

**Cyanosis.** A bluish color of the skin and the mucous membranes due to insufficient oxygen in the blood.

**Cyclins.** Cell cycle proteins.

**Cyst.** A sac or capsule containing fluid; usually harmless.

**Cystic fibrosis.** A disease that affects all the exocrine glands of the body, the glands of external secretion usually affecting children.

**Cystitis.** An inflammation of the urinary bladder, commonly called a bladder infection.

**Cystocele.** Urinary bladder is displaced into the vagina.

**Cystoscope.** An endoscope (lighted scope) through which the interior of the urinary bladder is made visible for observation.

**Cytotoxic T cells.** T cells, often called *killer cells* because of their capability to kill invading organisms.

**Decubitus ulcers.** Bedsores that typically occur on the bony areas of the body.

**Defibrillator.** A machine that delivers electrical shocks used to reestablish normal heart rhythm.

**Delirium tremens.** A medical emergency caused by heavy drinking over a long period of time; may occur after withdrawal from heavy alcohol intake.

**Delusion.** False beliefs associated with various mental illnesses.

**Dementia.** Organic loss of intellectual functions.

**Deoxyribonucleic acid (DNA).** The blueprint for protein synthesis within the cell.

**Dermatitis.** A noncontagious skin disorder.

**Dermatophytes.** Fungi that infect the skin and tend to live on the dead, top layer.

**Desensitize.** A procedure for causing tolerance to allergens so that they do not trigger allergic reactions.

**Diabetes insipidus.** A disease that results from a deficiency of ADH.

**Diabetes mellitus.** An endocrine disease in which the beta cells fail to secrete insulin or target cells fail to respond to insulin.

**Diabetic nephropathy.** A kidney disease resulting from diabetes mellitus.

**Diagnosis.** The determination of the nature of a disease based on many factors, including signs, symptoms, and, often, laboratory results.

**Diaphragm.** Primary muscle for inspiration that divides the thorax and abdominopelvic cavities.

**Diastole.** The period of the heartbeat when the heart relaxes and fills with blood.

**Diethylstilbestrol (DES).** A synthetic hormone used in the 1950s and early 1960s to prevent spontaneous abortion.

**Discoid.** The mild form of lupus erythematosus in which red, raised, itchy lesions develop.

**Disease.** A state of functional disequilibrium that may be resolved by recovery or death.

**Disinfection.** Reducing the risk of infection or contamination.

**Diuretic.** A substance that causes the kidneys to excrete water; can be administered as a drug to lower blood pressure.

**Diverticula.** Little pouches or sacs formed when the mucosal lining pushes through the underlying muscle layer.

**Diverticulitis.** Inflammation of the diverticula, usually occurring in the colon or small intestines.

**DNA repair genes.** Also known as caretaker genes, these are genes responsible for the repair of errors in normal DNA replication.

**Dominant.** A gene that is expressed when inherited.

**Dopamine.** A neuronal transmitter substance.

**Doppler echocardiography.** Instrument that uses echoes of moving blood columns to produce images of the vessel wall outline; the velocity of the blood is measured and the degree of carotid stenosis is determined.

**Down syndrome.** Chromosomal disorder that causes cognitive impairment; also called Trisomy 21.

**Duodenal ulcers.** Ulcers of the small intestine caused by an excessive secretion of hydrochloric acid and *Helicobacter pylori* infection.

**Duodenum.** First section of the small intestine; receives digested material from the stomach.

**Dysentery.** An acute inflammation of the colon, a colitis.

**Dysmenorrhea.** Painful or difficult menses.

**Dyspareunia.** Painful sexual intercourse.

**Dysphagia.** Difficult or painful swallowing.

**Dyspnea.** Air hunger resulting in labored or difficult breathing.

**Dysthymia.** Chronic, persistent depression for a period of at least two years.

**Dystrophin.** A skeletal protein that is missing in Duchenne's muscular dystrophy.

**Dystrophy.** Muscle degeneration that disables an individual.

**Dysuria.** Painful urination.

**Ecchymoses.** Hemorrhagic spots that develop on the skin and in mucous membranes, causing discoloration.

**Echocardiography.** A noninvasive procedure (ultrasound cardiography) that utilizes high-frequency sound waves to examine the size, shape, and motion of heart structures.

**Eclampsia.** Convulsions and coma that follow untreated pregnancy-induced hypertension.

**Ectopic pregnancy.** A pregnancy in which the fertilized ovum implants in a tissue other than the uterus, most commonly in the fallopian tubes.

**Eczema.** A noncontagious inflammatory skin disorder.

**Edema.** Swelling caused by leakage of plasma into tissues.

**Electrocardiogram (ECG).** An electrical recording of the heart action that aids in the diagnosis of coronary artery disease, myocardial infarction, valvular heart disease, and some congenital heart diseases.

**Electroencephalogram (EEG).** A recording of brain waves.

**Electrolyte balance.** The proper balance of salts, like potassium, and calcium.

**Electromyogram (EMG).** A testing procedure used to diagnose muscle and nerve disorders.

**Embolism.** A circulating blood clot.

**Emphysema.** A crippling, noncontagious disease of chronic lung obstruction and destruction.

**Encephalitis.** The inflammation of the brain and meninges, caused by a viral infection.

**Encephalomyelitis.** Acute inflammation of the brain and spinal cord.

**Endarterectomy.** A common surgical procedure used to treat a blockage in an artery by removing the thickened area of the inner vascular lining.

**Endemic.** Describes a disease that is always present at low levels in a population.

**Endocarditis.** Inflammation within the heart.

**Endocardium.** A smooth delicate membrane that lines chambers of the heart.

**Endogenous.** Originating or produced within an organism, tissue, or cell.

**Endometriosis.** Condition in which endometrial tissue from the uterus becomes embedded elsewhere.

**Endorphins.** Naturally occurring molecules made up of amino acids, the building blocks of proteins. Endorphins attach to special receptors in the brain and spinal cord to stop pain messages. These are the same receptors that respond to morphine and other opioid analgesics.

**Endoscope.** An instrument consisting of a hollow tube with a lens and light system used to view the inner surface of the digestive tract.

**Endoscopic sclerotherapy.** A procedure used to guide a retractable needle device through an area such as the esophagus to seal off vessels such as esophageal varices with a hardening agent.

**Endoscopy.** Imaging technique using flexible tubing mounted with camera and surgical tools.

**Endospores.** Structures produced by bacteria and formed to cope with harsh environmental conditions.

**Endotoxin.** A potent toxin from certain bacteria that causes life-threatening shock.

**Enkephalins.** Naturally occurring molecules in the brain that attach to special receptors in the brain and spinal cord to stop pain messages. These are the same receptors that respond to morphine and other opioid analgesics.

**Enuresis.** Commonly called bed-wetting; a disorder of elimination that involves the voluntary or involuntary release of urine into bedding, clothing, or other inappropriate places.

**Eosinophila-myalgia syndrome.** Multisystem disease with pain, fatigue, and elevations of circulating blood eosinophils.

**Eosinophils.** White blood cells that kill parasites and are involved in allergic responses.

**Ephylis.** Freckles.

**Epidemic.** The occurrence of a disease in unusually large numbers over a specific area.

**Epidemiological studies.** Population-based studies.

**Epididymis.** A coiled tube that lies along the outer wall of the testis and leads into the vas deferens.

**Epididymitis.** Inflammation of the epididymis.

**Epidural.** A hemorrhage between the dura mater and the skull.

**Epilepsy.** A group of uncontrolled cerebral discharges that recur at random intervals.

**Epinephrine.** The hormone secreted by the adrenal medulla in emergency situations or during periods of high stress; also used as a drug to dilate bronchioles in some asthma attacks.

**Erysipelas.** An inflammatory skin infection caused by streptococcus bacteria. Most commonly, the infections appear on the face, arm, or leg.

**Erythema.**   A reddened area of skin.

**Erythematous.**   An area of skin reddened by congested blood vessels resulting from injury or inflammation.

**Erythrocytes.**   Red blood cells.

**Erythropoiesis.**   The process of red cell formation that takes place in the red marrow of flat bones such as the sternum, hip bones, ribs, and skull bones.

**Erythropoietin.**   A hormone synthesized principally by the kidney that stimulates red blood cell development.

**Esophageal varices.**   Varicose veins of the esophagus.

**Esophagitis.**   Inflammation of the esophagus caused by acid reflux.

**Essential trace minerals.**   Minerals required in the diet in very low amounts.

**Estrogen.**   The sex hormone in females.

**Etiology.**   The cause of a disease.

**Exacerbation.**   The period of a chronic disease when signs and symptoms recur in all their severity.

**Exocrine glands.**   The glands of external secretion. They secrete mucus, perspiration, and digestive enzymes.

**Exophthalmos.**   The condition in which the eyeballs protrude outward, characteristic of a person with Graves' disease.

**Extradural.**   A hemorrhage between the dura mater and the skull.

**Familial hypercholesterolemia.**   An autosomal dominant disorder caused by a mutation in the gene encoding the receptor for low-density lipoproteins.

**Familial polyposis.**   A hereditary disease in which numerous polyps develop in the intestinal tract.

**Female arousal-orgasmic dysfunction.**   Lack of sexual desire or response in a female.

**Fibrillation.**   Quivering or spontaneously uncoordinated contraction of muscle fibers, such as heart ventricles.

**Fibrin.**   A plasma protein essential for blood clotting.

**Fibroblasts.**   Connective tissue cells that produce fibers to aid in healing damaged tissue.

**Fibrocystic disease.**   The formation of numerous fluid-filled lumps in the breast.

**Fimbriae.**   Fingerlike projections at the outer ends of the fallopian tubes, they propel ova into the tube.

**Flagella.**   Whip-like cell appendages used for locomotion.

**Flagellates.**   A type of protozoa that moves using whip-like appendages called flagella.

**Flatus.**   Intestinal gas.

**Flatworm.**   A wormlike animal that has a flattened body.

**Fluoroscopy.**   A diagnostic procedure that permits visualization of the lungs and diaphragm during respiration.

**Folliculitis.**   Inflammation of hair follicles caused by staphylococci.

**Foramen ovale.**   A small opening that allows blood from the right side of the heart to enter the left side directly, bypassing the nonfunctional fetal lungs.

**Fragile X syndrome.**   A sex-linked disorder associated with mental retardation. It is identified by a break or weakness on the long arm of the X chromosome.

**Free radicals.**   The molecules that may cause disease by injuring cells.

**Friable.**   Easily broken nodules or vegetations.

**Fulminating.**   Having a rapid or severe onset.

**Functional.**   Condition is one in which there is no organic change.

**Furuncles.**   Large, tender, swollen raised lesions, boils, caused by staphylococci.

**Gamma-aminobutyric acid (GABA).**   Inhibitory neurotransmitter associated with various mental illnesses, sleep, mood, and behavior.

**Galactosemia.**   An autosomal recessive disorder in which the enzyme necessary to convert galactose, a sugar derived from lactose in milk, to glucose is lacking.

**Gangrene.**   Condition in which bacteria infects and destroys dead tissue.

**Gastric ulcers.**   Ulcers of the stomach.

**Gastritis.**   Inflammation of the stomach caused by irritants such as aspirin, excessive coffee, tobacco, alcohol, or an infection.

**Gastroesophageal reflux disease.**   Regurgitation of acidic stomach contents into the esophagus.

**Gastroscopy.**   A procedure in which a camera is attached to a gastroscope, and the entire inner stomach is photographed.

**Genes.**   Found in chromosomes, each is responsible for the synthesis of one protein.

**Genital herpes.**   Sexually transmitted infection caused by herpes simplex virus type II.

**Genital warts.**   Sexually transmitted infection caused by the human papillomavirus.

**Gigantism.**   Usually the result of a tumor of the anterior pituitary.

**Glioblastomas.**   Highly malignant, rapid-growing tumors of the brain.

**Glioma.** A sarcoma of neuroglial tissue or glial cells.

**Glomerular capsule.** Structure surrounding the glomerular capillaries of the nephron.

**Glomerulonephritis.** A degenerative inflammation of the glomerulus of a nephron, which usually follows a prior streptococcal infection.

**Glomerulus.** A tuft of capillaries situated inside the glomerular capsule of a nephron.

**Glucagon.** A hormone that works antagonistically to insulin and is released when the blood sugar level falls below normal.

**Glucagon.** Hormone secreted by endocrine pancreas that raises blood glucose.

**Glucocorticoids.** The group of steroid hormones that helps regulate carbohydrate, lipid, and protein metabolism.

**Glycogen.** A form of glucose that is stored in the liver and muscle.

**Glycosuria.** The condition in which excess glucose is excreted in the urine, a major sign of diabetes mellitus.

**Gonadotropins.** Hormones of the anterior pituitary that regulate sexual development and function.

**Gonorrhea.** Sexually transmitted infection caused by *Neisseria gonorrhoeae.*

**Gout.** Often called "gouty arthritis," it affects the joints of the feet, particularly those of the big toe, and is very painful.

**Graafian follicles.** Ovarian follicles stimulated by a pituitary gonadotropic hormone at the beginning of each monthly cycle so that they begin to grow and develop.

**Gram stain.** The staining technique that permits the identification of bacteria.

**Grandiose delusion.** A false belief of having special power, influence, or wealth.

**Gynecomastia.** A condition in which the breasts become enlarged.

**Hallucination.** Disturbance in sensory perception in sight, sound, touch, or smell.

**Health.** A state of relative equilibrium in which the body's many organ systems function adequately and are free from disease.

**Heart block.** Impulses are prevented from flowing from the atria to the ventricles because of a damaged route (e.g., MI), and thus the heart rate and EKG are altered.

**Heart murmurs.** Characteristic sounds of the heart that indicate the presence of valve defects.

***Helicobacter pylori.*** A bacterium associated with ulcers.

**Helper T cells.** T cells that help the immune system by increasing the activity of killer cells and stimulating the suppressor T cells.

**Hemangioma.** Benign tumor made of small blood vessels that forms a red or purple birthmark.

**Hematemesis.** Vomiting of blood.

**Hematocrit.** The ratio of red-blood-cell-volume to whole blood.

**Hematoma.** A bruise caused by an injection.

**Hematuria.** Blood in the urine.

**Hemiplegia.** Paralysis on one side of the body.

**Hemodialysis.** Treatment for kidney failure; blood removed from the body is cleansed of metabolic waste, restored to physiological balance, and returned to the body.

**Hemoglobin.** A protein containing iron; serves as the oxygen-carrier protein that enables red blood cells to carry oxygen from the lungs to all body tissues.

**Hemolysis.** The rupture of red blood cells.

**Hemolytic streptococci.** A type of bacteria that cause a variety of infectious diseases, including infections of throat, skin, ear, and heart valves.

**Hemolyze.** Lysis of erythrocytes.

**Hemophilia.** Sex-linked inherited coagulation disorder cause by a deficiency of clotting factors.

**Hemoptysis.** Coughing blood.

**Hemorrhage.** A large loss of blood in a short period of time, either internally or externally.

**Hemorrhoids.** Varicose veins of the rectum or anus.

**Hemostasis.** Reduced blood flow.

**Heparin.** An anticoagulant.

**Hepatic coma.** Develops in the final stages of advanced liver disease; it is caused by an accumulation of ammonia in the blood, which has a toxic effect on the brain and may cause death.

**Hepatocarcinoma.** Cancer of the liver.

**Hepatomegaly.** Enlarged liver.

**Hereditary hemorrhagic telangiectasia.** Abnormal dilation of small vessels causing the appearance of red-violet lesions on the face, lips, and oral and nasal mucosa.

**Hermaphrodites.** Individuals who have both testes and ovaries.

**Heterozygous.** A person having two different alleles of a certain gene.

**Hiatal hernia.** The protrusion of part of the stomach through the diaphragm at the point where the esophagus joins the stomach.

**High-density lipoproteins (HDL).** The smallest lipoprotein particles containing the smallest amount of triglycerides; "good" cholesterol.

**Hippocampus.** Structure of the brain that processes and stores information to memory.

**Hirsutism.** Condition in which excess hair develops on the face of a woman.

**Histamine.** A substance that causes capillary walls to become more permeable.

**Histology.** The study of cells.

**Hodgkin's disease.** A type of lymphoma, distinguished by the presence of characteristic *Reed-Sternberg* cells in affected lymph nodes.

**Homeostasis.** The maintenance of a steady state within the body.

**Homozygous.** A person having the same two alleles of a particular gene.

**Hordeolum.** An infection of the sebaceous gland of the eyelid.

**Horizontal transmission.** The route by which an infectious disease is transmitted directly from an infected human to a susceptible human.

**Hormones.** Chemical messengers secreted by endocrine glands.

**Human chorionic gonadotropin (HCG).** Hormone secreted by the chorionic villi after implantation of the fertilized ovum in the uterus.

**Human immunodeficiency virus (HIV).** The causative agent of AIDS; a retrovirus—that is, it carries its genetic information as RNA rather than DNA.

**Human papillomavirus (HPV).** The type of virus responsible for genital warts that seems to be the causative agent in uterine cervical carcinoma.

**Humoral immunity.** Protection from infection provided by antibodies.

**Huntington's chorea.** A progressive degenerative disease of the brain that results in the loss of muscle control.

**Hydatidiform mole.** A benign tumor of the placenta, consisting of multiple cysts and resembling a bunch of grapes.

**Hydrocephalus.** The accumulation of cerebrospinal fluid in the brain.

**Hydrocortisone.** Anti-inflammatory agent.

**Hydrolithotripsy.** A procedure using sonic vibrations to crush kidney stones while the patient is immersed in a tank of water.

**Hydronephrosis.** A condition when the kidney is extremely dilated with urine.

**Hydroureters.** The condition caused when the ureters above a kidney obstruction dilate.

**Hymen.** A membranous fold that partly or completely closes the vaginal opening.

**Hyperactive.** The term used to describe when a gland produces an excessive amount of its secretion.

**Hypercalcemia.** A condition in which too much calcium occurs in the blood.

**Hyperemesis gravidarum.** Excessive vomiting during pregnancy.

**Hyperemia.** Increased blood flow to an injured area, causing heat and redness associated with inflammation.

**Hyperglycemia.** A condition resulting from deposits of calcium in organs such as kidneys, heart, lungs, and the walls of the stomach.

**Hyperkalemia.** An excess of potassium, which causes muscle weakness and can slow the heart to the point of cardiac arrest.

**Hypernephroma.** Carcinoma of the kidney; causes enlargement of kidney and destroys the organ.

**Hyperpituitarism.** Condition associated with hypersecretion of the pituitary, usually manifested as the effects of excessive growth hormone, which retards the normal closure of bones at puberty.

**Hypersensitivity.** An abnormal immune response and sensitivity to allergens such as pollens, dust, dog hair, and certain foods.

**Hypertension.** High blood pressure.

**Hypertrophy.** Abnormal enlargement of an organ.

**Hypoactive.** When a gland fails to secrete its hormone or secretes an inadequate amount.

**Hypoalbuminemia.** An albumin deficiency.

**Hypochromic.** Red blood cells appear lighter than normal, caused by an iron deficiency.

**Hypophysis.** Another name for the pituitary gland; has two parts, each of which acts as a separate gland.

**Hypothalamus.** The homeostatic center for the body, located just superior to the pituitary; controls thirst, temperature, and other functions, as well release of pituitary hormones.

**Hypovolemic shock.** Results from fluid volume loss after severe hemorrhage or loss of plasma in burn patients.

**Hypoxia.** Decreased concentration of oxygen in the blood due to low oxygen availability or blockages that prevent oxygen diffusing into the bloodstream.

**Hysterectomy.** Surgical removal of the uterus.

**Icterus.** Jaundiced, yellow coloration.

**Idiopathic.** Describes a disease for which the cause is not known.

**Idiopathic hypereosinophilic syndrome.** Mulitsystem disease associated with persistent increases in blood eosinophils.

**Immunity.** The ability of the body to defend itself against infectious agents, foreign cells, and abnormal body cells.

**Immunoglobulin.** Antibodies.

**Impetigo.** An acute, contagious skin infection common in children, most frequently affecting face and hands.

**Impotence.** Inability to achieve and maintain an erection sufficient for sexual intercourse.

**In situ.** In position; not disturbing surrounding tissues.

**Incidence.** The number of new cases of a disease in a population.

**Incontinence.** Inability to retain urine or feces due to loss of sphincter control or because of cerebral or spinal lesions.

**Infarct.** Dead tissue that occurs due to lack of blood flow in any organ or area, such as a coronary blockage in a heart vessel.

**Infectious diseases.** Diseases caused by pathogenic microorganisms.

**Infestations.** Infections involving wormlike animals called helminths.

**Inflammatory exudate.** Fluid composed of plasma and white cells that escape from capillaries.

**Influenza.** A viral infection of the upper respiratory system.

**Initiation.** The first stage of cancer in which there is a genetic change in a cell, an altering of the DNA by some agent, chemical, radiation, or an oncogenic virus.

**Insulin.** A hormone that is secreted when the blood sugar level rises.

**Insulin shock.** Hypoglycemic shock that results from too much insulin, not enough food, or excessive exercise.

**Interferon.** A group of substances that stimulates the immune system.

**Intrapleural pressure.** The pressure within the pleural cavity.

**Intravenous pyelogram.** Allows the visualization of the urinary system by means of contrast dyes injected into the veins, followed by an x-ray examination.

**Intrinsic factor.** Produced in the stomach, it carries vitamin $B_{12}$ to the small intestine, where it is absorbed into the bloodstream.

**Intussusception.** A type of organic obstruction in which a segment of intestine telescopes into the part forward of it.

**In-vitro research.** Research conducted in a laboratory.

**Irritable bowel.** A functional condition of the colon with diarrhea, constipation, abdominal pain, and gas.

**Irritable colon.** A functional disorder of the colon that results in diarrhea and cramping.

**Ischemia.** A deficiency of blood supply to any organ.

**Isolation.** Keeping an infected person in the hospital or staying at home in bed when suffering from a disease as a way of controlling the transmission of infectious diseases.

**Jaundice.** A yellow-orange discoloration of the skin, tissues, and the whites of the eyes caused when bilirubin (an orange pigment) accumulates in the plasma.

**Kaposi's sarcoma.** Purple neoplasm of the lower extremities.

**Karyotype.** The normal chromosomal composition of the nucleus of the cell that is characteristic of each species.

**Keloid.** The healing that occurs after surgery or a severe burn, consisting of a hard, raised scar.

**Keratin.** Protein in the epidermis produced by cells called keratinocytes; protects the skin from harmful substances.

**Ketone bodies.** Substances produced in diabetics' blood when insulin levels are low.

**Kidney dialysis.** Treatment for kidney failure; removes metabolic waste from blood and restores it to physiological balance.

**Klinefelter's syndrome.** A condition in which there is an extra sex chromosome resulting in a karyotype of 47,XXY.

**Kupffer cells.** Specialized cells that line the blood spaces within the liver. They engulf and digest bacteria and other foreign substances, thus cleansing the blood.

**Kwashiorkor.** Protein-calorie malnutrition that results from early weaning from breast milk.

**Laparoscopy.** A procedure in which an illuminated tube is inserted through a small incision or opening; used to diagnose endometriosis.

**Larynx.** The voice box located at the entrance of the trachea.

**Latent infection.** A condition caused when viruses insert themselves in cells and do not reproduce.

**Legionnaire's disease.**   A lung infection caused by the bacterium *Legionella pneumophila;* characterized by flulike symptoms.

**Leiomyomas.**   Benign tumors of the smooth muscle of the uterus, known as fibroid tumors.

**Lesion.**   An abnormal tissue structure or function. May be the result of a wound, injury, or pathologic condition.

**Lethargy.**   A condition of drowsiness.

**Leukemia.**   A cancer of white blood cells in which the bone marrow produces a large number of abnormal white blood cells.

**Leukocytes.**   White blood cells.

**Leukocytosis.**   The excessive production of white cells.

**Leukorrhea.**   White, foul-smelling vaginal discharge.

**Ligament.**   The substance that holds bones together.

**Lipase.**   A digestive enzyme that breaks down lipid or fat.

**Lipoma.**   Tumor that develops in adipose or fat tissue.

**Lipoprotein.**   A water-soluble lipid fat. It is packaged into particles that contain blood proteins, which do mix with water.

**Lithotripsy.**   A procedure using sonic vibrations to crush kidney stones; the patient is not immersed in water for the procedure.

**Low-density lipoproteins (LDL).**   The larger lipoprotein particles containing triglycerides; "bad" cholesterol.

**Lumbar puncture.**   Procedure in which a hollow needle is inserted into the spinal canal between vertebrae near the L-4, or lumbar region, to obtain and analyze cerebrospinal fluid; also known as a spinal tap.

**Lumen.**   The inner space of a hollow organ such as a blood vessel or intestine.

**Lumpectomy.**   Surgery to remove only the tumor from the breast.

**Lymphadenopathy.**   Enlarged lymph nodes.

**Lymphatic system.**   An important part of the body's immunity, it consists of nodes, organs, and a complex network of thin-walled capillaries carrying lymph fluid to help to maintain the internal fluid environment of the body.

**Lymphocytes.**   A type of white blood cell consisting of T lymphocytes and B lymphocytes.

**Lymphocytic.**   The type of leukemia that results from cancer of the lymphocytic stem cells, found in both the bone marrow and the lymph nodes.

**Lymphoma.**   Malignancy of the lymphatic system.

**Lyse.**   The infecting of cells by viruses.

**Macular.**   Flat lesions on the skin.

**Magnetic resonance imaging (MRI).**   A diagnostic-imaging technique that uses the behavior of protons when placed in powerful magnetic fields to make images of organs and tissues.

**Major depression.**   Mood disorder associated with sadness, hopelessness, and despair.

**Malabsorption.**   The inability of a person to absorb substances from the small intestines.

**Malignancy.**   A cancerous tumor that can invade and destroy nearby tissue, and that may metastasize to other organs or parts of the body.

**Malignant.**   Term used to describe a neoplasm or tumor that spreads and possibly causes death.

**Malignant melanoma.**   The most serious skin cancer; arises from the melanocytes.

**Malnutrition.**   Suboptimal supply of nutrients that results in decreased tissue mass and energy stores needed for proper growth and development.

**Mammography.**   Diagnostic x-ray for breast tissue that can detect even small, early cancers.

**Mania.**   An overly energetic elevated or irritable mood.

**Marfan syndrome.**   An autosomal dominant disorder that results from the dysfunction of the gene that codes for the connective tissue protein fibrillin.

**Marasmus.**   Protein-calorie malnutrition caused by near starvation.

**Mast cells.**   Cells found in connective tissue; they contain heparin, serotonin, bradykinin, and histamine.

**Mastectomy.**   Surgery to remove the breast due to cancer.

**Mastoiditis.**   Inflammation of the air cells in the mastoid process of the temporal bone.

**Medullary cavity.**   A hollow cavity found in the long bones of the arms and legs that is filled with yellow bone marrow primarily consisting of fat.

**Melanin.**   The dark pigment of the skin that protects the body from the harmful rays of the sun.

**Melanocytes.**   Cells at the bottom of the epidermis that produce melanin.

**Melanoma.**   Skin cancer.

**Melasma.**   Patches of dark skin on the cheeks that develop due to hormonal changes.

**Melena.**   Stool with a dark, tarry appearance caused by blood from the upper part of the digestive tract.

**Memory cells.**   B lymphocytes that do not become plasma cells but remain dormant until reactivated by the same antigen.

**Menarche.** The onset of menstruation, signalling the start of a woman's reproductive years; occurs generally between ages 10 and 15.

**Meninges.** Three coverings that protect the delicate nerve tissue of the spinal cord and brain.

**Meningioma.** A benign tumor that occurs in the membranes that surround the brain.

**Meningitis.** An acute inflammation of the first two meninges that cover the brain and spinal cord.

**Meningocele.** A form of spina bifida noticeable at birth; the spinal cord is not involved in this defect.

**Meningomyelocele.** A form of spina bifida in which the nerve elements protrude into the sac and are trapped, thus preventing proper placement and development.

**Menopause.** The cessation of menstrual periods, the ending of a woman's reproductive years; usually begins in the late 40s or early 50s.

**Menorrhagia.** Excessive or prolonged bleeding during menstruation.

**Mesothelioma.** Cancer of the membrane that covers and protects most of the internal organs of the body.

**Metastasis.** The spread of cancer to distant sites within the body.

**Metastasize.** To invade by metastasis.

**Metrorrhagia.** Bleeding between menstrual periods or extreme irregularity of the cycle.

**Mineralocorticoids.** A group of steroid hormones that regulate salt balance in the body.

**Mitral stenosis.** Occurs when the mitral valve opening is too small and the cusps that form the valve become rigid and fuse together.

**Mitral valve.** The valve between the left atrium and left ventricle; it has two flaps, or cusps, that meet when the valve is closed.

**Mixed cancers.** Cancer consisting of cells of different origins or tissue types.

**Monocyte.** A type of white blood cell that aids in clearing pus.

**Morbidity.** The number who become sick or disabled from a disease per 100,000 within a population.

**Mortality.** The number who die from a disease per 100,000 who have the disease within a population.

**Mucosa.** Secretes excessive mucus, causing a runny nose and congestion.

**Mucus.** Secretions from the mucous membranes; can be thick or watery.

**Mutagens.** Chemicals introduced to the lungs by cigarette smoking.

**Mutations.** Changes in DNA structure that may be inherited and cause disease.

**Myasthenia gravis.** An autoimmune neuromuscular disorder characterized by muscular fatigue that develops with repetitive muscle use and improves with rest.

**Mycelia.** Filaments in fungi specialized for absorption of nutrients.

**Mycoses.** Infectious diseases caused by fungi.

**Myelin.** A lipid covering that insulates the fibers of sensory and motor neurons.

**Myelocele.** The most severe form of spina bifida.

**Myelogenous.** The type of leukemia in which the cancer originates in the bone marrow.

**Myelomonocytic leukemia.** A type of myelogenous leukemia of malignant monocytes.

**Myocardial infarction.** A heart attack.

**Myocardium.** The cardiac muscle found in the chamber walls of the heart.

**Myoma.** A tumor of the muscle that develops in smooth or involuntary muscle.

**Myopia.** A visual defect in which distant objects appear blurred because their images are focused in front of the retina rather than on it.

**Myxedema.** The condition of severe hypothyroidism, an inadequate level of thyroxine.

**Natural killer cells.** A type of leukocyte that destroys cells with abnormal membranes.

**Nebulizer.** A device used to administer medication in a liquid mist to the airways.

**Necrotic.** Dead tissue caused by lack of blood flow to the area.

**Negative feedback.** Homeostatic control mechanism.

**Neoplasm.** A mass of new cells that grows in a haphazard fashion with no useful function; a tumor.

**Nephron.** The functional unit of the kidney.

**Neurofibrillatory tangle.** Abnormal collection of protein in the brain associated with Alzheimer's disease.

**Neurogenic bladder.** A condition in which the nerves of the urinary system don't work properly when the bladder is full and may allow urine leakage.

**Neurogenic shock.** Condition due to generalized vasodilation resulting from decreased vasomotor tone.

**Neuron.** Nerve cell.

**Neurotransmitter.** Chemical messengers that communicate in the synapse between nerve cells, or neurona.

**Neutropenia.** A reduction of circulating neutrophils, or white blood cells.

**Neutrophils.** White blood cells that fight against invading agents or injury.

**Nevus.** A small, dark skin growth that develops from pigment-producing cells, or melanocytes; a benign tumor.

**Nitroglycerin.** Medication used to dilate coronary arteries, permitting adequate bloodflow.

**Nocturia.** Urination at night, especially when excessive.

**Noncommunicable.** Infectious diseases that are not transmitted directly by humans.

**Nondisjunction.** The failure of two chromosomes to separate as the gametes, either the egg or the sperm, are being formed.

**Nonspecific defenses.** Defenses that are effective against any foreign agent that enters the body.

**Norepinephrine.** Neurotransmitter of the sympathetic nervous system.

**Notifiable diseases.** Diseases under surveillance that must be reported by physicians to the Centers for Disease Control and Prevention.

**Nucleic acid analogues.** Antiviral medications.

**Nutrient.** Chemical compound consumed in food that is required for vital cellular processes.

**Nystagmus.** Involuntary, rapid movement of the eyeball, characteristic of multiple sclerosis.

**Obesity.** A nutritional disorder in which an abnormal amount of fat accumulates in adipose tissue.

**Obesity-hypoventilation syndrome.** Also called pickwickian syndrome, a condition of recurrent episodes of apnea during sleep caused by airway occlusion due to excess weight or obesity.

**Obstructive sleep apnea syndrome.** Respiratory complication often associated with obesity.

**Occult blood.** Blood detected in stool by means of a chemical test but not apparent to the naked eye.

**Oliguria.** A reduced production of urine.

**Oncogene.** Any gene having the potential to induce a cancerous transformation.

**Oppositional defiant disorder.** Disruptive behavior disorder diagnosed in childhood.

**Orchitis.** Inflammation of the testes; can follow an injury or viral infection such as mumps.

**Organic obstructions.** A material blockage that prevents the contents of the intestinal tract from moving forward.

**Ossification.** Process by which bone tissue is formed.

**Osteitis fibrosa cystica.** In this disease, fibrous nodules and cysts form in the bones, which become very porous and decalcified.

**Osteoarthritis.** The most common form of arthritis, a chronic disease that accompanies aging and may affect only one joint.

**Osteoblasts.** A cell that works within the bone to form bone tissue.

**Osteoclasts.** A cell that works within the bone and resorbs bone.

**Osteocytes.** Mature cells in bone tissue.

**Osteogenic sarcoma.** A primary malignancy of the bone.

**Osteoma.** The most common benign tumor of the bone.

**Osteomalacia.** A bone disease in adults caused by the lack of vitamin D, which results in a softening of the bones.

**Osteomyelitis.** An inflammation of the bone, particularly of the bone marrow in the medullary cavity and in the spaces of spongy bone.

**Osteoporosis.** The increased porosity of the bone.

**Outbreak.** The sudden occurrence of a disease, in unexpected numbers in a limited area, which then subsides.

**Oxytocin.** One of two hormones secreted by the posterior pituitary; it causes smooth muscle, particularly that of the uterus, to contract and initiates milk secretions.

**Paget's disease.** A rare cancer involving inflammatory changes that affect the nipple and the areola.

**Pallor.** Whitening of the skin.

**Pancreatic islets.** Endocrine cells of the pancreas.

**Pancreatitis.** A potentially life-threatening inflammation of the pancreas.

**Pandemic.** Describes an epidemic that has spread to include several large areas worldwide.

**Papanicolaou test.** Screening test for cervical cancer based on observations of cells obtained in biopsies of the cervix.

**Papilloma.** Also known as a polyp; an epithelial tumor that grows as a projecting mass on the skin or from an inner mucous membrane. The common wart is an example.

**Pap smear.** A diagnostic technique for identifying cancer in the cervix by scraping cells from the cervix and examining them microscopically.

**Papular.** Raised lesions on the skin.

**Paralytic obstructions.** Caused when the contents of the intestinal tract are unable to move forward due to a decrease in peristalsis, preventing propulsion of intestinal contents.

**Parathormone.**  The hormone secreted by the parathyroids.

**Paresis.**  A general paralysis associated with organic loss of brain function; results in death if untreated.

**Paresthesia.**  Numbness, burning, or tingling sensation resulting from nerve injury.

**Passive immunity.**  Immunity transmitted through doses of preformed antibodies from immune serum of an animal, usually a horse. This type of immunity is short-lived but acts immediately.

**Patent ductus arteriosus (PDA).**  A common congenital disease in which the ductus arteriosus remains open and blood intended for the body flows from the aorta to the lungs, overloading the pulmonary artery.

**Pathogen.**  Microorganism that causes disease.

**Pathogenesis.**  The source or cause of an illness or abnormal condition and its development.

**Pathology.**  Study of the characteristics, causes, and effects of disease.

**Pathophysiology.**  Study of the physiological processes leading up to disease.

**Pediculosis.**  Louse infestations that are classified into three categories: head lice, pubic lice, and body lice.

**Pellagra.**  Niacin deficiency.

**Pelvic inflammatory disease (PID).**  Inflammation of the female reproductive organs due to bacterial, viral, fungal, or parasitic invasion.

**Peptic ulcers.**  Ulcers of the stomach and small intestine due, in part, to the action of pepsin, a proteolytic enzyme secreted by the stomach.

**Perforation.**  An ulcer that breaks through the intestinal or gastric wall, causing sudden and intense abdominal pain.

**Pericardium.**  The double membranous sac that encloses the heart.

**Periosteum.**  A highly vascular layer of fibrous connective tissue that covers the surface of bones.

**Peristalsis.**  Muscle contractions that propel food during the digestive process.

**Peritoneal dialysis.**  Treatment for kidney failure; fluid added to the peritoneal cavity draws metabolic waste from the blood and restores it to physiological balance.

**Peritonitis.**  Inflammation of the lining of the abdominal cavity. Usually results when the digestive contents enter the cavity, because this material contains numerous bacteria.

**Pernicious anemia.**  Anemia caused by a vitamin $B_{12}$ deficiency.

**Persecutory delusion.**  False belief that one is being followed, watched, or plotted against.

**Personality disorder.**  Mental disturbance characterized by inflexible patterns of behavior that affect interpersonal relationships. Includes three major categories or clusters based on symptoms: paranoid, schizoid (cluster A); antisocial, borderline, histrionic, narcissistic (cluster B); and avoidant, dependent, obsessive-compulsive (cluster C).

**Petechiae.**  Tiny red or purple spots caused by minute blood vessels that rupture in the skin.

**Phagocyte.**  Leukocyte that takes in and destroy foreign material.

**Phagocytosis.**  White blood cells taking in and destroying foreign material.

**Pharyngeoplasty.**  Surgical removal of the uvula to alleviate obstructive sleep apnea.

**Pharynx.**  The throat.

**Phenylketonuria (PKU).**  Caused by an autosomal recessive allele that lacks a specific enzyme that converts one amino acid, phenylalanine, to another, tyrosine.

**Pheochromocytoma.**  A neuroendocrine tumor of the adrenal gland.

**Phlebitis.**  An inflammation of a vein, usually in the leg.

**Phosphate.**  Compound containing phosphorous essential for bone and tooth structure as well as cell physiology.

**Physiology.**  Study of the normal function of the body.

**Pipestem colon.**  Term used to describe the colon in patients suffering from chronic ulcerative colitis; colon appears straight and rigid.

**Placenta.**  The interdigitation of embryonic and maternal tissue.

**Placenta previa.**  Abnormal positioning of the placenta in the lower uterus, often near the cervical opening.

**Plantar warts.**  Painful warts that form on the soles of the feet.

**Plaque.**  Fatty deposits in the walls of arteries.

**Plasma cells.**  Cells that develop from B cells and produce antibodies.

**Platelets.**  Clotting elements of blood.

**Pleura.**  A double membrane consisting of two layers that encases the lungs.

**Pleural cavity.**  The space between the two layers of the pleura containing a small amount of fluid that lubricates the surfaces, preventing friction as the lungs expand and contract.

**Pleurisy.**  The inflammation of the pleural membranes occurring as a complication of various lung diseases like pneumonia or tuberculosis.

**Pneumoconiosis.** A lung disease caused by the inhalation of a variety of organic or inorganic dusts or chemical irritants, usually over a prolonged period of time.

**Pneumonia.** An acute inflammation of the lung in which air spaces in the lungs become filled with an inflammatory exudate.

**Pneumothorax.** A collection of free air in the chest outside the lung.

**Poliomyelitis.** An infectious disease of the brain and spinal cord caused by a virus.

**Polydactyly.** An autosomal dominant disorder that causes extra fingers or toes.

**Polydipsia.** Extreme thirst.

**Polymorphs.** White blood cells specialized to fight against invading agents or injury.

**Polyp.** Benign epithelial tumor.

**Polysomnography.** Used in a sleep study to measure sleep cycles and stages by recording brain waves (EEG), electrical activity of muscles, and eye movement.

**Polyuria.** The excessive production of dilute urine.

**Postpartum depression.** Subcategory of depression that occurs 2 weeks to 6 months following the birth of a child.

**Premature ejaculation.** Ejaculation during foreplay or immediately after beginning intercourse.

**Premenstrual dysphoric disorder.** Subcategory of depression with cyclical symptoms prior to menstruation.

**Premenstrual syndrome (PMS).** Emotional, physical, and behavioral symptoms that are associated with the menstrual cycle.

**Prevalence.** The number of existing cases of a disease.

**Primary atypical pneumonia.** Also known as "walking pneumonia," it is caused by a variety of microorganisms, including viruses and an unusual bacterium called *Mycoplasma pneumoniae*.

**Primary follicle.** A single layer of cells that surround each ovum.

**Proctoscope.** An instrument consisting of a hollow tube with a lighted end used by physicians to observe the lining of the colon.

**Prognosis.** The predicted course and outcome of a disease.

**Progression.** The third stage of cancer development.

**Prolapse.** A falling or dropping down of an organ or internal structure, such as the uterus or rectum.

**Promotion.** The second stage of cancer development in which altered cells proliferate and resemble benign neoplasms, which can either regress to normal-appearing tissue or evolve into cancer.

**Prostate.** Produces alkaline fluid to help neutralize vaginal pH.

**Prostatitis.** Inflammation of the prostate.

**Prothrombin.** An enzyme synthesized by the liver with the aid of vitamin K that initiates the chain reaction in the blood-coagulation process.

**Pruritis.** Itching that accompanies many skin diseases.

**Pseudopodia.** Cell membrane extensions used for locomotion of phagocytosis.

**Psoriasis.** A superficial, recurring idiopathic skin disorder characterized by an abnormal rate of epidermal cell production and turnover.

**Psychiatric.** Pertaining to mental health.

**Psychiatry.** Medical field that studies and treats mental illness.

**Psychology.** Study of human behavior.

**Puerperal mastitis.** Bacterial infection of the breast.

**Puerperal sepsis.** An infection of the endometrium after childbirth or an abortion.

**Puerperium.** The time period after childbirth when the endometrium is open and particularly susceptible to infection.

**Pulmonary edema.** A buildup of fluid in the lungs, causing shortness of breath.

**Pulmonary stenosis.** The first cause of cyanosis in which the valve opening that leads into the pulmonary artery is too small and an inadequate amount of blood reaches the lungs to be oxygenated.

**Purging.** Self-induced, willful elimination of consumed food by vomiting or misuse of laxatives or diuretics.

**Purkinje fibers.** The specialized heart tissue that conducts the impulse for contraction to the myocardium of the ventricles.

**Purpura.** Small hemorrhages into the tissue beneath the skin or mucous membranes.

**Purpura simplex.** A condition of easy bruising.

**Pustules.** Lesions containing pus.

**Pyelitis.** An inflammation of the renal pelvis, the juncture between the ureter and the kidney, caused by *E. coli* or other pus-forming bacteria.

**Pyelonephritis.** A suppurative inflammation of the kidney and renal pelvis.

**Pyloric sphincter.** The sphincter muscle through which food passes from the stomach into the small intestine.

**Pyloric stenosis.**   A congenital obstruction of the intestinal tract.

**Pyogenic.**   Bacteria that cause the formation of a pus.

**Pyuria.**   This condition is caused when abscesses in the kidney rupture and pus enters the renal pelvis and then appears in urine.

**Quarantine.**   The separation of persons who may or may not be infected from healthy people until the period of infectious risk is passed.

**Rabies.**   An infectious disease of the brain and spinal cord caused by a virus that is transmitted by the saliva, urine, or feces of an infected animal.

**Rales.**   Abnormal respiratory sounds detected with a stethoscope.

**Raynaud's disease.**   The condition in which small arteries or arterioles in the fingers and toes constrict.

**Recessive.**   Term used to describe an allele that manifests itself when the person is homozygous for the trait.

**Rectocele.**   Protrusion of the rectum into the vagina.

**Reflux.**   The back-flow of the acid contents of the stomach causing inflammation of the esophagus.

**Regional enteritis.**   An inflammatory disease of the intestine that most frequently affects young adults, particularly females.

**Regurgitation.**   Passage of stomach contents into the esophagus.

**Relapse.**   Occurs when a disease returns weeks or months after its apparent cessation.

**Remission.**   The period of a chronic disease when signs and symptoms subside.

**Renal pelvis.**   The juncture between the kidneys and the ureters; final urine from all collecting ducts empties here.

**Renin.**   Secreted by cells that convert angiotensinogen to angiotensin, an active enzyme to help elevate blood pressure.

**Reservoirs.**   The sources of a pathogen and a potential source of disease.

**Respiratory epithelium.**   A mucous membrane that lines the entire respiratory tract.

**Resuscitation.**   Assisting or reviving respiration to a person with a myocardial infarction.

**Reticulocyte.**   The late stage of erythrocyte development.

**Reye's syndrome.**   A potentially devastating neurologic illness that sometimes develops in young children after a viral infection.

**Rh factor.**   Antigen on erythrocyte, used for blood typing.

**Rhabdomyosarcoma.**   A malignant tumor of the skeletal muscle.

**Rheumatoid factor.**   Antibodies in blood associated with rheumatoid arthritis.

**Rhodopsin.**   The pigment that absorbs light in the rods of the retina.

**Rickets.**   A disease of infancy and early childhood in which the bones do not properly ossify, or harden, generally caused by a vitamin D deficiency.

**Roundworm.**   A wormlike animal that is relatively round in cross section.

**Salpingitis.**   An inflammation of the fallopian tubes.

**Sarcoma.**   A less common type of cancer that spreads rapidly and is highly malignant.

**Scabies.**   A contagious skin disease associated with poor living conditions.

**Schizophrenia.**   Mental illness characterized by social withdrawal, delusions, hallucinations, and unpredictable behavior.

**Scleroderma.**   A chronic, progressive autoimmune disorder of the skin.

**Sclerosis.**   An abnormal hardening of a tissue.

**Sclerotherapy.**   Use of sclerosing or hardening agents to treat diseases like hemorrhoids or esophageal varices.

**Scurvy.**   Disease caused by vitamin C deficiency.

**Seasonal affective disorder.**   Subcategory of major depression associated with decreased sunlight exposure during the winter months.

**Sebaceous glands.**   Oil glands located within the dermis.

**Seborrheic dermatitis.**   The excessive secretion of sebum from the sebaceous glands; chronic dandruff.

**Seborrheic keratosis.**   Benign overgrowth of epithelial cells common in older adults.

**Sebum.**   Oily fluid released through the hair follicles.

**Secondary pneumonia.**   A pneumonia that develops as a secondary disorder from other diseases that weaken the lungs or the body's immune system.

**Seizures.**   An uncontrolled nervous-system activity manifested by uncoordinated motor action.

**Seminal vesicle.**   Produces fructose to nourish sperm.

**Seminiferous tubules.**   Highly coiled tubules contained within the testes in which sperm develop.

**Septic embolism.**   An embolism that contains infected material from pyogenic bacteria.

**Sequela.** The aftermath of a particular disease, such as permanent damage to the heart after rheumatic fever.

**Serotonin.** One of many neurotransmitters involved in regulating mood, emotions, and behavior.

**Sex-linked inheritance.** Diseases transmitted on the sex chromosomes.

**Serum.** Liquid portion of the blood.

**Shingles.** An acute inflammation of nerve cells caused by the chicken pox virus, herpes zoster.

**Sickle cell anemia.** An autosomal recessive disorder, in which hemoglobin is abnormal, resulting in deformed, sickle-shaped red blood cells.

**Signs.** The objective evidence of disease observed on physical examination, such as abnormal pulse or fever.

**Sinoatrial node.** The pacemaker of the heart, it is a small patch of tissue that initiates the heartbeat.

**Skeletal muscle.** Striated muscle attached to bone and that is under conscious control.

**Somatic.** False belief that something physical is occuring in one's body.

**Spastic colon (irritable colon).** A functional condition of the colon with diarrhea and cramping.

**Specific defenses.** Defenses that are effective against particular identified foreign agents.

**Somnoplasty.** A controlled delivery process of radio frequency energy; the tissue is heated in a limited area in order to trim or reduce its size.

**Spider veins.** Small, dense, red networks of veins close to the skin surface.

**Spina bifida.** A condition in which one or more vertebrae fail to fuse, leaving an opening in the vertebral canal. The word *bifid* means a cleft, or split into two parts, which is the condition of the vertebra in spina bifida.

**Spirilla.** Spiral-shaped bacterial cells.

**Spirochetes.** Corkscrew-shaped bacterial cells.

**Spirometer.** A simple instrument used to measure the movement of air in and out of the lungs.

**Spirometry.** A diagnostic procedure that measures and records changes in gas volume in the lungs, determining ventilation capacity and flow rate.

**Splenomegaly.** An enlarged spleen.

**Spongy bone.** Bone tissue with blood-filled spaces; found at ends of bones or in flat bones like those of the skull.

**Spores.** Microscopic fungal reproductive structures that can induce allergies.

**Sporozoans.** A form of protozoa; a single-celled, immobile, eukaryotic microorganism.

**Sprain.** The result of the wrenching or twisting of a joint such as an ankle that injures the ligaments.

**Spurs.** Spicules of abnormal new bone development.

**Squamous cell carcinoma.** A malignancy of the keratinocytes in the epidermis.

**Staghorn calculus.** A kidney stone that becomes so large it fills the renal pelvis completely, blocking the flow of urine.

**Staging.** Method used to establish the extent of disease, particularly cancer.

**Standard precautions.** Precautions such as gloves required of medical personnel when handling patients or bodily fluids.

**Stasis.** Slow blood flow that may lead to thrombosis or cause infection; slow urine flow that may promote kidney stones.

**Status asthmaticus.** Life-threatening form of an asthma attack.

**Stenosis.** Constriction or narrowing of a passage or orifice.

**Stent.** Rigid structure surgically inserted into arteries in order to hold them open.

**Stomatitis.** Inflammation of the lining of the mouth often caused by bacteria or fungi.

**Strabismus.** The condition of crossed eyes.

**Strains.** Pulled muscles that result from a tearing of a muscle and/or its tendon from excessive use or stretching.

**Streptococci.** A type of bacterium associated with infections of the ear, throat, skin, and heart valves.

**Stridor.** High-pitched breath sound.

**Stroke.** Common term to describe cerebral hemorrhages and blood-clot formation within cerebral blood vessels.

**Stye.** A red, tender bump on the eyelid that is caused by an acute infection of the oil glands of the eyelid.

**Subarachnoid.** A tear in the surface membrane of the brain, caused by a skull fracture.

**Subdural.** A hemorrhage under the dura mater, from large venous sinuses of the brain rather than an artery.

**Substance use disorders.** Includes alcohol and drug abuse and addiction.

**Suppressor T cells.** The type of T cell that controls the immune response.

**Suppurative.** A type of inflammation associated with pus formation.

**Symptom.** An indication of disease perceived by the patient, such as pain, dizziness, and itching.

**Syncope.** Fainting caused by insufficient blood supply to the brain.

**Syndrome.** Combination of symptoms.

**Synovial fluid.** Lubricating and shock-absorbing fluid found within joints.

**Synovial membrane.** The membrane that lines the joints.

**Syphilis.** STD caused by *Treponema pallidum.*

**Systemic lupus erythematosus (SLE).** An autoimmune disease that not only affects the skin but causes the deterioration of collagenous connective tissue.

**Systole.** The period of the heartbeat when the heart contracts and pumps the blood.

**T lymphocytes.** Provide cell-mediated immunity and are processed by the thymus gland.

**Tachycardia.** Heart rate of 100 beats per minute or more.

**Tay-Sachs.** An autosomal recessive disorder caused by the absence of the Hex A enzyme.

**Tachypnea.** Rapid respiration rate.

**Tendons.** Connective tissue that attaches skeletal or voluntary muscles firmly to bones.

**Terminal.** A disease ending in death.

**Tetanus toxoid.** A type of immunization that protects from the disease tetanus.

**Tetany.** A sustained muscular contraction.

**Tetralogy of Fallot.** One of the most serious congenital defects consisting of four (*tetra*) abnormalities.

**Thalassemia.** Group of inherited blood disorders in which there is deficient synthesis of one or more alpha or beta chains required for proper formation and optimal performance of the hemoglobin molecule.

**Thrombi.** Blood clots.

**Thrombocytopenia.** A disease of platelets resulting in gastrointestinal and urogenital hemorrhages as well as severe nosebleeds.

**Thrombolytic.** Agents that dissolve blood clots.

**Thrombophlebitis.** Thrombus formation in deep veins.

**Thrombosis.** The forming of blood clots on blood vessel walls.

**Thrombus.** A blood clot that forms in a blood vessel.

**Thyroxine.** One of the thyroid hormones.

**Tic.** Sudden, rapid, involuntary stereotyped movement or vocalization.

**Tinea.** Fungal skin infection.

**Toxic shock syndrome (TSS).** Caused by infection with *Staphylococcus aureus.*

**Toxoid.** A chemically altered toxin that stimulates an immune response.

**Trachea.** The "windpipe," which connects the larynx to the primary bronchi of the lungs.

**Tracheotomy.** Emergency procedure to maintain airway by cutting a hole in the trachea.

**Trachoma.** A chronic contagious form of conjunctivitis causing hypertrophy of the conjunctiva.

**Transformation.** A change from one tissue to another.

**Tremor.** A shakiness, particularly of the hands.

***Trichomonas vaginalis.*** A parasite that can be transmitted by sexual intercourse; one causative agent of vaginitis.

**Trichomoniasis.** Sexually transmitted disease caused by the protozoan *Trichomonas vaginalis.*

**Tricuspid valve.** The valve between the right atrium and right ventricle. It has three cusps.

**Triglycerides.** A lipid fat that is not water soluble and therefore cannot mix with blood plasma.

**Triiodothyronine.** A thyroid hormone.

**Trisomy 21.** The condition of having three, rather than two, copies of chromosome 21; causes Down syndrome.

**Tubercles.** Lesions that are formed when tissue infected with tuberculosis heals with fibrosis and calcification, walling off the bacteria for months or many years.

**Tuberculosis.** A chronic infectious disease characterized by necrosis of vital lung tissue, which can affect other body systems as well.

**Tumor.** A mass of new cells that grows in a haphazard fashion with no control or useful function.

**Tumor marker.** Abnormal levels or substances found in the blood of cancer patients; used to monitor the presence of cancer and the extent of disease.

**Turner's syndrome.** The condition caused when one of the sex chromosomes is missing, resulting in a karyotype of 45,XO.

**Ultrasound cardiography.** Shows the anatomy of arteries, particularly the carotid bifurcation and the internal carotid artery.

**Ultrasound.** Imaging technique utilizing low-frequency sound waves.

**Upper respiratory infections.** Disorders of the nose and throat, including common infections and allergies.

**Urea.** Nitrogen-containing waste products formed in the liver.

**Uremia.** A toxic condition of blood; the end result is kidney failure.

**Ureterocele.** Cyst-like dilation of the ureter near its opening to the urinary bladder.

**Ureter.** Muscular tube that passes urine from the kidney to the urinary bladder.

**Urethra.** The single tube through which urine empties to the outside from the urinary bladder.

**Urethritis.** Inflammation of the urethra.

**Urinalysis.** A simple diagnostic procedure that examines a urine specimen physically, chemically, and microscopically.

**Urinary calculi.** Stones formed primarily in the kidney when certain salts in the urine form a precipitate and grow in size.

**Urticaria.** Known as hives, results from a vascular reaction of the skin to an allergen.

**Uterine prolapse.** Uterus dropping downward into the vagina.

**Uvula.** Soft structure hanging from free edge of the soft palate in midline above the root of the tongue.

**Uvulopalatopharyngoplasty (UPPP).** A procedure that removes excess tissue in the throat (uvula and pharynx) to make the airway wider.

**Vaccine.** A low dose of dead or deactivated bacteria or virus that stimulates an immune response.

**Valvular insufficiency.** Occurs when a valve opening is too large and does not prevent backflow.

**Vas deferens.** A duct that passes through the inguinal canal into the abdominal cavity of males.

**Vascular dementia.** Degenerative memory disorder most often caused by physical insults to the brain.

**Vasopressin.** One of two hormones secreted by the posterior pituitary; also called antidiuretic hormone.

**Vectors.** Animals that transmit pathogenic microorganisms to humans.

**Vegetations.** Small nodular structures composed of bacteria and clots that form along the edge of cusps in a valve opening.

**Venae cavae.** The two largest veins of the body.

**Ventricular fibrillation.** Occurs when a series of uncoordinated impulses spread over the ventricles, causing them to twitch or quiver rather than contract.

**Verruca vulgaris.** Warts caused by viruses affecting the keratinocytes of the skin, causing them to proliferate.

**Vertical transmission.** The route by which an infectious disease is transmitted from one generation to the next.

**Vesicles.** Small, blisterlike eruptions on the skin.

**Vibrios.** Comma-shaped bacterial cells.

**Vitiligo.** A loss of melanin resulting in white patches of skin, which are usually well demarcated and may cover large parts of the body.

**Voluntary muscle.** Striated muscle attached to bone and that is under conscious control.

**Volvulus.** A condition in which the intestine is twisted on itself.

**Wernicke's encephalopathy.** A brain disease, often associated with chronic alcoholism, in which the patient becomes mentally confused and disoriented and may suffer delirium tremens.

**Wheals.** Rounded elevations on the skin known as lesions, with red edges and pale centers; extremely pruritic, or itchy.

**Wheezing.** The sound of labored breathing as a result of narrowed tubes in the lungs.

**Wilms' tumor.** A malignant tumor of the kidney that develops in very young children.

# Appendix B
# Interactive Exercises

## CHAPTER 1: INTRODUCTION TO DISEASE

### Answers to Cases for Critical Thinking

1. Abnormally high red blood cell counts can and do occur in well-trained athletes. Athletes develop increased cardiovascular efficiency and produce more red blood cells. Their hearts can handle the slightly increased viscosity of the blood and thus higher red blood cell levels may not be a sign of disease.
2. No. Many diseases share these symptoms. A simple history can determine if she ate recently or if she is under stress, depressed, or anxious, and a blood test can determine sugar levels and the presence of diabetes. The physician can consult a blood test to determine anemia or other blood disorders. A physical exam can determine whether she has hypertension. Cardiovascular abnormalities can be determined with a physical exam or with imaging techniques. In short, several diseases can explain these symptoms.
3. Many of the diseases are chronic. Education, screening, early diagnosis and treatment, and reduction of risk factors should have an impact on the prevalence of those diseases. Accidents are a significant cause of death. By applying the science of epidemiology to accidents, perhaps prevention can reduce mortality from accidents as well.

### Multiple Choice

1. a. sign
2. a. acute
3. d. etiology
4. a. homeostasis
5. b. exacerbation

### True or False

1. False
2. True
3. False
4. True
5. True

### Fill-Ins

1. prognosis
2. lesions
3. idiopathic
4. relapse
5. remission

## CHAPTER 2: IMMUNITY AND THE LYMPHATIC SYSTEM

### Answers to Cases for Critical Thinking

1. Antiserum containing preformed antibodies is given to act immediately, providing short-lived immunity.
2. Since identical twins have identical DNA, rejection of the organ is not an issue.

3. The bites happened after the women died because trauma is a trigger for inflammation and the bites were not inflamed.
4. Active immunity. The polio virus will trigger antibody production in the body. The baby will develop specific immunity against the virus.
5. IgA provides localized protection at mucosal surfaces like the respiratory system.
6. Helper CD4 T lymphocytes help the immune sytem in many ways. They increase the activity of cytotoxic T lyphocytes, they stimulate B lymphocytes, and they secrete lymphokines that increase the reponse of other types of lymphoid cells.

## Multiple Choice

1. a. preformed antibodies
2. d. memory lymphocytes
3. a. humoral immunity
4. d. all of the above
5. a. antigen
6. c. plasma
7. d. IV
8. a. IgE
9. c. helper or CD4 lymphocytes
10. d. helper cells

## True or False

1. False
2. False
3. False
4. True
5. False
6. False
7. True
8. True
9. False
10. False

## Fill-Ins

1. Pyrogenic
2. Interferon
3. antigen
4. vaccine
5. Nonspecific
6. histamine
7. M
8. Natural killer
9. HIV virus
10. passive

## CHAPTER 3: INFECTIOUS DISEASES

### Answers to Cases for Critical Thinking

1. Influenza is transmitted in respiratory droplets generated by coughing and sneezing. Isolation of flu patients would help decrease the transmission of the disease. Encouraging people to cover their noses and mouths when they sneeze or cough would also help decrease transmission. To control the spread of malaria we must control the vector, the mosquito.
2. Viruses do not have the targets of antibiotics, cell walls and membranes, metabolic and protein synthesis machinery. If antibiotics are used for viral infections, bacterial populations will more likely evolve resistance to those antibiotics.
3. Vaccines prevent disease, and prevention is a very effective method for controlling infectious disease.
4. Whooping cough is caused by *Bordetella pertussis*. The bacteria are spread by direct contact with respiratory droplets. Antibiotics would be the treatment for this bacterial infection. There is a vaccine; whooping cough is part of the diphtheria, tetanus, pertussis vaccine.
5. Chicken pox is caused by the varicella zoster virus. The virus is spread by direct contact, droplet transmission, and airborne transmission. Treatment is supportive and may include treatments to control scratching, pain relievers, and fever reducers. A vaccine is available for varicella zoster.
6. Diphtheria. Diagnosis is based on throat culture. Antibiotics would be the treatment for this bacterial infection.

## Multiple Choice

1. c. capsule
2. c. endospores
3. c. plasmid
4. c. binary fission
5. d. protozoa

6. c. rubella virus
7. a. *Bordetella pertussis*
8. b. capsid
9. a. Enterobius vermicularis
10. d. needle stick

## True or False

1. F
2. F
3. F
4. T
5. T

6. T
7. F
8. T
9. F
10. F

## Fill-Ins

1. normal flora
2. Re-emerging
3. rubeola
4. Nosocomial
5. horizontal

6. glycocalyx
7. Fimbriae
8. Prions
9. paramyxovirus
10. varicella zoster

## Labeling Exercise

1. Trypanosoma
2. Amoeba
3. Plasmodium

4. Tapeworm
5. Liver fluke
6. Ascaris

## CHAPTER 4: CANCER

### Answers to Cases for Critical Thinking

1. Diagnostic procedures used to rule out lung cancer include a chest x-ray, sputum analysis, bronchoscopy with a biopsy, and PET scan. Historical information should include: Have you smoked? (Smoking is the single most preventative cause of lung cancer.) How many packs of cigarettes per day/week? How many years have you smoked? What type of work does the patient do? Factory? (Potential for industrial chemicals to also cause symptoms of lung cancer.) Ask the patient about history of cancers in other parts of the body. The lung is a common site for cancer metastases. History of asthma, bronchitis, pneumonia? History of hoarseness of the voice?

2. Risk factors for breast cancer include age, female gender, genetics, overweight and obesity, post-menopausal hormone replacement therapy, physical inactivity, and consumption of alcohol. Mammography, breast ultrasound, and biopsy are common diagnostic tests and procedures; the definitive test for breast cancer is a biopsy.

### Multiple Choice

1. c. mutation
2. c. DNA repair genes
3. a. Tobacco use
4. d. colorectal
5. b. cervical

6. b. age (greater than 65 years)
7. d. germ cells
8. c. Cigarette smoking
9. b. Reed-Sternberg
10. d. 10

**True or False**

1. False
2. True
3. True
4. True
5. True

6. False
7. True
8. False
9. True
10. True

**Fill-Ins**

1. Sunlight
2. hepatitis B and hepatitis C
3. surgery
4. *Helicobacter pylori*
5. Hepatocellular

6. Pap
7. lymphoma
8. melanocytes
9. thyroid
10. glial

**Labeling Exercise**

1. Stomach cancer
2. Colon cancer

3. Liver cancer
4. Malignant melanoma

## CHAPTER 5: HEREDITY AND DISEASE

**Answers to Cases for Critical Thinking**

1. Turner's and Klinefelter's syndromes involve nondisjunction of an X sex chromosome, and either an egg or a sperm can donate an X sex chromosome. XXY involves nondisjunction of a Y sex chromosome; only the sperm donates a Y sex chromosome.
2. 50%
3. 50% of male children have hemophilia A. 0% of female children have hemophilia A but 50% will be carriers.
4. Hemochromatosis. Blood donation throughout normal life expectancy.

**Multiple Choice**

1. b. both are autosomal dominant traits
2. b. 46
3. a. recessive
4. c. men have one X chromosome
5. c. red and green

6. b. autosomal recessive
7. b. 50
8. c. 50
9. c. heterozygous
10. c. autosomes

**True or False**

1. True
2. True
3. False
4. False
5. False

6. False
7. False
8. True
9. True
10. False

## Fill-Ins

1. Congenital
2. Hermaphrodites
3. Recessive
4. Genes
5. Alleles
6. Polydactyly
7. Nondisjunction
8. 23
9. Phenylketonuria (PKU)
10. gene therapy

## CHAPTER 6: DISEASES OF THE CARDIOVASCULAR SYSTEM

### Answers to Cases for Critical Thinking

1. The heart or vascular diseases that should be considered for this patient include atherosclerosis, coronary heart disease, and myocarditis.
2. The heart diseases that should be considered for this patient include coronary heart disease, shock, and myocarditis.
3. Smoking increases risk of atherosclerosis, chronic venous insufficiency, and cardiac arrhythmia. Diabetes increases risk of atherosclerosis, hypercholsteremia, peripheral artery disease, and coronary heart disease.

### Multiple Choice

1. c. Lightheadedness
2. a. the filling of the heart
3. d. LDL
4. b. carotid artery
5. a. Atherosclerosis
6. b. angioplasty
7. b. Between the left atrium and the left ventricle
8. d. The sinoatrial node
9. a. Myocarditis
10. c. Autoimmune disease

### True or False

1. True
2. True
3. False
4. False
5. True
6. False
7. True
8. False
9. False
10. False

### Fill-Ins

1. thrombosis
2. atherosclerosis
3. restrictive cardiomyopathy
4. stenosis
5. rheumatic fever
6. ventricle to dilate
7. ectopic pacemaker
8. automated external defibrillator
9. tetrology of Fallot and transposition of the great arteries
10. coronary

### Labeling Exercise

1. Superior vena cava
2. Right pulmonary artery
3. Right pulmonary veins
4. Right atrium
5. Tricuspid valve
6. Chordae tendineae
7. Inferior vena cava
8. Aorta
9. Left pulmonary artery
10. Pulmonary semilunar valve
11. Left pulmonary veins
12. Left atrium
13. Bicuspid (mitral) valve
14. Aortic valve
15. Left ventricle
16. Right ventricle

## CHAPTER 7: DISEASES OF THE BLOOD

### Answers to Cases for Critical Thinking

1. Anemia should be considered with this patient. A blood test and health history will help confirm the diagnosis.
2. Thrombocytopenia, impaired synthesis of clotting factors, and vitamin K deficiency are to be considered. Symptoms to look for include prolonged bleeding, petechiae, and ecchymosis. Diagnostic tests include blood tests and bone marrow testing.

### Multiple Choice

1. d. hemoglobin
2. a. erythropoeisis
3. a. Vitamin $B_{12}$
4. d. 50
5. c. Hemoglobinopathy
6. b. Thalassemia
7. a. polycythemia vera
8. d. Idiopathic thrombocytopenic purpura
9. c. Hemophilia A
10. b. Neutropenia

### True or False

1. True
2. False
3. True
4. False
5. True
6. True
7. False
8. True
9. True
10. True

### Fill-Ins

1. leukocytes
2. erythrocytes
3. hemoglobin S
4. platelets
5. alpha thalassemia major and beta thalassemia major
6. iron deficiency
7. megaloblastic anemia
8. 90 to 120 days
9. polycythemia vera
10. thrombin

### Labeling Exercises

1. Ecchymosis
2. Petechiae

## CHAPTER 8: DISEASES OF THE RESPIRATORY SYSTEM

### Answers to Cases for Critical Thinking

1. In this case he should have a chest x-ray to determine if he has pneumonia and what type. A sputum sample can help identify bacteria.
2. These symptoms are typical of emphysema. It may have been triggered by years of exposure to irritating minute airborne particles at the grain mill.
3. Sara should be able to pursue track and enjoy running, because asthma can be managed with medicine and by avoiding triggers.

### Multiple Choice

1. d. emphysema
2. c. asthma
3. c. emphysema
4. c. tuberculosis
5. c. asthma
6. a. pneumonia
7. b. emphysema
8. d. bacteria
9. b. infant respiratory distress syndrome (IRDS)
10. c. pleurisy

## True or False

1. True
2. False
3. False
4. True
5. False
6. False
7. False
8. True
9. False
10. False

## Fill-Ins

1. Mantoux skin test
2. atelectasis
3. cigarette smoking
4. spirometry
5. viruses
6. pleurisy
7. lobar
8. emphysema
9. somnoplasty
10. cystic fibrosis

## Labeling Exercises

1. Pharyngitis
2. Tonsilitis
3. Laryngitis
4. Acute tracheobronchitis
5. Frontal sinus
6. Ethmoid sinus
7. Eustachian tube
8. Maxillary sinus

## CHAPTER 9: DISEASES OF THE GASTROINTESTINAL SYSTEM

### Answers to Cases for Critical Thinking

1. Gastroesophageal reflux disease (GERD) produces these symptoms. History should reveal a pattern of pain that follows meals and occurs at night or when prone. A physical exam can rule out little, but endoscopy can reveal abnormalities at the junction of the stomach and esophagus, such as a hiatal hernia. Treatment involves behavior changes such as taking smaller meals and avoiding food an hour before sleeping. Serious cases require surgical repair of the hiatal hernia.
2. Cholelithiasis (gallstones) causes these symptoms. If bile flow to the small intestine is blocked, dietary fat remains undigested and is not absorbed from the intestines. As a result, fat appears in the feces. Following a high fat meal the gallbladder secretes bile into the small intestine. Gallstones lodge in the bile ducts and cause pain in the upper right abdomen.
3. In cirrhosis, normal liver tissue is replaced by scar or fat tissue, which does not function as normal liver tissue. Thus, the liver does not process the hemoglobin that comes from dying erythrocytes and the orange and yellow-colored breakdown products build up in blood, tinting the skin and eyes yellow. Normal liver tissue processes carbohydrates and proteins and manufactures bile, which is used for fat absorption and the absorption of fat soluble vitamins. The normal liver also manufactures clotting proteins. Finally, as blood flow through the liver is restricted by cirrhosis, abdominal and esophageal venous pressure increases, which leads to the distortion of the esophageal veins.

### Multiple Choice

1. b. inflammation of stomach mucosa
2. b. ulcerative colitis
3. b. celiac disease/malabsorption syndrome
4. d. diverticulitis
5. d. prognosis is good, with an 85% cure rate
6. c. most often caused by diabetes
7. b. chronic alcoholism
8. a. cirrhosis
9. a. *Candida albicans*
10. c. cholecystitis

## True or False

1. False
2. True
3. False
4. True
5. True

6. False
7. False
8. False
9. False
10. True

## Fill-Ins

1. amoebic dysentery
2. Crohn's disease
3. hernia
4. endoscope
5. C

6. cholelithiasis
7. bile duct
8. ascites
9. mouth
10. large intestine

## Labeling Exercise

1. Hepatic duct
2. Liver
3. Gallbladder
4. Cystic duct
5. Stomach
6. Common bile duct

7. Pancreas
8. Duodenum
9. Mucous membrane lining gallbladder
10. Right and left hepatic ducts
11. Common hepatic duct

## CHAPTER 10: DISEASES OF THE URINARY SYSTEM

### Answers to Cases for Critical Thinking

1. Jane may occasionally notice blood in the urine because of the monthly menstrual cycle, but the pain is not normal. Because of a short urethra in females the urinary bladder is commonly contaminated by infection. The appropriate antibiotic agents like the fluoroquinolones (Cinobac) or older drugs like sulfonamides, e.g., Gantanol, may relieve the condition. If medication is ineffective, then a cystoscopic examination would be in order.

2. Britany had collected excess water for about two weeks because of a sequela-type event. Following the strep infection, it settled in the kidney glomerulus, causing glomerulonephritis. This inflammation is caused by an antigen-antibody complex that congests the glomerulus and reduces the filtration process.

   Treatment includes antibiotics like penicillin to reduce any underlying infection, ACE inhibitors and/or NSAIDs to reduce protein loss and antihypertensive medication if needed.

3. Because it is a young child, the suspicion is Wilm's tumor, a fast-acting malignant tumor. The symptoms and signs suggest a major problem and a biopsy confirms it. Surgery along with radiation and chemotherapy provide a positive prognosis, barring metastasis.

4. This patient has a renal tumor, and hematuria suggests tissue breakdown. A renalectomy rids the body of this organ and growth. Unfortunately, the tumor is usually advanced well before it is detected, and has had a chance to metastasize. Cancer therapy usually follows the surgery.

### Multiple Choice

1. a. diabetes mellitus
2. a. pyelonephritis
3. c. pyelitis
4. d. uremia
5. b. usually exhibit dysuria, urgency, and frequency

6. a. peritoneal dialysis
7. b. incontinence
8. a. protein
9. c. decreased plasma protein
10. b. aging

## True or False

1. False
2. True
3. True
4. True
5. True

6. True
7. True
8. False
9. False
10. True

## Fill-Ins

1. Pyuria
2. Diabetic nephropathy
3. kidney stones
4. Lithrotripsy
5. Polycystic kidney

6. oliguria
7. nocturia
8. bacteria
9. recessive
10. IVP

## Labeling Exercises

1. Kidney
2. Ureter

3. Urinary bladder
4. Urethra

## CHAPTER 11: DISEASES AND DISORDERS OF THE REPRODUCTIVE SYSTEM

### Answers to Cases for Critical Thinking

1. The condition is endometriosis; its cause is unknown. Treatments include pain relievers, hormone therapy, and surgery.
2. Trichomoniasis is a possible diagnosis. Tests and procedures would include pelvic examination, microscopic visualization, culture, and laboratory and pH tests. Antiparasitic medication is the available treatment.
3. Possible diagnoses include benign prostatic hyperplasia or prostate cancer. A digital-rectal examination, PSA test, and biopsy might be performed. Treatments include watchful waiting, surgery, and hormone therapy.
4. Decreasing transmission includes monogamy, use of condoms and dental dams, and regular pelvic exams. Taking anti-viral medication on a regular basis may decrease transmission of the virus.
5. Because prostate cancer often grows very slowly, some men (especially those who are older or who have other major health problems) may never need treatment for their cancer.
6. Cryptorchidism is the name of the disease, and complications can include infertility and testicular cancer. Hormone therapy or surgery are possible treatments.

### Multiple Choice

1. c. uterine fibroids
2. d. *Treponema pallidum*
3. c. syphilis is only transmitted by sexual contact
4. a. chlamydia
5. d. menorrhagia

6. c. rectocele
7. b. dysmenorrhea
8. c. cryptorchidism
9. b. fimbrae
10. c. human chorionic gonadotropin hormone

### True or False

1. True
2. False
3. True
4. False
5. True

6. True
7. True
8. True
9. False
10. False

## Fill-Ins

1. seminiferous tubules
2. Orchitis
3. chlamydia
4. prostate gland
5. Proststitis
6. Trichomoniasis
7. I; II
8. Cystocele
9. Amenorrhea
10. Erectile

## Labeling Exercise

1. Ovarian ligament
2. Myometrium
3. Endometrium
4. Fundus of uterus
5. Isthmus of uterine tube
6. Uterine (fallopian) tube
7. Ampulla
8. Ovarian follicles
9. Ovarian vessels
10. Corpus luteum
11. Fornix
12. External os
13. Vagina
14. Cervix
15. Cervical canal
16. Uterosacral ligament
17. Internal os
18. Ovary
19. Fimbriae
20. Infundibulum
21. Uterine cavity
22. Broad ligament

## CHAPTER 12: DISEASES OF THE ENDOCRINE SYSTEM

### Answers to Cases for Critical Thinking

1. Diabetes type 1 is consistent with age of onset, high urine production, and weight loss when the boy should be growing. It is possible that weight loss could be due to hyperthyroidism.
2. Cushing's syndrome occurs more commonly among women. High blood glucose and lipids, hypertension, and poor wound healing (the patient's bruise) are consistent with Cushing's syndrome.
3. Addison's disease is consistent with this history and these signs and symptoms.

### Multiple Choice

1. c. anterior pituitary
2. b. parathormone
3. b. Addison's disease
4. b. Cushing's disease
5. c. diabetes insipidus
6. a. Graves' disease
7. d. adrenal
8. a. Addison's disease
9. d. glucose
10. c. thyroxine

### True or False

1. True
2. False
3. False
4. False
5. False
6. False
7. False
8. True
9. True
10. True

## Fill-Ins

1. gigantism
2. acromegaly
3. oxytocin, vasopressin
4. diabetes
5. pheochromocytoma
6. islet cells
7. hyperparathyroidism
8. anterior pituitary
9. growth hormone
10. eunuchism

## Labeling Exercise

1. Thyroid gland
2. Follicle
3. Capillaries
4. Thyroid cartilage (Adam's apple)
5. Isthmus
6. Trachea
7. Follicular cells (site of hormone synthesis)
8. Colloidal material (storage of hormone)

## CHAPTER 13: DISEASES OF THE NERVOUS SYSTEM AND THE SPECIAL SENSES

### Answers to Cases for Critical Thinking

1. J.A. has bacterial meningitis, which is a very serious disease that may be acutely lethal. The signs and symptoms plus lumbar puncture fit the disease, and a course of action is to use a broad-spectrum antibiotic like cephalosporins given intravenously, analgesics for pain, antipyretics to reduce inflammation, and diuretics for cerebral edema.
2. Cataracts cause dimming of light and distortion of image formation on the retina. The lens should be replaced to prevent a potential blindness condition because the lens is too thick and ineffectual. The prognosis is very favorable following lens replacement surgery.
3. T.C. had a viral infection from the common cold that has spread into the middle ear (otitis media) and typically leads to a pus-forming bacterial infection. The doctor examines the ear drum externally using an otoscope to observe the tension on the tympanic membrane and notice any drainage. A warm heating pad gives some comfort and Tylenol (especially for children) is used to reduce pain and fever. Antibiotics kill bacteria and stop bacterial growth, and this (combination) regimen approach is usually a successful treatment process.

### Multiple Choice

1. b. virus
2. d. all of these
3. d. heart rate and breathing
4. b. meningitis
5. a. is caused by a virus
6. c. damaged myelin sheath
7. b. TPA
8. c. epilepsy
9. a. no dopamine
10. c. conjunctivitis

### True or False

1. True
2. True
3. False
4. True
5. False
6. True
7. False
8. True
9. False
10. False

## Fill-Ins

1. Tetanus
2. electromyography
3. Multiple sclerosis
4. Essential tremor
5. L-dopa

6. Cluster
7. trigeminal neuralgia
8. Bell's palsy
9. ALS
10. Myelocele

## Labeling Exercise

1. Foresight, abstract thinking judgment
2. Motor area
3. Central sulcus
4. Sensory area
5. Speech

6. Hearing
7. Pain, temp., touch, pressure, position, body image
8. Memory, visual and auditory association
9. Vision
10. Equilibrium, muscle tone, coordination

## CHAPTER 14: MENTAL ILLNESS AND COGNITIVE DISORDERS

### Answers to Cases for Critical Thinking

1. A full mental health evaluation would provide appropriate diagnoses and recommendations for JR. These would include various personality tests, IQ tests, symptom inventory, a complete physical examination with neurological testing, and a complete evaluation by a psychiatrist. JR's symptoms are suggestive of Attention Deficit Hyperactivity Disorder. As adolescents, untreated patients with ADHD may abuse drugs or exhibit impulsive behaviors. ADHD has a genetic basis, however, and without treatment the symptoms can continue to escalate.
2. AM has signs of both depression and anxiety that may be due to her current set of circumstances. If AM has had a significant weight loss, one would also have to consider anorexia nervosa as a possible diagnosis. AM would benefit from a mental health evaluation. Further treatment may include medication for her depression and anxiety and psychotherapy.
3. DT is displaying symptoms of PTSD and depression. Symptoms of mental illness include withdrawal, regret, loss of interest in activities that he previously found enjoyable, history of abuse. Recommendations include: approaching DT with the subject of mental health counseling, stress management, and/or a complete physical and mental health examination. A supportive spouse, counselor, and medication can often assist in healing from PTSD.

### Multiple Choice

1. b. Franz Mesmer
2. c. DSM
3. d. dopamine
4. a. ADHD is limited to children
5. c. acetylcholine

6. a. persecutory
7. b. bulimia nervosa
8. b. bipolar I
9. c. stimulant medications
10. d. obsessions

### True or False

1. False
2. False
3. True
4. True
5. True

6. True
7. False
8. True
9. False
10. False

## Fill-Ins

1. Psychiatry
2. neurotransmitters
3. dopamine
4. mental retardation
5. tic disorders
6. acetylcholine
7. compulsive use, cravings, tolerance, and withdrawal
8. affect
9. Seasonal affective disorder
10. mania

## CHAPTER 15: DISEASES OF THE MUSCULOSKELETAL SYSTEM

### Answers to Cases for Critical Thinking

1. Osteoporosis is common in elderly women. Pain and height loss and kyphosis may all be due to vertebral fractures and bone loss. Calcium supplements and mild exercise such as walking with a cane or walker may increase muscle strength and thus prevent falls and fractures. Calcium-supplemented diet and weight-bearing exercise throughout adolescence and adulthood can reduce risk of developing osteoporosis later in life.
2. History, physical exam, and occupation suggests osteoporosis. X-ray can show joint damage.
3. This young woman reports pain in her bone, not in her joint. This could be shin splints, which require rest. Bone infection would be accompanied by fever and systemic symptoms such as weakness. A tumor would also cause pain and weakness. An x-ray can rule out tumors and blood work can rule out infections.

### Multiple Choice

1. c. vitamin D
2. d. the bones of adults
3. c. median nerve
4. d. Duchenne's MD
5. b. Osteoarthritis
6. a. rheumatoid arthritis
7. d. gout
8. c. osteogenic sarcoma
9. c. myasthenia gravis
10. c. osteomyelitis

### True or False

1. False
2. False
3. False
4. True
5. True
6. True
7. True
8. False
9. True
10. True

### Fill-Ins

1. Pott's disease
2. rickets
3. osteoporosis
4. gout
5. calcium, phosphate
6. osteoblasts
7. synovial
8. myasthenia gravis
9. gout
10. calcium

## Labeling Exercise

1. Closed fracture
2. Open fracture
3. Comminuted fracture
4. Depressed fracture
5. Spiral fracture
6. Greenstick fracture

## CHAPTER 16: DISEASES OF THE INTEGUMENTARY SYSTEM

### Answers to Cases for Critical Thinking

1. Impetigo is the diagnosis; staphylococcus aureus or Streptococcus pyogenes are potential causes. Treatment is antibiotic medication.
2. Possible causes of the rash include tinea cruris, candidiasis, pediculosis, and scabies. Visual examination and culture are the diagnostic tests performed.
3. Basal cell carcinoma or squamous cell carcinoma are possible diagnoses; treatment includes a visual examination and biopsy.
4. Hormones, overproduction of sebum, bacteria, lack of or uneven exfoliation of skin cells. Treament may include topical antibiotics and antibacterials, retinoid, oral antibiotics, oral contraceptives, and isotretinoin. Prevention of acne includes not overcleansing the skin, not using harsh scrubs, avoiding products with high concentrations of alcohol, and keeping the hands away from the face.
5. Cold sores caused by the herpes simplex type I virus. HSV-1 is spread by kissing, close contact with herpetic lesions, or contact with skin that is shedding the virus. Antiviral drugs.
6. The hard, thick patches are likely plantar warts, caused by human papillomavirus.

### Multiple Choice

1. c. staphylococci
2. b. macule
3. b. cyst
4. a. epidermis
5. c. white
6. c. subcutaneous tissue
7. c. papule
8. c. hair follicles
9. a. parasitic
10. c. Sebum

### True or False

1. False
2. False
3. False
4. False
5. False
6. True
7. False
8. False
9. True
10. False

### Fill-Ins

1. Melanin
2. Keratin
3. dermis
4. Herpes
5. Pediculosis
6. Psoriasis
7. Contusions
8. Hemangioma
9. Vitiligo
10. Tinea pedis

### Labeling Exercises

1. Folliculitis
2. Furuncle (boil)
3. Wart
4. Psoriasis
5. Vitiligo

| Test | Normal Value Range (Conventional) | Normal Value Range (SI units) | Possible Indications |
|---|---|---|---|
| Ammonia ($NH_3$) diffusion | 20–120 mcg/dl | 12–70 mcmol/L | Abnormal levels of ammonia in the body are used to investigate severe changes in mood and consciousness and to help diagnose the cause of a coma of unknown origin. |
| Ammonia nitrogen | 15–45 µg/dl | 11–32 µmol/L | The test for ammonia nitrogen is nonspecific and does not indicate a cause. Higher than normal levels simply indicate the body is not effectively metabolizing and eliminating ammonia. |
| Amylase | 35–118 IU/L | 0.58–1.97 mckat/L | The normal level of amylase will depend on the method used to collect the data. An increase level may indicate several disorders of the digestive and reproductive systems or cancer of the pancreas. Tubal pregnancies will also cause a rise in the amylase levels. Decreased amylase levels may indicate damage to the pancreas and kidneys. |
| Anion gap ($Na^+-[Cl^- + HCO_3^-]$) (P) | 7–16 mEq/L | 7–16 mmol/L | A determination of electrolytes in the blood fluid. Abnormal readings indicate a variety of factors. The test is non-specific and only tells the physician that there is cause for additional testing. Some factors that cause an abnormal anion gap reading are uncontrolled diabetes, starvation, kidney damage, and ingestion of potentially toxic substances such as antifreeze, excessive amounts of aspirin, or methanol. |
| Bicarbonate<br>Arterial<br>Venous | <br>21–28 mEq/L<br>22–29 mEq/L | <br>21–28 mmol/L<br>22–29 mmol/L | See *Carbon dioxide content* below |
| Bilirubin:<br>Conjugated (direct)<br>Total | <br>0.2 mg/dl<br>0.1–1 mg/dl | <br>4 mcmol/L<br>2–18 mcmol/L | Increased levels of bilirubin may be an indication of some kind of blockage of the liver or bile duct, hepatitis, trauma to the liver, a drug reaction, or long-term alcohol abuse or some inherited disorders, such as Gilbert's, Rotor's, Dubin-Johnson, Crigler-Najjar, which will cause an increase in levels. Increased levels of bilirubin in newborns is a critical situation as excessive levels kill developing brain cells and may lead to mental retardation. |
| Calcitonin | < 100 pg/ml | < 100 ng/L | Increased levels of calcitonin in combination with a thyroid biopsy may be an indication of C-cell hyperplasia. |

*(continued)*

| Test | Normal Value Range (Conventional) | Normal Value Range (SI units) | Possible Indications |
|------|-----------------------------------|-------------------------------|----------------------|
| Calcium, total: <br> Calcium, ionized: | 8.6–10.3 mg/dl <br> 4.4–5.1 mg/dl | 2.2–2.74 mmol/L <br> 1–1.3 mmol/L | Increased levels of calcium in the body indicate an inability to metabolize the intake. This can be due to several factors: hyperthyroidism, sarcoidosis, tuberculosis, excess Vitamin D intake, kidney transplant, and high protein levels (for example, if a tourniquet is used for too long while blood is collected). In this case, free or ionized calcium remains normal. |
| Carbon dioxide content (plasma) | 21–32 mmol/L | 21–32 mmol/L | Higher or lower than normal $CO_2$ levels indicate a problem losing or retaining fluid—disrupting the acid-base balance, which can be an indication of several disorders. |
| Carcinoembryonic antigen | < 3 ng/ml | < 3 mcg/L | CEA is a protein that is found in embryonic tissues. Increased CEA levels can indicate some non-cancer-related conditions of inflammation of internal organs. Pregnant women who smoke tend to have embryos that have increased levels of CEA. <br><br> In a normally healthy infant all detectable levels of CEA are gone by birth. |
| Chloride | 95–110 mEq/L | 95–110 mmol/L | Increased levels of chloride may indicate dehydration or increased blood sodium. Decreased levels of chloride occurs with prolonged vomiting, chronic diarrhea, emphy[[check]]sema, or other chronic lung disease, and with loss of acid from the body. |
| Coagulation screen <br>  Bleeding time <br>  Prothrombin time <br>  Partial thrombo- <br>  plastin <br>  time (activated) <br>  Protein C <br>  Protein S | <br> 3–9.5 min <br> 10–13 sec <br> 22–37 sec <br> 0.7–1.4 µ/ml <br> 0.7–1.4 µ/ml | <br> 180–570 sec <br> 10–13 sec <br> 22–37 sec <br> 700–1400 U/ml <br> 700–1400 U/ml | Indicates an inability of the body to develop adequate clotting factors or the inability to produce the correct amount of clotting factors. |
| Copper, total | 70–160 mcg/dl | 11–25 mcmol/L | Indication of liver disease |
| Corticotropin (ACTH: adreno-corticotropic hormone)—0800 hr | < 60 pg/ml | < 13.2 pmol/L | This test is used in conjunction with cortisol to determine if a patient has Cushing's syndrome or Addison's disease. |
| Cortisol 0800 hr <br> 1800 hr <br> 2000 hr | 5–30 mcg/dl <br> 2–15 mcg/dl <br> 50% of 0800 hr | 138–810 nmol/L <br> 50–410 nmol/L <br> 50% of 0800 hr | Abnormal levels in coritsol may indicate Cushing's syndrome or Addison's disease. |

| Test | Normal Value Range (Conventional) | Normal Value Range (SI units) | Possible Indications |
|---|---|---|---|
| Creatine kinase<br>    Female<br>    Male | 20–170 IU/L<br>30–220 IU/L | 0.33–2.83 mckat/L<br>0.5–3.67 mckat/L | Creatine kinase is an enzyme found in the heart, brain, skeletal muscle, and other tissues. The body has specific types of CK to indicate which muscles are affected. |
| Creatinine kinase isoenzymes, MB fraction | 0–12 IU/L | 0–0.2 mckat/L | Depending on the ratio, the CK-MB fraction will indicate some form of muscle damage. The specific ratio can indicate if the muscle damage is cardiac or skeletal. |
| Creatinine | 0.5–1.7 mg/dl | 44–150 mcmol/L | Increased creatinine levels indicate a disorder with kidney function. Creatinine can also increase temporarily as a result of muscle injury. |
| | | | Low levels of creatinine are not common. They may been seen in persons with decreased muscle mass, such as comatose patients. Normal pregnancy will cause the creatinine levels to drop and are not a cause for concern. |
| Follicle-stimulating hormone (FSH)<br>    Female<br>    Midcycle<br>    Men | <br>2–13 mlU/ml<br>5–22 mlU/ml<br>1–8 mlU/ml | <br>2–13 IU/L<br>5–22 IU/L<br>1–8 IU/L | Increased levels of FSH and LH (luteinizing hormone) are consistent with primary ovarian failure, which is when ovaries themselves fail. In men this may be an indication of testicular developmental defects or injury. |
| | | | Decreased levels of FSH and LH are an indication of secondary ovarian failure, which results in a problems with the pituitary or hypothalamic gland. In men this may be an indication of hypothalamic disorders. |
| Glucose, fasting | 65–115 mg/dl | 3.6–6.3 mmol/L | Indicates diabetes or pre-diabetes. |
| Glucose tolerance test (oral) 2 hour | (mg/dl)<br>Normal fasting | | Indicates diabetes or pre-diabetes. |
| Post-drink:<br>Impaired tolerance<br>Indicates diabetes | 65–99<br>< 140 mg/dl<br>140–199 mg/dl<br>> 200 mg/dl | | |
| Haptoglobin | 44–303 mg/dl | 0.44–3.03 g/L | If the haptoglobin levels are decreased in combination with several other tests, it may be an indication of hemolytic anemia. |
| | | | Haptoglobin will be elevated in many inflammatory diseases, such as ulcerative colitis, acute rheumatic disease, heart attack, and severe infection. |

(*continued*)

| Test | Normal Value Range (Conventional) | Normal Value Range (SI units) | Possible Indications |
|---|---|---|---|
| Fibrinogen | 200–400 mg/dl | 2–4 g/L | Lower than normal fibrinogen levels indicate that the person may not be able to form a stable blood clot after injury. Chronically low levels may indicate an inherited condition such as afibrinogenemia, or to an acquired condition such as liver disease, malnutrition, or some types of cancer. Higher than normal levels of fibrinogen may indicate acute infections, breast, kidney, or stomach cancer, chronic DIC, inflammatory disorders, myocardial infarction, stroke, or trauma. Fibrinogen concentrations may rise sharply in any condition that causes inflammation or tissue damage. |
| Hematocrit (Hct)<br>  Female<br>  Male | <br>35%–46%<br>40.0%–50.0% | <br>0.36–0.446<br>0.4–0.503 | Decreased hematocrit level indicates anemia, such as iron deficiency, but may have other causes such as vitamin or mineral deficiencies, recent bleeding, liver cirrhosis, and malignancies. |
| Hemoglobin A$_{1C}$ | 40.0%–50.0% of total | 0.053–0.075 | Abnormally high levels of hematocrit may be an indication of dehydration and can be easily cured by increased fluid intake.<br><br>*Polycythemia vera*—greater than normal number of red blood cells in a person can also cause a pro- longed increase in the hematocrit levels. Higher than normal hematocrit levels are also seen in persons with chronic pulmonary conditions or lung damage. The person's bone marrow will in crease production of red blood cells to supply the body with oxygen in response to a lacking pulmonary system. |
| Hemoglobin (Hb)<br>  Female<br>  Male | <br>11.6–15.5 g/dl<br>13.7–16.7 g/dl | <br>121–153 g/L<br>138–175 g/L | Low levels of Hb are an indication of anemia. Some types of anemia are treated with iron, folic acid, or vitamin B$_{12}$ or B$_6$ supplements.<br><br>It is normal for women of childbearing age to have temporary decreases during menstrual periods and pregnancy. |
| Leukocyte count (WBC) | 3800–9800/mcl | $3.8–9.8 \times 10^9$/L | Infections usually cause increased WBC counts and may be treated with antibiotics. Leukemias (blood cancer) require chemotherapy and other treatments. |
| Erythrocyte count (RBC)<br>  Female<br>  Male | <br>$3.8–5.2 \times 10^6$/mcl<br>$4.3–5.7 \times 10^6$/mcl | <br>$3.8–5.2 \times 10^{12}$/L<br>$4.3–5.7 \times 10^{12}$/L | A low ESR can indicate polycythemia, extreme leukocytosis, and some protein abnormalities. |
| Erythrocyte sedimentation rate (sedrate, ESR)<br>  Female<br>  Male | <br><br><br>30 mm/hr<br>mm/hr | <br><br><br>30 mm/hr<br>20 mm/hr | Elevated ESR level is an indication of inflammation, anemia, infection, pregnancy, and advanced age. |

| Test | Normal Value Range (Conventional) | Normal Value Range (SI units) | Possible Indications |
|---|---|---|---|
| Leukocytes (WBC)<br>Men<br>Women | 5000-10000/mcL<br>4500-11000/mcL<br>(higher during pregnancy) | 5-10 x $10^9$L<br>4.5-11 x $10^9$L | Raised levels may indicate infections, inflammation, or cancer. Decreased levels may indicate autoimmune conditions, some severe infections, bone marrow failure, and congenital marrow aplasia. Decreased levels may also occur with certain medications such as methotrexate. |
| Lymphocytes | of WBC | | Chronic high levels may indicate lymphocytic leukemia. |
| Lipase | 7–60 units/L @ 37°C | 7–60 units/L @ 37°C | High lipase levels, with abdominal pain, may indicate acute pancreatitis, slightly raised levels can indicate kidney disease, salivary gland inflammation, or peptic ulcer disease. |
| Lipids<br>  Total cholesterol<br>    Borderline high<br>    High | < 200 mg/dl<br>200–239 mg/dl<br>240–above | | A person with high cholesterol has more than twice the risk of coronary heart disease as someone whose cholesterol is below 200 mg/dL. |
|   HDL<br>    High | > 60 mg/dl<br>< 40 mg/dl (men)<br>< 50 mg/dl (women) | | Low HDL is considered a major risk factor for heart disease. |
|   LDL<br>    High | < 100 mg/dl<br>> 130 mg/dl | | If you don't have coronary heart disease or diabetes and have one or no risk factors, your LDL goal is less than 160 mg/dL.<br><br>If you don't have coronary heart disease or diabetes and have two or more risk factors, your LDL goal is less than 130 mg/dL.<br><br>If you do have coronary heart disease or diabetes, your LDL goal is less than 100 mg/dL. |
| Triglycerides<br>  High | >150 mg/dl<br>> 200 mg/dl and above | | Normal triglyceride levels vary by age and sex. A high triglyceride level combined with low HDL cholesterol or high LDL cholesterol seems to speed up atherosclerosis (the buildup of fatty deposits in artery walls). Atherosclerosis increases the risk for heart attack and stroke. (Info on lipids from the American Heart Association) |
| PSA<br>  0–54 yrs<br>  55–59 yrs<br>  60–64 yrs<br>  65–69 yrs<br>  70 plus yrs | 0.00–2.50 ng/ml<br>0.00–3.40 ng/ml<br>0.00–4.10 ng/ml<br>0.00–5.10 ng/ml<br>0.00–5.60 ng/ml | | PSA is a test indicating the level of protein cells the prostate is producing. The higher the PSA number, the more likely prostate cancer is present. Age, hormonal factors, and medications can alter the test results so a high PSA alone is not a cancer indicator. |
| TSH | 0.40–5.00 IU/ml | | A high TSH result is often due to some type of acute or chronic thyroid dysfunction that causes the thyroid to be underactive. Although rare, a high TSH can be an indication of secondary hyperthyroidism, which is a problem with the pituitary gland.<br><br>A low TSH result can indicate an overactive thyroid gland. |

*(continued)*

| Test | Normal Value Range (Conventional) | Normal Value Range (SI units) | Possible Indications |
|---|---|---|---|
| Urea, plasma (BUN) | 8.5–25 mg/dl | 2.9–8.9 mmol/liter | Increased BUN levels may be due to acute or chronic kidney disease, damage, or failure. Conditions that result in reduced blood flow to the kidneys, such as a recent heart attack, will also result in an increased BUN. Low BUN level are rarely detected because they result from diseases or symptoms, such as dehydration or starvation, that do not warrant a BUN test. |
| Urinalysis pH Specific gravity | 5.0–7.5 1.001–1.030 | 5.0–7.5 1.001–1.030 | Specific gravity is an indication of how well the kidneys are filtering waste products. Reduced specific gravity can indicate diabetes insipidus, certain renal diseases, excess fluid intake, or diabetes mellitus. Raised specific gravity can indicate dehydration, adrenal insufficiency, nephrosis, congestive cardiac failure, or liver disease. |

# Index

Page references followed by *t* represent tables, those followed by *f* represent figures, and those followed by *b* represent boxes.

# Pearson Education, Inc.

## YOU SHOULD CAREFULLY READ THE TERMS AND CONDITIONS BEFORE USING THE CD-ROM PACKAGE. USING THIS CD-ROM PACKAGE INDICATES YOUR ACCEPTANCE OF THESE TERMS AND CONDITIONS.

Pearson Education, Inc. provides this program and licenses its use. You assume responsibility for the selection of the program to achieve your intended results, and for the installation, use, and results obtained from the program. This license extends only to use of the program in the United States or countries in which the program is marketed by authorized distributors.

### LICENSE GRANT

You hereby accept a nonexclusive, nontransferable, permanent license to install and use the program ON A SINGLE COMPUTER at any given time. You may copy the program solely for backup or archival purposes in support of your use of the program on the single computer. You may not modify, translate, disassemble, decompile, or reverse engineer the program, in whole or in part.

### TERM

The License is effective until terminated. Pearson Education, Inc. reserves the right to terminate this License automatically if any provision of the License is violated. You may terminate the License at any time. To terminate this License, you must return the program, including documentation, along with a written warranty stating that all copies in your possession have been returned or destroyed.

### LIMITED WARRANTY

THE PROGRAM IS PROVIDED "AS IS" WITHOUT WARRANTY OF ANY KIND, EITHER EXPRESSED OR IMPLIED, INCLUDING, BUT NOT LIMITED TO, THE IMPLIED WARRANTIES OR MERCHANTABILITY AND FITNESS FOR A PARTICULAR PURPOSE. THE ENTIRE RISK AS TO THE QUALITY AND PERFORMANCE OF THE PROGRAM IS WITH YOU. SHOULD THE PROGRAM PROVE DEFECTIVE, YOU (AND NOT PRENTICE-HALL, INC. OR ANY AUTHORIZED DEALER) ASSUME THE ENTIRE COST OF ALL NECESSARY SERVICING, REPAIR, OR CORRECTION. NO ORAL OR WRITTEN INFORMATION OR ADVICE GIVEN BY PRENTICE-HALL, INC., ITS DEALERS, DISTRIBUTORS, OR AGENTS SHALL CREATE A WARRANTY OR INCREASE THE SCOPE OF THIS WARRANTY.

SOME STATES DO NOT ALLOW THE EXCLUSION OF IMPLIED WARRANTIES, SO THE ABOVE EXCLUSION MAY NOT APPLY TO YOU. THIS WARRANTY GIVES YOU SPECIFIC LEGAL RIGHTS AND YOU MAY ALSO HAVE OTHER LEGAL RIGHTS THAT VARY FROM STATE TO STATE.

Pearson Education, Inc. does not warrant that the functions contained in the program will meet your requirements or that the operation of the program will be uninterrupted or error-free.

However, Pearson Education, Inc. warrants the diskette(s) or CD-ROM(s) on which the program is furnished to be free from defects in material and workmanship under normal use for a period of ninety (90) days from the date of delivery to you as evidenced by a copy of your receipt.

The program should not be relied on as the sole basis to solve a problem whose incorrect solution could result in injury to person or property. If the program is employed in such a manner, it is at the user's own risk and Pearson Education, Inc. explicitly disclaims all liability for such misuse.

### LIMITATION OF REMEDIES

Pearson Education, Inc.'s entire liability and your exclusive remedy shall be:

1. the replacement of any diskette(s) or CD-ROM(s) not meeting Pearson Education, Inc.'s "LIMITED WARRANTY" and that is returned to Pearson Education, or

2. if Pearson Education is unable to deliver a replacement diskette(s) or CD-ROM(s) that is free of defects in materials or workmanship, you may terminate this agreement by returning the program.

IN NO EVENT WILL PRENTICE-HALL, INC. BE LIABLE TO YOU FOR ANY DAMAGES, INCLUDING ANY LOST PROFITS, LOST SAVINGS, OR OTHER INCIDENTAL OR CONSEQUENTIAL DAMAGES ARISING OUT OF THE USE OR INABILITY TO USE SUCH PROGRAM EVEN IF PRENTICE-HALL, INC. OR AN AUTHORIZED DISTRIBUTOR HAS BEEN ADVISED OF THE POSSIBILITY OF SUCH DAMAGES, OR FOR ANY CLAIM BY ANY OTHER PARTY.

SOME STATES DO NOT ALLOW FOR THE LIMITATION OR EXCLUSION OF LIABILITY FOR INCIDENTAL OR CONSEQUENTIAL DAMAGES, SO THE ABOVE LIMITATION OR EXCLUSION MAY NOT APPLY TO YOU.

### GENERAL

You may not sublicense, assign, or transfer the license of the program. Any attempt to sublicense, assign or transfer any of the rights, duties, or obligations hereunder is void.

This Agreement will be governed by the laws of the State of New York.

Should you have any questions concerning this Agreement, you may contact Pearson Education, Inc. by writing to:

Director of New Media
Higher Education Division
Pearson Education, Inc.
One Lake Street
Upper Saddle River, NJ 07458

**Should you have any questions concerning technical support you may contact:**

**Product Support Department: Monday–Friday 8:00 A.M. –8:00 P.M. and Sunday 5:00 P.M.-12:00 A.M. (All times listed are Eastern). 1-800-677-6337**

**You can also get support by filling out the web form located at http://247.prenhall.com**

YOU ACKNOWLEDGE THAT YOU HAVE READ THIS AGREEMENT, UNDERSTAND IT, AND AGREE TO BE BOUND BY ITS TERMS AND CONDITIONS. YOU FURTHER AGREE THAT IT IS THE COMPLETE AND EXCLUSIVE STATEMENT OF THE AGREEMENT BETWEEN US THAT SUPERSEDES ANY PROPOSAL OR PRIOR AGREEMENT, ORAL OR WRITTEN, AND ANY OTHER COMMUNICATIONS BETWEEN US RELATING TO THE SUBJECT MATTER OF THIS AGREEMENT.